Urological Cancer 2020

Urological Cancer 2020

Editors

José I. López
Claudia Manini

MDPI • Basel • Beijing • Wuhan • Barcelona • Belgrade • Manchester • Tokyo • Cluj • Tianjin

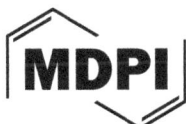

Editors
José I. López
Cruces University Hospital
Spain

Claudia Manini
Ospedale San Giovanni Bosco
Italy

Editorial Office
MDPI
St. Alban-Anlage 66
4052 Basel, Switzerland

This is a reprint of articles from the Special Issue published online in the open access journal *Cancers* (ISSN 2072-6694) (available at: https://www.mdpi.com/journal/cancers/special_issues/UC).

For citation purposes, cite each article independently as indicated on the article page online and as indicated below:

LastName, A.A.; LastName, B.B.; LastName, C.C. Article Title. *Journal Name* **Year**, *Volume Number*, Page Range.

ISBN 978-3-0365-0270-0 (Hbk)
ISBN 978-3-0365-0271-7 (PDF)

Cover image courtesy of Jose I. Lopez.

© 2021 by the authors. Articles in this book are Open Access and distributed under the Creative Commons Attribution (CC BY) license, which allows users to download, copy and build upon published articles, as long as the author and publisher are properly credited, which ensures maximum dissemination and a wider impact of our publications.

The book as a whole is distributed by MDPI under the terms and conditions of the Creative Commons license CC BY-NC-ND.

Contents

About the Editor ix

Claudia Manini and José I. López
Insights into Urological Cancer
Reprinted from: *Cancers* 2021, *13*, 204, doi:10.3390/cancers13020204 1

Matthias Schnetz, Julia K. Meier, Claudia Rehwald, Christina Mertens, Anja Urbschat, Elisa Tomat, Eman A. Akam, Patrick Baer, Frederik C. Roos, Bernhard Brüne and Michaela Jung
The Disturbed Iron Phenotype of Tumor Cells and Macrophages in Renal Cell Carcinoma Influences Tumor Growth
Reprinted from: *Cancers* 2020, *12*, 530, doi:10.3390/cancers12030530 7

Tsu-Ming Chien, Ti-Chun Chan, Steven Kuan-Hua Huang, Bi-Wen Yeh, Wei-Ming Li, Chun-Nung Huang, Ching-Chia Li, Wen-Jeng Wu and Chien-Feng Li
Role of Microtubule-Associated Protein 1b in Urothelial Carcinoma: Overexpression Predicts Poor Prognosis
Reprinted from: *Cancers* 2020, *12*, 630, doi:10.3390/cancers12030630 27

Juan Li, Baotong Zhang, Mingcheng Liu, Xing Fu, Xinpei Ci, Jun A, Changying Fu, Ge Dong, Rui Wu, Zhiqian Zhang, Liya Fu and Jin-Tang Dong
KLF5 Is Crucial for Androgen-AR Signaling to Transactivate Genes and Promote Cell Proliferation in Prostate Cancer Cells
Reprinted from: *Cancers* 2020, *12*, 748, doi:10.3390/cancers12030748 47

Megan Crumbaker, Eva K. F. Chan, Tingting Gong, Niall Corcoran, Weerachai Jaratlerdsiri, Ruth J. Lyons, Anne-Maree Haynes, Anna A. Kulidjian, Anton M. F. Kalsbeek, Desiree C. Petersen, Phillip D. Stricker, Christina A. M. Jamieson, Peter I. Croucher, Christopher M. Hovens, Anthony M. Joshua and Vanessa M. Hayes
The Impact of Whole Genome Data on Therapeutic Decision-Making in Metastatic Prostate Cancer: A Retrospective Analysis
Reprinted from: *Cancers* 2020, *12*, 1178, doi:10.3390/cancers12051178 67

Michelle D. Bardis, Roozbeh Houshyar, Peter D. Chang, Alexander Ushinsky, Justin Glavis-Bloom, Chantal Chahine, Thanh-Lan Bui, Mark Rupasinghe, Christopher G. Filippi and Daniel S. Chow
Applications of Artificial Intelligence to Prostate Multiparametric MRI (mpMRI): Current and Emerging Trends
Reprinted from: *Cancers* 2020, *12*, 1204, doi:10.3390/cancers12051204 95

Chandrani Sarkar, Sandeep Goswami, Sujit Basu and Debanjan Chakroborty
Angiogenesis Inhibition in Prostate Cancer: An Update
Reprinted from: *Cancers* 2020, *12*, 2382, doi:10.3390/cancers12092382 113

Meredith Mihalopoulos, Zachary Dovey, Maddison Archer, Talia G. Korn, Kennedy E. Okhawere, William Nkemdirim, Hassan Funchess, Ami Rambhia, Nihal Mohamed, Steven A. Kaplan, Reza Mehrazin, Dara Lundon, Che-Kai Tsao, Ketan K. Badani and Natasha Kyprianou
Repurposing of α1-Adrenoceptor Antagonists: Impact in Renal Cancer
Reprinted from: *Cancers* 2020, *12*, 2442, doi:10.3390/cancers12092442 135

Sirin Saranyutanon, Sachin Kumar Deshmukh, Santanu Dasgupta, Sachin Pai, Seema Singh and Ajay Pratap Singh
Cellular and Molecular Progression of Prostate Cancer: Models for Basic and Preclinical Research
Reprinted from: *Cancers* **2020**, *12*, 2651, doi:10.3390/cancers12092651 147

Shyama U. Tetar, Omar Bohoudi, Suresh Senan, Miguel A. Palacios, Swie S. Oei, Antoinet M. van der Wel, Berend J. Slotman, R. Jeroen A. van Moorselaar, Frank J. Lagerwaard and Anna M. E. Bruynzeel
The Role of Daily Adaptive Stereotactic MR-Guided Radiotherapy for Renal Cell Cancer
Reprinted from: *Cancers* **2020**, *12*, 2763, doi:10.3390/cancers12102763 173

Manuela A. Hoffmann, Hans-Georg Buchholz, Helmut J Wieler, Florian Rosar, Matthias Miederer, Nicolas Fischer and Mathias Schreckenberger
Dual-Time Point [^{68}Ga]Ga-PSMA-11 PET/CT Hybrid Imaging for Staging and Restaging of Prostate Cancer
Reprinted from: *Cancers* **2020**, *12*, 2788, doi:10.3390/cancers12102788 185

Jennifer Kubon, Danijel Sikic, Markus Eckstein, Veronika Weyerer, Robert Stöhr, Angela Neumann, Bastian Keck, Bernd Wullich, Arndt Hartmann, Ralph M. Wirtz, Helge Taubert and Sven Wach
Analysis of CXCL9, PD1 and PD-L1 mRNA in Stage T1 Non-Muscle Invasive Bladder Cancer and Their Association with Prognosis
Reprinted from: *Cancers* **2020**, *12*, 2794, doi:10.3390/cancers12102794 201

Carlo Cattrini, Davide Soldato, Alessandra Rubagotti, Linda Zinoli, Elisa Zanardi, Paola Barboro, Carlo Messina, Elena Castro, David Olmos and Francesco Boccardo
Epidemiological Characteristics and Survival in Patients with De Novo Metastatic Prostate Cancer
Reprinted from: *Cancers* **2020**, *12*, 2855, doi:10.3390/cancers12102855 215

Mathieu Roumiguié, Evanguelos Xylinas, Antonin Brisuda, Maximillian Burger, Hugh Mostafid, Marc Colombel, Marek Babjuk, Joan Palou Redorta, Fred Witjes and Bernard Malavaud
Consensus Definition and Prediction of Complexity in Transurethral Resection or Bladder Endoscopic Dissection of Bladder Tumours
Reprinted from: *Cancers* **2020**, *12*, 3063, doi:10.3390/cancers12103063 227

Molishree Joshi, Jihye Kim, Angelo D'Alessandro, Emily Monk, Kimberley Bruce, Hanan Elajaili, Eva Nozik-Grayck, Andrew Goodspeed, James C. Costello and Isabel R. Schlaepfer
CPT1A Over-Expression Increases Reactive Oxygen Species in the Mitochondria and Promotes Antioxidant Defenses in Prostate Cancer
Reprinted from: *Cancers* **2020**, *12*, 3431, doi:10.3390/cancers12113431 247

Niklas Klümper, Marthe von Danwitz, Johannes Stein, Doris Schmidt, Anja Schmidt, Glen Kristiansen, Michael Muders, Michael Hölzel, Manuel Ritter, Abdullah Alajati and Jörg Ellinger
Downstream Neighbor of SON (DONSON) Expression Is Enhanced in Phenotypically Aggressive Prostate Cancers
Reprinted from: *Cancers* **2020**, *12*, 3439, doi:10.3390/cancers12113439 267

Claudia Manini and José I. López
Unusual Faces of Bladder Cancer
Reprinted from: *Cancers* **2020**, *12*, 3706, doi:10.3390/cancers12123706 279

Sofia Karkampouna, Maria R. De Filippo, Charlotte K. Y. Ng, Irena Klima, Eugenio Zoni, Martin Spahn, Frank Stein, Per Haberkant, George N. Thalmann and Marianna Kruithof-de Julio
Stroma Transcriptomic and Proteomic Profile of Prostate Cancer Metastasis Xenograft Models Reveals Prognostic Value of Stroma Signatures
Reprinted from: *Cancers* **2020**, *12*, 3786, doi:10.3390/cancers12123786 . . . . **293**

About the Editors

José I. López is head of Department of Pathology at the Hospital Universitario Cruces and principal investigator of the Biomarker in Cancer Unit at the Biocruces-Bizkaia Health Research Institute. He graduated at the Faculty of Medicine, University of the Basque Country, Leioa, Spain, and trained in Pathology at the Hospital Universitario 12 de Octubre, Madrid, Spain. He received his PhD degree at the Universidad Complutense of Madrid, Spain. Dr. López has served as pathologist for more than 30 years in several hospitals in Spain, and is subspecialized in Uropathology, where he has published more than 180 peer-reviewed articles and reviews. Dr. López is interested in translational uropathology in general and in renal cancer in particular, and collaborates with several international research groups unveiling the genomic landscape of urological cancer. Intratumor heterogeneity, tumor sampling, tumor microenvironment, tumor ecology, immunotherapy, and basic mechanisms of carcinogenesis are his main topics of interest.

Claudia Manini is head of the Department of Pathology at San Giovanni Bosco Hospital in Turin, Italy. She graduated from the Faculty of Medicine and Surgery and post-graduated in Surgical Pathology at the University of Turin, Turin, Italy. Dr. Manini has served as pathologist for more than 25 years in several hospitals in Italy developing an expertise in diagnostic uropathology, neuropathology and gynecopathology. Her main interest is translational pathology.

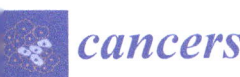

Editorial

Insights into Urological Cancer

Claudia Manini [1,*] and José I. López [2,*]

1 Department of Pathology, San Giovanni Bosco Hospital, 10154 Turin, Italy
2 Department of Pathology, Cruces University Hospital, Biocruces-Bizkaia Health Research Institute, 48903 Barakaldo, Spain
* Correspondence: claudiamaninicm@gmail.com (C.M.); jilpath@gmail.com (J.I.L.)

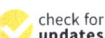

Citation: Manini, C.; López, J.I. Insights into Urological Cancer. *Cancers* **2021**, *13*, 204. https://doi.org/10.3390/cancers13020204

Received: 5 January 2021
Accepted: 6 January 2021
Published: 8 January 2021

Publisher's Note: MDPI stays neutral with regard to jurisdictional claims in published maps and institutional affiliations.

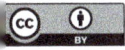

Copyright: © 2021 by the authors. Licensee MDPI, Basel, Switzerland. This article is an open access article distributed under the terms and conditions of the Creative Commons Attribution (CC BY) license (https://creativecommons.org/licenses/by/4.0/).

The year the Covid-19 pandemic appeared has been quite prolific in urological cancer research, and the collection of articles, perspectives, and reviews on renal, prostate, and urinary tract tumors merged in this *Urological Cancer 2020* issue is just a representative sample of this assertion. Urological malignancies nowadays remain a hot topic of translational oncologic research. These are quite common neoplasms in clinical practice, with a high impact on the economy. All of them rank in the top-ten list of human cancers and account for up to 33% of malignancies affecting the male population [1]. In addition, kidney, prostate, and bladder tumors display different pathogenetic mechanisms, and their varied diagnostic and therapeutic approaches represent a challenge for multidisciplinary clinical teams.

Finding useful biomarkers to manage these diseases represents a key point in modern oncology. A relevant advance in the field, i.e., the importance and limits of analyzing the extracellular vesicles as potential biomarkers in urological neoplasms, has been reviewed this year, illustrating the promising therapeutic expectancies of this approach in the near future [2]. Since most biomarkers currently focused on in the research in the bladder, kidney, and prostate cancer (DNA, microRNA, proteins, etc.) travel packaged within exosomes and ectosomes in the bloodstream, these cellular structures remain as promising potential targets for testing both in urine [3] and liquid biopsies [4].

The European Association of Urology, in some instances, together with other international associations, such as the European Association of Nuclear Medicine, European Society for Radiotherapy and Oncology, European Society of Urogenital Radiology, and International Society of Geriatric Oncology, has recently updated the guidelines for the management of kidney [5], prostate [6,7], and bladder [8] tumors. On the other hand, pathological updates in tumor staging [9] and grading [10] of genitourinary tumors also appeared in 2020.

The pathogenesis, histological spectrum, molecular alterations, prognosis, and therapy of renal cancer is a maze for urologists, oncologists, pathologists, and basic researchers [11]. Under the term "renal cancer", several different diseases coexist, each one of them being heterogeneous by itself. In this complex context, an exhaustive and systematic update of renal cancer classification based on morphological, immunohistochemical, and molecular data was performed during 2020 by a panel of international experts belonging to the Genitourinary Pathology Society (GUPS) [12,13]. While the most efficient treatment for the non-clear cell renal cell carcinomas group remains poorly defined, recent trials advise for the use of nivolumab/cabozantinib alone or in combination with immune checkpoint inhibition as the elective strategy for advanced clear cell renal cell carcinomas (CCRCC) [5].

CCRCC is a paradigm of unpredictable intratumor heterogeneity, and this fact makes it especially difficult to find a successful therapeutic response for every patient [5]. The decision to use immune checkpoint inhibitors depends on the immunohistochemical evaluation of the PD-1/PD-L1 axis status in the intratumor inflammatory infiltrates, a subject that is controversial since insufficient or partial tumor analysis may provide inconclusive results [14]. A recent study, however, has obtained much more sensitive results in its evaluation using a new methodology called Förster Resonance Energy Transfer (FRET), which is based on the physical properties of the intervening molecules [15].

This *Urological Cancer 2020* Special Issue includes two articles and one perspective on renal neoplasia [16–18]. Schnetz et al. [16] analyzed the role of macrophage-secreted iron in tumor progression of patients with CCRCC, papillary renal cell carcinomas (PRCC), and chromophobe renal cell carcinoma (ChRCC). They have found that genes regulating iron homeostasis are associated with tumor stage and grade through the pro-tumorigenic activity of a specialized subset of macrophages present in the local microenvironment. The iron chelator EC1 seems to reverse the pro-tumorigenic effect of these macrophages scavenging iron in the local extracellular matrix. Mihalopoulos et al. [17] hypothesized that the quinazoline-based α1-adrenoreceptor-antagonists may have a direct therapeutic action in renal cancer and reviewed its mechanism of action in human disease, their antitumor effects in several neoplasms, and its potential therapeutic usefulness in renal cancer. Finally, Tetar et al. [18] described their results using the stereotactic magnetic-resonance-guided radiotherapy (MRgRT) in 36 patients with large renal tumors and concluded that this technique shows low toxicity and high local control of the disease.

Two large groups of patients with urothelial carcinomas are distinguished in the clinical practice, non-muscle invasive and muscle invasive, each one of them displaying a specific clinical approach and management. Apart from the classical prognostic parameters, such as tumor Stage and Grade [19], still valid, pathologists distinguish basal and luminal phenotypes in muscle-invasive urothelial carcinomas based on immunohistochemical and molecular profiles, which correlate with different molecular tumorigenic pathways, clinical evolution, and prognosis [20]. Some patients with advanced urothelial carcinoma may benefit from immune checkpoint blockade [21].

Two articles [22,23] and two reviews [24,25] dealing with urothelial tumors have been included in this collection of urological neoplasia. Chien et al. [22] described in a study of 635 patients, how the overexpression of the microtubule-associated protein 1b (*MAP1B*) is an independent prognostic factor with adverse clinical outcomes and shorter survival in both upper urinary tract and bladder urothelial carcinomas. The authors concluded that MAP1B could be used as an additional biomarker and then potentially targeted in the future. Kubon et al. [23] analyzed the mRNA of three immune markers (*CXCL9*, *PD-1*, and *PD-L1*) in a series of non-muscle invasive bladder urothelial carcinomas and demonstrated that increased levels of *CXCL9* mRNA are associated with longer overall and disease-free survivals. In addition, they have confirmed the survival benefit of high levels of *PD-L1* mRNA.

The two reviews come directly from the clinical perspective. A multi-institutional and international group of urologists achieved a consensus to define and predict the complexity of transurethral resection and dissection of bladder tumors, a crucial issue to optimize and adapt human and technical resources to every clinical setting [24]. Most urothelial carcinomas are composed of clearly recognizable, though more or less differentiated, transitional cells. Manini and López [25] reviewed the varied morphology that urothelial tumors may eventually display with their respective characteristic pictures. The importance of its correct recognition relies on that some of them carry prognostic implications per se, a point that every pathologist should know.

Prostate cancer usually presents as a localized (organ-confined) disease. Depending on several factors, radical surgery or radiotherapy are the two recommended treatments [26], but active surveillance [27] and focal therapy [28] have also been proposed in selected low-grade/low-volume cases. Another subset of patients presents with aggressive and disseminated disease at diagnosis [29]. In between these two extreme clinical settings, the third subset of patients is characterized by the development of only a few metastases (<5) along the clinical course of the disease, the so-called oligometastatic prostate adenocarcinoma. Oligometastatic prostate cancers are usually under-diagnosed because they do not present any specific clinical or histologic feature [30]. As a result, the on-time identification and application of any eventual treatment exclusively directed to the metastases remain a difficult challenge.

Urological Cancer 2020 contains three reviews [31–33] and seven articles [34–40] about prostate cancer. Sarkar et al. [31] reviewed the intimate mechanisms of angiogenesis in prostate cancer and their possible blockade to maximize benefits minimizing toxicity. Another interesting review revisited the cellular and molecular progression pathways of prostate cancer in different cell lines [32]. The prostate cancer associated with *PTEN*-deficiency deserves a special mention. It is well-known that *PTEN* loss is a key factor for cancer initiation in many organs, the prostate included. In this sense, a recent study showed that *PTEN* heterozygosity in *LKB1*-mutant mice promotes the development of a metastatic aggressive form of prostate cancer [41]. Bardis et al. [33] reviewed the applications of Artificial Intelligence to multiparametric magnetic resonance imaging in prostate cancer and its interaction with radiologists' algorithms.

Cattrini et al. [34] analyzed the epidemiological characteristics of more than 26,000 patients collected in 17 years to understand the effect on survival provided by the advances in therapy in de novo metastatic prostate cancer better. A dual-time point hybrid imaging [^{68}Ga]Ga-PSMA-11 PET/CT has been implemented for staging and restaging 233 prostate cancer patients [35], showing a potential benefit to define improved algorithms with clinical applicability to detect the primary, recurrent, and metastatic cases better. Crumbaker et al. [36] performed a retrospective deep whole-genome sequencing in a series of 13 patients with prostate cancer, highlighting the extreme genomic complexity and heterogeneity. This information may be of help when making therapeutic decisions, for example, unveiling cases with alterations in PI3K, MAPK, and Wnt pathways or detecting losses in genes related to sensitivity to immunotherapy or with resistance to androgen therapy. As in many other cancers, the local microenvironment greatly influences prostate cancer cell evolution. In this sense, Karkampouna et al. [37] analyzed the importance of the stromal signatures found in xenograft models of metastatic prostate cancer, which correlated with clinical parameters, such as the Gleason score, metastasis progression, and progression-free survival.

DONSON (downstream neighbor of SON) mRNA expression was analyzed by Klümper et al. [38] in aggressive variants of prostate cancer. Upregulation of this gene related to cell cycle progression and genomic stability maintenance has been associated with clinical aggressiveness, metastases development, and androgen-deprivation resistance. The authors stressed that DONSON expression could be considered a robust prognostic biomarker in prostate cancer [38]. Androgen deprivation resistance is the final common step of many advanced prostate cancers. Li et al. [39] identified the key promoting role of KLF5, the transcription factor Krüppel-like factor 5, in the androgen-AR signaling of LNCaP and C4-2B prostate cell lines. The authors considered this effect as a potential target to develop new therapeutic strategies in castration-resistant prostate cancers. Transcriptomic and metabolomic analyses of LNCaP-C4-2 cell lines with depleted and increased CPT1A (carnitine palmitoyl transferase 1) expression, respectively, were investigated [40]. CPT1A plays an important role in the adaptation to stress and antioxidant production and is an enzyme involved in lipid catabolism and may be critically involved in promoting neuroendocrine differentiation in prostate cancer cells. The authors concluded that an excess of CPT1A is associated with prostate cancer progression and propose to target lipid catabolic pathways as an alternative therapeutic tool.

To summarize, this *Urological Cancer 2020* collection contains a set of multidisciplinary contributions to the extraordinary heterogeneity of tumor mechanisms, diagnostic approaches, and therapies of the renal, urinary tract, and prostate cancers, with the intention of offering a representative snapshot of the current urological research.

Author Contributions: C.M. and J.I.L. conceived, designed, and wrote the manuscript. All authors have read and agreed to the published version of the manuscript.

Funding: This study received no external funding.

Conflicts of Interest: The authors declare no conflict of interest.

References

1. Siegel, R.L.; Miller, K.D.; Jemal, A. Cancer statistics, 2020. *CA Cancer J. Clin.* **2020**, *70*, 7–30. [CrossRef] [PubMed]
2. Linxweiler, J.; Junker, K. Extracellular vesicles in urological malignancies: An update. *Nat. Rev. Urol.* **2020**, *17*, 11–27. [CrossRef] [PubMed]
3. Solé, C.; Goicoechea, I.; Goñi, A.; Schramm, M.; Armesto, M.; Arestín, M.; Manterola, L.; Tellaetxe, M.; Alberdi, A.; Nogueira, L.; et al. The urinary transcriptome as a source of biomarkers for prostate cancer. *Cancers* **2020**, *12*, 513. [CrossRef] [PubMed]
4. Bryant, R.J.; Pawlowski, T.; Catto, J.W.F.; Marsden, G.; Vessella, R.L.; Rhees, B.; Kuslich, C.; Visakorpi, T.; Hamdy, F.C. Changes in circulating microRNA levels associated with prostate cancer. *Br. J. Cancer* **2012**, *106*, 768–774. [CrossRef] [PubMed]
5. Bedke, J.; Albiges, L.; Capitanio, U.; Giles, R.H.; Hora, M.; Lam, T.B.; Ljungberg, B.; Marconi, L.; Klatte, T.; Volpe, A.; et al. Updated European Association of Urology guidelines on renal cell carcinoma: Nivolumab plus cabozantinib joins immune checkpoint inhibition combination therapies for treatment-naïve metastatic clear-cell renal cell carcinoma. *Eur. Urol.* **2020**. [CrossRef] [PubMed]
6. Mottet, N.; van den Bergh, R.C.N.; Briers, E.; Van den Broeck, T.; Cumberbatch, M.G.; De Santis, M.; Fanti, S.; Fossati, N.; Gandaglia, G.; Gillessen, S.; et al. EAU-EANM-ESTRO-ESUR-SIOG Guidelines on Prostate Cancer-2020 Update. Part 1: Screening, Diagnosis, and Local Treatment with Curative Intent. *Eur. Urol.* **2020**. [CrossRef]
7. Cornford, P.; van den Bergh, R.C.N.; Briers, E.; Van den Broeck, T.; Cumberbatch, M.G.; De Santis, M.; Fanti, S.; Fossati, N.; Gandaglia, G.; Gillessen, S.; et al. EAU-EANM-ESTRO-ESUR-SIOG Guidelines on Prostate Cancer. Part II-2020 Update: Treatment of Relapsing and Metastatic Prostate Cancer. *Eur. Urol.* **2020**. [CrossRef]
8. Witjes, J.A.; Bruins, H.M.; Cathomas, R.; Compérat, E.M.; Cowan, N.C.; Gakis, G.; Hernández, V.; Espinós, E.L.; Lorch, A.; Neuzillet, Y.; et al. European Association of Urology guidelines on muscle-invasive and metastatic bladder cancer: Summary of the 2020 guidelines. *Eur. Urol.* **2021**, *79*, 82–104. [CrossRef]
9. Cornejo, K.M.; Rice-Stitt, T.; Wu, C.L. Updates in staging and reporting of genitourinary malignancies. *Arch. Pathol. Lab. Med.* **2020**, *144*, 305–319. [CrossRef]
10. Rice-Stitt, T.; Valencia-Guerrero, A.; Cornejo, K.M.; Wu, C.L. Updates in histologic grading of urologic malignancies. *Arch. Pathol. Lab. Med.* **2020**, *144*, 335–343. [CrossRef]
11. Manini, C.; López, J.I. The labyrinth of renal cell carcinoma. *Cancers* **2020**, *12*, 521. [CrossRef] [PubMed]
12. Trpkov, K.; Hes, O.; Williamson, S.; Adeniram, A.J.; Agaimy, A.; Alaghebandan, R.; Amin, M.B.; Argani, P.; Chen, Y.B.; Cheng, L.; et al. New developments in existing WHO entities and evolving molecular concepts: The Genitourinary Pathology Society (GUPS) Update on Renal Neoplasia. *Mod. Pathol.* in press.
13. Trpkov, K.; Hes, O.; Williamson, S.; Adeniram, A.J.; Agaimy, A.; Alaghebandan, R.; Amin, M.B.; Argani, P.; Chen, Y.B.; Cheng, L.; et al. Novel, emerging and provisional renal entities: The Genitourinary Pathology Society (GUPS) Update on Renal Neoplasia. *Mod. Pathol.* in press.
14. Nunes-Xavier, C.E.; Angulo, J.C.; Pulido, R.; López, J.I. A critical insight into the clinical translation of PD-1/PD-L1 blockade therapy in clear cell renal cell carcinoma. *Curr. Urol. Rep.* **2019**, *20*, 1. [CrossRef]
15. Sánchez-Magraner, L.; Miles, J.; Baker, C.; Applebee, C.J.; Lee, D.J.; Elsheikh, S.; Lashin, S.; Withers, K.; Watts, A.; Parry, R.; et al. High PD-1/PD-L1 checkpoint interaction infers tumor selection and therapeutic sensitivity to anti-PD1/PD-L1 treatment. *Cancer Res.* **2020**, *80*, 4244–4257. [CrossRef]
16. Schnetz, M.; Meier, J.K.; Rehwald, C.; Mertens, C.; Urbschat, A.; Tomat, E.; Akam, E.A.; Baer, P.; Roos, F.C.; Brüne, B.; et al. The disturbed iron phenotype of tumor cells and macrophages in renal cell carcinoma influences tumor growth. *Cancers* **2020**, *12*, 530. [CrossRef]
17. Mihalopoulos, M.; Dovey, Z.; Archer, M.; Korn, T.G.; Okhawere, K.E.; Nkemdirim, W.; Funchess, H.; Rambhia, A.; Mohamed, N.; Kaplan, S.A.; et al. Repurposing of α1-adrenoreceptor antagonists: Impact in renal cancer. *Cancers* **2020**, *12*, 2442. [CrossRef]
18. Tetar, S.U.; Bohoudi, O.; Senan, S.; Palacios, M.A.; Oei, S.S.; van der Wel, A.M.; Slotman, B.J.; van Moorselaar, R.J.A.; Lagerwaard, F.J.; Bruynzeel, M.E. The role of daily adaptative stereotactic MR-guided radiotherapy for renal cell cancer. *Cancers* **2020**, *12*, 2763. [CrossRef]
19. Angulo, J.C.; López, J.I.; Flores, N.; Toledo, J.D. The value of tumour spread, grading and growth pattern as morphological predictive parameters in bladder carcinoma. A critical revision of the 1987 TNM Classification. *J. Cancer Res. Clin. Oncol.* **1993**, *119*, 578–593. [CrossRef]
20. Guo, C.C.; Bondaruk, J.; Yao, H.; Wang, Z.; Zhang, L.; Lee, S.; Lee, J.G.; Cogdell, D.; Zhang, M.; Yang, G.; et al. Assessment of luminal and basal phenotypes in bladder cancer. *Sci. Rep.* **2020**, *10*, 9743. [CrossRef]
21. Rouanne, M.; Radulescu, C.; Adam, J.; Allory, Y. PD-L1 testing in urothelial bladder cancer: Essentials of clinical practice. *World J. Urol.* **2020**. [CrossRef] [PubMed]
22. Chien, T.M.; Chan, T.C.; Huang, S.K.H.; Yeh, B.W.; Li, W.M.; Huang, C.N.; Li, C.C.; Wu, W.J.; Li, C.F. Role of microtubule-associated protein 1b in urothelial carcinoma: Overexpression predicts poor prognosis. *Cancers* **2020**, *12*, 630. [CrossRef] [PubMed]

23. Kubon, J.; Sikic, D.; Eckstein, M.; Weyerer, V.; Stöhr, R.; Neumann, A.; Keck, B.; Wullich, B.; Hartmann, A.; Wirtz, R.M.; et al. Analysis of CXCL9, PD1, and PD-L1 mRNA in stage T1 non-muscle invasive bladder cancer and their association with prognosis. *Cancers* **2020**, *12*, 2794. [CrossRef] [PubMed]
24. Roumiguié, M.; Xylinas, E.; Brisuda, A.; Burger, M.; Mostafid, H.; Colombel, M.; Babjuk, M.; Palou Redorta, J.; Witjes, F.; Malavaud, B. Consensus definition and prediction of complexity in transurethral resection or bladder endoscopic dissection of bladder tumours. *Cancers* **2020**, *12*, 3063. [CrossRef]
25. Manini, C.; López, J.I. Unusual faces of bladder cancer. *Cancers* **2020**, *12*, 3706. [CrossRef]
26. Hamdy, F.C.; Donovan, J.L.; Lane, J.A.; Mason, M.; Metcalfe, C.; Holding, P.; Davis, M.; Peters, T.J.; Turner, E.L.; Martin, R.M.; et al. 10-year outcomes after monitoring, surgery, or radiotherapy for localized prostate cancer. *N. Eng. J. Med.* **2016**, *375*, 1415–1424. [CrossRef]
27. Kasivisvanathan, V.; Giganti, F.; Emberton, M.; Moore, C.M. Magnetic resonance imaging should be used in the active surveillance of patients with localised prostate cancer. *Eur. Urol.* **2020**, *77*, 318–319. [CrossRef]
28. Kluytmans, A.; Fütterer, J.J.; Emberton, M.; Sedelaar, M.; Grutters, J. Exploring the risk-reward balance in focal therapy for prostate cancer-a contribution to the debate. *Prostate Cancer Prostatic. Dis.* **2019**, *22*, 382–384. [CrossRef]
29. Yadav, S.S.; Stockert, J.A.; Hackert, V.; Yadav, K.K.; Tewari, A.K. Intratumor heterogeneity in prostate cancer. *Urol. Oncol.* **2018**, *36*, 349–360. [CrossRef]
30. Manini, C.; González, A.; Büchser, D.; García-Olaverri, J.; Urresola, A.; Ezquerro, A.; Fernández, I.; Llarena, R.; Zabalza, I.; Pulido, R.; et al. Oligometastatic prostate adenocarcinoma. A clinical-pathologic study of a histologically under-recognized prostate cancer. *J. Pers. Med.* **2020**, *10*. [CrossRef]
31. Sarkar, C.; Goswami, S.; Basu, S.; Chakroborty, D. Angiogenesis inhibition in prostate cancer: An update. *Cancers* **2020**, *12*, 2382. [CrossRef]
32. Saranyutanon, S.; Deshmukh, S.K.; Dasgupta, S.; Pai, S.; Singh, S.; Singh, A.P. Cellular and molecular progression of prostate cancer: Models for basic and preclinical research. *Cancers* **2020**, *12*, 2651. [CrossRef]
33. Bardis, M.D.; Houshyar, R.; Chang, P.D.; Ushinsky, A.; Glavis-Bloom, J.; Chahine, C.; Bui, T.L.; Rupasinghe, M.; Filippi, C.G.; Chow, D.S. Applications of artificial intelligence to prostate multiparametric MRI (mpMRI): Current and emerging trends. *Cancers* **2020**, *12*, 1204. [CrossRef]
34. Cattrini, C.; Soldato, D.; Rubagotti, A.; Zinoli, L.; Zanardi, E.; Barboro, P.; Messina, C.; Castro, E.; Olmos, D.; Boccardo, F. Epidemiological characteristics and survival in paients with de novo metastatic prostate cancer. *Cancers* **2020**, *12*, 2855. [CrossRef]
35. Hoffmann, M.A.; Buchholz, H.G.; Wieler, H.J.; Rosar, F.; Miederer, M.; Fisher, N.; Schreckenberger, M. Dual-time point [^{68}Ga]Ga-PSMA-11 PET/CT hybrid imaging for staging and restaging of prostate cancer. *Cancer* **2020**, *12*, 2788. [CrossRef]
36. Crumbaker, M.; Chan, E.K.F.; Gong, T.; Corcoran, N.; Jaratlerdsiri, W.; Lyons, R.J.; Haynes, A.M.; Kulidjian, A.A.; Kalsbeek, A.M.F.; Petersen, D.C.; et al. The impact of whole genome data on therapeutic decision-making in metastatic prostate cancer: A retrospective analysis. *Cancers* **2020**, *12*, 1178. [CrossRef] [PubMed]
37. Karkampouna, S.; de Filippo, M.R.; Ng, C.K.Y.; Klima, I.; Zoni, E.; Spahn, M.; Stein, F.; Haberkant, P.; Thalmann, G.N.; Kruithof-de Julio, M. Stroma transcriptomic and proteomic profile of prostate cancer metastasis xenograft models reveals prognostic value of stroma signatures. *Cancers* **2020**, *12*, 3786. [CrossRef] [PubMed]
38. Klümper, N.; von Danwitz, M.; Stein, J.; Schmidt, D.; Schmidt, A.; Kristiansen, G.; Muders, M.; Hölzel, M.; Ritter, M.; Alajati, A.; et al. Downstream neighbor of SON (DONSON) expression in enhanced in phenotypically aggressive prostate cancers. *Cancers* **2020**, *12*, 3439. [CrossRef] [PubMed]
39. Li, J.; Zhang, B.; Liu, M.; Fu, X.; Ci, X.; Fu, C.; Dong, G.; Wu, R.; Zhang, Z.; Fu, L.; et al. KLF5 is crucial for androgen-AR signaling to transactivate genes and promote cell proliferation in prostate cancer cells. *Cancers* **2020**, *12*, 748. [CrossRef] [PubMed]
40. Joshi, M.; Kim, J.; D'Alessandro, A.; Monk, E.; Bruce, K.; Elajaili, H.; Nozik-Grayck, E.; Goodspeed, A.; Costello, J.C.; Schlaepfer, I.R. CPT1A over-expression increases reactive oxygen species in the mitochondria and promotes antioxidant defenses in prostate cancer. *Cancers* **2020**, *12*, 3431. [CrossRef]
41. Hermanova, I.; Zúñiga-García, P.; Caro-Maldonado, A.; Fernández-Ruiz, S.; Salvador, F.; Martín-Martín, N.; Zabala-Letona, A.; Nuñez-Olle, M.; Torrano, V.; Camacho, L.; et al. Genetic manipulation of LKB1 elicits lethal metastatic prostate cancer. *J. Exp. Med.* **2020**, *217*, e20191787. [CrossRef] [PubMed]

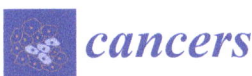

Article

The Disturbed Iron Phenotype of Tumor Cells and Macrophages in Renal Cell Carcinoma Influences Tumor Growth

Matthias Schnetz [1], Julia K. Meier [1], Claudia Rehwald [1], Christina Mertens [1], Anja Urbschat [2], Elisa Tomat [3], Eman A. Akam [3], Patrick Baer [4], Frederik C. Roos [5], Bernhard Brüne [1,6,7,8] and Michaela Jung [1,*]

- [1] Institute of Biochemistry I, Goethe-University Frankfurt, Theodor-Stern-Kai 7, 60590 Frankfurt am Main, Germany; matthias.schnetz@t-online.de (M.S.); meier@biochem.uni-frankfurt.de (J.K.M.); rehwald@biochem.uni-frankfurt.de (C.R.); c.mertens86@gmail.com (C.M.); B.Bruene@biochem.uni-frankfurt.de (B.B.)
- [2] Institute for Biomedicine, Aarhus University, C. F. Møllers Allé 6, 8000 Aarhus, Denmark; anja.urbschat@staff.uni-marburg.de
- [3] Department of Chemistry and Biochemistry, University of Arizona, 1306 E. University Blvd., Tucson, AZ 85721-0041, USA; tomat@email.arizona.edu (E.T.); EAKAM@mgh.harvard.edu (E.A.A.)
- [4] Division of Nephrology, Department of Internal Medicine III, Goethe-University Frankfurt, Theodor-Stern-Kai 7, 60590 Frankfurt am Main, Germany; p.baer@em.uni-frankfurt.de
- [5] Clinic of Urology, Goethe-University Frankfurt, Theodor-Stern-Kai 7, 60590 Frankfurt am Main, Germany; Frederik.Roos@kgu.de
- [6] German Cancer Consortium (DKTK), partner site Frankfurt/Mainz, 60590 Frankfurt am Main, Germany
- [7] Frankfurt Cancer Institute, Goethe-University Frankfurt, 60596 Frankfurt am Main, Germany
- [8] Project Group Translational Medicine and Pharmacology TMP, Fraunhofer Institute for Molecular Biology and Applied Ecology, 60596 Frankfurt am Main, Germany
- * Correspondence: m.jung@biochem.uni-frankfurt.de; Tel.: +49-69-6301-6931; Fax: +49-69-6301-4203

Received: 11 December 2019; Accepted: 23 February 2020; Published: 25 February 2020

Abstract: Accumulating evidence suggests that iron homeostasis is disturbed in tumors. We aimed at clarifying the distribution of iron in renal cell carcinoma (RCC). Considering the pivotal role of macrophages for iron homeostasis and their association with poor clinical outcome, we investigated the role of macrophage-secreted iron for tumor progression by applying a novel chelation approach. We applied flow cytometry and multiplex-immunohistochemistry to detect iron-dependent markers and analyzed iron distribution with atomic absorption spectrometry in patients diagnosed with RCC. We further analyzed the functional significance of iron by applying a novel extracellular chelator using RCC cell lines as well as patient-derived primary cells. The expression of iron-regulated genes was significantly elevated in tumors compared to adjacent healthy tissue. Iron retention was detected in tumor cells, whereas tumor-associated macrophages showed an iron-release phenotype accompanied by enhanced expression of ferroportin. We found increased iron amounts in extracellular fluids, which in turn stimulated tumor cell proliferation and migration. In vitro, macrophage-derived iron showed pro-tumor functions, whereas application of an extracellular chelator blocked these effects. Our study provides new insights in iron distribution and iron-handling in RCC. Chelators that specifically scavenge iron in the extracellular space confirmed the importance of macrophage-secreted iron in promoting tumor growth.

Keywords: renal cell carcinoma; iron; macrophages; chelation therapy

1. Introduction

Iron is the most abundant transition metal in the human body and drives a variety of mechanisms considered as hallmarks of cancer. Due to its role as critical cofactor for the rate-limiting step of DNA synthesis, iron controls cell division, DNA repair, and chromatin remodeling [1]. Iron is essential for basic cellular processes such as mitochondrial respiration and the enhanced metabolic turnover under cancerous conditions is controlled by iron-sulfur cluster proteins [2]. Considering the poor bioavailability of iron and its potent role in tumorigenesis, the interplay of different proteins important for iron import, storage, and export has to be tightly regulated through the interplay of various proteins, including the major iron storage protein ferritin with its subunits ferritin light chain (FTL) and ferritin heavy chain (FTH), the iron exporter ferroportin (FPN), transferrin receptor 1 (TfR1) for iron uptake, and iron-regulatory proteins 1 and 2 (IRP1/2) [3].

The kidney plays a unique role in systemic iron homeostasis by filtering and reabsorbing iron as well as providing the main body source of erythropoietin, which promotes hemoglobin synthesis [4]. It was previously shown that renal iron overload in anemic patients requiring chronic transfusions enhanced the incidence of renal cell carcinoma (RCC) development [5]. Repeated injections of iron led to RCC development with increased metastasis to the lungs and lymph nodes in experimental models [6]. Recently, the expression of TfR1 was associated with progression and mortality in clear cell RCC (ccRCC), identifying TfR1 as a novel RCC biomarker and potential therapeutic target [7]. Despite these compelling observations and the fact that RCC is one of the 15 most common cancers in humans as well as the third most common cause of death among urological cancers in 2018 [8], the role of iron for renal cancer was not investigated in detail so far. As RCC is considered to be resistant against conventional chemo- and radiation therapy, medical therapeutic options are currently still limited, thus making nephrectomy the first treatment approach in localized disease [9]. For metastatic disease state, treatment options include systemic therapy with multitarget tyrosine kinase inhibitors (TKIs), including sunitinib, cabozantinib, and pazopanib as well as mammalian target of rapamycin (mTOR) inhibitors such as everolimus or temsirolimus, offering only modest benefits [10]. Novel promising approaches for the treatment of metastatic RCC include immunotherapy and immune checkpoint inhibitors (ICI) targeting the cytotoxic-T-lymphocyte-associated antigen 4 (CTLA-4) and programmed death-1 (PD-1) with monoclonal antibodies [11]. Herein, besides to monotherapy a combinatory immunotherapy with checkpoint inhibitors has recently been approved on the base of a clinical phase-3 trial [12]. However, it is clear that there is still an urgent need for a deeper understanding of the molecular processes underlying RCC, which could provide new strategies to interfere during cancer therapy or might help to better determine patient prognosis.

Based on its concentration-dependent toxicity under physiological conditions, cellular iron homeostasis has to be strictly regulated [13]. This balance is shown to be compromised in the tumor microenvironment [14]. The malignant state of cancer cells is associated with a deregulation in cellular iron homeostasis, particularly in the expression of iron-regulated genes to fuel their higher metabolic iron demand needed for division, growth, and survival [14]. Cancer cells of various tumor entities develop an iron retaining phenotype by upregulating FTL, FTH [15,16], TfR1 [7,17], and IRP1/2 [18], while downregulating the iron exporter FPN [17]. These alterations result in increased tumor growth, aggressiveness and a poor patient outcome [14,19]. However, it still remains partly unclear how cancer cells acquire iron from the tumor microenvironment. One of the key players of iron homeostasis are macrophages (MΦ), which play a dual, activation-dependent role in iron homeostasis [20]. While classical, pro-inflammatory MΦ sequester iron to restrict iron availability for bacterial growth [21], alternatively activated anti-inflammatory MΦ recycle iron from dying cells by enhanced phagocytic activity [22]. Due to their physiological function, alternatively activated MΦ promote tissue repair, cell proliferation, and angiogenesis [23]. In the context of carcinogenesis, tumor associated MΦ (TAM) are major players when looking at abundance [24] and pro-tumoral function [25]. TAMs show characteristics of both pro-inflammatory MΦ that create an inflammatory environment during early stages of tumor development as well as anti-inflammatory MΦ [25,26] during later stages that suppress anti-tumor immunity and stimulate tumor neovascularization as well as metastasis [27,28]. Accordingly, TAMs were shown to positively associate with tumor progression and worse patient prognosis [29–31].

Although the control of iron availability in the tumor microenvironment seems to be crucial for tumor development, the distribution of iron within cellular compartments of the tumor, in particular tumor cells and TAMs, as well their association with tumor outcome have not been investigated so far in renal cancer. In the present study, we provide evidence that iron-dependent genes are highly expressed in renal cancer and are associated with tumor pT-stage (tumor size and invasion as defined by UICC) and tumor grade. We further show that TAMs adopt an iron-release phenotype with increased expression of the iron exporter FPN, whereas tumor cells retain intracellular iron. *In vitro* assays with patient-derived extracellular fluids as well as novel extracellular iron chelators showed the iron-dependence of renal tumor growth and metastasis.

2. Results

2.1. Iron Homeostasis Is Altered in RCC

In order to determine whether renal iron homeostasis is altered in RCC, we first analyzed mRNA expression of several iron-dependent genes, including *FPN*, *FTL*, *FTH*, *IRP2*, and *TfR1* in whole tissue homogenates of our patient cohort (Table 1).

Table 1. Patient cohort. The patient cohort is composed of 64 patients, grouped into three major renal tumor types ccRCC, pRCC, and chRCC. Patient parameters age, sex, pT-stage and grade are depicted in the table.

Number of Patients	ccRCC	pRCC	chRCC
	56	7	7
Age (years)			
mean	64 ± 10	68 ± 11	63 ± 10
median	64 ± 10	71 ± 11	62 ± 10
range	44–85	48–79	48–75
sex			
female	24%	29%	80%
male	76%	71%	20%
pT-stage			
pT1-pT2	55%		
pT3-pT4	45%		
Grade			
G1-G2	84%		
G3-G4	16%		

We found a significantly increased mRNA expression in tumor tissue compared to adjacent healthy tissue for all genes (Figure 1A–E). We performed hematoxylin staining in both healthy adjacent tissue and RCC subtypes of clear cell RCC (ccRCC), papillary RCC (pRCC) as well as chromophobe RCC (chRCC) that were included in our patient cohort (Figure S1A), and analyzed the *CAIX* mRNA expression, which was shown to be upregulated in more than 90% of RCC cases [32] (Figure S1B). Accordingly, *CAIX* mRNA expression was significantly upregulated in ccRCC and pRCC tumor subtypes, whilst varying in chRCC compared to adjacent healthy tissue. We next analyzed the mRNA expression of iron-dependent genes in relation to tumor grade (G1-G2 vs. G3-G4) and tumor pT-stage (pT1 pT2 vs. pT3-pT4). *FPN* mRNA expression was significantly increased in all tumor pT-stages and tumor grades compared to adjacent healthy tissue with the notion of enhanced expression in higher tumor pT-stage (Figure 1F). This expression pattern was also observed for mRNA expression of *TfR1* (Figure 1G).

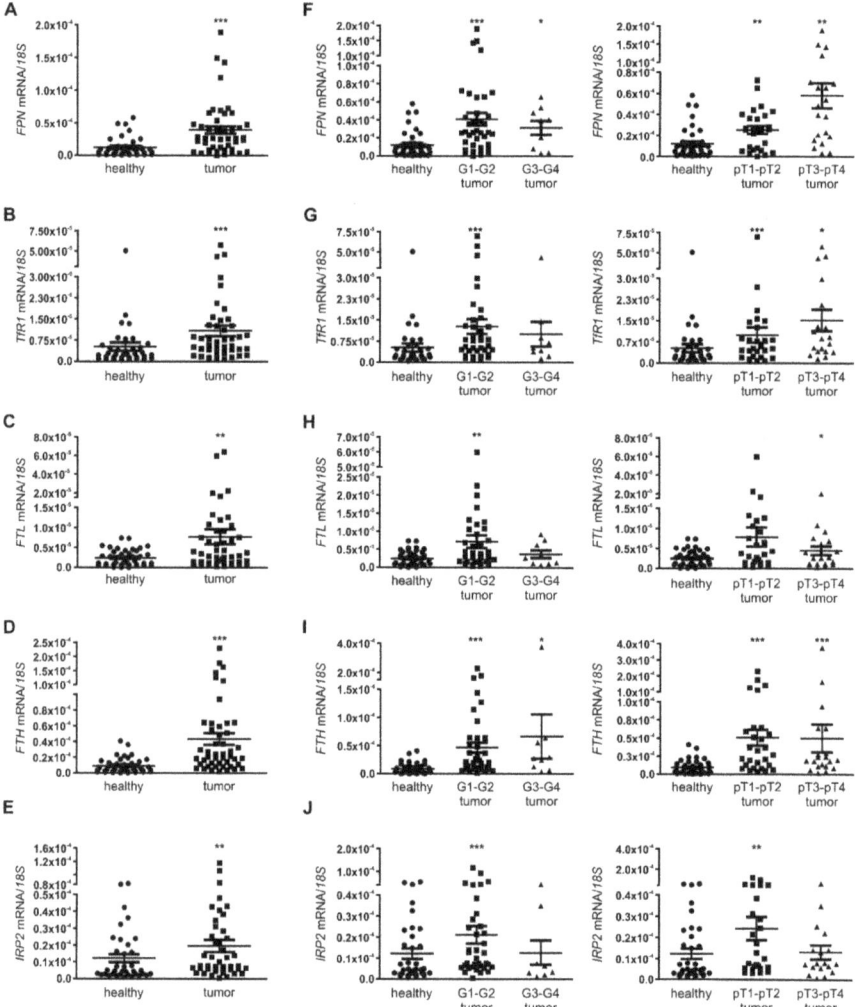

Figure 1. Expression of iron-regulated genes in human renal cancer samples. mRNA expression normalized to the housekeeping gene *18S* in whole tissue homogenates of renal tumor tissue and adjacent healthy tissue of (**A**) *FPN* (n = 48), (**B**) *TfR1* (n = 47), (**C**) *FTL* (n = 48), (**D**) *FTH* (n = 48), and (**E**) *IRP2* (n = 46). (**F–J**) Left: mRNA expression of (**F**) *FPN*, (**G**) *TfR1*, (**H**) *FTL*, (**I**) *FTH*, and (**J**) *IRP2* correlated to low (G1-G2) and high (G3-G4) tumor grade. Right: mRNA expression of (**F**) *FPN*, (**G**) *TfR1*, (**H**) *FTL*, (**I**) *FTH*, and (**J**) *IRP2* correlated to low (pT1–pT2) and high (pT3–pT4) tumor pT-stage. Number of tested patients differ between genes due to patients with failed measurements of initially low sample RNA amount. No samples have been excluded as outliers. Graphs are displayed as means ± SEM with * $p < 0.05$, ** $p < 0.01$, *** $p < 0.001$.

For *FTL*, *FTH*, and *IRP2*, we found an increased mRNA expression in lower tumor grades (G1-G2) and lower tumor pT-stage (pT1–pT2), but either similar or lower expression within the group of higher tumor grades (G3-G4) and higher tumor pT-stage (pT3–pT4; Figure 1H–J).

Since RCC subtypes significantly differ regarding in the prognosis and treatment [33], we analyzed the mRNA expression of iron-dependent gene expression in patients with ccRCC, pRCC, or chRCC of our cohort (Figure 2A–E, left panel). While the defined iron-dependent genes were significantly upregulated within the ccRCC subgroup in comparison to adjacent healthy tissue, mRNA expression in the pRCC and the chRCC subtype varied, depending on the analyzed gene. Expression of *FPN*, *FTH*, and *IRP2* was higher in all RCC subtypes compared to adjacent healthy tissue, whereas *FTL* remained unaltered in the chRCC subtype and *TfR1* was lower in pRCC subtypes. In order to verify our data, especially regarding patients diagnosed with pRCC and chRCC, where less patients were included in our cohort, we analyzed publically available TCGA KIRC (ccRCC), KIRP (pRCC), and KICH (chRCC) data sets (Figure 2A–E, right panel). RNA expression in the TCGA data sets confirmed a significant upregulation of *FPN*, *FTL*, and *FTH* in ccRCC. In pRCC, *FPN*, *FTL*, and *FTH* are significantly higher expressed, while *IRP2* remained unaltered. Our data regarding reduced *TfR1* expression in pRCC and unaltered *FTL* expression in chRCC was corroborated using the TCGA data analysis.

As we showed an altered iron homeostasis in all histopathological subtypes, we next aimed at looking into the iron distribution in RCC tissue. We first analyzed the iron amount of tumor and adjacent healthy tissues by AAS measurements. Tumor tissue showed an overall significantly higher iron amount than adjacent healthy renal tissue (Figure 3A). When analyzing the histopathological subtypes, both ccRCC and chRCC showed a higher iron amount compared to adjacent healthy tissue, whereas in pRCC the total iron amount remained nearly unaltered (Figure 3B). To address the question of iron localization within the tissues, Perl's staining of tumor versus adjacent healthy tissue slides was used. In line with our AAS analysis, healthy renal tissue showed a low amount of iron deposits appearing in blue. Compared to the healthy adjacent tissue, a more intense staining in ccRCC was observed, whereas iron deposits in pRCC remained low (Figure 3C and Figure S2A–D). Intriguingly, the iron load in chRCC varies considerably between different patients (Figure S2D) with the notion of overall enhanced iron deposits in tumor tissue compared to adjacent healthy tissue. In ccRCC tissue, we hypothesize that the highly intense blue-colored cells might be tumor cells, whereas the diffuse positive staining around long-shaped cells in the stroma might be iron secreted by MΦ. There are also other positive-stained cells in the stroma that appear much smaller, which we believe might be lymphocytes that are also able to handle iron in the tumor stroma as previously described by Marques et al. in mammary carcinoma [34]. For pRCC we only detect low amounts of overall Perl's staining, with localized positive staining mostly in tumor cells, whereas we observed high amounts of iron deposits in chRCC, mostly within the tumor stroma. We and others previously showed that tumor cells are prone to adopt an iron retaining phenotype, whereas cells from the tumor stroma such as MΦ rather adopt an iron mobilization and iron releasing phenotype [34,35]. In order to verify the location of iron within different tumor compartments in RCC tissues, we sorted both tumor cells and tumor-associated MΦ from tumor tissue of all histopathological RCC subtypes and compared them to sorted epithelial cells and MΦ isolated from adjacent healthy tissue (Figure 3D,E). A significantly reduced intracellular iron amount in MΦ isolated from ccRCC and pRCC tissues was observed, whereas MΦ from chRCC tissues showed similar intracellular iron levels as cells from adjacent healthy tissue (Figure 3D). In contrast, tumor cells showed a significant increased iron amount in ccRCC and pRCC compared to adjacent renal epithelial cells. In chRCC, iron amount in tumor cells showed a larger variation resulting in a non-significant increase compared to renal epithelial cells isolated from adjacent healthy tissue (Figure 3E).

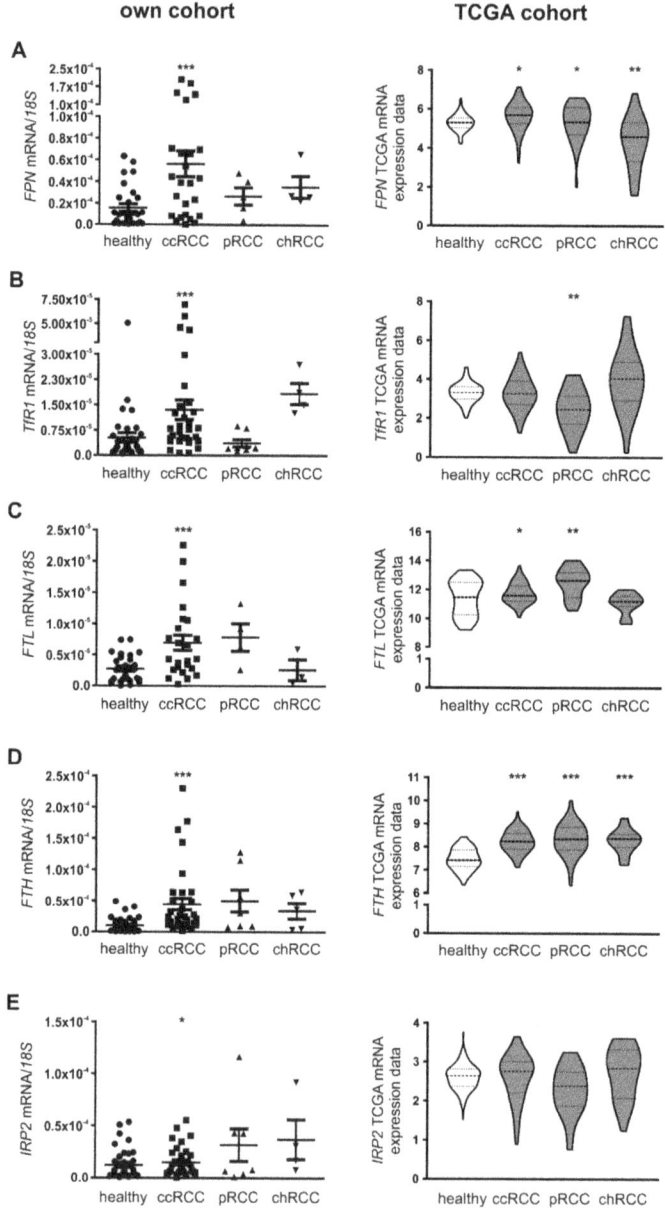

Figure 2. Profile of iron-regulated genes in histopathologically distinct RCC subtypes. mRNA expression of renal tumor and adjacent healthy samples in clear cell (ccRCC), papillary (pRCC), and chromophobe (chRCC) RCC of own patient cohort (left) compared to mRNA expression acquired from the TCGA database applying the ccRCC-KIRC ($n = 70$), pRCC-KIRP ($n = 31$), and chRCC-KICH ($n = 23$) datasets (right). Analyzed genes include (**A**) *FPN*, (**B**) *TfR1*, (**C**) *FTL*, (**D**) *FTH*, and (**E**) *IRP2*. Own cohort is normalized to housekeeping gene *18S* expression. Graphs are displayed as means ± SEM with * $p < 0.05$, ** $p < 0.01$, *** $p < 0.001$.

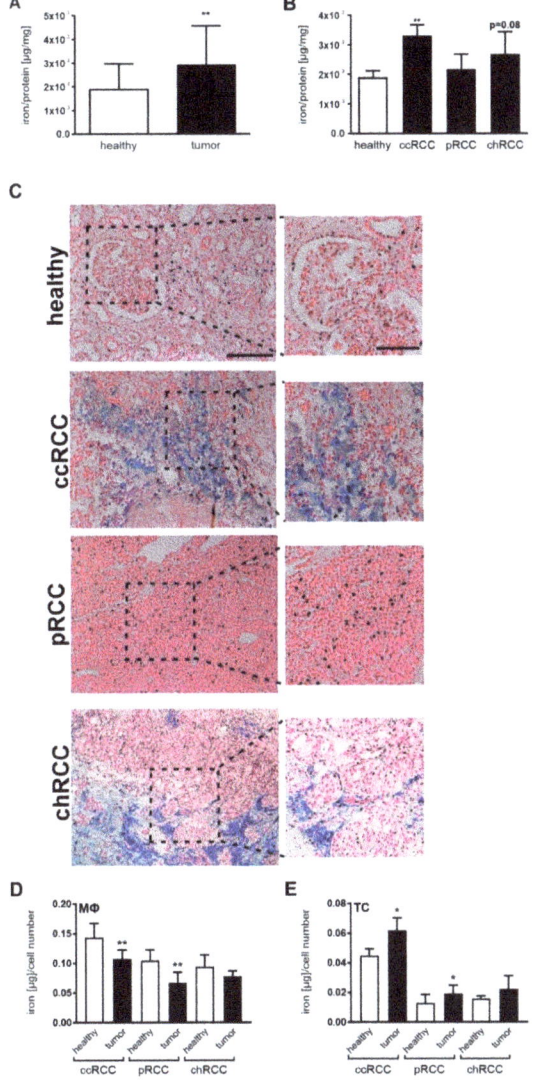

Figure 3. Iron homeostasis and distribution is altered in RCC. (**A**) Iron load normalized to protein amount in whole tissue homogenates of renal cancer tissue in comparison to adjacent healthy renal tissue measured by AAS ($n = 31$). (**B**) Iron load in whole tissue homogenates of clear cell (ccRCC; $n = 17$), papillary (pRCC; $n = 7$), and chromophobe (chRCC; $n = 7$) RCC in comparison to corresponding healthy renal tissue measured by AAS. (**C**) Representative pictures of Perl's staining of RCC tissue and adjacent healthy renal tissue of ccRCC, pRCC, and chRCC. Representative pictures (scale bar: 200 μm) with corresponding detailed pictures (scale bar: 100 μm) are given. (**D,E**) Macrophages (MΦ) and CD326+ cells were isolated by FACS-sorting from RCC tissue and adjacent healthy tissue. Intracellular iron load of (**D**) MΦ and (**E**) either tumor cells (TC) or epithelial cells from adjacent healthy tissue of ccRCC ($n = 7$), pRCC ($n = 13$), and chRCC ($n = 4$) measured by AAS. Statistical analysis was performed comparing tumor to adjacent healthy tissue within the histopathological subtypes. Graphs are displayed as means ± SEM. * $p < 0.05$, ** $p < 0.01$.

2.2. Iron Promotes Renal Tumor Cell Growth

In order to test the role of iron released into the tumor stroma, we generated extracellular fluids (EC fluids) from both tumor tissue as well as adjacent healthy tissue (Figure 4A). First, we analyzed the iron amount in EC fluids by AAS and observed significantly higher iron amounts in EC fluids isolated from tumor tissue as compared to EC fluids from adjacent healthy tissue (Figure 4B). We then stimulated renal tumor cells CAKI-1 (Figure 4C) and 786-O (Figure 4D) as well as primary patient-derived tumor tubular epithelial cells (TTEC; Figure 4E) with tumor EC fluids. Cellular proliferation was analyzed applying xCELLigence real-time measurements. Results showed that all tested cell lines as well as primary tumor cells positively responded to treatments with tumor EC fluids and augmented cellular proliferation upon stimulation.

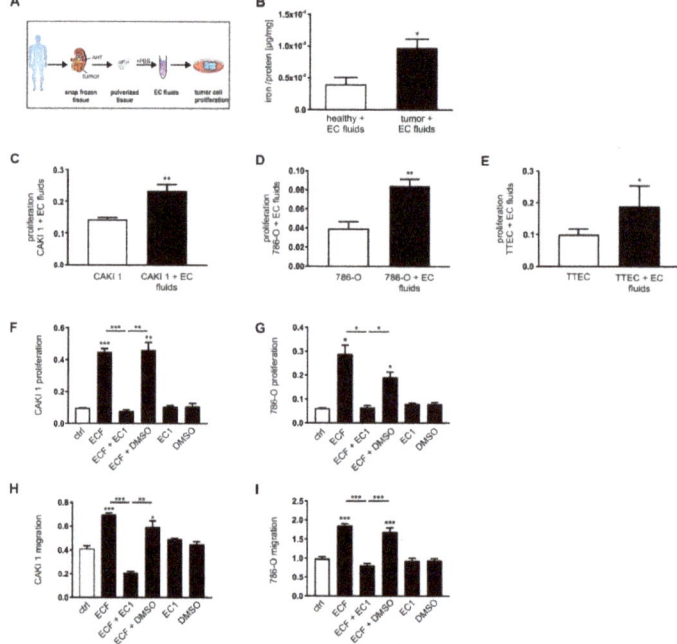

Figure 4. Extracellular iron induces proliferation and migration of tumor cells in vitro. (**A**) Schematic overview of how to generate extracellular (EC) fluids (ECF) from primary human renal tumor and adjacent healthy tissue. (**B**) Iron load measured by AAS relative to the total protein amount of EC fluids of ccRCC tissue compared to adjacent healthy renal tissue ($n = 8$). Proliferation of (**C**) CAKI-1 ($n = 7$), (**D**) 786-O ($n = 8$), and (**E**) primary human tumor tubular epithelial cells (TTEC) upon stimulation with EC fluids in vitro measured with the xCELLigence system ($n = 8$). Proliferation of (**F**) CAKI 1 ($n = 4$) and (**G**) 786-O ($n = 4$) cells as well as migration of (**H**) CAKI 1 ($n = 4$) and (**I**) 786-O cells ($n = 4$) upon stimulation with EC fluids in the presence or absence of an extracellular chelator (EC1, 100µM) or dimethyl sulfoxide (DMSO) as negative control measured with the xCELLigence system. Graphs are displayed as means ± SEM with * $p < 0.05$, ** $p < 0.01$, *** $p < 0.001$.

To further verify the role of extracellular iron on tumor proliferation and migration, we stimulated tumor cells with EC fluids in the presence of a specific extracellular chelator (EC1). This novel compound was designed for extracellular chelation as it features an established iron-binding unit as well as a negatively charged group to hinder cell membrane permeation (Figure S3A). In particular, the tridentate chelating unit of EC1 includes a thiosemicarbazone moiety that is common to many anti-proliferative iron chelators [36,37]; however, the incorporation of a negatively charged sulfonate group significantly limits the ability of EC1 to cross cellular membranes. As a result, EC1 is expected to chelate iron only in the extracellular space without affecting intracellular iron levels. The iron binding abilities were validated using optical absorption spectroscopy (Figure S3B). The effects of EC1 on cellular viability and proliferation were tested in vitro in CAKI-1 and 786-O cells in comparison to the unspecific chelator 2,2'-dipyridine (2'2-DPD) and the intracellularly activated prochelator (TC3-S)$_2$ [38–40]. Whereas EC1 showed no effect at concentrations up to 100 µM with regard to both, viability (Figure S3C,D) and cellular proliferation (Figure S3E,F) under basal growth conditions, both 2'2-DPD and (TC3-S)$_2$ showed increasingly adverse effects at higher concentrations regarding cellular viability and anti-proliferative capacity due to the fact that both are able to chelate intracellular iron. In contrast, EC1 showed toxicity effects only at very high concentrations (500 µM), which might be due to non-specific side effects. Supplementation of EC fluids with EC1 (100 µM) in order to specifically block iron secreted to the supernatant resulted in a significant inhibition of cellular proliferation and migration of both CAKI-1 (Figure 4F,H) and 786-O cells (Figure 4G,I).

2.3. Tumor Proliferation by Macrophage-Secreted Iron Is Suppressed by EC1

According to our previous observation that tumor-associated MΦ adopt an iron releasing phenotype (Figure 3D), we further established an in vitro setting to analyze the role of macrophage-secreted iron in conferring renal tumor cell growth (Figure 5A).

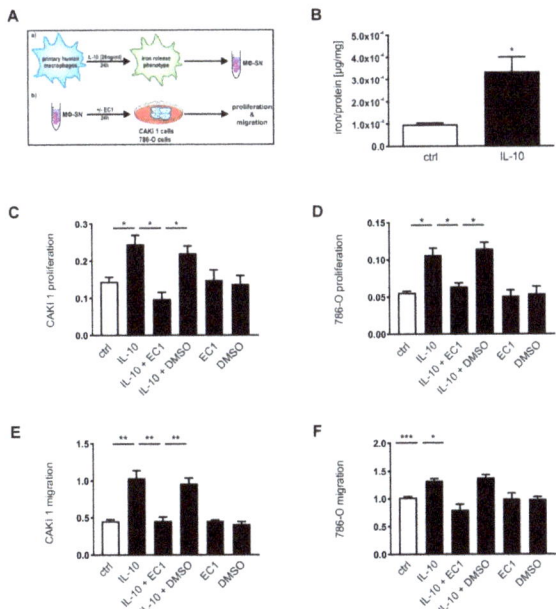

Figure 5. Macrophage-secreted iron induces proliferation and migration of tumor cells in vitro. (**A**) Schematic overview of how to generate conditioned medium from iron-releasing human MΦ. (**B**) Iron amount measured by AAS relative to the total protein amount in the supernatant of primary human MΦ, either left untreated (ctrl) or stimulated with IL-10 (20 ng/mL; 24 h) ($n = 5$). Proliferation of (**C**) CAKI 1 ($n = 4$) and (**D**) 786-O ($n = 4$) cells as well as migration of (**E**) CAKI 1 ($n = 4$) and (**F**) 786-O cells ($n = 4$) upon stimulation with the supernatant of IL-10-stimulated MΦ in the presence or absence of an extracellular chelator (EC1, 100 µM) or dimethyl sulfoxide (DMSO) as negative control measured with the xCELLigence system. Graphs are displayed as means ± SEM with * $p < 0.05$, ** $p < 0.01$, *** $p < 0.001$.

As previously published [41,42], IL-10 stimulation of primary human MΦ induced the release of iron into the supernatant measured by AAS (Figure 5B). We next applied macrophage-conditioned supernatants to renal tumor cells CAKI-1 (Figure 5C,E) and 786-O (Figure 5D,F) and observed enhanced proliferation (Figure 5C,D) as well as tumor cell migration (Figure 5E,F) measured by xCELLigence in real-time upon stimulation with IL-10-conditioned media.

To further verify the effect of EC1 on tumor proliferation and migration in the presence of macrophage-secreted iron, we stimulated tumor cells with MΦ-conditioned media supplemented by EC1 (100 µM). In line with our previous observations using EC fluids (Figure 4F–I), EC1 was able to significantly inhibit cellular proliferation and migrations of both CAKI-1 (Figure 5C,E) and 786-O cells (Figure 5D,F).

2.4. Macrophage-Derived Iron Is Exported Via the Iron Exporter FPN, Which Is Positively Associated with Poor Patient Outcome

We next asked whether the iron exporter FPN was expressed in tumor-associated MΦ. Therefore, FPN protein expression in MΦ by flow cytometry (Figure 6A) was measured, showing higher FPN expression in both tumor stroma (Figure 6B) as well as tumor-associated MΦ (Figure 6C) compared to stroma and MΦ from adjacent healthy tissue. In order to localize FPN protein within the tissue, multiplex-immunohistochemistry was applied, combining CD163 as macrophage marker, FPN, and DAPI as nuclear stain (Figure 6D), showing enhanced co-localization of CD163 and FPN in tumor tissue compared to adjacent healthy tissue. Taking our previous FPN mRNA data into consideration that showed enhanced FPN expression in tumor tissue compared to adjacent healthy tissue (Figures 1A and 2A), we next questioned the association of FPN expression with tumor grade (Figure 6E) and tumor (Figure 6F) of our own cohort (upper part) compared to the TCGA data set (lower part). In line with the TCGA data set, we observed association of FPN mRNA expression only with lower tumor grade (Figure 6E). For tumor pT-stage (Figure 6F), a positive association with lower tumor pT-stages (pT1–pT2) was noticed, which was more pronounced in higher tumor pT-stages (pT3–pT4). However, TCGA data suggests higher FPN expression in patients with low tumor grade (G1–G2) and tumor pT-stage (pT1–pT2). Accordingly, low tissue FPN expression correlated with a lower overall survival probability analyzed by the R2: Genomics Analysis and Visualization Platform applying the 'Tumor Kidney Renal Clear Cell Carcinoma—TCGA-533' data set (Figure 6G).

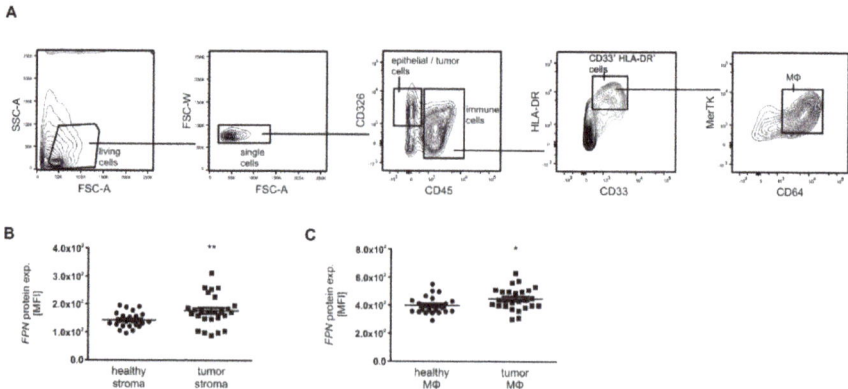

Figure 6. Cont.

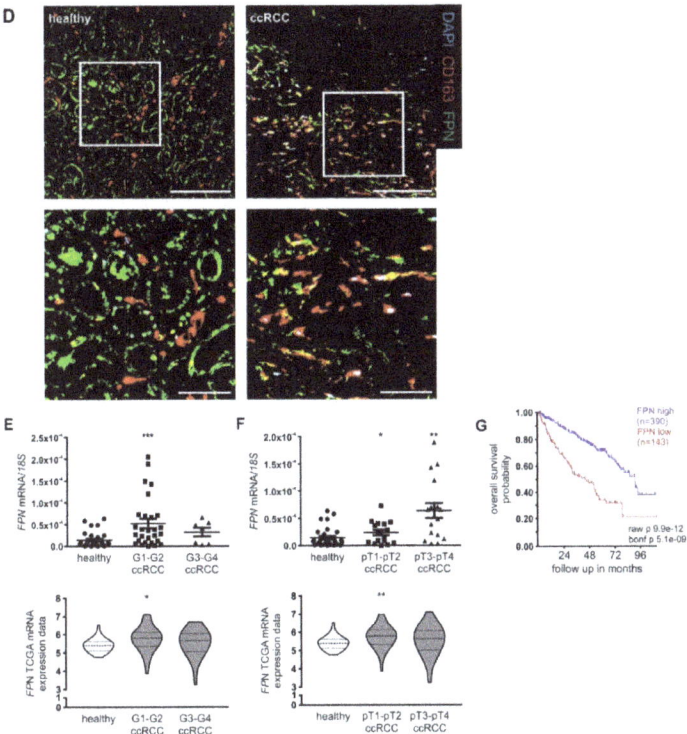

Figure 6. Tumor-associated MΦ express enhanced FPN protein. (**A**) FACS panel how to gate CD45$^+$ immune cells and CD326$^+$ epithelial/tumor cells. Immune cells were further gated for CD33$^+$/HLA-DR$^+$ cells of which CD64$^+$ and MerTK$^+$ MΦ were sub-selected. Cells were subsequently analyzed for their FPN protein expression, displayed as MFI (mean fluorescence intensity). (**B**) FPN protein expression as MFI of CD45$^-$/CD326$^-$ stroma cells ($n = 26$). (**C**) FPN protein expression as MFI of MΦ in tumor tissue compared to adjacent healthy tissue ($n = 26$). (**D**) Representative pictures for the MΦ marker CD163 and FPN protein expression in tumor tissue compared to healthy adjacent tissue applying confocal laser scanning miscroscopy. DAPI was used as nuclear stain. Scale bar: 200 μm. *FPN* mRNA expression normalized to *18S* expression correlated to (**E**) low (G1–G2) and high (G3–G4) tumor grade and (**F**) low (pT1–pT2) and high (pT3–pT4) tumor pT-stage in our patient cohort (upper panels; $n = 48$) compared to the TCGA data base, applying the ccRCC-KIRC data set (lower panels; $n = 70$). (**G**) Kaplan-Meier curve of high or low *FPN* expression from the R2 bioinformatics platform using the ccRCC-KIRC data set. Graphs are displayed as means ± SEM with * $p < 0.05$, ** $p < 0.01$, *** $p < 0.001$.

3. Discussion

We present evidence that iron metabolism is significantly altered in renal cancer. We observed elevated iron deposits in renal tumor tissue compared to adjacent healthy tissue as well as enhanced expression of iron-regulated genes in tumor tissue isolated from patients with renal cancer compared to adjacent healthy tissue. As iron is of importance for essentially all tumor hallmarks, we further investigated the role of iron in determining tumor cell proliferation and migration. In this setting, we also described and characterized the use of a novel extracellular iron chelator that scavenges iron in the extracellular space, thereby providing a valuable tool to investigate its role in the tumor microenvironment.

Numerous studies support a positive association between increased iron levels and cancer development, whereby cancer cells evolved specialized mechanisms for iron acquisition, storage, and mobilization in order to ensure their enhanced metabolic turnover [43]. Despite the fact that both availability as well as distribution of iron is strictly regulated under healthy conditions, cancers exert a profoundly dysregulated iron-handling capacity with altered expression of iron-regulated genes [15–17,44,45]. These observations are corroborated by the present study, detecting enhanced expression of iron-regulated genes in renal tumor tissue as compared to adjacent healthy tissue, which was most prominent in ccRCC. This effect was further confirmed by TCGA data base analysis. In this regard, we also found that cancer cells isolated from patients with renal cancer showed enhanced iron sequestration compared to their healthy counterparts.

Taking the unique role of the kidney in iron physiology into consideration [4], several markers, including erythropoietin [46] have been tested in RCC. Regardless of the initial promising effects, they only showed low predictive value. There are still no specific and reliable tumor markers neither for RCC diagnosis nor for monitoring post-operative disease outcome. Despite the apparent association of RCC with the development of systemic anemia in RCC patients [47], the role of iron in human RCC carcinogenesis is largely unknown and was only scarcely investigated so far. Because of the growing evidence on their tumor-promoting effects, the expression of iron-regulated genes could become an important factor among the markers of tumorigenesis. Along these lines, Greene at al. recently showed an association of TfR1 expression and RCC progression [7], with TfR1 levels being highest in benign primary tumors, subsequently dropping during the course of disease progression. TfR1 levels were therefore inversely associated with worse survival, but independent of tumor pathology. In line, we observed overall enhanced iron amounts in tumor tissue as compared to adjacent healthy tissue for all investigated renal cancer subtypes. Interestingly, iron amounts in chRCC varied considerably between different patients and needs to be further addressed in follow-up studies including higher patient number. Intriguingly, we also found initial differences in iron levels in adjacent healthy tissue for each histopathological subtype. These observations might arise both from the original localization of the tissue for individual samples as well as result from different basal iron levels of each individual patient. Therefore, healthy control tissue has to be controlled carefully to avoid misleading interpretation.

Nonetheless, modulating the iron-retaining tumor phenotype reduced growth and progression of both human and mouse carcinomas [48]. The use of iron chelators in the treatment of cancer inhibited DNA synthesis and caused a G1-S-phase cell cycle arrest, attenuated epithelial-mesenchymal-transition, and promoted cancer cell apoptosis [39]. Furthermore, chemically-induced and oncogene-driven cancer models corroborated these findings and stressed the relevance of iron for tumor development [49,50]. Numerous studies investigated methods to interfere with iron-handling in cancer cells, either by directly modulating iron-regulated genes [43] or by the use of iron chelators [37]. Nevertheless, a detailed knowledge of the effects of chelators within the tumor microenvironment (and on potential iron sources thereof) is still lacking [43]. In this study, we identified enhanced iron levels in extracellular fluids of tumor tissue in comparison to healthy adjacent tissue, suggesting that cells of the tumor microenvironment secreted iron in extracellular fluids. Due to their important role in tumor development and iron handling, we proposed that MΦ might adopt a pro-tumorigenic iron-releasing phenotype, whereby tumor growth is favored. Since MΦ are central players in systemic iron homeostasis, they have evolved unique mechanisms to recycle, store, and release iron to their local microenvironment. However, our data suggest differences in total tissue iron levels versus iron amounts of both MΦ and tumor cells for histopathological renal cancer subtypes. We hypothesize that even if the overall amount of iron is not changed in tumor tissue compared to adjacent healthy tissue in pRCC patients, the different distribution of iron within the tissue and in cells of the tumor mass, i.e. MΦ or tumor cells might add to the characteristics of iron as a pro-tumoral factor.

Macrophage iron homeostasis is functionally coupled to their heterogeneity and plasticity, with their polarization status being reflected also by their expression profiles of iron-regulated genes. We previously showed that treatment of MΦ with LPS/IFNγ enhanced the retention of iron within the cell, whereas stimulation with anti-inflammatory cytokines such as IL-10 or IL-4 induced the release of iron [41]. This observation falls in line with a typical cytokine/chemokine profile of differentially polarized MΦ. We used this setting also in the present study to generate supernatant from IL-10-polarized iron-releasing MΦ. We tested the effect of iron, which was released by MΦ, in combination with an iron chelator that specifically binds iron in the extracellular space. EC1, which was designed and synthesized specifically for this study, is a thiosemicarbazone chelator featuring a sulfonate group that is negatively charged near neutral pH. While the tridentate (O,N,S) binding unit (see Figure S3A) ensures high-affinity iron coordination, the negative charge on the scaffold was incorporated to limit or hamper cellular membrane permeability. This strategy is particularly advantageous for the study of iron with respect to the crosstalk between TAMs and cancer cells. We found that the addition of EC1 reversed the positive effect of macrophage-conditioned media on the proliferation and migration of cancer cells. Although the exact molecular speciation of iron released in the macrophage supernatant remains to be determined, these experiments indicated that this iron pool is accessible by small-molecule chelators and could represent a hitherto unrecognized effect of these antiproliferative compounds in the tumor microenvironment.

Our previous studies using intracellularly active pro-chelators underscore the importance of macrophage-released iron for tumor cell proliferation [41]. Intriguingly, current research focuses primarily on the role of iron and iron-chelation therapy in tumor cells, whereas detailed knowledge on the crosstalk between tumor cells and tumor-associated MΦ as a possible source of iron is lacking. Taking into account that the presence of MΦ in tumor tissue is closely linked to tumor progression, we further analyzed the expression of the iron exporter FPN as a determinant of the iron releasing capacity of MΦ. We found enhanced expression of FPN in tumor MΦ compared to MΦ of adjacent healthy tissues, which was significantly associated with tumor pT-stage. However, these data could not be corroborated by TCGA data base analysis regarding overall patient survival. This discrepancy might arise from low cohort size of analyzed patients. Furthermore, it might also be necessary to distinguish FPN expression in stromal cells versus tumor cells as compared to whole tissue analysis. Recently, it was shown that tumor-associated MΦ also secrete iron in form of FT, which, in turn, stimulated tumor cell proliferation [44]. FTL expression in MΦ was further described as an independent prognostic marker in node-negative breast cancer. However, in the present study, we did not observe significant changes in FT protein expression in tumor-associated MΦ compared to MΦ isolated from adjacent healthy tissue. Recently, Marques et al. observed that FT expression was elevated in tumor-infiltrating lymphocytes, whereas no changes were detected for FT expression in tumor-associated MΦ [34]. The crucial implication of MΦ in tumor development and their role in iron distribution within the tumor microenvironment represents an important area of investigation in contemporary cancer biology.

Collectively, the results of the present study indicate that iron homeostasis is significantly disturbed in renal cancer with most of the investigated iron-regulated genes being associated with tumor grade and tumor pT-stage. Moreover, we observed that iron availability in the tumor microenvironment might be controlled by tumor-associated MΦ, which adopt an iron-release phenotype through increased expression of FPN. Application of chelators that are able to specifically scavenge iron in the extracellular space confirmed the importance of macrophage-secreted iron in promoting tumor cell proliferation and migration.

Future experimental in vivo studies should address the possibility to either interfere with iron availability in the tumor microenvironment or use macrophage-targeted chelation strategies. Moreover, more research is needed with regard to the questions of: i) the molecular networks that allow tumor cells to actually take up, store, and utilize iron and ii) the release of tumor cell-derived mediators that re-program stromal cells, i.e., MΦ, to serve as an iron source in order to maintain their enhanced metabolism and growth.

4. Materials and Methods

4.1. Ethics

Investigations were conducted in accordance with the ethical standards according to the Declaration of Helsinki and to national and international guidelines. Primary human tumor and adjacent healthy tissues were obtained from 64 patients with the approval of the ethics committees of the Goethe-University Hospital Frankfurt am Main (04/09 UGO 03/10) and the Philipps-University Hospital Marburg (122/14). Patients gave their written informed consent prior to surgery (UCT 122/14 and 04/09 UGO 03/10).

4.2. Participants

Patients included in this study underwent nephrectomy or partial nephrectomy for renal lesions histopathologically diagnosed with renal cancer between 2016 and 2019 at University Hospitals Frankfurt am Main and Marburg (see Table 1). Patients underwent preoperative staging either by computed tomography or Magnetic resonance imaging and surgery was performed before receiving other therapy. Tissue was collected immediately after surgery and processed for single cell suspensions, fixed in 4% paraformaldehyde (PFA) or stored at −80 °C. Pathological examination was performed by independent pathologists applying the UICC TNM classification of malignant tumors [51].

4.3. RNA Extraction and Quantitative Real-Time PCR (qRT-PCR)

Total RNA was extracted from homogenized tissue samples using peqGold RNAPure (VWR, Darmstadt, Germany, 732-3312) and transcribed using Maxima First Strand cDNA synthesis kit (Thermo Fisher, Dreieich, Germany, K1642). Gene expression profiles were determined by qPCR using the SYBR Green Supermix (Bio-Rad, Munich, Germany, 1725006CUST) on a CFX-Connect real-time-PCR detection system (Bio-Rad). Results were quantified using the Bio-Rad CFX-Manager (Bio-Rad, version 3) with 18S mRNA expression as housekeeping control. All primers except TfR1 Primer (Qiagen, Hilden, Germany, QT00094850) are listed in the supplemental information file and were purchased from Biomers (Ulm, Germany).

4.4. Data baSe Analysis

To show mRNA expression of *FPN*, *FTL*, *FTH*, *TfR1* and *IRP2* in different renal cancer subtypes, gene expression data of the Cancer Genome Atlas were analyzed (https://portal.gdc.cancer.gov/). Expression data of TCGA files were used of the following data sets: "Tumor Kidney Renal Clear Cell Carcinoma" (KIRC, $n = 533$), "Tumor Kidney Renal Papillary Cell Carcinoma" (KIRP, $n = 290$), and "Tumor Kidney Chromophobe" (KICH, $n = 66$). Cases with tumor and adjacent renal healthy tissue data available were included in the analysis (KIRC: $n = 70$; KIRP: $n = 31$; KICH: $n = 23$).

Kaplan-Meier plots were generated using the R2 Genomics Analysis and Visualization Platform (http://r2.amc.nl). The dataset "Tumor Kidney Renal Clear Cell Carcinoma" ($n = 533$) was chosen. Default settings of the KaplanScan including a log rank comparison between the groups were used to determine an optimum survival cut-off as described in the portal. The resulting p-value as well as the Bonferroni correction of the log rank comparison are included in the plots.

4.5. Atomic Absorption Spectroscopy (AAS)

Iron measurements were performed as previously described [35]. Whole tissue homogenates where either measured as whole homogenates and normalized to total protein amount or underwent FACS sorting with the final cell suspension being analyzed for its iron content and normalized to the total number of sorted cells.

4.6. Perl's Stain

Tissue slides were dewaxed in xylene and rehydrated in a series of alcohol solutions using decreasing concentrations. Perl's stain was performed using the Iron Stain Kit (Sigma Aldrich, Taufkirchen, Germany, HT20) according to the manufacturer's protocol. Slides were then washed in distilled water, counterstained with Nuclear Fast Red solution (Sigma Aldrich, N3020), rapidly dehydrated, and mounted in Entellan (Merck, Darmstadt, Germany, 107961). Pictures were acquired using an Axioskop 40 (Zeiss, Oberkochen, Germany).

4.7. Flow Cytometric Analyses

Tumors and adjacent healthy renal tissues were dissociated using the human Tumor Dissociation Kit (Miltenyi Biotec, Bergisch-Gladbach, Germany, 130-095-929) and GentleMACS System (Miltenyi Biotec). Samples were acquired with a LSRII/Fortessa flow cytometer (BD, Heidelberg, Germany) expressed as mean fluorescence intensity (MFI). CompBeads (BD) were used for single color compensation to create multi-color compensation matrices. For gating, fluorescence minus one (FMO) controls were used. Prior to experiments, all antibodies and secondary reagents were titrated to determine optimal concentrations.

For staining of FPN, extracellular staining of patient-derived single cell suspensions was performed, containing CD33 BV510 (BD, 563257), MerTK BV421 (Biolegend, San Diego, CA, USA, 367603), CD45 AF700 (Biolegend, 368513), CD 64 BV605 (Biolegend, 305033), CD206 PE-Cy7 (Biolegend, 321124), CD326 PE-CF594 (BD, 565399), HLA-DR APC-Cy7 (Biolegend, 307658), and FPN PE (Novus, Wiesbaden, Germany, NBP1-21502).

4.8. FACS Sorting and Processing of Sorted Cells

Single cell suspensions of tumor and adjacent healthy renal tissue were stained with an antibody cocktail containing CD33 BV510 (BD, 563257), MerTK BV421 (Biolegend, 367603), CD45 AF700 (Biolegend, 368513), CD64 BV605 (Biolegend, 305033), CD326 PE-CF594 (BD, 565399), HLA-DR APC-Cy7 (Biolegend, 307658). Cell suspensions were sorted using a FACS Aria (BD) FACS sorter, resulting in $CD45^-/CD326^+$ epithelial cells and $CD45^+/CD33^+/HLA\text{-}DR^+/CD64^+/MerTK^+$ MΦ from tumor and healthy tissue.

Cells were harvested for AAS (5000 cells) or used for RNA isolation (1000 cells). RNA isolation and transcription were performed using the RNeasy Micro Kit (Qiagen, 74004) and Sensiscript RT Kit (Qiagen, 205211) according to the manufacturer's kit protocols.

4.9. Cell Culture

Human renal cancer cell lines CAKI-1 and 786-O cells (kindly provided by PD Dr. Anja Urbschat) were cultured in Dulbecco's modified Eagle's medium (Gibco, Dreieich, Germany, 41965) supplemented with penicillin 100 U/mL (Sigma-Aldrich, P4333), streptomycin 100 mg/mL (Sigma-Aldrich, S8636), and 10% FCS (Capricorn Scientific, Ebersdorfergrund, Germany FBS-11A). Cells were regularly tested for mycoplasma contamination using Venor GeM Classic (Minerva Biolabs, Berlin, Germany, 11-1100).

4.10. Tumor Tubular Epithelial Cell Isolation

Human tubular epithelial cells (TTEC) were isolated as previously described [52]. Briefly, tumor tissue was minced, digested with collagenase/dispase (1 mg/mL), and passed through a 106 μm mesh. The tumor tissue solution was then incubated with collagenase (1 mg/mL), DNase (0.1 mg/mL) and $MgCl_2$ (5 mmol/L). Cells were seeded on FCS-precoated plates and grown in M199 medium (Sigma Aldrich, M4530), supplemented with penicillin (100 U/mL), streptomycin (100 mg/mL), and 10% FBS. Meropenem (100 μg/mL, Sigma Aldrich, M2574) was added to the culture medium for the first 2–3 days after isolation. Passages from two to four were used for experiments.

4.11. EC Fluids Generation

Frozen tumor and adjacent healthy renal tissues were crushed into fragments <2 mm in diameter and suspended in 1:2 weight/volume of 2× phosphate-buffered saline (PBS). The solution was rotated at 4 °C for 3 h. The samples were then vortexed, and the centrifugation-cleared supernatants were used for experiments.

4.12. Generation of Conditioned Medium (CM) from Human MΦ

Human monocytes were isolated from commercially available, anonymized buffy coats (DRK-Blutspendedienst Baden-Württemberg-Hessen, Frankfurt, Germany) using Ficoll-Hypaque gradients (PAA Laboratories, Cölbe, Germany) as previously described [41]. Briefly, monocytes were differentiated into primary human MΦ with RPMI-1640 containing 5% AB-positive human serum (DRK-Blutspendedienst Baden-Württemberg-Hessen, Frankfurt, Germany). Prior to stimulation, cells were serum-starved for 24 h and stimulated with 20 ng/mL IL-10 (Peprotech, Hamburg, Germany) for 24 h to generate conditioned-media of polarized MΦ [41]. Conditioned-media from iron-releasing MΦ were collected and used for following proliferation and migration assays. Supernatant of unstimulated MΦ served as control.

4.13. Proliferation and Migration Assays

Proliferation and migration assays were performed using the xCELLigence RTCA DP instrument (OLS, Bremen, Germany) as previously described [53]. Proliferation was recorded continuously for 3 days and migration for 24 h. Data were acquired as a measure for time-dependent impedance changes. RTCA Software 1.2 (OLS) was used for acquisition and analysis.

4.14. Immunohistochemistry

Immunohistochemical staining was adapted from previously described protocols [35]. Formalin-fixed and paraffin-embedded patient tissues were stained with antibodies against FPN (Novus, NBP1-21502) and CD163 (Abcam, Cambridge, UK, ab182422) according to the manufacturer's protocol using the Opal 4-color-automation IHC-kit (PerkinElmer, Rodgau, Germany, NEL820001KT). Images were acquired using the LSM 800 microscope (Zeiss) and edited using ImageJ software.

4.15. Hematoxylin and Eosin Stain

For hematoxylin and eosin staining, formalin-fixed and paraffin-embedded tissues were rehydrated, stained using Mayer's hemalum solution (Merck, 109249), washed, counter-stained using Eosin (Merck, 102439), and mounted in Entellan (Merck, 107961). An Axioskop 40 (Zeiss) was used to acquire images.

4.16. XTT

Cytotoxicity of iron chelators was tested by a photometric XTT assay (Panreac, Darmstadt, Germany, A8088). Briefly, sub-confluent cells were exposed to iron chelators for 12 h. Subsequently, XTT reagent was added and absorbance was measured at 450 nm vs. 630 nm according to manufacturer's protocol. Experiments were conducted in quintuplicates. Cell viability was normalized to the untreated control.

4.17. Synthesis and Chemical Characterization of the Extracellular Chelator EC1

2-Hydroxybenzaldehyde (125 mg, 1.0 mmol) was added to a solution of sodium 4-(hydrazinecarbothioamido) benzenesulfonate (426 mg, 1.5 mmol) in water (1 mL). Ethanol (2 mL) was added and the solution was brought to reflux and stirred for 30 min. The reaction mixture was then allowed to cool to room temperature and the formed precipitate was filtered, washed with ethanol, and dried under vacuum. The identity and purity of the desired product (311 mg, 81% yield) were confirmed by high-resolution mass spectrometry via electrospray ionization (HRMS-ESI) and nuclear magnetic resonance (NMR) spectroscopy. HRMS-ESI (*m/z*): [M − Na]$^-$ calcd for [C$_{14}$H$_{12}$N$_3$O$_4$S$_2$]$^-$, 350.02747; found, 350.02741; [M + H]$^+$ calcd for [C$_{14}$H$_{13}$N$_3$NaO$_4$S$_2$]$^+$, 374.02397; found, 374.02401. ^{1}H NMR (500 MHz, DMSO-d_6) δ 11.79 (s, 1H), 10.07 (s, 1H), 9.98 (bs, 1H), 8.50 (s, 1H), 8.09 (bd, 1H), 7.64–7.44 (m, 4H), 7.24 (m, 1H), 6.95–6.78 (m, 2H). ^{13}C NMR (125 MHz, DMSO-d_6) δ 176.21, 157.17, 145.37, 140.65, 139.76, 131.86, 127.55, 125.85, 125.12, 120.69, 119.70, 116.53.

4.18. Chelator Solutions

2,2′-Dipyridine (2′2-DPD) was obtained commercially (Sigma Aldrich, D216305) and the intracellular prochelator (TC3-S)$_2$ was prepared as previously reported [54]. Extracellular chelator EC1 was synthesized as described above. For experiments in cell cultures, stock solutions were prepared at a standard concentration of 100 µM in dimethyl sulfoxide (DMSO) and were always prepared freshly in degassed DMSO.

4.19. Statistical Analysis

Statistical analysis was performed applying GraphPad Prism software (GraphPad Inc., San Diego, CA, USA, version 8.2.1). Variable distribution was tested for normality using the Kolmogorov-Smirnov test. Respectively, Gaussian distributed, and non-Gaussian distributed patient samples were statistical analyzed using two-tailed paired student's *t*-test or Wilcoxon matched-pairs signed-ranks test. In vitro experiments were analyzed using one-way ANOVA. Cell culture experiments were performed at least three times (independent experiments using technical replicates). Patient samples were used in experiments upon availability. P values were considered significant at * $p < 0.05$, ** $p < 0.01$, *** $p < 0.001$.

5. Conclusions

This study provides new insights of a significantly altered iron metabolism in renal cell carcinoma. Most of the studied iron-regulated genes are associated with tumor grade and tumor pT-stage. Moreover, our results suggest that tumor-associated macrophages adopt a pro-tumorigenic iron-releasing phenotype through increased expression of FPN. These tumor-associated macrophages are then able to fuel the increased iron demands of tumor cells by secreting iron in the tumor microenvironment.

EC1, a novel iron chelator, specifically scavenges iron in the extracellular space and was able to reverse pro-tumorigenic effects of macrophage-conditioned media on proliferation and migration of cancer cells, including primary patient-derived renal cancer cells. These results might pave the way towards further in vivo studies addressing the possibility to interfere with iron availability in the tumor microenvironment by targeted chelation strategies.

6. Patents

Issued patent: Tomat E.; Chang, T. M. "Redox-Directed Chelators Targeting Intracellular Metal Ions" U.S. Patent No. 9,486,423, November 8th, 2016.

Pending patent application: Tomat, E.; Chang, T.; Akam, E. A. "Redox-activated Pro-chelators" U.S. Patent Appl. No.: 16/200,286, November 26th, 2018.

Supplementary Materials: The following are available online at http://www.mdpi.com/2072-6694/12/3/530/s1, Figure S1: Primary human renal tissue verification, Figure S2: Perl's staining of histopathological renal cell carcinoma subtypes. Figure S3: Characterization of the extracellular iron chelator EC1.

Author Contributions: Conceptualization: M.J.; Methodology: M.S., C.R., C.M., E.T., E.A.A., M.J.; Software: M.S.; Validation: M.S., C.R., C.M., J.K.M., M.J.; Formal analysis: M.S., C.R., A.U., C.M., E.T., E.A.A., M.J.; Investigation: M.S., C.R., A.U., C.M., J.K.M., E.T., E.A.A., P.B., F.C.R., M.J.; Resources: A.U., P.B., F.R., B.B., M.J.; Data curation: M.J.; Writing—original draft preparation: M.S., E.T., B.B., M.J.; Writing—review and editing, M.S., E.T., B.B., M.J.; Visualization: M.S., M.J.; Supervision: M.J.; Project administration: M.J.; Funding acquisition: E.T., B.B., M.J. All authors have read and agreed to the published version of the manuscript.

Funding: MS—PhD scholarship from the Faculty of Medicine, Goethe-University Frankfurt; CR—PhD scholarship from EKFS (Else Kröner-Fresenius-Graduiertenkolleg); BB—Else Kröner-Fresenius Foundation (EKFS), Research Training Group Translational Research Innovation–Pharma (TRIP); MJ—Wilhelm Sander-Stiftung (2017.130.1); ET—U.S. National Institutes of Health (GM127646).

Acknowledgments: The authors thank Aline Kraus and Yu-Shien Sung for assistance on the chemical characterization of EC1.

Conflicts of Interest: The authors declare no conflict of interest.

References

1. White, M.F.; Dillingham, M.S. Iron-sulphur clusters in nucleic acid processing enzymes. *Curr. Opin. Struct. Biol.* **2012**, *22*, 94–100. [CrossRef] [PubMed]
2. Wang, Y.; Yu, L.; Ding, J.; Chen, Y. Iron Metabolism in Cancer. *Int. J. Mol. Sci.* **2018**, *20*, 95. [CrossRef] [PubMed]
3. Pantopoulos, K.; Porwal, S.K.; Tartakoff, A.; Devireddy, L. Mechanisms of mammalian iron homeostasis. *Biochemistry* **2012**, *51*, 5705–5724. [CrossRef] [PubMed]
4. Haase, V.H. Hypoxic regulation of erythropoiesis and iron metabolism. *Am. J. Physiol. Ren. Physiol.* **2010**, *299*, F1–F13. [CrossRef] [PubMed]
5. Seminog, O.O.; Ogunlaja, O.I.; Yeates, D.; Goldacre, M.J. Risk of individual malignant neoplasms in patients with sickle cell disease: English national record linkage study. *J. R. Soc. Med.* **2016**, *109*, 303–309. [CrossRef] [PubMed]
6. Vargas-Olvera, C.Y.; Sánchez-González, D.J.; Solano, J.D.; Aguilar-Alonso, F.A.; Montalvo-Muñoz, F.; Martínez-Martínez, C.M.; Medina-Campos, O.N.; Ibarra-Rubio, M.E. Characterization of N-diethylnitrosamine-initiated and ferric nitrilotriacetate-promoted renal cell carcinoma experimental model and effect of a tamarind seed extract against acute nephrotoxicity and carcinogenesis. *Mol. Cell. Biochem.* **2012**, *369*, 105–117. [CrossRef] [PubMed]
7. Greene, C.J.; Attwood, K.; Sharma, N.J.; Gross, K.W.; Smith, G.J.; Xu, B.; Kauffman, E.C. Transferrin receptor 1 upregulation in primary tumor and downregulation in benign kidney is associated with progression and mortality in renal cell carcinoma patients. *Oncotarget* **2017**, *8*, 107052–107075. [CrossRef]
8. Bray, F.; Ferlay, J.; Soerjomataram, I.; Siegel, R.L.; Torre, L.A.; Jemal, A. Global cancer statistics 2018: GLOBOCAN estimates of incidence and mortality worldwide for 36 cancers in 185 countries. *CA Cancer J. Clin.* **2018**. [CrossRef]
9. Makhov, P.; Joshi, S.; Ghatalia, P.; Kutikov, A.; Uzzo, R.G.; Kolenko, V.M. Resistance to Systemic Therapies in Clear Cell Renal Cell Carcinoma: Mechanisms and Management Strategies. *Mol. Cancer Ther.* **2018**, *17*, 1355–1364. [CrossRef]
10. Gill, D.M.; Agarwal, N.; Vaishampayan, U. Evolving Treatment Paradigm in Metastatic Renal Cell Carcinoma. *Am. Soc. Clin. Oncol. Educ. Book* **2017**, *37*, 319–329. [CrossRef]
11. Amin, A.; Hammers, H. The Evolving Landscape of Immunotherapy-Based Combinations for Frontline Treatment of Advanced Renal Cell Carcinoma. *Front. Immunol.* **2018**, *9*, 3120. [CrossRef] [PubMed]
12. Cella, D.; Grünwald, V.; Escudier, B.; Hammers, H.J.; George, S.; Nathan, P.; Grimm, M.-O.; Rini, B.I.; Doan, J.; Ivanescu, C.; et al. Patient-reported outcomes of patients with advanced renal cell carcinoma treated with nivolumab plus ipilimumab versus sunitinib (CheckMate 214): A randomised, phase 3 trial. *Lancet Oncol.* **2019**, *20*, 297–310. [CrossRef]
13. Kohgo, Y.; Ikuta, K.; Ohtake, T.; Torimoto, Y.; Kato, J. Body iron metabolism and pathophysiology of iron overload. *Int. J. Hematol.* **2008**, *88*, 7–15. [CrossRef] [PubMed]
14. Torti, S.V.; Torti, F.M. Iron and cancer: More ore to be mined. *Nat. Rev. Cancer* **2013**, *13*, 342–355. [CrossRef]
15. Kirkali, Z.; Esen, A.A.; Kirkali, G.; Güner, G. Ferritin: A tumor marker expressed by renal cell carcinoma. *Eur. Urol.* **1995**, *28*, 131–134. [CrossRef]
16. Jézéquel, P.; Campion, L.; Spyratos, F.; Loussouarn, D.; Campone, M.; Guérin-Charbonnel, C.; Joalland, M.-P.; André, J.; Descotes, F.; Grenot, C.; et al. Validation of tumor-associated macrophage ferritin light chain as a prognostic biomarker in node-negative breast cancer tumors: A multicentric 2004 national PHRC study. *Int. J. Cancer* **2012**, *131*, 426–437. [CrossRef]

17. Brookes, M.J.; Hughes, S.; Turner, F.E.; Reynolds, G.; Sharma, N.; Ismail, T.; Berx, G.; McKie, A.T.; Hotchin, N.; Anderson, G.J.; et al. Modulation of iron transport proteins in human colorectal carcinogenesis. *Gut* **2006**, *55*, 1449–1460. [CrossRef]
18. Wang, W.; Deng, Z.; Hatcher, H.; Miller, L.D.; Di, X.; Tesfay, L.; Sui, G.; D'Agostino, R.B.; Torti, F.M.; Torti, S.V. IRP2 regulates breast tumor growth. *Cancer Res.* **2014**, *74*, 497–507. [CrossRef]
19. Ludwig, H.; Müldür, E.; Endler, G.; Hübl, W. Prevalence of iron deficiency across different tumors and its association with poor performance status, disease status and anemia. *Ann. Oncol.* **2013**, *24*, 1886–1892. [CrossRef]
20. Corna, G.; Campana, L.; Pignatti, E.; Castiglioni, A.; Tagliafico, E.; Bosurgi, L.; Campanella, A.; Brunelli, S.; Manfredi, A.A.; Apostoli, P.; et al. Polarization dictates iron handling by inflammatory and alternatively activated macrophages. *Haematologica* **2010**, *95*, 1814–1822. [CrossRef]
21. Cairo, G.; Recalcati, S.; Mantovani, A.; Locati, M. Iron trafficking and metabolism in macrophages: Contribution to the polarized phenotype. *Trends Immunol.* **2011**, *32*, 241–247. [CrossRef] [PubMed]
22. Recalcati, S.; Locati, M.; Marini, A.; Santambrogio, P.; Zaninotto, F.; De Pizzol, M.; Zammataro, L.; Girelli, D.; Cairo, G. Differential regulation of iron homeostasis during human macrophage polarized activation. *Eur. J. Immunol.* **2010**, *40*, 824–835. [CrossRef] [PubMed]
23. Murray, P.J.; Wynn, T.A. Protective and pathogenic functions of macrophage subsets. *Nat. Rev. Immunol.* **2011**, *11*, 723–737. [CrossRef] [PubMed]
24. Chevrier, S.; Levine, J.H.; Zanotelli, V.R.T.; Silina, K.; Schulz, D.; Bacac, M.; Ries, C.H.; Ailles, L.; Jewett, M.A.S.; Moch, H.; et al. An Immune Atlas of Clear Cell Renal Cell Carcinoma. *Cell* **2017**, *169*, 736–749. [CrossRef] [PubMed]
25. Chanmee, T.; Ontong, P.; Konno, K.; Itano, N. Tumor-associated macrophages as major players in the tumor microenvironment. *Cancers* **2014**, *6*, 1670–1690. [CrossRef] [PubMed]
26. Ikemoto, S.; Yoshida, N.; Narita, K.; Wada, S.; Kishimoto, T.; Sugimura, K.; Nakatani, T. Role of tumor-associated macrophages in renal cell carcinoma. *Oncol. Rep.* **2003**. [CrossRef]
27. Toge, H.; Inagaki, T.; Kojimoto, Y.; Shinka, T.; Hara, I. Angiogenesis in renal cell carcinoma: The role of tumor-associated macrophages. *Int. J. Urol.* **2009**, *16*, 801–807. [CrossRef]
28. Lewis, C.E.; Pollard, J.W. Distinct role of macrophages in different tumor microenvironments. *Cancer Res.* **2006**, *66*, 605–612. [CrossRef]
29. Komohara, Y.; Hasita, H.; Ohnishi, K.; Fujiwara, Y.; Suzu, S.; Eto, M.; Takeya, M. Macrophage infiltration and its prognostic relevance in clear cell renal cell carcinoma. *Cancer Sci.* **2011**, *102*, 1424–1431. [CrossRef]
30. Xu, L.; Zhu, Y.; Chen, L.; An, H.; Zhang, W.; Wang, G.; Lin, Z.; Xu, J. Prognostic value of diametrically polarized tumor-associated macrophages in renal cell carcinoma. *Ann. Surg. Oncol.* **2014**, *21*, 3142–3150. [CrossRef]
31. Sangaletti, S.; Di Carlo, E.; Gariboldi, S.; Miotti, S.; Cappetti, B.; Parenza, M.; Rumio, C.; Brekken, R.A.; Chiodoni, C.; Colombo, M.P. Macrophage-derived SPARC bridges tumor cell-extracellular matrix interactions toward metastasis. *Cancer Res.* **2008**, *68*, 9050–9059. [CrossRef] [PubMed]
32. Sandlund, J.; Oosterwijk, E.; Grankvist, K.; Oosterwijk-Wakka, J.; Ljungberg, B.; Rasmuson, T. Prognostic impact of carbonic anhydrase IX expression in human renal cell carcinoma. *BJU Int.* **2007**, *100*, 556–560. [CrossRef] [PubMed]
33. Nguyen, D.P.; Vertosick, E.A.; Corradi, R.B.; Vilaseca, A.; Benfante, N.E.; Touijer, K.A.; Sjoberg, D.D.; Russo, P. Histological subtype of renal cell carcinoma significantly affects survival in the era of partial nephrectomy. *Urol. Oncol.* **2016**, *34*, 259.e1–259.e8. [CrossRef] [PubMed]
34. Marques, O.; Porto, G.; Rêma, A.; Faria, F.; Cruz Paula, A.; Gomez-Lazaro, M.; Silva, P.; Martins da Silva, B.; Lopes, C. Local iron homeostasis in the breast ductal carcinoma microenvironment. *BMC Cancer* **2016**, *16*, 187. [CrossRef]
35. Mertens, C.; Mora, J.; Ören, B.; Grein, S.; Winslow, S.; Scholich, K.; Weigert, A.; Malmström, P.; Forsare, C.; Fernö, M.; et al. Macrophage-derived lipocalin-2 transports iron in the tumor microenvironment. *Oncoimmunology* **2018**, *7*, e1408751. [CrossRef]
36. Jung, M.; Weigert, A.; Tausendschön, M.; Mora, J.; Ören, B.; Sola, A.; Hotter, G.; Muta, T.; Brüne, B. Interleukin-10-induced neutrophil gelatinase-associated lipocalin production in macrophages with consequences for tumor growth. *Mol. Cell. Biol.* **2012**, *32*, 3938–3948. [CrossRef]

37. Mertens, C.; Akam, E.A.; Rehwald, C.; Brüne, B.; Tomat, E.; Jung, M. Intracellular Iron Chelation Modulates the Macrophage Iron Phenotype with Consequences on Tumor Progression. *PLoS ONE* **2016**, *11*, e0166164. [CrossRef]
38. Yu, Y.; Kalinowski, D.S.; Kovacevic, Z.; Siafakas, A.R.; Jansson, P.J.; Stefani, C.; Lovejoy, D.B.; Sharpe, P.C.; Bernhardt, P.V.; Des Richardson, R. Thiosemicarbazones from the old to new: Iron chelators that are more than just ribonucleotide reductase inhibitors. *J. Med. Chem.* **2009**, *52*, 5271–5294. [CrossRef]
39. Utterback, R.D.; Tomat, E. Developing Ligands to Target Transition Metals in Cancer. *Encycl. Inorg. Bioinorg. Chem.* **2019**. [CrossRef]
40. Akam, E.A.; Chang, T.M.; Astashkin, A.V.; Tomat, E. Intracellular reduction/activation of a disulfide switch in thiosemicarbazone iron chelators. *Metallomics* **2014**, *6*, 1905–1912. [CrossRef]
41. Akam, E.A.; Utterback, R.D.; Marcero, J.R.; Dailey, H.A.; Tomat, E. Disulfide-masked iron prochelators: Effects on cell death, proliferation, and hemoglobin production. *J. Inorg. Biochem.* **2018**, *180*, 186–193. [CrossRef] [PubMed]
42. Greene, B.T.; Thorburn, J.; Willingham, M.C.; Thorburn, A.; Planalp, R.P.; Brechbiel, M.W.; Jennings-Gee, J.; Wilkinson, J.; Torti, F.M.; Torti, S.V. Activation of caspase pathways during iron chelator-mediated apoptosis. *J. Biol. Chem.* **2002**, *277*, 25568–25575. [CrossRef] [PubMed]
43. Jung, M.; Mertens, C.; Tomat, E.; Brüne, B. Iron as a Central Player and Promising Target in Cancer Progression. *Int. J. Mol. Sci.* **2019**, *20*, 273. [CrossRef] [PubMed]
44. Alkhateeb, A.A.; Han, B.; Connor, J.R. Ferritin stimulates breast cancer cells through an iron-independent mechanism and is localized within tumor-associated macrophages. *Breast Cancer Res. Treat.* **2013**, *137*, 733–744. [CrossRef]
45. Kukulj, S.; Jaganjac, M.; Boranic, M.; Krizanac, S.; Santic, Z.; Poljak-Blazi, M. Altered iron metabolism, inflammation, transferrin receptors, and ferritin expression in non-small-cell lung cancer. *Med. Oncol.* **2010**, *27*, 268–277. [CrossRef]
46. Nseyo, U.O.; Williams, P.D.; Murphy, G.E. Clinical significance of erythropoietin levels in renal carcinoma. *Urology* **1986**, *28*, 301–306. [CrossRef]
47. Dowd, A.A.; Ibrahim, F.I.; Mohammed, M.M. Renal cell carcinoma as a cause of iron deficiency anemia. *Afr. J. Urol.* **2014**, *20*, 25–27. [CrossRef]
48. Jiang, X.P.; Elliott, R.L.; Head, J.F. Manipulation of iron transporter genes results in the suppression of human and mouse mammary adenocarcinomas. *Anticancer Res.* **2010**, *30*, 759–765.
49. Coombs, G.S.; Schmitt, A.A.; Canning, C.A.; Alok, A.; Low, I.C.C.; Banerjee, N.; Kaur, S.; Utomo, V.; Jones, C.M.; Pervaiz, S.; et al. Modulation of Wnt/β-catenin signaling and proliferation by a ferrous iron chelator with therapeutic efficacy in genetically engineered mouse models of cancer. *Oncogene* **2012**, *31*, 213–225. [CrossRef]
50. Hrabinski, D.; Hertz, J.L.; Tantillo, C.; Berger, V.; Sherman, A.R. Iron repletion attenuates the protective effects of iron deficiency in DMBA-induced mammary tumors in rats. *Nutr. Cancer* **1995**, *24*, 133–142. [CrossRef]
51. Brierley, J.; Gospodarowicz, M.K.; Wittekind, C. *TNM Classification of Malignant Tumours*, 8th ed.; Brierley, J., Gospodarowicz, M.K., Wittekind, C., O'Sullivan, B., Eds.; John Wiley & Sons, Inc: Oxford, UK, 2017; ISBN 9781119263562.
52. Baer, P.C.; Nockher, W.A.; Haase, W.; Scherberich, J.E. Isolation of proximal and distal tubule cells from human kidney by immunomagnetic separation. Technical note. *Kidney Int.* **1997**, *52*, 1321–1331. [CrossRef] [PubMed]
53. Jung, M.; Ören, B.; Mora, J.; Mertens, C.; Dziumbla, S.; Popp, R.; Weigert, A.; Grossmann, N.; Fleming, I.; Brüne, B. Lipocalin 2 from macrophages stimulated by tumor cell-derived sphingosine 1-phosphate promotes lymphangiogenesis and tumor metastasis. *Sci. Signal.* **2016**, *9*, ra64. [CrossRef] [PubMed]
54. Chang, T.M.; Tomat, E. Disulfide/thiol switches in thiosemicarbazone ligands for redox-directed iron chelation. *Dalton Trans.* **2013**, *42*, 7846–7849. [CrossRef] [PubMed]

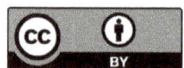

© 2020 by the authors. Licensee MDPI, Basel, Switzerland. This article is an open access article distributed under the terms and conditions of the Creative Commons Attribution (CC BY) license (http://creativecommons.org/licenses/by/4.0/).

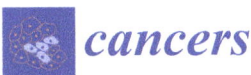

Article

Role of Microtubule-Associated Protein 1b in Urothelial Carcinoma: Overexpression Predicts Poor Prognosis

Tsu-Ming Chien [1,2,3], Ti-Chun Chan [4,5], Steven Kuan-Hua Huang [6], Bi-Wen Yeh [3,5], Wei-Ming Li [1,2,3,7], Chun-Nung Huang [2,3], Ching-Chia Li [1,2,3,8], Wen-Jeng Wu [1,2,3,8,9,10] and Chien-Feng Li [4,5,11,12,13,*]

1. Graduate Institute of Clinical Medicine, College of Medicine, Kaohsiung Medical University, Kaohsiung 807, Taiwan; u108801005@kmu.edu.tw (T.-M.C.); u8401067@yahoo.com.tw (W.-M.L.); ccli1010@hotmail.com (C.-C.L.); wejewu@kmu.edu.tw (W.-J.W.)
2. Department of Urology, Kaohsiung Medical University Hospital, Kaohsiung 807, Taiwan; cnhuang.uro@gmail.com
3. Department of Urology, School of Medicine, College of Medicine, Kaohsiung Medical University, Kaohsiung 807, Taiwan; bewen90@yahoo.com.tw
4. Institute of Biomedical Science, National Sun Yat-sen University, Kaohsiung 80424, Taiwan; ibosaa@mail.nsysu.edu.tw
5. Department of Pathology, Chi Mei Medical Center, Tainan 710, Taiwan
6. Department of Urology, Chi Mei Medical Center, Tainan 710, Taiwan; skhsteven@gmail.com
7. Department of Urology, Ministry of Health and Welfare Pingtung Hospital, Pingtung 900, Taiwan
8. Department of Urology, Kaohsiung Municipal Ta-Tung Hospital, Kaohsiung 801, Taiwan
9. Center for Infectious Disease and Cancer Research, Kaohsiung Medical University, Kaohsiung 807, Taiwan
10. Center for Stem Cell Research, Kaohsiung Medical University, Kaohsiung 807, Taiwan
11. Institute of Medical Science and Technology, National Sun Yat-sen University, Kaohsiung 80424, Taiwan
12. Department of Biotechnology, Southern Taiwan University of Science and Technology, Tainan 71005, Taiwan
13. National Cancer Research Institute, National Health Research Institutes, Tainan 70456, Taiwan
* Correspondence: angelo.p@yahoo.com.tw; Tel.: +886-6-281-2811 (ext. 53680); Fax: +886-6-251-1235

Received: 6 February 2020; Accepted: 6 March 2020; Published: 9 March 2020

Abstract: We sought to examine the relationship between microtubule-associated proteins (MAPs) and the prognosis of urothelial carcinoma by assessing the microtubule bundle formation genes using a reappraisal transcriptome dataset of urothelial carcinoma (GSE31684). The result revealed that microtubule-associated protein 1b (*MAP1B*) is the most significant upregulated gene related to cancer progression. Real-time reverse-transcription polymerase chain reaction was used to measure *MAP1B* transcription levels in urothelial carcinoma of the upper tract (UTUC) and the bladder (UBUC). Immunohistochemistry was conducted to detect *MAP1B* protein expression in 340 UTUC and 295 UBUC cases. Correlations of *MAP1B* expression with clinicopathological status, disease-specific survival, and metastasis-free survival were completed. To assess the oncogenic functions of *MAP1B*, the RTCC1 and J82 cell lines were stably silenced against their endogenous *MAP1B* expression. Study findings indicated that *MAP1B* overexpression was associated with adverse clinical features and could independently predict unfavorable prognostic effects, indicating its theranostic value in urothelial carcinoma.

Keywords: urothelial carcinoma; transcriptome; microtubule; MAP1B; prognosis

---

1. Introduction

Urothelial carcinoma (UC) is the most common malignancy of the urinary tract and includes UC of the urinary bladder (UBUC) and upper urinary tract (UTUC). UBUC is a major UC, with an estimated

429,800 new cases and 165,100 deaths annually worldwide [1]. When first diagnosed, UBUC presents in most patients as a non–muscle-involved invasive disease with an estimated five-year survival rate of 88%, but this rate dramatically decreases to 15% in patients with tumor metastasis [2]. The prevalence of UTUC accounts for approximately 5% to 10% of all UC cases [3]; however, in Taiwan, the rate of UTUC is as high as 30% of affected cases. Furthermore, there is a slight predominance toward females, and ureteral tumors are attributed to greater than half of all cases of UTUC [4,5].

Transurethral resection of the bladder and radical nephroureterectomy with bladder cuff excision remain the gold-standard treatments in UBUC and UTUC for adequate local tumor control and improved long-term survival. However, despite proper surgical treatment, the mortality rate remains high [2,6,7]. Clinical prognostic factors, such as pathological tumor stage and grade, have diverse impacts in patients with identical findings; therefore, they are insufficient means for detailed risk stratification and are difficult to define before treatment [5].

UBUC staging starts from papillary (Ta) and superficial (T1) stages and extends to muscle-invasive advanced stages (T2–T4). Although the recurrence rate of superficial tumors following surgical resection of the bladder is high, it is associated with a markedly better prognosis than that of muscle-invasive tumors [8]. There is a growing pool of evidence to suggest a pathophysiological distinction exists between superficial and muscle-invasive cases of UBUC [9]. It is also important to distinguish a particular variant that may be associated with the administration of a therapy distinctive from that used in conventional invasive UC [10]. A previous study demonstrated that the gene expression profiles of UC from renal pelvis, ureter and bladder were highly similar, indicating that a common functional molecular pathway likely underlies the carcinogenesis [11]. A larger, follow-up study to elucidate better genomics-based predictors for UC is warranted, the results of which could lead to improvements in neoadjuvant/adjuvant therapy and provide suitable follow-up strategies.

Microtubules are a critical component of the cytoskeleton and are important and indispensable in several cellular processes. They are located throughout the cytoplasm and are dynamically unstable (i.e., coexisting in a state of assembly and disassembly). Microtubule-associated proteins (MAPs) are a large family of proteins involved in microtubule assembly, which is an essential step in stabilizing microtubules. MAPs are divided into two classical families: type I, which includes the MAP1 (MAP1A, MAP1B, and MAP1S) proteins [12] and type II, which includes MAP2, MAP4, and MAPT/TAU proteins [13]. Disrupting microtubule dynamics is one of the most successful and widely considered targets of cancer chemotherapy agents [14,15]. Microtubule agents target the aberrant expression of MAPs in a variety of malignancies, and their resistant phenotypes have been documented. Herein, we aimed to examine the relationship between MAPs and the prognosis of urothelial carcinoma by assessing the microtubule bundle formation genes using a reappraisal transcriptome dataset of urothelial carcinoma (GSE31684). Moreover, to our knowledge, this study is the first to examine *MAP1B* expression and the prognosis and intrinsic biologic aggressiveness of UC.

2. Results

2.1. MAP1B Is the Most Significantly Upregulated Gene Associated with Microtubule Bundle Formation in UBUC Transcriptomes

The UBUC transcriptome dataset includes 93 tissue samples, with 78 categorized as deeply invasive tissues (pT2–pT4) and 15 categorized as noninvasive or superficial (pTa and pT1) tissues. Metastasis was detected in 28 patients and absent in 49 patients. Through transcriptome profiling, we identified 11 probes spanning six transcripts associated with microtubule bundle formation (GO:0001578). Among these expressed genes, we found that tumors with increased *MAP1B* expression and decreased *MARK4* had a more advanced pT status and a higher incidence of metastatic events (Figure 1A). Our main goal was to find the most significant upregulated genes associated with advanced disease. Therefore, we choose *MAP1B* for further validation. Table 1 shows the *MAP1B* gene (Probe: 226084_at, 214577_at) upregulation with up to 1.2832-, 0.3773- and 0.9436-, 0.3943- fold log ratios in advanced and metastatic UC, respectively. Furthermore, we found through survival analysis that increased *MAP1B* expression was significantly related to poor prognosis in patients with UBUC (Figure 1B). As shown in Figure 1c,d, the *MAP1B* transcripts level was significantly higher among tumors with high pT status (pT2–pT4) than in noninvasive tumors (pTa–pT1) in both the UTUC and UBUC groups (both $p < 0.01$). Our findings indicate that *MAP1B* is associated with tumor aggressiveness.

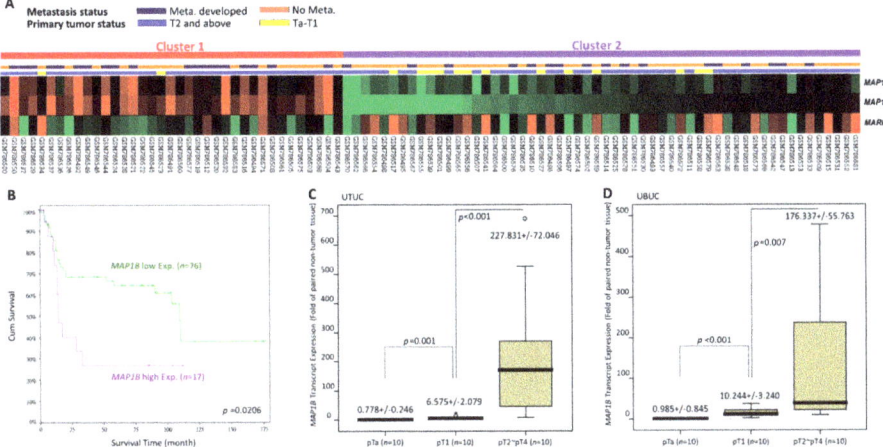

Figure 1. Analysis of gene expression in urinary bladder urothelial carcinoma (UBUC) using a published transcriptome dataset (GSE31684). (**A**) Cluster analysis of genes focusing on the GO microtubule bundle formation class (GO:0001578) revealed that *MAP1B* was one of the most significantly upregulated genes associated with more advanced pT status and metastatic disease. Tissue specimens from cancers with a distinct pT status are illustrated at the top of the heat map, and the expression levels of upregulated and downregulated genes are represented as a continuum of brightness of red or green, respectively. Specimens with no change in messenger RNA (mRNA) expression are shown in black. (**B**) Kaplan–Meier plots showing the prognostic significance of *MAP1B* expression for the survival of UBUC. Using a QuantiGene assay, *MAP1B* mRNA expression was significantly increased in both (**C**) upper tract urothelial carcinoma (UTUC) and (**D**) UBUC at advanced primary pT stages.

Table 1. Summary of differentially expressed genes associated with microtubule bundle formation (GO: 0001578) and showing positive associations to cancer invasiveness and metastasis in the transcriptome of UBUC (GSE31684).

Probe Title 1	Comparing T2-4 to Ta-T1		Comparing Meta. to Non-Meta. #		Gene Symbol	Gene Title	Biological Process	Molecular Function
	Log ratio	p-Value	Log ratio	p-Value				
214577_at	0.3773	0.0029	0.3943	<0.0001	MAP1B	Microtubule-associated protein 1B	Dendrite development, microtubule bundle formation	Protein binding, structural molecule activity
221560_at	−0.3436	0.0058	−0.0115	0.9048	MARK4	MAP/microtubule affinity-regulating kinase 4	G1/S transition of mitotic cell cycle, G2/M transition of mitotic cell cycle, Wnt receptor signaling pathway, microtubule bundle formation, microtubule cytoskeleton organization and biogenesis, nervous system development, positive regulation of cell proliferation, positive regulation of programmed cell death, protein amino acid phosphorylation	ATP binding, gamma-tubulin binding, kinase activity, microtubule-binding, nucleotide-binding, protein-binding, protein kinase activity, protein serine/threonine kinase activity, protein-tyrosine kinase activity, tau-protein kinase activity, transferase activity, ubiquitin-binding
226084_at	1.2832	<0.0001	0.9436	<0.0001	MAP1B	Microtubule-associated protein 1B	Dendrite development, microtubule bundle formation	Protein-binding, structural molecule activity

#, Meta., distal metastasis developed during follow-up; Non-Meta.: no metastatic event developed.

2.2. MAP1B Immunoexpression and Clinicopathological and Genomic Correlations in UTUC and UBUC

The association of clinicopathological characteristics with *MAP1B* immunoreactivity is shown in Table 2. We found, in UTUC cases, that high *MAP1B* expression was markedly associated with synchronous multiple tumors ($p = 0.024$), advanced pT status ($p = 0.005$) (Figure 2A–C), positive lymph node metastasis ($p = 0.002$), the presence of vascular invasion ($p < 0.001$), and an increased mitotic rate ($p < 0.001$) (Table 2 and Figure 2D). Similarly, in cases with UBUC, we found evidence of associations between increased *MAP1B* expression and advanced pathological tumor stage ($p < 0.001$), positive lymph node metastasis ($p = 0.012$), a high histological tumor grade ($p = 0.016$), the presence of vascular invasion ($p = 0.045$), and an increased mitotic rate ($p = 0.006$) (Table 2 and Figure 2E). Of note, none of the 30 cases displaying high *MAP1B* expression enrolled for mutational analysis were positive for *MAP1B* mutation, suggesting a mutation-independent expression of *MAP1B*.

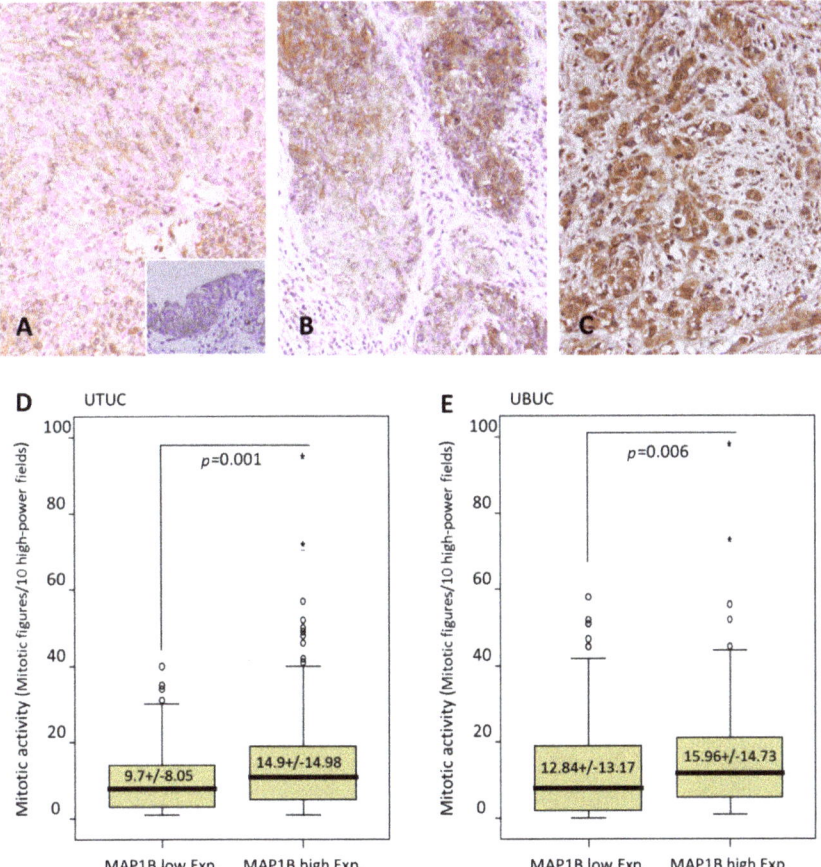

Figure 2. Representative sections of *MAP1B* immunostaining. Note the stepwise increments in *MAP1B* immunoreactivity from the nontumoral urothelial epithelium (inlet) and (**A**) noninvasive papillary UCs to (**B**) non–muscle-invasive (pT1), and (**C**) muscle-invasive (pT2–pT4) UCs. A comparison of mitotic activity showed significantly higher mitotic rates in (**D**) UTUC and (**E**) UBUC cells with increased *MAP1B* expression than in cells with low expression.

Table 2. Correlations between MAP1B expression and other important clinicopathological parameters in UCs.

Parameter	Category	Upper Urinary Tract Urothelial Carcinoma				Urinary Bladder Urothelial Carcinoma			
		Case no.	MAP1B Expression		p-value	Case no.	MAP1B Expression		p-value
			Low	High			Low	High	
Gender &	Male	158	79	79	1.000	216	103	113	0.223
	Female	182	91	91		79	44	35	
Age (years) #		340	65.2+/−9.87	65.9+/−9.92	0.409	295	65.76+/−12.02	66.33+/−12.44	0.759
Tumor location	Renal pelvis	141	64	77	0.023 *	-	-	-	-
	Ureter	150	87	63		-	-	-	-
	Renal pelvis & ureter	49	19	30		-	-	-	-
Multifocality &	Single	278	144	134	0.160	-	-	-	-
	Multifocal	62	26	36		-	-	-	-
Primary tumor (T) &	Ta	89	54	35	0.005 *	84	56	28	<0.001 *
	T1	92	51	41		88	45	43	
	T2	159	65	94		123	46	77	
Nodal metastasis &	Negative (N0)	312	164	148	0.002 *	266	139	127	0.012 *
	Positive (N1-N2)	28	6	22		29	8	21	
Histological grade &	Low grade	56	34	22	0.079	56	36	20	0.016 *
	High grade	284	136	148		239	111	128	
Vascular invasion &	Absent	234	132	102	<0.001 *	246	129	117	0.045 *
	Present	106	38	68		49	18	31	
Perineural invasion &	Absent	321	162	159	0.479	275	140	135	0.169
	Present	19	8	11		20	7	13	

&, Chi-squared test; #, Mann–Whitney U test; * Statistically significant.

2.3. Survival Analysis in UTUC and UBUC

During follow-up, we found in our UTUC cohort that 61 (17.9%) patients died because of their cancer and 70 (20.6%) patients experienced disease progression. During univariate analysis, we observed that multifocal tumors, advanced pathological tumor stage, positive lymph node metastasis, high histological tumor grade, the presence of vascular invasion, perineural invasion, and high MAP1B expression (Figure 3A,B) were associated with worse disease-specific survival (DSS) and metastasis-free survival (MFS) (all $p < 0.05$). In multivariate analysis, multifocal tumors, advanced pathological tumor stage, positive lymph node metastasis, high histological tumor grade, perineural invasion, and MAP1B expression were independently predictive for both DSS and MFS (all $p < 0.05$) (Table 3).

In our follow-up of UBUC patients, we found that 52 (17.6%) patients died due to the cancer and 76 (25.8%) patients experienced disease progression. During univariate analysis, we determined that advanced pT status, positive lymph node metastasis, high histological tumor grade, the presence of vascular invasion, perineural invasion, an increased mitotic rate, and increment of MAP1B expression (Figure 3C,D) were associated with worse DSS and MFS (all $p < 0.05$). Using multivariate analysis, we confirmed that advanced pathological tumor stage, an increased mitotic rate, and MAP1B expression remained significant in predicting reduced DSS and MFS (all $p < 0.05$) (Table 4).

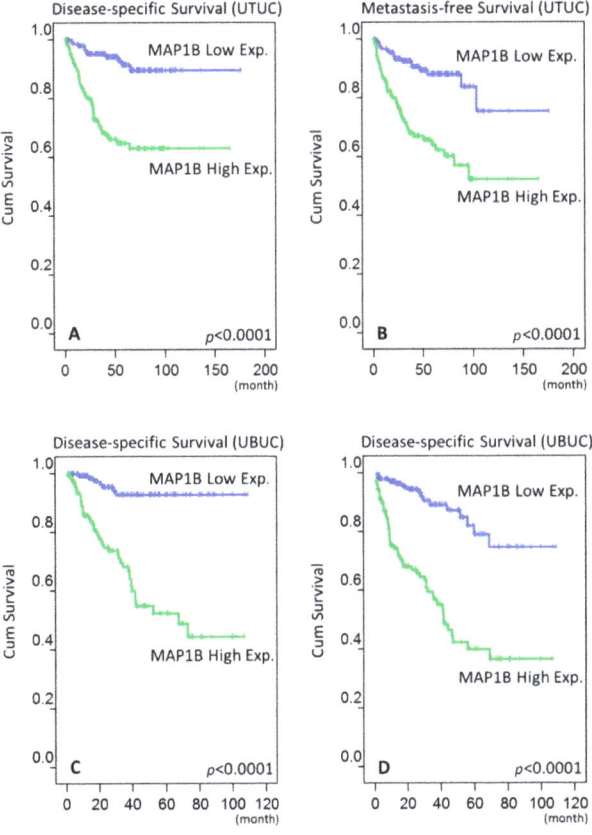

Figure 3. Kaplan–Meier survival analysis showing the prognostic significance of MAP1B expression for the DSS and MFS outcomes of UTUC (**A** and **B**) and UBUC (**C** and **D**).

Table 3. Univariate log-rank and multivariate analyses for DSS and MFS in UTUC.

Parameter	Category	Case No.	Disease-Specific Survival					Metastasis-Free Survival				
			Univariate Analysis		Multivariate Analysis			Univariate Analysis		Multivariate Analysis		
			No. of Event	p-value	R.R.	95% C.I.	p-value	No. of Event	p-value	R.R.	95% C.I.	p-value
Gender	Male	158	28	0.8730	-	-	-	32	0.8307	-	-	-
	Female	182	33		-	-	-	38		-	-	-
Age (years)	<65	138	26	0.9728	-	-	-	30	0.8667	-	-	-
	≥65	202	35		-	-	-	40		-	-	-
Tumor side	Right	177	34	0.7188	-	-	-	38	0.3903	-	-	-
	Left	154	26		-	-	-	32		-	-	-
	Bilateral	9	1		-	-	-	0		-	-	-
Tumor location	Renal pelvis	141	24	0.0100 *	1	-	0.562	31	0.0752	-	-	-
	Ureter	150	22		1.167	0.618–2.203		25		-	-	-
	Renal pelvis & ureter	49	15		1.261	0.345–4.615		14		-	-	-
Multifocality	Single	273	48	0.0031 *	1	-	0.050 *	52	0.0144 *	1	-	0.001 *
	Multifocal	62	18		2.238	0.998–5.017		18		2.648	1.496–4.687	
Primary tumor (T)	Ta	89	2	<0.0001 *	1	-	0.008 *	4	<0.0001 *	1	-	0.036 *
	T1	92	9		2.641	0.561–12.419		15		2.643	0.563–12.410	
	T2–T4	159	50		5.667	1.250–25.699		51		5.538	1.236–24.817	
Nodal metastasis	Negative (N0)	312	42	<0.0001 *	1	-	<0.001 *	55	<0.0001 *	1	-	<0.001 *
	Positive (N1–N2)	28	19		4.188	2.244–7.819		15		4.421	2.415–8.094	
Histological grade	Low	56	4	0.0177 *	1	-	0.008 *	3	0.0022 *	1	-	0.008 *
	High	284	57		4.746	1.514–14.881		67		4.770	1.509–15.077	
Vascular invasion	Absent	234	24	<0.0001 *	1	-	0.139	26	<0.0001 *	1	-	0.147
	Present	106	37		1.571	0.863–2.859		44		1.565	0.855–2.868	
Perineural invasion	Absent	321	50	<0.0001 *	1	-	<0.001 *	61	<0.0001 *	1	-	<0.001 *
	Present	19	11		4.768	2.251–10.102		9		4.865	2.294–10.318	
Mitotic rate (per 10 high power fields)	<10	173	27	0.1442	-	-	-	30	0.0739	-	-	-
	≥10	167	34		-	-	-	40		-	-	-
MAP1B expression	Low	170	11	<0.0001 *	1	-	0.001 *	17	<0.0001 *	1	-	<0.001 *
	High	170	50		4.115	2.077–8.154		53		3.962	2.022–7.763	

* Statistically significant.

Table 4. Univariate log-rank and multivariate analyses for DSS and MFS in UBUC.

| Parameter | Category | Case No. | Disease-Specific Survival ||||| Metastasis-Free Survival |||||
| | | | Univariate Analysis || Multivariate Analysis ||| Univariate Analysis || Multivariate Analysis |||
			No. of Event	p-value	R.R.	95% C.I.	p-value	No. of Event	p-value	R.R.	95% C.I.	p-value
Gender	Male	216	41	0.4404	-	-	-	60	0.2786	-	-	-
	Female	79	11		-	-	-	16		-	-	-
Age (years)	<65	121	17	0.1010	-	-	-	31	0.6285	-	-	-
	≥65	174	35		-	-	-	45		-	-	-
Primary tumor (T)	Ta	84	1	<0.0001 *	1	-	<0.001 *	4	<0.0001 *	1	-	<0.001 *
	T1	88	9		6.493	0.696–60.560		23		5.044	1.469–17.327	
	T2–T4	123	42		27.783	3.011–256.370		49		7.845	2.239–27.484	
Nodal metastasis	Negative (N0)	266	41	0.0001 *	1	-	0.729	61	<0.0001 *	1	-	0.100
	Positive (N1–N2)	29	11		1.132	0.560–2.288		15		1.685	0.905–3.137	
Histological grade	Low grade	56	2	0.0010 *	1	-	0.714	5	0.0005*	1	-	0.572
	High grade	239	50		0.744	0.153–3.610		71		0.729	0.244–2.179	
Vascular invasion	Absent	246	37	0.0017 *	1	-	0.174	54	0.0001 *	1	-	0.798
	Present	49	15		0.624	0.316–1.231		22		1.083	0.590–1.985	
Perineural invasion	Absent	275	44	<0.0001 *	1	-	0.099	66	0.0006 *	1	-	0.339
	Present	20	8		2.990	0.878–4.510		10		1.422	0.690–2.930	
Mitotic rate (per 10 high power fields)	<10	139	12	<0.0001 *	1	-	0.021 *	23	<0.0001 *	1	-	0.045 *
	≥10	156	40		2.184	1.124–4.246		53		1.697	1.012–2.846	
MAP1B expression	Low	147	7	<0.0001 *	1	-	<0.001 *	16	<0.0001 *	1	-	<0.001 *
	High	148	45		5.551	2.466–12.498		60		3.770	2.146–6.622	

* Statistically significant.

2.4. MAP1B Promotes the Cell Proliferation, Migration, and Invasion of UC Cell Lines

To investigate the biological effects of MAP1B, we first characterized endogenous MAP1B expression in eight UC cell lines and noticed RTCC1 and J82 cells had the most abundant MAP1B transcripts and protein expression (Figure 4A). We next successfully knocked down MAP1B in both the RTCC1 (Figure 4B, left) and J82 (Figure 4B, right) cell lines using short hairpin RNA (shRNA). We found significantly attenuated proliferation (viability) in stable MAP1B-silenced RTCC1 (Figure 4C1) and J82 (Figure 4C2) cells. Due to the positive relationship between MAP1B expression and the development of metastasis, we evaluated the effect of MAP1B in UC cell migration and invasion. MAP1B knockdown significantly decreased the migratory and invasive abilities of RTCC1 (Figure 4C3,C5) and J82 (Figure 4C4,C6) cells.

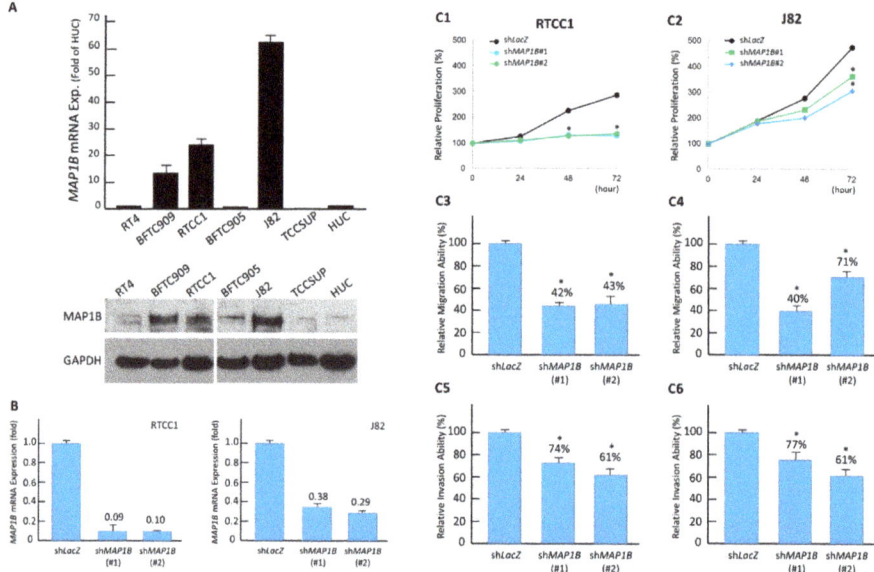

Figure 4. *MAP1B* expression promotes the growth of UC cells in vitro. (**A**) As compared with RT4 cells, endogenous *MAP1B* mRNA (upper) and protein (lower) expressions were increased in cells from the J82 and RTCC1 cell lines. (**B**) The two cell lines with high endogenous *MAP1B* expression were stably silenced against *MAP1B* expression by a lentiviral vector bearing one of the two clones of *MAP1B* shRNA with different sequences for both RTCC1 (left panel) and J82 (right panel) cells. Using an ELISA-based colorimetric assay to assess the rate of BrdU uptake, cell proliferation was significantly reduced in stable *MAP1B*-knockdown (**C1**) RTCC1 and (**C2**) J82 cell lines compared with that in the corresponding shLacZ controls. Similar trends were found for cell migration and invasion among cells from the (**C3** and **C5**) RTCC1 and (**C4** and **C6**) J82 cell lines. (* $p<0.05$). More details of western blot, please view at the supplementary materials.

2.5. MAP1B Expression Correlates with Chemoresistance In Vitro and In Vivo

Flow cytometric analysis of stable *MAP1B* knockdown RTCC1 and J82 cell lines showed stable *MAP1B* knockdown significantly increased the sub-G1 population, indicating induced cell apoptosis (Figures 5 and 6). Further analysis of vinblastine-treated RTCC1 and J82 cell lines also disclosed induced cell apoptosis (Figures 7 and 8). In other words, MAP1B expression might lead to a resistance to anti-mitotic chemotherapeutics. In the independent UBUC patient cohort receiving adjuvant chemotherapy, Kaplan–Meier survival analysis showed high MAP1B expression correlated with inferior DFS (Figure 9), further supporting the role of MAP1B in chemoresistance.

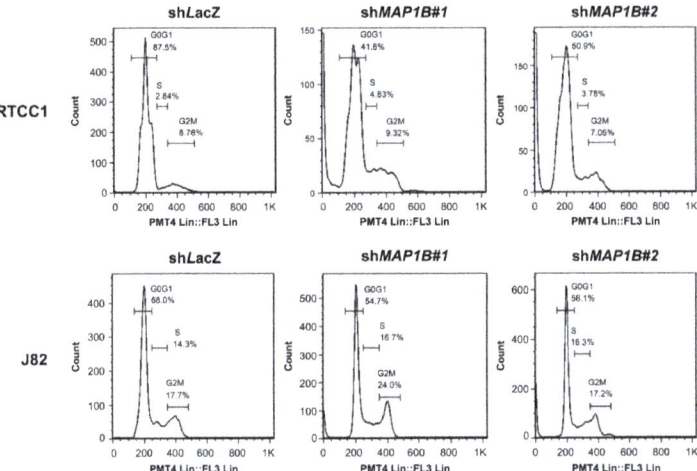

Figure 5. Stable *MAP1B* knockdown increases the sub-G1 population with significantly altered cell-cycle progression. Cell-cycle analysis as conducted by flow cytometry identified a remarkable increment of sub-G1 population indicating cell death in *MAP1B*-knockdown RTCC1 (upper panel) and J82 (lower panel) cells.

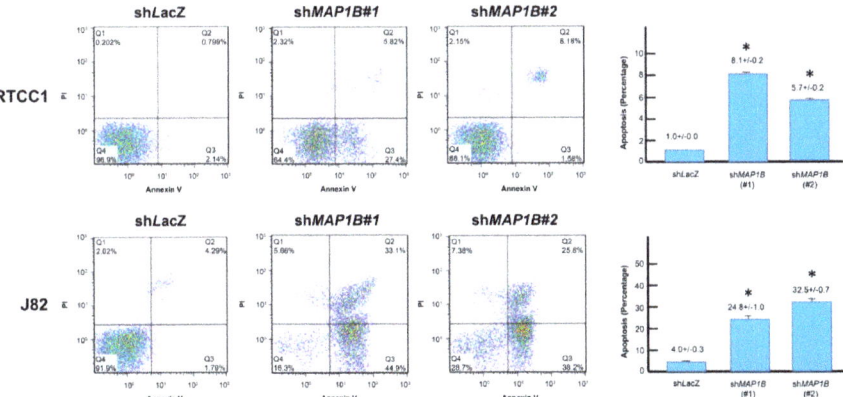

Figure 6. *MAP1B* knockdown induces apoptosis. Flow cytometric analysis of annexin V/propidium iodide-stained RTCC1 (upper panel) and J82 (lower panel) cell lines disclosed *MAP1B* knockdown significantly increased percentage of apoptosis. (* $p < 0.05$).

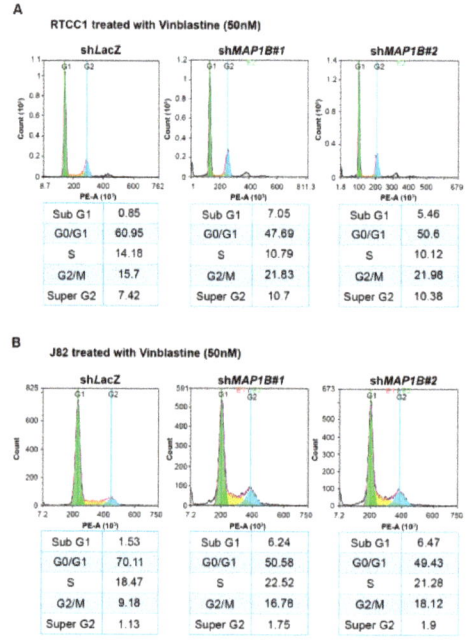

Figure 7. Stable *MAP1B* knockdown increased vinblastine-induced apoptosis. Flow cytometric analysis of vinblastine-treated RTCC1 (upper panel) and J82 (lower panel) cell lines disclosed that *MAP1B* knockdown significantly increased the sub-G1 population, indicating induced cell apoptosis.

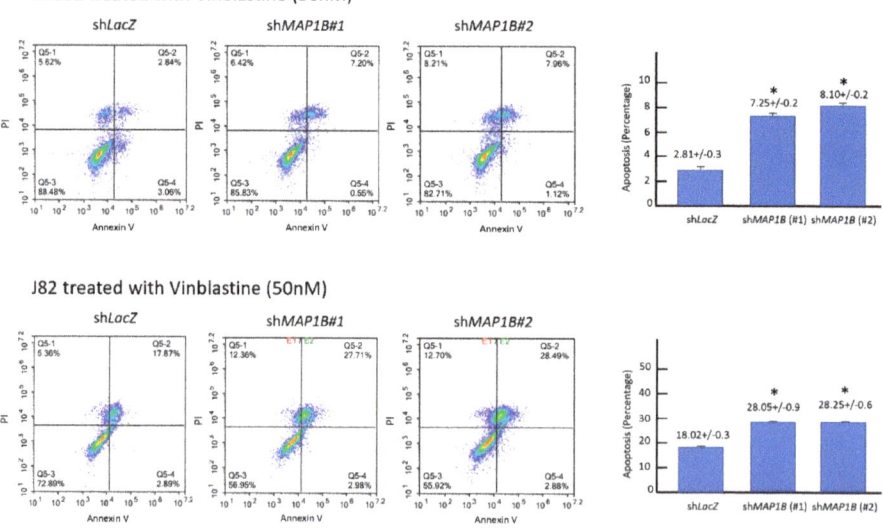

Figure 8. Stable *MAP1B* knockdown increase vinblastine-induced apoptosis. Flow cytometric analysis of annexin V/propidium iodide-stained RTCC1 (upper panel) and J82 (lower panel) cell lines demonstrated *MAP1B* knockdown significantly increased percentage of vinblastine-induced apoptosis. (* $p < 0.05$).

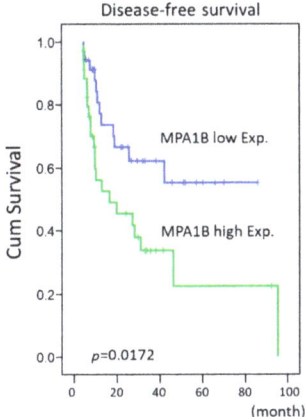

Figure 9. Kaplan–Meier survival analysis of *MAP1B* expression for the DFS of the UBUC patient cohort receiving adjuvant chemotherapy. Kaplan–Meier survival analysis showing the prognostic significance of *MAP1B* expression for the DFS of the UBUC patient cohort receiving adjuvant chemotherapy.

3. Discussion

It is estimated that one-third of patients with UBUC have advanced disease at presentation [16]. A similar poor prognosis was found among patients with advanced UTUC in that the DSS has not changed significantly during the last two decades [17]. Regardless of the high initial response, the therapeutic effects of current treatment were insufficient and resulted in recurrence and death. Currently, there are no effective salvage regimens for treating metastatic UC. Metastasis requires the inherent dynamic instability of microtubules for cell motility, and many changes in the microtubule network have been identified in various cancers [14]. There is accumulating evidence that MAPs are associated with changes in microtubule dynamics, that they can determine the effects of microtubule-targeting agents, and that they play a role in cancer resistance [14]. However, reliable tumor markers that predict the sensitivity to chemotherapy and resistance to tumor metastasis remain elusive.

MAPs contain products of oncogenes, tumor suppressors, and apoptosis regulators thought to be involved in microtubule assembly. On the other hand, vinblastine, listed in the World Health Organization's List of Essential Medicines, binds tubulin and inhibits the assembly of microtubules [18]. It causes M-phase–specific cell-cycle arrest by breaking microtubule assembly and proper formation of the mitotic spindle and the kinetochore, which were essential for the separation of chromosomes during the anaphase of mitosis. Due to the possibility of sharing a common function, the rational microtubule-targeting cancer therapeutic approaches should preferably include proteomic profiling of tumor MAPs before the administration of antimicrotubule agents preferentially in combination with agents that modulate the expression of relevant MAPs [14].

Histologically, MAPs were originally related to the development of the nervous system, based on their very early detection in neurons. However, the aberrant expression of primarily neuronal MAPs has since been detected in non-neural cancer tissues [14]. We also assessed MAP1B expression across various cancer types using Oncomine™ Platform (Thermo Fisher, Ann Arbor, MI). Data revealed a diverse expression of MAP1B in various cancers. Of these, CNS tumor has highest MAP1B expression; bladder tumor has moderate expression. In our present results and using a published transcriptome dataset (GSE31684), we first found that *MAP1B* was significantly upregulated in UC and associated with more advanced pT status and metastatic disease in UBUC. Next, we found using immunohistochemistry that *MAP1B* overexpression markedly correlated with disease status in affected patients. In patients with UTUC, *MAP1B* overexpression was positively associated with synchronous multiple tumors, advanced pathological tumor stage, positive lymph node metastasis, the presence of vascular invasion, and an increased mitotic rate. However, in patients with UBUC, *MAP1B* overexpression was associated with advanced pathological tumor stage, positive lymph node metastasis, high histological tumor grade, the presence of vascular invasion, and an increased mitotic rate. Furthermore, using survival analysis, we demonstrated an association between *MAP1B* and aggressive clinical progression, whereby *MAP1B* overexpression independently predicted poor DSS and MFS rates for all patients with UC. These findings indicate that standard clinical practices may benefit from evaluating the *MAP1B* status to improve the risk stratification of patients with UC.

Different *MAP1B* interactors can be grouped into seven different categories, including signaling, cytoskeleton, transmembrane proteins, RNA-binding proteins, apoptosis, neurodegeneration-linked proteins, and neurotransmitter receptors [19]. *MAP1B* is translated as a precursor polypeptide that undergoes proteolytic processing to cleave into an N-terminal heavy chain (*MAP1B* HC) and a C-terminal light chain (*MAP1B* LC1). *MAP1B* LC1 overexpression, which can generate protein aggregates, has been observed in endoplasmic reticulum-related stress-induced cell apoptosis. This effect is blocked by DJ-1, a Parkinson's disease–related protein that has been proposed to act like a molecular chaperone, and inhibits α-synuclein aggregation [20]. However, in contrast to the proapoptotic effects caused by LC1 overexpression, *MAP1B* overexpression is not related to cell death related to *p53*, a tumor-suppressor gene; in fact, *MAP1B* overexpression reduces *p53* transcriptional activity and inhibits doxorubicin-induced apoptosis [21]. In addition, we found that the percentages of cells in the early and late stages of apoptosis were significantly increased between shLacZ controls and shMAP1B-treated cells. Further in vivo studies are warranted to confirm our findings and to determine whether such results may lead to new therapeutic targets for UC.

Recent studies have found that changes in the expression of MAPs are associated with chemotherapy resistance and cancer progression [14,22]. For example, stathmin plays a role in regulating neuroblastoma cell migration and invasion [22]. Silencing stathmin expression using RNAi gene silencing significantly reduced lung metastasis in neuroblastoma in vivo. Similarly, we demonstrated using UC cell lines with high endogenous *MAP1B* expression that silencing by *MAP1B* shRNA significantly reduced cell proliferation, migration, and invasion ability. Based on these findings, we posit that *MAP1B* may be a clinically valuable diagnostic marker for early cancer detection and a promising prognostic marker.

Further, *MAP1B* interacts with several other proteins associated with cancer. For example, Ras-association domain family 1 isoform A (RASSF1A), a tumor suppressor whose inactivation is implicated in the development of many human cancers, interacts with *MAP1B* to influence microtubule dynamics in the cell cycle and is involved in the inhibition of cancer cell growth [23]. Through distinct bifunctional structural domains, C19ORF5, a sequence homolog of *MAP1B*, mediates the communication between the microtubular cytoskeleton and mitochondria in the control of cell death and defective genome destruction. In addition, it has been proposed that the accumulation of C19ORF5 results in microtubule hyperstability, which may be involved in the tumor suppression activity of RASSF1A [24]. In the mammary cancer susceptibility 1 (*Mcs1*) region in chromosome 2 (a region that expresses centromeric proteins), Laes et al. analyzed candidate genes in the region and found that *MAP1B* was expressed in the mammary glands of rats [25]. Interactions with other proteins not related to its role in stabilizing microtubules suggest that *MAP1B* may be part of a "signaling protein" that regulates molecular pathways [19]. We propose that *MAP1B* has multiple functions, and whether the main function of *MAP1B* is microtubule stabilization or whether it has many cellular functions warrants further investigation.

A recent study that focused on kidney glomerular development and function found that *MAP1B* was specifically expressed in podocytes in human and murine adult kidney tissues [26]. In a mouse model, *MAP1B* was not essential for glomerular filtration function but may play a role in the development and differentiation of the kidney tubular system. The authors hypothesize that *MAP1B* may be related to either stress maintenance or the aging process in the kidney. It is clear that the overall effects of *MAP1B* on UC are complex, with reports of associations between *MAP1B* and survival and metastasis. Research aimed at decoding the functional consequences of *MAP1B* and signaling cross-talk with other proteins in different cancers is needed in the future. However, due to a slight predominance toward females, it is unclear if the results can easily be transferred to the rest of the world.

4. Materials and Methods

4.1. Data Mining of GSE31684 to Identify Altered Gene Expression in UC

The transcriptome dataset GSE31684 (http://www.ncbi.nlm.nih.gov/geo/query/acc.cgi?acc=GSE31684), which includes 93 patients with UBUC who underwent radical cystectomy, was obtained from the Gene Expression Omnibus repository at the National Center for Biotechnology Information. Raw data were imported by Nexus Expression 3 (BioDiscovery, El Segundo, CA, USA) to quantify the gene expression level. No pre-selection or filtering was conducted during the analysis of the data for all probes. Comparative analyses were performed to determine the significant differences in the expressed genes by comparing the primary tumor (pT) status (high-stage to low-stage) and the presence or absence of metastatic events.

4.2. Patients and Tumor Specimens

Between 1996 and 2004, 340 patients with UTUC and 295 with UBUC who underwent surgery with curative intent at the Chi Mei Medical Center were enrolled. This study was reviewed and approved by the institutional review board (105-01-005). Informed patient consent was obtained from all participants. Demographic characteristics and clinical information including pathological features, oncological follow-up, and cause of mortality were retrospectively collected. Patients who underwent neoadjuvant chemotherapy or radiotherapy; who had concurrent muscle-invasive bladder tumor, acute blood disorders, or bone marrow diseases; and those with incomplete clinical information were excluded from our study. The tumor stage was defined in accordance with the 2002 American Joint Committee Cancer (AJCC)'s Tumor, Node, Metastasis system. Two pathologists reviewed tumor tissues and reclassified then as low- or high-grade using the seventh edition of the AJCC staging system. As a rule, all patients were treated initially by surgery with curative intent. All UBUC patients with pT3 or pT4 diseases or with nodal involvement received cisplatin-based adjuvant chemotherapy. However, of the 106 UTUC patients with pT3 or pT4 and nodal positive diseases, only 29 received cisplatin-based adjuvant chemotherapy. One expert pathologist (CFL) re-evaluated the hematoxylin and eosin–stained sections of all cases. To determine the *MAP1B* transcript level, a pilot batch of 30 UTUC and 30 UBUC snap-frozen tissues with a high tumor percentage (> 70%) was retrieved. Each group included 10 tumor tissues of the pTa stage, 10 of the pT1 stage, and 10 that were muscle-invasive (pT2–pT4).

4.3. Immunohistochemical Staining

Immunohistochemistry was conducted to detect *MAP1B* protein expression in 340 UTUC and 295 UBUC cases. One representative slide of a tumor with most invasive area was evaluated by two pathologists manually. Tumor tissue slide preparation was performed as described in our previous study [27]. Slides were incubated with the primary antibody against *MAP1B* (1:100, clone AA6; Millipore, Beverly, MA, USA). We quantified *MAP1B* protein expression levels by combining the intensity and percentage of immunostaining in the cytoplasm of UC cells to generate an H score using the following equation: H score = $\Sigma P_i (i + 1)$, where P_i is the percentage of stained tumor cells (0–100%) and i represents the intensity of immunoreactivity (0–3+). The resulting scores ranged from 100 to 400 points, where a score of 100 points indicated that 100% of cancer cells were nonreactive and a score of 400 points meant that 100% of the cancer cells examined were strongly immunoreactive (3+).

4.4. Real-Time Reverse-Transcription Polymerase Chain Reaction (RT-PCR) to Assess the Transcription Levels of MAP1B in Cell Lines and UC Samples

We calculated the fold change in *MAP1B* gene expression of UC tumors relative to that of normal tissues as previously described [27]. We extracted total RNA from cell lines and a pilot batch of cases consisting of 30 UTUCs and 30 UBUCs to quantify the transcription level of *MAP1B* using real-time RT-PCR. Predesigned TaqMan assay reagents (Applied Biosystems, Waltham, MA, USA) were used to assess the mRNA abundance of *MAP1B* (Hs00195485_m1) using the ABI StepOnePlus™ system (Applied Biosystems, Waltham, MA, USA), for which *POLR2A* (Hs01108291_m1) was used as the internal control for normalization.

4.5. Cell Culture

The cell lines RT4, TCCSUP, J82, and HUC were purchased from the American Type Culture Collection (Manassas, VA, USA). The cell lines BFTC 909, and BFTC 905 were obtained from the Food Industry Research and Development Institute (Hsinchu, Taiwan). RTCC1 cells were kindly provided by Professor Lien-Chai Chiang at Kaohsiung Medical University [28]. Short-tandem repeat profiling cell authentication had been performed in all cell lines (Mission Biotech, Taipei, Taiwan).

4.6. RNA Interference

The lentiviral vectors pLKO.1-*shLacZ* (TRCN0000072223: 5′-TGTTCGCATTATCCGAACCAT-3′) and pLKO.1-*shMAP1B* (#1, TRCN0000116621: 5′-GCCTGGAATAAACAGCATGTT-3′; #2, TRCN0000290688: 5′- CCCTGACTTAGGAGTTGTATT-3′) were obtained from the Taiwan National RNAi Core Facility (Taipei, Taiwan) and used to establish stable *MAP1B*-silenced clones of RTCC1 and J82 cell lines using shRNAs against *MAP1B* (*shMAP1B*).Viruses were produced by transfecting HEK293 cells with the above three vectors using Lipofectamine 2000 (Thermo Fisher Scientific, Waltham, MA, USA) [29]. For viral infection, 3×10^6 RTCC1 and J82 cells were incubated with 8 mL of lentivirus in the presence of polybrene, followed by puromycin selection of the stable clones of lentivirus-transduced cells.

4.7. Western Blotting

Our previously published western blotting assay procedure was used to evaluate endogenous *MAP1B* expression and the *MAP1B*-knockdown efficiency in RTCC1 and J82 cell lines using primary antibodies against *MAP1B* (1:500, clone AA6; Millipore, Beverly, MA, USA) and glyceraldehyde 3-phosphate dehydrogenase (GADPH) (6C5, 1:10,000; Millipore, Beverly, MA, USA). Cell lysates with 25 μg of protein were separated using a 4% to 12% gradient NuPAGE gel (Invitrogen, Carlsbad, CA, USA), then transferred onto polyvinylidene difluoride membranes (Amersham Biosciences, Buckinghamshire, UK) for the immobilization of proteins. Membranes were incubated with tris-buffered saline containing Tween 20 (TBST) buffer and 5% skimmed milk at room temperature for one hour for blocking, followed by exposure to primary antibodies at 4 °C overnight against *MAP1B* (1:500, clone AA6; Millipore, Beverly, MA, USA) using GADPH as a loading control (6C5, 1:10,000; Millipore, Beverly, MA, USA). Membranes were incubated with the secondary antibody at room temperature for 1.5 h, and proteins were detected using a chemiluminescence system (Amersham Biosciences, Buckinghamshire, UK).

4.8. Bromodeoxyuridine (BrdU) Assay to Assess DNA Synthesis

DNA synthesis was measured using an enzyme-linked immunosorbent assay (ELISA)-based and colorimetric bromodeoxyuridine (BrdU) assay (Roche Holding AG, Basel, Switzerland). *MAP1B*-knockdown or *shLacA* control RTCC1 and J82 cell lines were plated into a 96-well plate at a density of 3000 cells per well. At 24, 48, and 72 h, we measured the amount of DNA synthesis. The labeling medium was removed after three hours of incubation with BrdU at 37 °C under 5% CO_2, followed by fixation and a final incubation with an anti-BrdU-POD solution. An ELISA reader

(Promega Corp., Madison, WI, USA) was used to measure the absorbance at 450 nm, and the reference was set at an absorbance of 690 nm.

4.9. Pharmacological Assays

The colorimetric 2,3-bis-(2-methoxy-4-nitro-5-sulfophenyl)-2H-tetrazolium-5-carboxanilide (XTT) assay (Sigma-Aldrich, St. Louis, MO, USA) was used to assess cell viability as previously described [30]. Vinblastine sulfate (Hospira UK Ltd., Maidenhead, UK) was obtained and suspended in normal saline. RTCC1 and J82 cells were seeded in 96-well plates at a density of 5×10^3 cells per well the day before treatment at the indicated time points with vehicle control (0.9% saline) or increasing concentrations of vinblastine sulfate. The length of treatment interval was 72 h. After incubation with XTT reaction mixture for three hours at 37 °C under 5% CO_2, the absorbance of the samples was determined using an ELISA reader (Promega Corp., Madison, WI, USA) at 450 nm, with the absorbance set at 630 nm as reference.

4.10. Migration and Invasion Assays

Cell migration assay was performed using Falcon HTS FluoroBlok 24-well inserts (BD Biosciences, Franklin Lakes, NJ, USA) and the cell invasion assay was performed using the 24-well Collagen-based Cell Invasion Assay (Millipore, Beverly, MA, USA). Briefly, we added serum-free medium to rehydrate each insert, then replaced it with a serum-free suspension with equal numbers of cells in the upper chamber, followed by a 12- to 24-h incubation period to allow cells to migrate toward (i.e., invade) the lower chamber, which contained medium with 10% fetal bovine serum. After removal of the noninvading cells in the upper chamber, cells that invaded through the inserts were stained, lysed in extraction buffer, and transferred to 96-well plates for colorimetric readings at 560 nm.

4.11. Flow Cytometry Analysis of Cell-Cycle Kinetics

Stable pools of *MAP1B* knockdown versus the corresponding *shLacZ* control of the RTCC1 and J82 cell lines were pelleted and fixed overnight in 75% cold ethanol at −20 °C. The cells were washed twice using cold phosphate-buffered saline with 10 mg/mL of DNase-free RNase. Next, the cells were labeled with 0.05 mg/mL of propidium iodide and analyzed using a NovoCyte flow cytometer (ACEA Biosciences, San Diego, CA, USA) to determine the different proportions of cells at each phase of the cell cycle. Our lower limit of the number of sorted cells after gating out fixation artifacts and cell debris was 10^4 cells for all experiments.

4.12. Flow Cytometry Analysis of Apoptosis

Cell apoptosis was evaluated by plating RTCC1 and J82 cells (10^5 cells each) with sh*LacZ* or sh*MAP1B* for 24 h, followed by 15 min of incubation using an Annexin V-FITC kit (BD Biosciences, Franklin Lakes, NJ, USA) that contained propidium iodide. The percentages of cells at late apoptosis were calculated from three independent experiments.

4.13. Mutation Analysis

To explore potential *MAP1B* mutation in UC, we randomly selected 15 UTUC and 15 UBUC cases (Table S1) with high protein expressions of *MAP1B* for mutation analysis. Mutation analyses were performed by using an ABI3100 sequencer targeting eight pathogenic point mutations occurring in other cancer types according to the database of COSMIC repository (https://cancer.sanger.ac.uk/cosmic/gene/analysis?ln=HSD11B1#variants). Validated *MAP1B* mutations and primers sets are shown in Table S2. The PCR amplification started with an initial denaturation step at 95 °C for 15 min, followed by 35 cycles of 95 °C for 30 s, 58 °C for 30 s, and 72 °C for 30 s, and a final extension step at 72 °C for 10 min. Then, these amplicons generated in individual PCR reactions were analyzed by direct sequencing.

4.14. Postoperative Adjuvant Chemotherapy in UBUC

To evaluate the role of *MAP1B* expression in the response to adjuvant chemotherapy in UBUC patients, an independent cohort containing 70 patients with pT3 or pT4 disease or with nodal involvement received cisplatin-based adjuvant chemotherapy combined with vinblastine and were enrolled for further survival analysis (Table S3).

4.15. Statistical Analyses

The Statistical Package for the Social Sciences version 12.0 software program (IBM Corp., Armonk, NY, USA) was used for all statistical analyses. Differences between categorical parameters were assessed using the chi-squared or Fisher's exact test. The median H scores of *MAP1B* immunoreactivity were used as cutoff values to separate UTUC and UBUC into two subgroups of high and low *MAP1B* expression. Pearson's chi-squared test was used to compare the association between *MAP1B* expression and clinicopathological parameters. The Kaplan–Meier method was applied to estimate the effect of *MAP1B* expression on DSS and MFS. The survival curves were compared using the log-rank test. We used a Cox proportional-hazards model to identify independent predictors for DSS and MFS. In all figure legend, continuous parameters (such as MAP1B transcript expression in Figure 1, mitotic activity in Figure 2, *MAP1B* mRNA expression, relative proliferation, migration and invasion in Figure 4, apoptosis rate in Figure 6) were assessed using a t-test or Mann–Whitney–Wilcoxon test. Survival analysis (DSS and MFS) were performed using Kaplan-Meier plots and compared by the log-rank test. Statistical significance was set at $p < 0.05$.

5. Conclusions

In summary, the present study demonstrated that MAP1B overexpression was not only an indicator of unfavorable clinicopathological parameters, but also an independent prognostic factor able to predict poor DSS and MFS rates in patients with UTUC or UBUC. Additional studies must be conducted to elucidate the details of the biological significance of MAP1B and its encoded protein in UC oncogenesis for exploring possible MAP1B-targeted therapy for both kinds of UC.

Supplementary Materials: The following are available online at http://www.mdpi.com/2072-6694/12/3/630/s1, Table S1: Urothelial carcinoma enrolled to explore potential MAP1B mutation, Table S2: MAP1B mutations validated and primer sets, Table S3: Characters of independent UBUC patient cohorts receiving postoperative adjuvant chemotherapy.

Author Contributions: Conceptualization, T.-M.C., S.K.-H.H., W.-J.W., C.-F.L.; Methodology, B.-W.Y.; Formal analysis, T.-C.C.; Data curation, T.-C.C., S.K.-H.H., W.-J.W., C.-F.L.; Writing—original draft preparation, T.-M.C.; Writing—review and editing, C.-N.H.; Supervision, W.-M.L., C.-C.L.; Project administration, C.-F.L. All authors have read and agreed to the published version of the manuscript.

Funding: This study was supported by Kaohsiung Medical University "Aim for the Top Universities," grant nos. KMU-TP104E31, KMU-TP105G00, KMU-TP105G01, and KMU-TP105G02; the Health and Welfare Surcharge of Tobacco Products, Ministry of Health and Welfare, grant no. MOHW105-TDU-B-212-134007l the Ministry of Science and Technology, grant no. MOST103-2314-B-037-067-MY3; Kaohsiung Medical University Hospital, grant nos. KMUH101-1R47 and KMUH102-2R42. KMU-KI109002 to WM.Li, WJ. Wu and CF. Li.

Acknowledgments: The authors gratefully acknowledge the assistance of all the members in our group and the BioBank of Chi Mei Medical center. The authors would like to thank Enago (www.enago.tw) for the English language review.

Conflicts of Interest: The authors declare no conflict of interest.

References

1. Torre, L.A.; Bray, F.; Siegel, R.L.; Ferlay, J.; Lortet-Tieulent, J.; Jemal, A. Global cancer statistics, 2012. *CA Cancer J. Clin.* **2015**, *65*, 87–108. [CrossRef] [PubMed]
2. Lynch, C.F.; Davila, J.A.; Platz, C.E. Cancer of the urinary bladder. In *SEER Survival Monograph: Cancer Survival Among Adults: US SEER Program, 1988–2001, Patient and Tumor Characteristics, National*; Ries, Y.J., Keel, G.E., Eisner, M.P., Eds.; Cancer Institute, SEER Program: Bethesda, MD, USA, 2007; pp. 193–202.

3. Margulis, V.; Shariat, S.F.; Matin, S.F.; Kamat, A.M.; Zigeuner, R.; Kikuchi, E.; Lotan, Y.; Weizer, A.; Raman, J.D.; Wood, C.G. Outcomes of radical nephroureterectomy: A series from the Upper Tract Urothelial Carcinoma Collaboration. *Cancer* **2009**, *115*, 1224–1233. [CrossRef] [PubMed]
4. Lai, M.N.; Wang, S.M.; Chen, P.C.; Chen, Y.Y.; Wang, J.D. Population-based case-control study of Chinese herbal products containing aristolochic acid and urinary tract cancer risk. *J. Natl. Cancer Inst.* **2010**, *102*, 179–186. [CrossRef]
5. Li, C.C.; Chang, T.H.; Wu, W.J.; Ke, H.L.; Huang, S.P.; Tsai, P.C.; Chang, S.J.; Shen, J.T.; Chou, Y.H.; Huang, C.H. Significant predictive factors for prognosis of primary upper urinary tract cancer after radical nephroureterectomy in Taiwanese patients. *Eur. Urol.* **2008**, *54*, 1127–1134. [CrossRef] [PubMed]
6. Ploussard, G.; Xylinas, E.; Lotan, Y.; Novara, G.; Margulis, V.; Rouprêt, M.; Matsumoto, K.; Karakiewicz, P.I.; Montorsi, F.; Remzi, M.; et al. Conditional survival after radical nephroureterectomy for upper tract carcinoma. *Eur. Urol.* **2015**, *67*, 803–812. [CrossRef] [PubMed]
7. Raman, J.D.; Scherr, D.S. Management of patients with upper urinary tract transitional cell carcinoma. *Nat. Clin. Pract. Urol.* **2007**, *4*, 432–443. [CrossRef] [PubMed]
8. Knowles, M.A. What we could do now: Molecular pathology of bladder cancer. *Mol. Pathol.* **2001**, *54*, 215–221. [CrossRef] [PubMed]
9. McConkey, D.J.; Lee, S.; Choi, W.; Tran, M.; Majewski, T.; Lee, S.; Siefker-Radtke, A.; Dinney, C.; Czerniak, B. Molecular genetics of bladder cancer: Emerging mechanisms of tumor initiation and progression. *Urol. Oncol.* **2010**, *28*, 429–440. [CrossRef]
10. Amin, M.B. Histological variants of urothelial carcinoma: Diagnostic, therapeutic and prognostic implications. *Mod. Pathol.* **2009**, *22* (Suppl. 2), S96–S118. [CrossRef]
11. Zhang, Z.; Furge, K.A.; Yang, X.J.; Teh, B.T.; Hansel, D.E. Comparative gene expression profiling analysis of urothelial carcinoma of the renal pelvis and bladder. *BMC Med. Genom.* **2010**, *3*, 58. [CrossRef]
12. Halpain, S.; Dehmelt, L. The MAP1 family of microtubule-associated proteins. *Genome Biol.* **2006**, *76*, 224. [CrossRef] [PubMed]
13. Dehmelt, L.; Halpain, S. The MAP2/Tau family of microtubule-associated proteins. *Genome Biol.* **2005**, *6*, 204. [CrossRef] [PubMed]
14. Bhat, K.M.; Setaluri, V. Microtubule-associated proteins as targets in cancer chemotherapy. *Clin. Cancer Res.* **2007**, *13*, 2849–2854. [CrossRef] [PubMed]
15. Parker, A.L.; Kavallaris, M.; McCarroll, J.A. Microtubules and their role in cellular stress in cancer. *Front. Oncol.* **2014**, *4*, 153. [CrossRef] [PubMed]
16. Niegisch, G.; Lorch, A.; Droller, M.J.; Lavery, H.J.; Stensland, K.D.; Albers, P. Neoadjuvant chemotherapy in patients with muscle-invasive bladder cancer: Which patients benefit? *Eur. Urol.* **2013**, *64*, 355–357. [CrossRef] [PubMed]
17. Adibi, M.; Youssef, R.; Shariat, S.F.; Lotan, Y.; Wood, C.G.; Sagalowsky, A.I.; Zigeuner, R.; Montorsi, F.; Bolenz, C.; Margulis, V. Oncological outcomes after radical nephroureterectomy for upper tract urothelial carcinoma: Comparison over the three decades. *Int. J. Urol.* **2012**, *19*, 1060–1066. [CrossRef] [PubMed]
18. Altmann, K.H. Preclinical Pharmacology and Structure-Activity Studies of Epothilones. In *The Epothilones: An Outstanding Family of Anti-Tumor Agents. Fortschritte der Chemie Organischer Naturstoffe/Progress in the Chemistry of Organic Natural Products*; Springer: Vienna, Austria, 2009; Volume 90. [CrossRef]
19. Villarroel-Campos, D.; Gonzalez-Billault, C. The MAP1B case: An old MAP that is new again. *Dev. Neurobiol.* **2014**, *74*, 953–971. [CrossRef]
20. Wang, Z.; Zhang, Y.; Zhang, S.; Guo, Q.; Tan, Y.; Wang, X.; Xiong, R.; Ding, J.; Chen, S. DJ-1 can inhibit microtubule associated protein 1 B formed aggregates. *Mol. Neurodegener.* **2011**, *6*, 38. [CrossRef]
21. Lee, S.Y.; Kim, J.W.; Jeong, M.H.; An, J.H.; Jang, S.M.; Song, K.H.; Choi, K.H. Microtubule-associated protein 1B light chain (MAP1B-LC1) negatively regulates the activity of tumor suppressor p53 in neuroblastoma cells. *FEBS Lett.* **2008**, *582*, 2826–2832. [CrossRef]
22. Byrne, F.L.; Yang, L.; Phillips, P.A.; Hansford, L.M.; Fletcher, J.I.; Ormandy, C.J.; McCarroll, J.A.; Kavallaris, M. RNAi-mediated stathmin suppression reduces lung metastasis in an orthotopic neuroblastoma mouse model. *Oncogene* **2014**, *33*, 882–890. [CrossRef]
23. Dallol, A.; Agathanggelou, A.; Fenton, S.L.; Ahmed-Choudhury, J.; Hesson, L.; Vos, M.D.; Clark, G.J.; Downward, J.; Maher, E.R.; Latif, F. RASSF1A interacts with microtubule-associated proteins and modulates microtubule dynamics. *Cancer Res.* **2004**, *64*, 4112–4116. [CrossRef]

24. Liu, L.; Vo, A.; Liu, G.; McKeehan, W.L. Distinct Structural Domains within C19ORF5 Support Association with Stabilized Microtubules and Mitochondrial Aggregation and Genome Destruction. *Cancer Res.* **2005**, *65*, 4191–4201. [CrossRef] [PubMed]
25. Laes, J.F.; Quan, X.; Ravoet, M.; Stieber, D.; Van Vooren, P.; Van Reeth, T.; Szpirer, J.; Szpirer, C. Analysis of candidate genes included in the mammary cancer susceptibility 1 (Mcs1) region. *Mamm. Genome* **2001**, *12*, 199–206. [CrossRef] [PubMed]
26. Gödel, M.; Temerinac, D.; Grahammer, F.; Hartleben, B.; Kretz, O.; Riederer, B.M.; Propst, F.; Kohl, S.; Huber, T.B. Microtubule associated protein 1b (MAP1B) is a marker of the microtubular cytoskeleton in podocytes but is not essential for the function of the kidney filtration barrier in mice. *PLoS ONE* **2015**, *10*, e0140116. [CrossRef] [PubMed]
27. Fan, E.W.; Li, C.C.; Wu, W.J.; Huang, C.N.; Li, W.M.; Ke, H.L.; Yeh, H.C.; Wu, T.F.; Liang, P.I.; Ma, L.J.; et al. FGF7 Over expression is an independent prognosticator in patients with urothelial carcinoma of the upper urinary tract and bladder. *J. Urol.* **2015**, *194*, 223–229. [CrossRef] [PubMed]
28. Chiang, L.C.; Chiang, W.; Chang, L.L.; Wu, W.J.; Huang, C.H. Characterization of a new human transitional cell carcinoma cell line from the renal pelvis, RTCC-1/KMC. *Kaohsiung J. Med. Sci.* **1996**, *12*, 448–452. [PubMed]
29. Li, C.F.; Chen, L.T.; Lan, J.; Chou, F.F.; Lin, C.Y.; Chen, Y.Y.; Chen, T.J.; Li, S.H.; Yu, S.; Fang, F.M.; et al. AMACR amplification and overexpression in primary imatinib-naïve gastrointestinal stromal tumors: A driver of cell proliferation indicating adverse prognosis. *Oncotarget* **2014**, *5*, 11588–11630. [CrossRef]
30. Li, C.F.; Fang, F.M.; Chen, Y.Y.; Chen, Y.Y.; Liu, T.T.; Chan, T.C.; Yu, S.C.; Chen, L.T.; Huang, H.Y. Overexpressed fatty acid synthase in gastrointestinal stromal tumors: Targeting a progression-associated metabolic driver enhances the antitumor effect of imatinib. *Clin. Cancer Res.* **2017**, *23*, 4908–4918. [CrossRef]

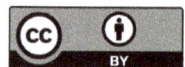

© 2020 by the authors. Licensee MDPI, Basel, Switzerland. This article is an open access article distributed under the terms and conditions of the Creative Commons Attribution (CC BY) license (http://creativecommons.org/licenses/by/4.0/).

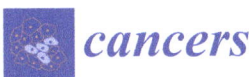

Article

KLF5 Is Crucial for Androgen-AR Signaling to Transactivate Genes and Promote Cell Proliferation in Prostate Cancer Cells

Juan Li [1,2], Baotong Zhang [3], Mingcheng Liu [1,2], Xing Fu [1,2], Xinpei Ci [4], Jun A [1,2], Changying Fu [1,2], Ge Dong [1], Rui Wu [1,2], Zhiqian Zhang [2], Liya Fu [1] and Jin-Tang Dong [2,3,*]

1. Department of Genetics and Cell Biology, College of Life Sciences, Nankai University, 94 Weijin Road, Tianjin 300071, China; 1120150354@mail.nankai.edu.cn (J.L.); 1120170388@mail.nankai.edu.cn (M.L.); 1120140347@mail.nankai.edu.cn (X.F.); 1120170387@mail.nankai.edu.cn (J.A.); 1120160365@mail.nankai.edu.cn (C.F.); 1120160366@mail.nankai.edu.cn (G.D.); 1120160367@mail.nankai.edu.cn (R.W.); fuchu12@nankai.edu.cn (L.F.)
2. School of Medicine, Southern University of Science and Technology, 1088 Xueyuan Road, Shenzhen, Guangdong 518055, China; zhangzq@sustc.edu.cn
3. Emory Winship Cancer Institute, Department of Hematology and Medical Oncology, Emory University School of Medicine, 1365-C Clifton Road, Atlanta, GA 30322, USA; baotong.zhang@emory.edu
4. Vancouver Prostate Centre, Department of Urologic Sciences, University of British Columbia, Vancouver, BC V6H 3Z6, Canada; xci@prostatecentre.com
* Correspondence: j.dong@emory.edu

Received: 26 February 2020; Accepted: 17 March 2020; Published: 21 March 2020

Abstract: Androgen/androgen receptor (AR) signaling drives both the normal prostate development and prostatic carcinogenesis, and patients with advanced prostate cancer often develop resistance to androgen deprivation therapy. The transcription factor Krüppel-like factor 5 (KLF5) also regulates both normal and cancerous development of the prostate. In this study, we tested whether and how KLF5 plays a role in the function of AR signaling in prostate cancer cells. We found that KLF5 is upregulated by androgen depending on AR in LNCaP and C4-2B cells. Silencing *KLF5*, in turn, reduced AR transcriptional activity and inhibited androgen-induced cell proliferation and tumor growth in vitro and in vivo. Mechanistically, KLF5 occupied the promoter of *AR*, and silencing *KLF5* repressed *AR* transcription. In addition, KLF5 and AR physically interacted with each other to regulate the expression of multiple genes (e.g., *MYC*, *CCND1* and *PSA*) to promote cell proliferation. These findings indicate that, while transcriptionally upregulated by AR signaling, KLF5 also regulates the expression and transcriptional activity of AR in androgen-sensitive prostate cancer cells. The KLF5-AR interaction could provide a therapeutic opportunity for the treatment of prostate cancer.

Keywords: KLF5; androgen receptor; cell proliferation; tumorigenesis; prostate cancer

1. Introduction

Prostate cancer (PCa) is prevalent among older men; and is one of the common causes of cancer-related death in men. While genetic and epigenetic alterations of multiple genes, including loss of *PTEN* [1–3], fusion between *TMPRSS2* and *ERG* [4,5], amplification and over-expression of *MYC*, and inactivation of *P53* and *RB* [3], initiate and promote prostatic carcinogenesis [6–8], androgen/androgen receptor (AR) signaling is the driving force in the process [9,10]. AR is thus a major therapeutic target, and androgen deprivation therapy (ADT) via surgical or chemical castration, including abiraterone and enzalutamide treatment, is thus the most commonly used effective therapy for patients with PCa. Unfortunately, PCa often develop resistance to ADT and become castration-resistant prostate cancers (CRPCs), which usually maintain AR activity by different mechanisms, such as generating AR splice variants, gain-of-function mutations in *AR*, and functional alterations leading to androgen independence [11–13].

AR is a member of the nuclear steroid receptor superfamily that is predominantly activated by testosterone and di-hydrotestosterone [14,15]. AR signaling is essential not only for postnatal development and maintenance of normal prostates but also for the regeneration of prostates after androgen deprivation. AR signaling also promotes the development and progression of PCa via enhanced cell proliferation and survival [16]. Many PCa driver genes alter the activity or structure of AR or are regulated by AR signaling during prostatic carcinogenesis.

KLF5 is a basic transcription factor that belongs to the Krüppel-like factor (KLF) family. It regulates a variety of biological processes including cell proliferation, apoptosis, angiogenesis, stemness and the epithelial-mesenchymal transition (EMT) [17,18]. KLF5 also functions in multiple pro- and anti-proliferative signaling pathways, including the RAS/ERK and PI3K/AKT proliferative pathways and the TGF-β anti-proliferative signaling to regulate different cancer cell behaviors [19–21]. As a transcription factor, KLF5 interacts with other transcription factors such as c-Jun [22], p53 [23], and ERα [24] to regulate the transcription of many genes involved in cell proliferation and tumorigenesis [25], including *CCND1* and *MYC* [26–28]. In the prostate, KLF5 also plays crucial roles in postnatal development, regeneration after castration, and PCa. In both human and mouse prostates, Klf5 is expressed in both basal and luminal cells, and basal cells preferentially express acetylated Klf5 [29,30]. Androgen ablation by castration in mice increases both Klf5 expression level and the number of KLF5-expressing cells [29], and both Klf5 and acetylated Klf5 are indispensable for the maintenance of basal progenitors and their luminal differentiation [30]. Klf5 and its acetylation are also necessary for the survival and regeneration of basal progenitor-derived luminal cells following castration and subsequent androgen restoration [30]. During tumorigenesis, the deletion of *Klf5* promotes *Pten* loss-induced prostate tumors, and the $Klf5^{-/-}/Pten^{-/-}$ tumors also have increased basal to luminal differentiation [31].

Taken together with the facts that androgen/AR signaling is the driving force in both normal prostate development and regeneration and PCa development, both KLF5 and AR are transcription factors, and androgen appears to induce the expression of *KLF5* in PCa cells [32,33], we propose that KLF5 and AR could be functionally associated with each other in prostatic carcinogenesis. We tested this hypothesis in this study. We demonstrated that silencing *KLF5* inhibited cell proliferation and tumor growth of PCa cells. In addition, as a transcription factor, KLF5 occupied the promoter of *AR* to promote its transcription; and KLF5 was also required for AR's transcriptional activity. Furthermore, KLF5 and AR interacted with each other to regulate transcription of AR target genes (e.g., *MYC*, *CCND1*, and *PSA*) to promote cell proliferation and tumor growth. These findings suggest that specific targeting of the AR-KLF5 interaction could be a potential therapeutic strategy for disrupting androgen signaling in PCa treatment.

2. Results

2.1. Androgen/AR Signaling Upregulates KLF5 Transcription in PCa cells

To test the role of androgen/AR signaling in KLF5 transcription, we measured KLF5 expression in two androgen-responsive PCa cell lines, LNCaP and C4-2B, in hormone-free medium (RIPA1640 medium supplemented with charcoal-stripped bovine fetal serum) treated with varying concentrations of R1881, a synthetic androgen, specifically binds to AR with higher affinity than dihydrotestosterone (DHT), and R1881-bound AR dimerizes and translocates to the nucleus to interact with coregulators to regulate gene transcription [34,35]. Androgen treatment caused a dose-dependent increase in KLF5 expression at both protein and mRNA levels (Figure 1a–d). As expected, R1881 treatment also increased the expression of known AR targets *PSA*, *TMPRSS2*, and *FKBP5* at the mRNA level (Figure 1b). Treatment of C4-2B cells with R1881 at 10 nM for different times increased KLF5 expression in a time-dependent manner (Figure 1e,f).

The same two cell lines grown in normal medium, which contains hormones to activate AR signaling, were treated with enzalutamide to block androgen/AR signaling. Enzalutamide is an AR antagonist that binds with AR to block its nuclear translocation and subsequent interactions with its coactivators in regulation target gene transcription [36,37]. Enzalutamide is widely used in the treatment of PCa [38,39]. Enzalutamide treatment at varying concentrations caused a dose-dependent decrease in KLF5 expression at both protein and mRNA levels in both cell lines (Figure 1g–j), while decreasing the expression of AR and its target genes (*PSA*, *TMPRSS2*, and *FKBP5*) as expected (Figure 1h). Consistently, treatment of C4-2B cells with 10 µM enzalutamide for different times decreased the expression of both KLF5 and AR in a time-dependent manner (Figure 1k,l).

To test whether R1881-induced KLF5 expression depends on AR, we knocked down AR by siRNA in C4-2B cells cultured in hormone-free medium in the presence of R1881 (10 nM) or enzalutamide (10 µM) and analyzed KLF5 expression. AR silencing by siRNA, which was confirmed by western blotting (Figure 1m), eliminated the induction of KLF5 by R1881 at both protein and mRNA levels (Figure 1m,n). Although cells were cultured in hormone-free medium, enzalutamide treatment still reduced AR protein (Figure 1m) and KLF5 mRNA levels (Figure 1n). Further supporting a role of AR in R1881-induced KLF5 expression, the promoter-luciferase reporter assay demonstrated that, in C4-2B cells cultured in hormone-free media, R1881 induced a significant KLF5 promoter activity while enzalutamide decreased the activity, and AR silencing eliminated these effects (Figure 1o). These findings indicate that androgen/AR signaling upregulates KLF5 transcription.

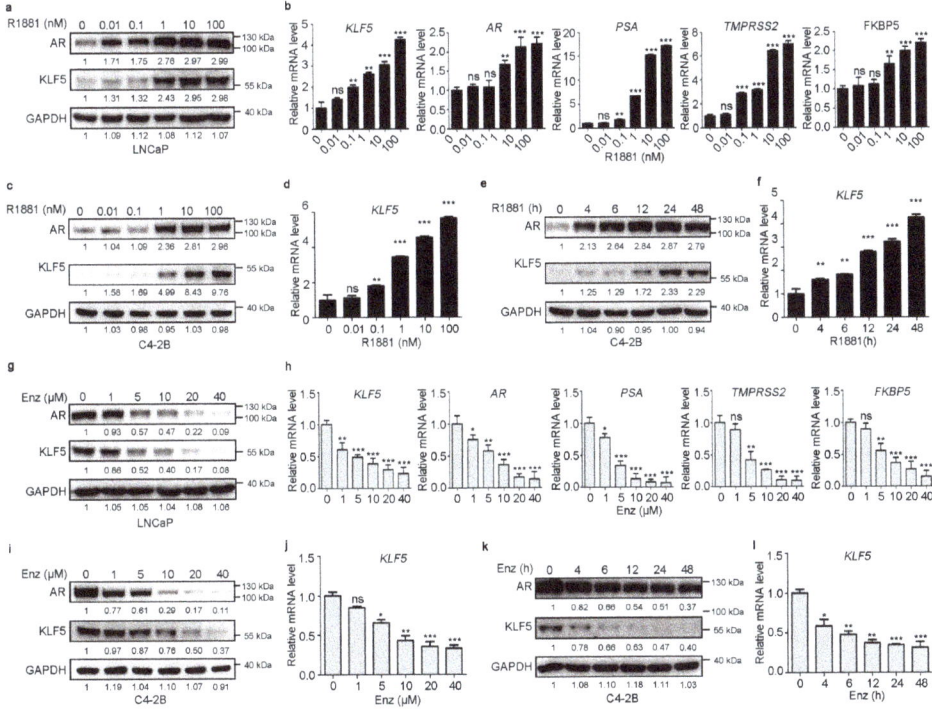

Figure 1. *Cont.*

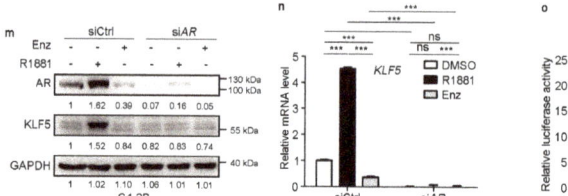

Figure 1. Androgen-androgen receptor (AR) signaling upregulates the transcription of KLF5 in PCa cells. (**a–d**) R1881 induced the expression of KLF5 at both protein (a, c) and RNA (b, d) levels in LNCaP (a, b) and C4-2B (c, d) cells. After 24-hour culture in phenol red–free RPMI-1640 medium containing 10% charcoal-stripped (CS) FBS, cells were treated with R1881 for 24 h at the indicated concentrations. Western blotting and real-time qPCR were performed to detect protein and mRNA respectively. (**e,f**) R1881 induced the expression of KLF5 at both protein (e) and RNA (f) levels at the indicated times in C4-2B cells. Cell culture conditions and the detection of KLF5 protein and mRNA were the same as in panels a-d. After 24-hour culture, cells were treated with R1881 (10 nM) for the indicated times. (**g–j**) Enzalutamide inhibited the expression of KLF5 at both protein (g, i) and RNA (h, j) levels in LNCaP (g, h) and C4-2B (i, j) cells. Cells were cultured in complete media for 24 h and treated with enzalutamide at the indicated concentrations for 24 h. (**k,l**) Enzalutamide inhibited the expression of KLF5 at both protein (k) and RNA (l) levels at the indicated times in C4-2B cells. Cell culture conditions and the detection of KLF5 protein and mRNA were the same as in panels g-j. After 24-hour culture, cells were treated with enzalutamide (Enz, 10 µM) for the indicated times. (**m,n**) RNAi-mediated silencing of AR prevented R1881 from upregulating KLF5 expression at both protein (m) and mRNA (n) levels in C4-2B cells. Cell culture conditions and the detection of KLF5 protein and mRNA were the same as in panels a-d. Transfection of siRNAs was for 6 h before R1881 treatment (10 nM). Enzalutamide (Enz, 10 µM) was used as a control. siCtrl, control siRNA; siAR, AR siRNA. (**o**) Knockdown of AR also prevented R1881 from inducing transcriptional activity of the KLF5 promoter in C4-2B cells, as detected by the promoter luciferase reporter activity assay. Experimental conditions were the same as in panels i and j except that the reporter plasmid was co-transfected with siRNAs. ns, not significant; *, $p < 0.05$; **, $p < 0.01$; ***$p < 0.001$.

2.2. KLF5 is Crucial for Maintaining the Transcriptional Activity of AR in PCa Cells

To determine whether androgen-upregulated KLF5 has a functional role in androgen/AR signaling, we evaluated whether knockdown of KLF5 affects AR's transcriptional activity in LNCaP cells with KLF5 silencing by siRNA and C4-2B cells with KLF5 silencing by shRNA. Cells were cultured in regular media, which contains hormones as regular FBS was used. Enzalutamide treatment was applied to inhibit AR signaling activity. KLF5 silencing clearly decreased the expression of PSA, a classic transcriptional target of AR [40], at both protein and mRNA levels in both LNCaP and C4-2B cell lines (Figure 2a,b). With enzalutamide treatment, expression of both PSA and AR was dramatically reduced, and the effect of KLF5 knockdown on PSA expression was weakened at the protein and mRNA level (Figure 2a–d). The mRNA expression of two additional AR target genes, *TMPRSS2* and *FKBP5* [41,42], was also decreased by KLF5 silencing, as detected by real-time qPCR (Figure 2c,d). We noticed that KLF5 silencing also decreased AR expression in both cell lines (Figure 2a,b), which is further addressed in Figure 3.

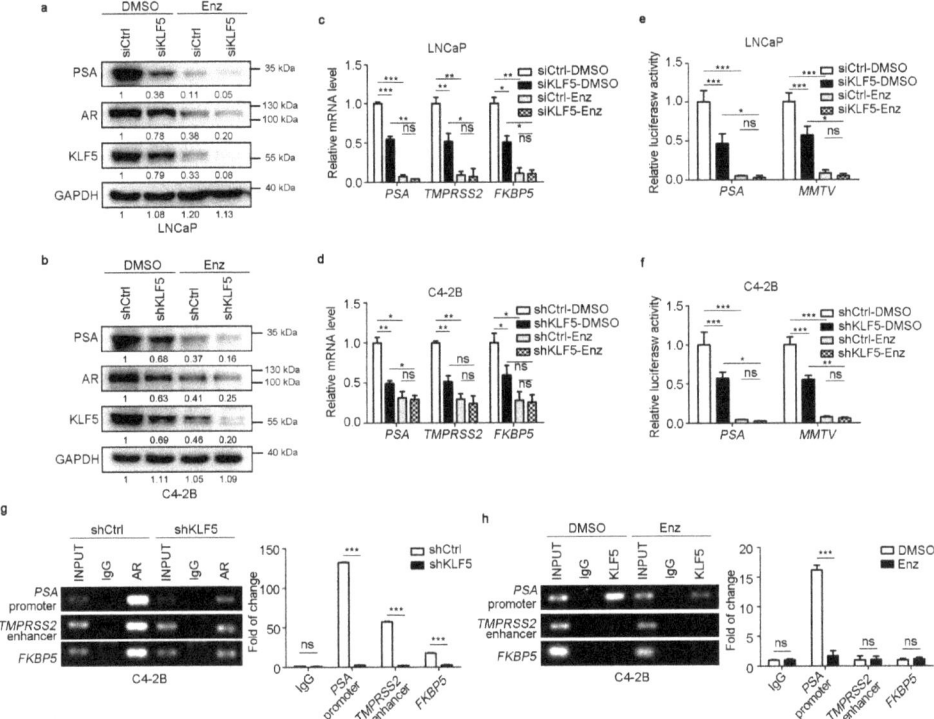

Figure 2. KLF5 is crucial for the transcriptional activity of AR in PCa cells. (**a–d**) Knockdown of KLF5 reduced the expression of AR transcriptional target genes *PSA*, *TMPRSS2*, and *FKBP5*. Gene expression was detected for protein by western blotting (a, b) and real-time qPCR for mRNA (c, d). LNCaP (a, c) and C4-2B (b, d) cells in full medium were transfected with siRNAs (a, c) or infected with shRNA lentiviruses (b, d) to silence KLF5. One group of cells were treated with enzalutamide (10 μM, 24 h) to inhibit AR function, which served as a control. siCtrl and shCtrl are control siRNA and shRNA respectively. (**e,f**) Knockdown of KLF5 reduced the activities of two androgen-responsive promoters, *PSA* and *MMTV*, in the same cells with the same treatments as in panels a-d, except that the PSA– or MMTV–luciferase reporter plasmid and Renilla-luciferase reporter plasmid were transfected for 24 h before enzalutamide treatment. (**g**) Binding of AR to the promoters of *PSA* and *FKBP5* and the enhancer of *TMPRSS2* was detected after the knockdown of KLF5 in C4-2B cells, as detected by ChIP and regular PCR (left) or real-time qPCR (right). Cells were infected with lentiviruses expressing shRNAs against KLF5 (shKLF5) or control (shCtrl) to knock down KLF5. (**h**) KLF5 binds to the promoter of *PSA* but not the promoter of *FKBP5* or the enhancer of *TMPRSS2* in C4-2B cells in full medium, as detected by ChIP and regular PCR (left) or real-time qPCR (right). Cells were treated with enzalutamide (10 μM, 24 h), with DMSO as a control. ns, not significant; *, $p < 0.05$; **, $p < 0.01$; ***$p < 0.001$.

We also analyzed the activities of two androgen-responsive promoters, *PSA* and *MMTV* [43], in the same cells with the same treatments. The activities of both *PSA* and *MMTV* promoters were significantly decreased by KLF5 knockdown, and enzalutamide treatment eliminated both the promoter activities and the effect of KLF5 silencing on promoter activities (Figure 2e,f).

To test whether KLF5 directly binds to the promoters and enhancer of AR target genes, we performed ChIP assay using both AR and KLF5 antibodies. In AR-precipitated DNA, the *PSA* and *FKBP5* promoters and the *TMPRSS2* enhancer were detected by PCR in C4-2B cells, as expected, and KLF5 silencing reduced the promoter and enhancer DNA (Figure 2g). In KLF5-precipitated DNA, while the promoter DNA of *PSA* was detected, neither the *FKBP5* promoter nor the *TMPRSS2* enhancer was detected (Figure 2g), and the *PSA* promoter was eliminated by the inhibition of AR signaling by enzalutamide (Figure 2h). These results suggest that KLF5 is crucial for the transcriptional activity of AR.

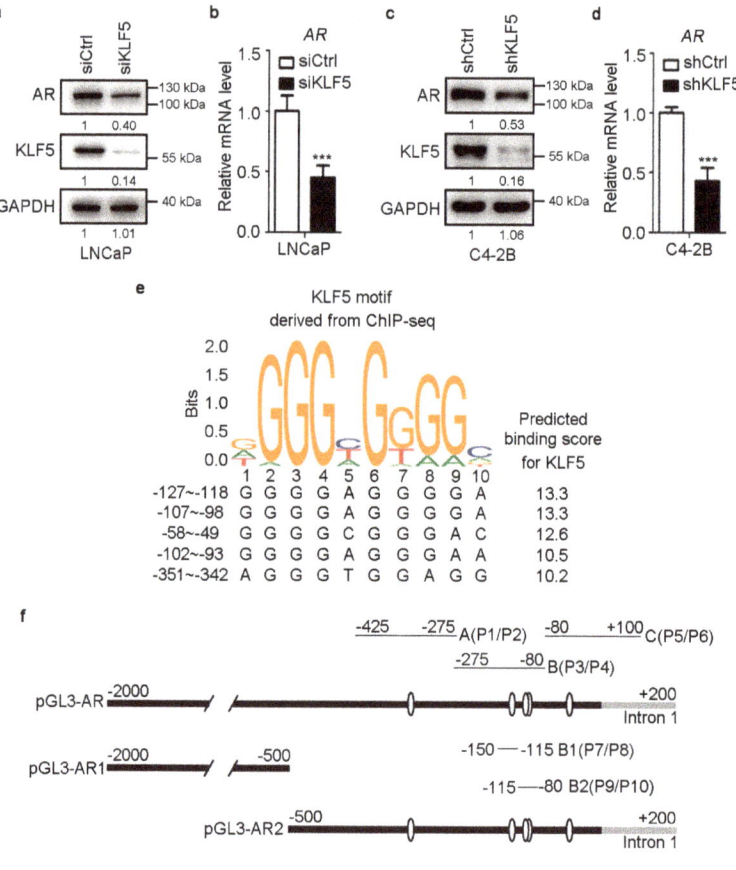

Figure 3. *Cont.*

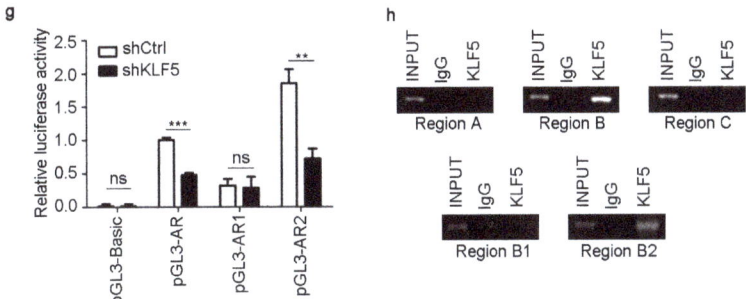

Figure 3. KLF5 is required for the transcription of AR in PCa cells. (**a–d**) Knockdown of KLF5 decreased AR expression at both protein (a, c) and RNA (b, d) levels in LNCaP (a-b) and C4-2B cells (c–d). Cells were cultured in complete media for 24 h and transfected with siRNAs for 48 h in LNCaP cells or infected with lentiviruses expressing shRNA targeting KLF5 (shKLF5) in C4-2B cells. Western blotting and real-time qPCR were performed to detect protein and mRNA respectively. (**e**) The AR promoter contains multiple potential KLF5 binding sites, as predicted by aligning the 2-Kb immediate promoter sequence of AR to the consensus KLF5 binding sequence (top) defined in the JASPAR database. Location of these sequences relative to the transcription initiation site (+1) is shown at left. (**f**) Schematic of the AR promoter region (−2000 to +200) with the locations of predicted KLF5 binding sites (empty oval) and primers used for PCR amplification of 5 regions (A, B, C, B1, B2) of the AR promoter spanning the potential binding sites. (**g**) Knockdown of KLF5 decreased AR promoter activity in C4-2B cells, as detected by the luciferase activity assay. The pGL3 vector was used to express full-length AR promoter (g, pGL3-AR, from −2000 to +200) and two shorter AR promoter fragments (pGL3-AR-1, −2000 to −500; pGL3-AR-2, −500 to +200), with their luciferase readings normalized by that of the pGL3-Basic vector control. (**h**) Detection of KLF5-bound AR promoter DNA in C4-2B cells using ChIP and PCR. ns, not significant; *, $p < 0.05$; **, $p < 0.01$; ***$p < 0.001$.

2.3. KLF5 also Promotes Transcription of the AR Gene in PCa Cells

Analyzing the effect of KLF5 on AR's gene transactivating function, we noticed that knockdown of KLF5 reduced AR expression in both LNCaP and C4-2B cells (Figure 2a,b). We thus tested whether KLF5 modulates the expression of AR. Knockdown of KLF5 by siRNA in LNCaP cells or by shRNA in C4-2B cells clearly reduced AR expression at both protein and mRNA levels (Figure 3a–d).

To further test whether KLF5 directly promotes AR transcription, we analyzed the 2-Kb immediate AR promoter sequence for potential KLF5 binding sites using the JASPAR database, in which the consensus KLF5 binding sequences were defined by ChIP-Seq study [40]. Multiple such sites were predicted, and the 5 with the highest binding scores were all located within the immediate 350-bp AR promoter (Figure 3e).

We then constructed a promoter-luciferase reporter plasmid with the entire 2-Kb immediate AR promoter sequence in the pGL3 vector (pGL3-AR, Figure 3f). Two additional AR promoter luciferase reporter plasmids were also constructed, one with the upper 1.5-Kb and the other with the lower 0.5-Kb of the full 2-kb promoter sequence (pGL3-AR1 and pGL3-AR2, Figure 3f). Both pGL3-AR and pGL3-AR2 also contained 0.2-Kb sequence of exon 1 (Figure 3f). Interestingly, knockdown of KLF5 significantly decreased the activities of pGL3-AR and pGL3-AR2, both of which contained potential KLF5 binding sites, but not that of pGL3-AR1, which did not contain a KLF5 binding site (Figure 3g). Therefore, it is likely that KLF5 directly promotes AR transcription via promoter binding.

To test whether KLF5 directly binds to AR promoter, ChIP was performed with KLF5 antibody in C4-2B cells and PCR performed with primers to amplify the AR promoter in pGL3-AR2 in three fragments, A, B, and C (Figure 3f). Fragment B, which contained three potential KLF5 binding sites (Figure 3f), was detected in the DNA pulled down by KLF5 antibody, but fragments A and C were not (Figure 3h). Further analysis showed that fragment B2, containing the sites from −107 to −93, was detected in the DNA pulled down by KLF5 antibody, but fragment B1 was not. Therefore, KLF5 can directly bind the AR promoter via the sites from −107 to −93.

2.4. KLF5 Physically Associates with AR in Prostate Epithelial Cells

Considering that KLF5 is crucial for AR function and that both KLF5 and AR are transcription factors, it is likely that KLF5 and AR could physically associate with each other to regulate gene transcription. We transfected FLAG-tagged KLF5 (Flag-KLF5) with pSG5-AR or FLAG-tagged AR (Flag-AR) with HA-tagged KLF5 (HA-KLF5) into HEK293T cells, and performed IP with anti-Flag antibody. Western blotting detected AR in the KLF5 precipitate (Figure 4a) and KLF5 in the AR precipitate (Figure 4b), supporting a physical association between KLF5 and AR. We noticed that enzalutamide treatment reduced AR in the KLF5 precipitate (Figure 4c), which could suggest a role of AR's ligand binding domain in the AR-KLF5 interaction.

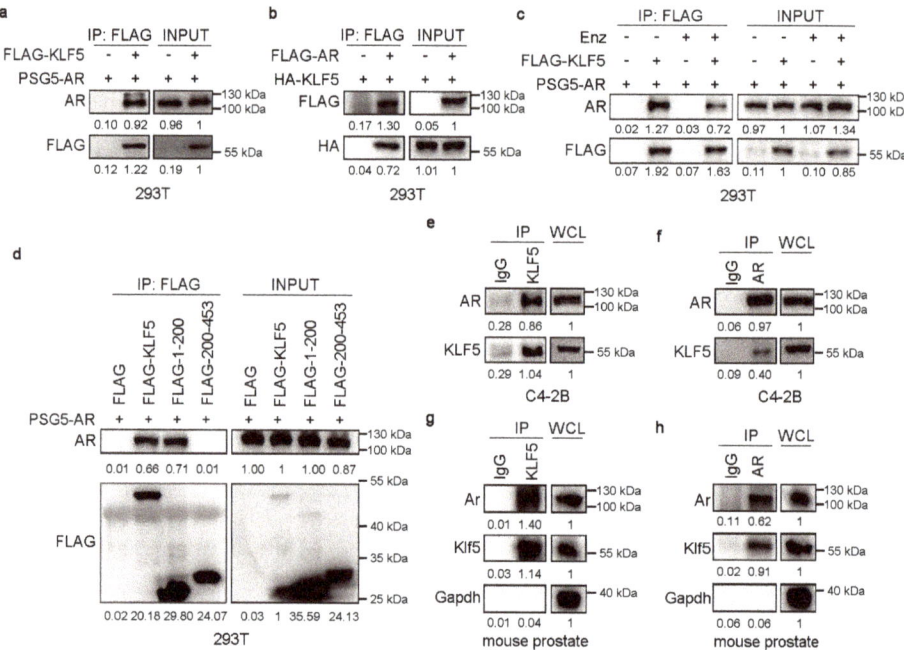

Figure 4. KLF5 physically associates with AR in epithelial cells. (**a,b**) HEK293T cells were transiently transfected with expression plasmids of vector control, Flag-tagged (a) or HA-tagged KLF5 (b), and pSG5-AR (a) or FLAG-tagged AR (b), and then subjected to co-IP with FLAG antibody and western blotting with indicated antibodies. (**c**) HEK293T cells transfected with KLF5 and/or AR as in panel a for 24 h were treated with 10 μM enzalutamide for 24 h, and then subjected to co-IP and western blotting with indicated antibodies. (**d**) Mapping of interacting KLF5 regions that interact with AR by co-IP with Flag antibody and western blotting with indicated antibodies in HEK293T cells expressing AR and different fragments of KLF5. (**e,f**) Detection of endogenous KLF5-AR association in C4-2B cells by co-IP with KLF5 (e) or AR antibody (f) and western blotting with indicated antibodies. WCL is whole cell lysates before IP. IgG was used as a negative control for co-IP. (**g,h**) Detection of the Klf5-Ar association in mouse prostates by co-IP with KLF5 (g) or AR antibody (h) and western blotting with indicated antibodies.

We also divided KLF5 into two fragments, one with residues 1–200 and the other with 201–453, and tested which fragment mediates KLF5's association with AR using the same approaches as in

Figure 4a,b. The domain of KLF5 mediating the KLF5-AR interaction was restricted residues 1 to 200 (Figure 4d).

We also performed IP with anti-KLF5 or anti-AR antibody to pull down their respective protein complexes in C4-2B cells. Western blotting detected AR in the KLF5 complex and KLF5 in the AR complex (Figure 4e,f), indicating a physical association between the endogenous KLF5 and AR. This set of experiments was repeated with mouse prostate lysates, and the endogenous Ar-Klf5 association was again detected (Figure 4g,h). Therefore, KLF5 physically associates with AR in prostate cells.

2.5. KLF5 Is also Crucial for AR-Mediated MYC and Cyclin D1 Expression in PCa Cells

In PCa cells, AR promotes cell proliferation via the upregulation of a subset of genes such as *MYC* and *CCND1*, and KLF5 has also been shown to upregulate the same two genes in epithelial cells [26–28,44–47]. We thus tested whether KLF5 is also required for AR to upregulate *MYC* and *CCND1* in androgen-responsive PCa cells. In LNCaP and C4-2B cells cultured in normal medium, knockdown of KLF5 decreased the expression MYC and cyclin D1 at both protein (Figure 5a,b) and mRNA levels (Figure 5c,d). When AR activity was inhibited by enzalutamide at 10 µM for 24 h, both MYC and cyclin D1 were significantly downregulated, and silencing KLF5 had little or no effect on the expression of MYC and cyclin D1 (Figure 5a–d). ChIP-PCR demonstrated that the amount of AR bound to the promoters of *CCND1* and *MYC* was apparently reduced by the knockdown of KLF5 (Figure 5e), and similarly, the amount of KLF5 bound to the same two promoters was also reduced by inhibiting AR signaling with enzalutamide treatment in C4-2B cells (Figure 5f).

2.6. KLF5 Is Crucial for Androgen/AR to Promote Cell Proliferation and Tumor Growth in PCa Cells

Based on the necessity of KLF5 for AR to regulate genes including *MYC* and *CCND1*, we tested whether KLF5 is indeed involved in the pro-proliferative function of AR in PCa cells. In LNCaP or C4-2B cells, colony and sphere formation assays demonstrated that silencing KLF5 by RNAi in normal medium significantly reduced colony-forming efficiency in 2-D culture (Figure 6a,b) and sphere formation in Matrigel (Figure 6c,d). Inhibition of AR signaling by enzalutamide treatment strongly suppressed both colony and sphere formation (Figure 6a–d). Further, under the condition of AR inhibition, KLF5 silencing had a weaker yet detectable effect (Figure 6a–d).

We also tested whether KLF5 is necessary for AR to promote xenograft tumorigenesis. C4-2B cells with stable knockdown of KLF5 were inoculated into immunosuppressed female BABL/c nude mice, with or without enzalutamide treatment (10 mg/kg, administered via oral gavage once a day for up to 21 days, for the tumorigenesis assays). Consistent with colony and sphere formation results, KLF5 silencing reduced tumor growth, as indicated by tumor images and tumor weights at excision (Figure 6e,f). Enzalutamide treatment also reduced tumor growth, and KLF5 silencing and enzalutamide had an additive effect on tumor growth (Figure 6e,f).

In the tumor xenografts, IHC staining demonstrated enzalutamide treatment reduced the expression of both KLF5 and AR, which is consistent with in vitro findings (Figure 1g–l), and KLF5 silencing also downregulated AR expression (Figure 6g,h). Similarly, IHC staining demonstrated that both KLF5 silencing and enzalutamide treatment reduced the expression of Ki67, a cell proliferation marker; the number of Ki67-positive cells; and the expression of cyclin D1 and MYC (Figure 6i,j). These results indicate that KLF5 is crucial for AR to function in PCa cells.

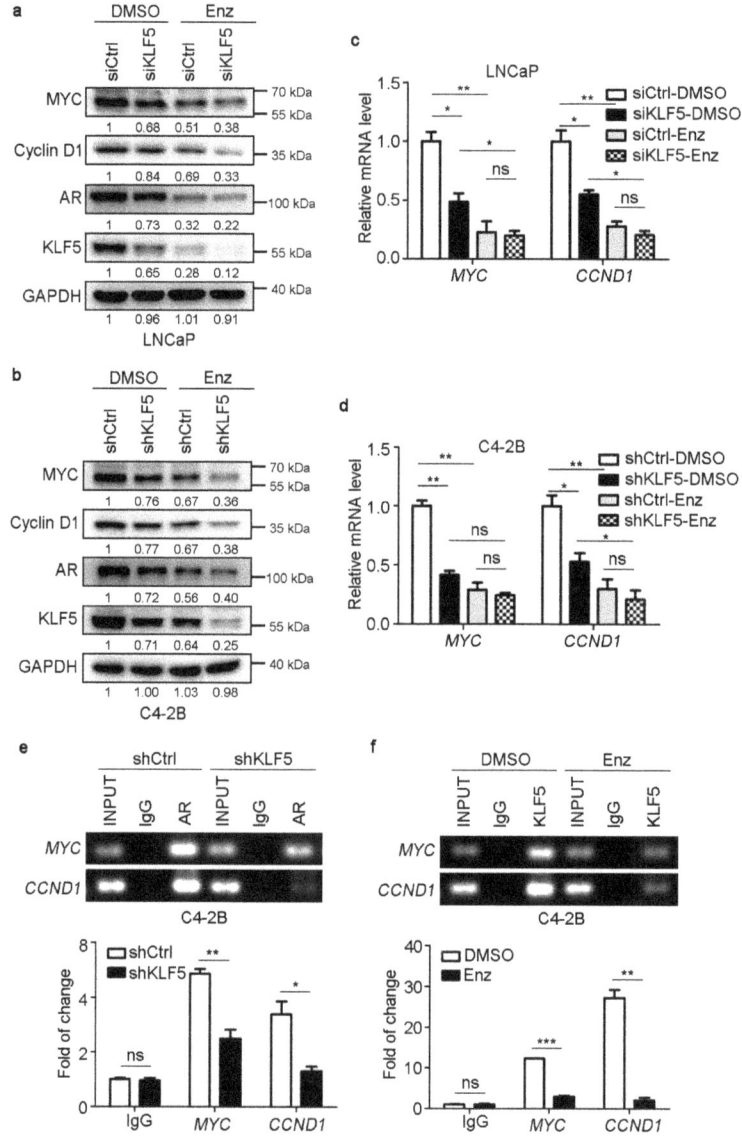

Figure 5. Knockdown of KLF5 attenuates AR-mediated expression of MYC and cyclin D1 in androgen-responsive PCa cells. (**a–d**) RNAi-mediated KLF5 silencing attenuated R1881-promoted expression of cyclin D1 and MYC in LNCaP (a) and C4-2B (b) cells, as detected by western blotting for protein (a, b) and by real-time qPCR for mRNA (c, d). One group of cells were treated with 10 μM enzalutamide for 72 h. (**e**) Binding of AR to the promoters of *MYC* and *CCND1* was detected by ChIP and PCR (top) or real-time qPCR (bottom) in C4-2B cells expressing shRNAs against KLF5 (shKLF5) and control (shCtrl). (**f**) Binding of KLF5 to the promoters of *MYC* and *CCND1* was detected by ChIP and PCR (top) or real-time qPCR (bottom) in C4-2B cells treated with or without enzalutamide (10 μM, 24 h). ns, not significant; *, $p < 0.05$; **, $p < 0.01$; ***$p < 0.001$.

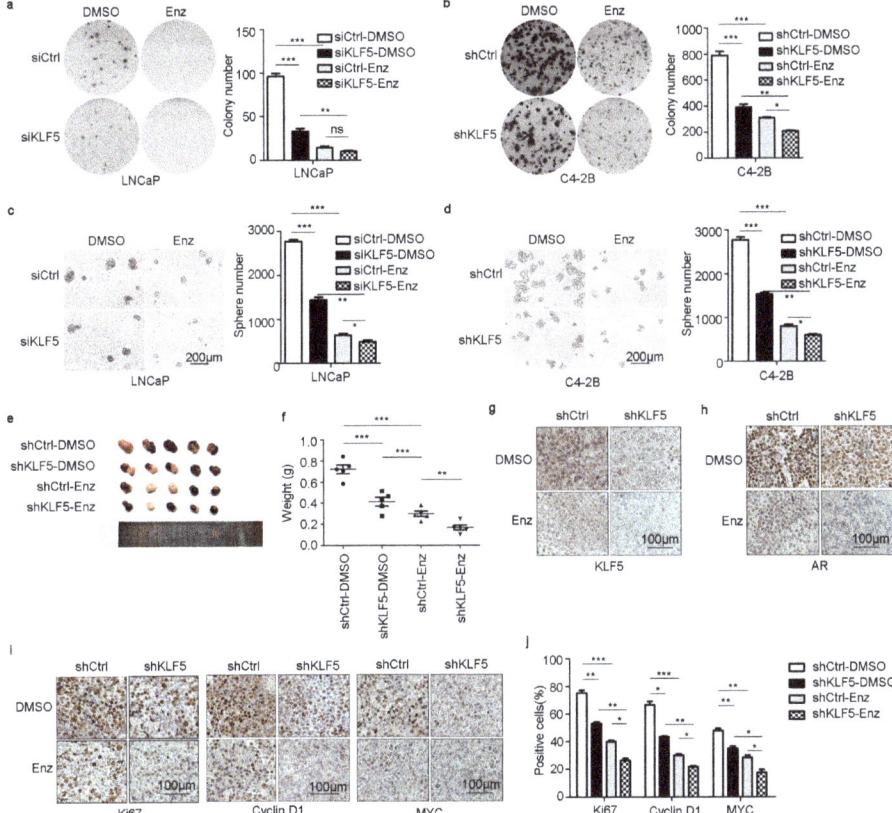

Figure 6. KLF5 is also crucial for androgen/AR signaling to promote cell proliferation and tumor growth in PCa cells. (**a–d**) Knockdown of KLF5 by siRNA in LNCaP cells or by shRNA in C4-2B cells reduced colony forming efficiency in 2-D culture (a, b) and sphere formation in Matrigel (c, d). Cells with KLF5 knockdown were seeded onto 6-well plates at 2000 cells/well for LNCaP and 1000 cells/well for C4-2B in regular medium for colony formation assay, and at 4000 cells/well for LNCaP and 2000 cells/well for C4-2B cells for sphere formation assay. Regular media were used, and enzalutamide (10 μM) treatment was applied. The culture time was 2 weeks for C4-2B and 3 weeks for LNCaP in both assays. Images of colonies or spheres were taken (left), and their numbers were counted (right). Only spheres with a diameter greater than 80 μm were counted. Scale bars, 200 μm. (**e,f**) Knockdown of KLF5 attenuated tumor growth of C4-2B cells in nude mice, as indicated by tumor images (e) and tumor weights at excision (f). (**g,h**) Knockdown of KLF5 reduced AR expression in xenograft tumors of C4-2B cells, as detected by immunohistochemical (IHC) staining with anti-KLF5 (g) and anti-AR (h) antibodies. (**i–j**) Knockdown of KLF5 reduced cell proliferation, as indicated by the Ki67 index, and the expression of cyclin D1 and MYC in tumor xenografts of C4-2B cells, as detected by IHC staining (i) and quantitation of positive cells (j). Scale bars, 100 μm. ns, not significant; *, $p < 0.05$; **, $p < 0.01$; ***$p < 0.001$.

3. Discussion

Our findings in this study indicate that KLF5 is crucial for androgen/AR signaling to function in PCa cells. The first line of evidence is that the transcriptional activity of AR depended on the expression of KLF5. For example, *KLF5* silencing decreased the expression of *PSA*, a classic transcriptional target gene of AR in the prostate [41], and *TMPRSS2* and *FKBP5*, two other AR target genes [42,43], in LNCaP and C4-2B cells (Figure 2). The necessity of KLF5 for AR's transcriptional activity was also demonstrated by promoter luciferase reporter assays using two androgen responsive promoters (i.e., *PSA* and *MMTV* [48]) (Figure 2) and by the expression of two genes that mediate AR's pro-proliferative function, i.e., *MYC* and *CCND1* [26–28,44–47], in the same cells with *KLF5* silencing (Figure 5). We have also presented evidence from cellular analyses, in which androgen/AR signaling also required KLF5 to maintain a steady proliferation of PCa cells. Specifically, *KLF5* silencing significantly attenuated the functions of AR in the maintenance of colony and sphere formation in vitro and xenograft tumor growth in nude mice (Figure 6a). Consistently, *KLF5* silencing also reduced the number of Ki67-positive cells and the expression of cyclin D1 and MYC (Figure 6). We noticed that, after blocking AR activity with enzalutamide, which had a profound effect (Figures 5 and 6), *KLF5* silencing still had a detectable effect in both the expression of MYC and cyclin D1 and cell proliferation (Figures 5 and 6), which suggests that, while crucial for AR to function, KLF5 can still function when AR is inhibited. Indeed, in androgen-independent PCa cell lines including PC-3 and DU 145, KLF5 is clearly pro-proliferative, even though when TGF-β is activated, TGF-β and KLF5 slow but do not stop cell proliferation [49,50].

Molecularly, the enhancing effect of KLF5 on AR function in cell proliferation is mediated by at least three distinct mechanisms. For example, via direct promoter binding, AR promotes the transcription of *KLF5* to increase its expression [32]. As expected, the upregulation of *KLF5* by androgen was mediated by AR (Figure 1), since inhibition of AR by RNAi-mediated *AR* silencing or enzalutamide treatment eliminated the induction of *KLF5* transcription (Figure 1).

The second molecular mechanism by which KLF5 facilitates AR function is that KLF5 also activates *AR* transcription in PCa cells. For example, *KLF5* silencing by RNAi reduced AR expression in both LNCaP and C4-2B cells (Figure 3). In addition, the *AR* promoter indeed contained multiple consensus KLF5 binding elements that were necessary not only for the *AR* promoter's activities in the promoter-reporter assay and but also for the binding of KLF5 to the *AR* promoter in the ChIP-PCR analysis (Figure 3), and two adjacent KLF5 binding elements in the *AR* promoter have been confirmed to be essential for KLF5 binding and promoter activity (Figure 3).

The third mechanism is that KLF5 and AR coordinate to regulate gene transcription, which is supported by multiple lines of evidence. Firstly, KLF5 and AR depend on each other in their binding to the promoters of *PSA*, *MYC* and *CCND1*, as *KLF5* silencing reduced the amount of promoter/enhancer DNA of these genes in AR-precipitated DNA (Figure 2) while inhibition of AR reduced this DNA in KLF5-precipitated DNA (Figure 5). Nevertheless, the details of KLF5 and AR binding to gene promoters are unclear (e.g., the chromatin landscape for the binding). Secondly, KLF5 and AR, both of which are transcription factors, physically associate with each other to regulate gene transcription. AR was detected in the KLF5 protein complex and KLF5 in the AR complex (Figure 4). In addition, the KLF5-AR interaction occurred not only for ectopically expressed KLF5 and AR in HEK293T cells but also for endogenous KLF5 and AR in both human cells and mouse prostates (Figure 4). Furthermore, the KLF5-AR interaction was mediated by a sequence within residues 1-200 of KLF5 (Figure 4) and was attenuated by enzalutamide treatment (Figure 4).

Therefore, androgen/AR signaling activates *KLF5* expression via the binding of AR to *KLF5* promoter, KLF5 in turn enhances the transcription of *AR* by promoter binding, and AR and KLF5 then coordinate to transactivate a subset of genes to promote the proliferation of PCa cells.

We noticed that, for AR target genes *PSA*, *TMPRSS2*, and *FKBP5*, while *KLF5* silencing reduced their induction by AR (Figure 2a–d), which supports the necessity of KLF5 for AR function in their transcription, AR-bound promoter DNA was detected in KLF5-precipitated promoter DNA only for *PSA* but not for *TMPRSS2* and *FKBP5* (Figure 2). The reason for this discrepancy is unknown. Neither is it known whether the KLF5-AR association depends on promoter DNA or cofactors of AR.

In mouse prostates, castration-mediated androgen depletion increased Klf5-positive cells [29], which is seemingly inconsistent with the induction of KLF5 by androgen in PCa cells (Figure 1). Compared to luminal cells in the prostate, basal cells preferentially express Klf5, particularly acetylated Klf5 [30], castration causes massive death in luminal cells but much less so in basal cells, and basal cells express much less AR and are androgen insensitive. LNCaP and C4-2B cells are AR-positive and androgen-dependent/sensitive, and thus have a different lineage from basal cells.

The role of KLF5 in androgen-induced cell proliferation and tumor growth could also involve KLF5's function in tumor microenvironment (TME) and immune responses. For example, pro-inflammatory TNFα and lipopolysaccharide (LPS) induce KLF5 expression, and TNFα depends on KLF5 to induce MCP-1 [51]. In addition, KLF5 directly interacts with NF-κB [52], a potent inflammatory factor, and interruption of this interaction inhibits LPS-induced macrophage proliferation [53]. Knockdown of KLF5 also reduces the expression of p50 and p65 subunits of NF-κB and its downstream target genes TNFα and IL-6 in response to LPS [54]. This and other potential mechanisms for KLF5 function remain to be examined.

During late stages of tumor progression, AR becomes activated even when androgen levels are low, causing CRPC [9,10]. Further studying how KLF5 and AR coordinate to regulate the expression of genes, particularly those mediating cell proliferation/survival and thus likely affecting PCa progression, will facilitate our understanding of AR activation in CRPC and the development of therapeutic approaches for the treatment of CRPCs. For example, in advanced PCa, the *KLF5* locus often undergoes hemizygous deletion [21,55], which downregulates *KLF5* expression because the gene is haploinsufficient [31]. As KLF5 is necessary for AR function in PCa cells, as discussed above, downregulation of KLF5 could generate a feedback signal that leads to the upregulation of AR or functional compensation of AR activity. This hypothesis remains to be tested.

4. Materials and Methods

4.1. Cell Lines, Cell Culture, and RNA Interference

Human PCa cell line LNCaP was purchased from American Type Cell Culture (Manassas, VA) and cultured in RPMI-1640 medium supplemented with 10% fetal bovine serum (FBS, Gibco, Waltham, MA). The C4-2B cell line, originally derived from a bone metastasis of a LNCaP clone in mice [56], was kindly provided by Dr. Leland W. K. Chung of Cedars-Sinai Medical Center and cultured in the same medium as LNCaP. Cells were maintained at 37 °C with 5% CO_2. During experiments, cells recovered from a liquid nitrogen freezer were used within two months (<20 passages) with no noticeable morphological changes. All cell lines were authenticated by STR profiling before experiments were started. For all experiments involving R1881 (Melonepharma, Dalian, China, catalog number: MB5484) treatments, the medium was replaced with phenol red-free medium containing 10% charcoal-stripped FBS.

For RNA interference (RNAi) with shRNA, C4-2B cells were infected with lentiviruses expressing an shRNA specifically targeting human *KLF5*, which was developed and validated in a previous study with various PCa cell lines [57], to establish the cell population in which *KLF5* is stably knocked down. For RNAi with siRNAs, siRNA (si*AR*: 5′-CAAGGGAGGUUACACCAAA-3′; si*KLF5*: 5′-AAGCUCACCUGAGGACUCA-3′) oligos against human *KLF5* and *AR* were synthesized by Sagon Biotech (Guangzhou, China) and transfected into cells using the Lipofectamine RNAiMAX reagent (Invitrogen, Carlsbad, CA) according to the manufacturer's protocol.

4.2. Western Blot Analysis

Cultured cells were lysed in lysis buffer (50 mM Tris pH 7.4, 150 mM NaCl, 2 mM EDTA, 0.8% NP-40, 0.2% Triton X-100, 3% glycerol). Cell lysates were subjected to polyacrylamide gel electrophoresis (PAGE), and proteins were transferred onto a polyvinylidene fluoride (PVDF) membrane. Membranes were soaked in 5% nonfat milk or 5% BSA solution for one hour to block nonspecific binding of proteins, and then incubated with primary antibodies overnight at 4 °C. On the following day, membranes were incubated with secondary antibodies for 2 h at room temperature, and WesternBright ECL (Advansta, Menlo Park, CA) was used with the luminescent image analyzer (Jun Yi Dong Fang, Beijing, China) to capture images. Uncropped scans can be found in Figure S1.

Antibodies used in western blotting were: KLF5 (1:1000, 21017-1-AP, Proteintech), AR (1:1000, 5153S, Cell Signaling), PSA (1:3000, 10679-1-AP, Proteintech), MYC (1:1000, 9402, Cell Signaling), cyclin D1 (1:10000, ab134175, Abcam), FLAG (1:3000, SAB4200071, Sigma), HA (1:3000, 3724S, Cell Signaling), GAPDH (1:3000, 60004-1-Ig, Proteintech).

4.3. RNA Extraction and Real-time qPCR

Total RNA was extracted from cells using the Trizol reagent (Invitrogen) and 2 μg total RNA reverse-transcribed using the PrimeScript™ RT reagent Kit with gDNA Eraser (TaKaRa, Tokyo, Japan). Real-time qPCR was performed with the SYBR Green MasterMix reagent (Takara) using the Mastercycler Realplex real time PCR system (Eppendorf, Hamburg, Germany). Human *GAPDH* gene served as an internal control. The comparative $2^{-\Delta\Delta Ct}$ method was used to calculate gene expression levels. Each sample was analyzed in triplicate. Primer sequences for real-time qPCR are listed in Supplementary Table S1.

4.4. Construction of Expression and Luciferase Report Plasmids

Mammalian expression plasmids for Flag-KLF5, HA-KLF5, pSG5-AR, Flag-AR, and luciferase reporter plasmids for pGL3-KLF5, pGL3-PSA, and pGL3-MMTV were generated in our laboratory. For promoter-luciferase plasmids, pGL3-AR, pGL3-AR1, and pGL3-AR2, primers were respectively designed with the entire 2-Kb immediate AR promoter sequence (AR), the upper 1.5-Kb (AR1) and the lower 0.5-Kb (AR2). PCR and cloning of PCR products were used to generate luciferase reporter plasmids for AR, AR1, and AR2 in pGL3-Basic vector following standard procedures. Primer sequences for gene cloning are listed in Supplementary Table S1.

4.5. Luciferase Reporter Assay

LNCaP and C4-2B cells were transiently transfected with pGL3-Basic, pGL3-KLF5, or pGL3-PSA, or pGL3-MMTV and pRL-TK (Renilla luciferase, Promega, Madison, WI) as an internal control. After 48 h of transfection and enzalutamide (Beyotime Biotechnology, Shanghai, China, catalog number: SC0074) treatment, cells were lysed in 5 × lysis buffer (Promega) for 30 min and luciferase activity was measured using a luminometer (Tristar LB941, Berthold Technologies, BadWild, Germany). Firefly luciferase activity was normalized to Renilla luciferase activities in each reaction. Experiments were performed in triplicate.

4.6. Colony Formation Assay

One thousand C4-2B cells/well or 2000 LNCaP cells/well were seeded in 6-well plates and cultured in the presence of RPMI-1640 medium containing 10% FBS with DMSO or 10 μM enzalutamide (Beyotime Biotechnology,). The plates were incubated for 2 (C4-2B) or 3 (LNCaP) weeks, after which cultures were fixed with 4% paraformaldehyde for 30 min and stained by 0.05% crystal violet (BBI life sciences, Shanghai, China) for 1 h at room temperature and then photographed. In a single experiment, assays were conducted in triplicate and then as three independent experiments.

4.7. 3D Matrigel Assay

In 8-well chamber slides (BD Bioscience, Shanghai, China, catalog number: 354108), 30 μL growth factor reduced BD Matrigel (BD Biosciences, catalog number: 354230) was added per well. Slides were placed in a cell culture incubator for at least 15 min to solidify the Matrigel. Next, 2000 C4-2B cells/well or 4000 LNCaP cells/well were seeded in RPMI-1640 medium containing 10% FBS with DMSO or 10 μM enzalutamide (Beyotime Biotechnology) and 2% Matrigel. Media were replenished every 3 days. Chamber slides were incubated for 2 (C4-2B) or 3 (LNCaP) weeks, and then photographed. Image J program (NIH, USA) was used to measure the diameter of each sphere. Spheres with a diameter larger than 80 μm were counted.

4.8. Immunoprecipitation

For exogenous immunoprecipitation, HEK293T cells were cotransfected with pcDNA3.0-Flag or Flag-KLF5 in the same vector with pSG5-AR plasmid using the Lipofectamine 2000 Transfection Reagent (Invitrogen) according to the manufacturer's protocol. After 48 h, the cells were collected and resuspended in cell lysis buffer containing 50 mM Tris (pH 7.4), 150 mM NaCl, 2 mM EDTA, 0.8% NP-40, 0.2% Triton X-100, and 3% glycerol. EDTA-free Protease Inhibitor Cocktail (Roche, Indianapolis, IN) and PMSF (Sangon Biotech) were added to the cell lysis buffer. Cell lysates were incubated with anti-FLAG-agarose beads at 4 °C for 2 h (Sigma). Beads were washed and eluted and supernatants analyzed by western blotting. For endogenous immunoprecipitation, C4-2B cells or mouse prostate were collected and resuspended in lysis buffer and then rabbit or mouse normal IgG, KLF5 antibody (self-made) or AR antibody (06-680-AF488, Millipore) added to the lysate, followed by overnight incubation at 4 °C. Lysates coupled with antibody were incubated with magnetic Dynabeads (Invitrogen) for 2 h. Beads were washed extensively and eluted and supernatants analyzed by western blotting as above.

4.9. Mouse Xenograft Studies

C4-2B (2×10^7) cells in 100 μL PBS-Matrigel (1:1) (BD Biosciences, catalog number: 354248) were implanted via subcutaneous injection into the flanks of mice. Cells were left to grow for one week. Mice were randomly divided into control or enzalutamide (10 mg/kg) (MedChemExpress, New Jersey, USA, catalog number: HY-70002) [58] groups, which were given once a day via oral gavage for up to 21 days (n=6/group). Mice were euthanized and tumors were surgically dissected, immediately weighed and fixed in 10% formalin for standard histopathological evaluation.

4.10. Immunohistochemistry (IHC)

IHC staining was performed to detect protein expression of KLF5 (1:400, Proteintech), AR (1:800, 06-680-AF488, Millipore), Ki67 (1:2000, ab15580, Abcam), cyclin D1 (1:2000, ab134175, Abcam) and MYC (1:1000, 9106, Abcam) in tumor xenografts. Formalin-fixed paraffin embedded tissues were sectioned at 4 μm, deparaffinized in xylene, rehydrated in graded ethanol (100–75%) and repaired antigen by boiling the slides in a citrate buffer (10 mM trisodium citrate, pH 6.0) for 3 min using a pressure cooker. After treatment with 3% H_2O_2 for 10 min, tissue sections were blocked with 10% normal goat serum, incubated with primary antibodies at 4 °C overnight, and then with EnVision PolymerHRP secondary antibodies (MXB Biotechnologies, Fuzhou, China) at room temperature for 30 min. After chromogenic reaction using DAB (MXB Biotechnologies), nuclei were stained with hematoxylin (MXB Biotechnologies). Finally, tissue sections were dehydrated and mounted.

4.11. Chromatin Immunoprecipitation (ChIP)

C4-2B cells were grown for 3 days in RPMI-1640 medium supplemented with 10% FBS. ChIP was performed using the Simple ChIP Enzymatic Chromatin IP Kit (Cell Signaling Technology, Danvers, MA, catalog number: #9003) according to the manufacturer's instructions. Firstly, cells were cross-linked with 1% formaldehyde for 10 min and quenched with glycine at room temperature. Samples were collected and digested using micrococcal nuclease for 20 min at 37 °C; reactions were stopped by the addition of 0.5 M EDTA and incubated in ChIP buffer with protease inhibitors on ice for 10 min. After sonication, chromatin extracts were immunoprecipitated using anti-AR (06-680-AF488, Millipore), anti-KLF5 (AF3758, R&D Systems) or anti-IgG antibody. ChIP products were detected by regular PCR (with input loading quantity of one fourth of IgG or AR) or real-time qPCR (each gene in triplicate). Sequences of PCR primers are described in Supplementary Table S1.

4.12. Statistical Analysis

All in vitro experiments were repeated at least three times. All numerical results are expressed as mean ± SD. Two group comparisons were compared using Student's t test by SPSS 21 (IBM corporation, Armonk, NY, USA). A value of $p < 0.05$ was considered statistically significant.

5. Conclusions

In summary, we demonstrated that KLF5 is crucial for androgen/AR signaling to activate the transcription of specific genes, including some that mediate cell proliferation, and to promote cell proliferation and tumor growth in PCa cells. Mechanistically, androgen promotes the expression of KLF5 via AR, KLF5 in turn promotes the transcription of AR by binding to AR promoter, and KLF5 and AR coordinate to transactivate the target genes of AR. These findings not only suggest that KLF5 is a crucial factor for the function of AR in PCa cells, they will also further the understanding of how AR signaling is sustained in CRPC. In addition, they will likely facilitate the development of therapeutic strategies for the treatment of CRPC.

Supplementary Materials: The following are available online at http://www.mdpi.com/2072-6694/12/3/748/s1, Figure S1: Unprocessed blot images for western blotting results, Table S1: Primer sequences used in various PCRs in the study.

Author Contributions: Data curation, J.L. and J.A.; Funding acquisition, J.-T.D.; Investigation, J.L., M.L., X.F. and X.C.; Methodology, B.Z., M.L., X.F., X.C., C.F., G.D., R.W., Z.Z. and L.F.; Writing – original draft, J.L.; Writing – review & editing, B.Z., Z.Z. and J.-T.D. All authors have read and agreed to the published version of the manuscript.

Funding: This research received no external funding.

Acknowledgments: We thank Anthea Hammond of Emory University for editing the manuscript. We also thank Qiao Wu, Gui Ma and Qingxia Hu, Xiawei Li, and Na An of Nankai University for advice and help throughout the study.

Conflicts of Interest: All authors declare no conflict of interest to this work.

References

1. El Sheikh, S.S.; Romanska, H.M.; Abel, P.; Domin, J.; Lalani el, N. Predictive value of PTEN and AR coexpression of sustained responsiveness to hormonal therapy in prostate cancer—A pilot study. *Neoplasia* **2008**, *10*, 949–953. [CrossRef]
2. Reid, A.H.; Attard, G.; Ambroisine, L.; Fisher, G.; Kovacs, G.; Brewer, D.; Clark, J.; Flohr, P.; Edwards, S.; Berney, D.M.; et al. Molecular characterisation of ERG, ETV1 and PTEN gene loci identifies patients at low and high risk of death from prostate cancer. *Br. J. Cancer* **2010**, *102*, 678–684. [CrossRef]
3. Taylor, B.S.; Schultz, N.; Hieronymus, H.; Gopalan, A.; Xiao, Y.; Carver, B.S.; Arora, V.K.; Kaushik, P.; Cerami, E.; Reva, B.; et al. Integrative genomic profiling of human prostate cancer. *Cancer Cell* **2010**, *18*, 11–22. [CrossRef]
4. Tomlins, S.A.; Rhodes, D.R.; Perner, S.; Dhanasekaran, S.M.; Mehra, R.; Sun, X.W.; Varambally, S.; Cao, X.; Tchinda, J.; Kuefer, R.; et al. Recurrent fusion of TMPRSS2 and ETS transcription factor genes in prostate cancer. *Science* **2005**, *310*, 644–648. [CrossRef]
5. Tu, J.J.; Rohan, S.; Kao, J.; Kitabayashi, N.; Mathew, S.; Chen, Y.T. Gene fusions between TMPRSS2 and ETS family genes in prostate cancer: Frequency and transcript variant analysis by RT-PCR and FISH on paraffin-embedded tissues. *Mod. Pathol.* **2007**, *20*, 921–928. [CrossRef]
6. Bavik, C.; Coleman, I.; Dean, J.P.; Knudsen, B.; Plymate, S.; Nelson, P.S. The gene expression program of prostate fibroblast senescence modulates neoplastic epithelial cell proliferation through paracrine mechanisms. *Cancer Res.* **2006**, *66*, 794–802. [CrossRef]
7. Bethel, C.R.; Chaudhary, J.; Anway, M.D.; Brown, T.R. Gene expression changes are age-dependent and lobe-specific in the brown Norway rat model of prostatic hyperplasia. *Prostate* **2009**, *69*, 838–850. [CrossRef]
8. Begley, L.; Monteleon, C.; Shah, R.B.; Macdonald, J.W.; Macoska, J.A. CXCL12 overexpression and secretion by aging fibroblasts enhance human prostate epithelial proliferation in vitro. *Aging Cell* **2005**, *4*, 291–298. [CrossRef]

9. Hammerer, P.; Madersbacher, S. Landmarks in hormonal therapy for prostate cancer. *BJU Int.* **2012**, *110* (Suppl. 1), 23–29. [CrossRef]
10. Pagliarulo, V.; Bracarda, S.; Eisenberger, M.A.; Mottet, N.; Schroder, F.H.; Sternberg, C.N.; Studer, U.E. Contemporary role of androgen deprivation therapy for prostate cancer. *Eur. Urol.* **2012**, *61*, 11–25. [CrossRef]
11. Antonarakis, E.S.; Lu, C.; Wang, H.; Luber, B.; Nakazawa, M.; Roeser, J.C.; Chen, Y.; Mohammad, T.A.; Chen, Y.; Fedor, H.L.; et al. AR-V7 and resistance to enzalutamide and abiraterone in prostate cancer. *N. Engl. J. Med.* **2014**, *371*, 1028–1038. [CrossRef]
12. Chandrasekar, T.; Yang, J.C.; Gao, A.C.; Evans, C.P. Mechanisms of resistance in castration-resistant prostate cancer (CRPC). *Transl. Androl. Urol.* **2015**, *4*, 365–380. [CrossRef]
13. Sarwar, M.; Semenas, J.; Miftakhova, R.; Simoulis, A.; Robinson, B.; Gjorloff Wingren, A.; Mongan, N.P.; Heery, D.M.; Johnsson, H.; Abrahamsson, P.A.; et al. Targeted suppression of AR-V7 using PIP5K1alpha inhibitor overcomes enzalutamide resistance in prostate cancer cells. *Oncotarget* **2016**, *7*, 63065–63081. [CrossRef]
14. Evans, R.M. The steroid and thyroid hormone receptor superfamily. *Science* **1988**, *240*, 889–895. [CrossRef]
15. Itkonen, H.; Mills, I.G. Chromatin binding by the androgen receptor in prostate cancer. *Mol. Cell. Endocrinol.* **2012**, *360*, 44–51. [CrossRef]
16. Shen, M.M.; Abate-Shen, C. Molecular genetics of prostate cancer: New prospects for old challenges. *Genes Dev.* **2010**, *24*, 1967–2000. [CrossRef]
17. Evan, G.I.; Vousden, K.H. Proliferation, cell cycle and apoptosis in cancer. *Nature* **2001**, *411*, 342–348. [CrossRef]
18. Sogawa, K.; Imataka, H.; Yamasaki, Y.; Kusume, H.; Abe, H.; Fujii-Kuriyama, Y. cDNA cloning and transcriptional properties of a novel GC box-binding protein, BTEB2. *Nucleic Acids Res.* **1993**, *21*, 1527–1532. [CrossRef]
19. Ci, X.; Xing, C.; Zhang, B.; Zhang, Z.; Ni, J.J.; Zhou, W.; Dong, J.T. KLF5 inhibits angiogenesis in PTEN-deficient prostate cancer by attenuating AKT activation and subsequent HIF1alpha accumulation. *Mol. Cancer* **2015**, *14*, 91. [CrossRef]
20. Diakiw, S.M.; D'Andrea, R.J.; Brown, A.L. The double life of KLF5: Opposing roles in regulation of gene-expression, cellular function, and transformation. *IUBMB Life* **2013**, *65*, 999–1011. [CrossRef]
21. Dong, J.T.; Chen, C. Essential role of KLF5 transcription factor in cell proliferation and differentiation and its implications for human diseases. *Cell. Mol. Life Sci.* **2009**, *66*, 2691–2706. [CrossRef]
22. David, C.J.; Huang, Y.H.; Chen, M.; Su, J.; Zou, Y.; Bardeesy, N.; Iacobuzio-Donahue, C.A.; Massague, J. TGF-beta tumor suppression through a lethal EMT. *Cell* **2016**, *164*, 1015–1030. [CrossRef]
23. Zhu, N.; Gu, L.; Findley, H.W.; Chen, C.; Dong, J.T.; Yang, L.; Zhou, M. KLF5 interacts with P53 in regulating survivin expression in acute lymphoblastic leukemia. *J. Biol. Chem.* **2006**, *281*, 14711–14718. [CrossRef]
24. Guo, P.; Dong, X.Y.; Zhao, K.W.; Sun, X.; Li, Q.; Dong, J.T. Estrogen-induced interaction between KLF5 and estrogen receptor (ER) suppresses the function of ER in ER-positive breast cancer cells. *Int. J. Cancer* **2010**, *126*, 81–89. [CrossRef]
25. Sun, R.; Chen, X.; Yang, V.W. Intestinal-enriched kruppel-like factor (kruppel-like factor 5) is a positive regulator of cellular proliferation. *J. Biol. Chem.* **2001**, *276*, 6897–6900. [CrossRef]
26. McConnell, B.B.; Bialkowska, A.B.; Nandan, M.O.; Ghaleb, A.M.; Gordon, F.J.; Yang, V.W. Haploinsufficiency of Kruppel-like factor 5 rescues the tumor-initiating effect of the Apc(Min) mutation in the intestine. *Cancer Res.* **2009**, *69*, 4125–4133. [CrossRef]
27. Chen, C.; Benjamin, M.S.; Sun, X.; Otto, K.B.; Guo, P.; Dong, X.Y.; Bao, Y.; Zhou, Z.; Cheng, X.; Simons, J.W.; et al. KLF5 promotes cell proliferation and tumorigenesis through gene regulation in the TSU-Pr1 human bladder cancer cell line. *Int. J. Cancer* **2006**, *118*, 1346–1355. [CrossRef]
28. Guo, P.; Dong, X.Y.; Zhao, K.; Sun, X.; Li, Q.; Dong, J.T. Opposing effects of KLF5 on the transcription of MYC in epithelial proliferation in the context of transforming growth factor beta. *J. Biol. Chem.* **2009**, *284*, 28243–28252. [CrossRef]
29. Xing, C.; Fu, X.; Sun, X.; Guo, P.; Li, M.; Dong, J.T. Different expression patterns and functions of acetylated and unacetylated Klf5 in the proliferation and differentiation of prostatic epithelial cells. *PLoS ONE* **2013**, *8*, e65538. [CrossRef]

30. Zhang, B.; Ci, X.; Tao, R.; Ni, J.J.; Xuan, X.; King, J.L.; Xia, S.; Li, Y.; Frierson, H.F.; Lee, D.K.; et al. Klf5 acetylation regulates luminal differentiation of basal progenitors in prostate development and regeneration. *Nat. Commun.* **2020**, *11*, 997. [CrossRef]
31. Xing, C.; Ci, X.; Sun, X.; Fu, X.; Zhang, Z.; Dong, E.N.; Hao, Z.Z.; Dong, J.T. Klf5 deletion promotes Pten deletion-initiated luminal-type mouse prostate tumors through multiple oncogenic signaling pathways. *Neoplasia* **2014**, *16*, 883–899. [CrossRef]
32. Frigo, D.E.; Sherk, A.B.; Wittmann, B.M.; Norris, J.D.; Wang, Q.; Joseph, J.D.; Toner, A.P.; Brown, M.; McDonnell, D.P. Induction of Kruppel-like factor 5 expression by androgens results in increased CXCR4-dependent migration of prostate cancer cells in vitro. *Mol. Endocrinol.* **2009**, *23*, 1385–1396. [CrossRef]
33. Lee, M.Y.; Moon, J.S.; Park, S.W.; Koh, Y.K.; Ahn, Y.H.; Kim, K.S. KLF5 enhances SREBP-1 action in androgen-dependent induction of fatty acid synthase in prostate cancer cells. *Biochem. J.* **2009**, *417*, 313–322. [CrossRef]
34. Ai, J.; Wang, Y.; Dar, J.A.; Liu, J.; Liu, L.; Nelson, J.B.; Wang, Z. HDAC6 regulates androgen receptor hypersensitivity and nuclear localization via modulating Hsp90 acetylation in castration-resistant prostate cancer. *Mol. Endocrinol.* **2009**, *23*, 1963–1972. [CrossRef]
35. Koochekpour, S. Androgen receptor signaling and mutations in prostate cancer. *Asian J. Androl.* **2010**, *12*, 639–657. [CrossRef]
36. Tran, C.; Ouk, S.; Clegg, N.J.; Chen, Y.; Watson, P.A.; Arora, V.; Wongvipat, J.; Smith-Jones, P.M.; Yoo, D.; Kwon, A.; et al. Development of a second-generation antiandrogen for treatment of advanced prostate cancer. *Science* **2009**, *324*, 787–790. [CrossRef]
37. Watson, P.A.; Chen, Y.F.; Balbas, M.D.; Wongvipat, J.; Socci, N.D.; Viale, A.; Kim, K.; Sawyers, C.L. Constitutively active androgen receptor splice variants expressed in castration-resistant prostate cancer require full-length androgen receptor. *Proc. Natl. Acad. Sci. USA* **2010**, *107*, 16759–16765. [CrossRef]
38. Ferraldeschi, R.; Pezaro, C.; Karavasilis, V.; de Bono, J. Abiraterone and novel antiandrogens: Overcoming castration resistance in prostate cancer. *Annu. Rev. Med.* **2013**, *64*, 1–13. [CrossRef]
39. Scher, H.I.; Fizazi, K.; Saad, F.; Taplin, M.E.; Sternberg, C.N.; Miller, K.; de Wit, R.; Mulders, P.; Chi, K.N.; Shore, N.D.; et al. Increased survival with enzalutamide in prostate cancer after chemotherapy. *N. Engl. J. Med.* **2012**, *367*, 1187–1197. [CrossRef]
40. Pattison, J.M.; Posternak, V.; Cole, M.D. Transcription Factor KLF5 Binds a Cyclin E1 Polymorphic Intronic Enhancer to Confer Increased Bladder Cancer Risk. *Nat. Commun.* **2016**, *14*, 1078–1086. [CrossRef] [PubMed]
41. Chu, T.M. Prostate-specific antigen in screening of prostate cancer. *J. Clin. Lab. Anal.* **1994**, *8*, 323–326. [CrossRef] [PubMed]
42. Yu, J.; Yu, J.; Mani, R.S.; Cao, Q.; Brenner, C.J.; Cao, X.; Wang, X.; Wu, L.; Li, J.; Hu, M.; et al. An integrated network of androgen receptor, polycomb, and TMPRSS2-ERG gene fusions in prostate cancer progression. *Cancer Cell* **2010**, *17*, 443–454. [CrossRef] [PubMed]
43. Magee, J.A.; Chang, L.W.; Stormo, G.D.; Milbrandt, J. Direct, androgen receptor-mediated regulation of the FKBP5 gene via a distal enhancer element. *Endocrinology* **2006**, *147*, 590–598. [CrossRef] [PubMed]
44. Kim, Y.C.; Chen, C.; Bolton, E.C. Androgen Receptor-Mediated Growth Suppression of HPr-1AR and PC3-Lenti-AR Prostate Epithelial Cells. *PLoS ONE* **2015**, *10*, e0138286. [CrossRef]
45. Petre-Draviam, C.E.; Cook, S.L.; Burd, C.J.; Marshall, T.W.; Wetherill, Y.B.; Knudsen, K.E. Specificity of cyclin D1 for androgen receptor regulation. *Cancer Res.* **2003**, *63*, 4903–4913.
46. Maina, P.K.; Shao, P.; Liu, Q.; Fazli, L.; Tyler, S.; Nasir, M.; Dong, X.; Qi, H.H. c-MYC drives histone demethylase PHF8 during neuroendocrine differentiation and in castration-resistant prostate cancer. *Oncotarget* **2016**, *7*, 75585–75602. [CrossRef]
47. Yang, S.; Jiang, M.; Grabowska, M.M.; Li, J.; Connelly, Z.M.; Zhang, J.; Hayward, S.W.; Cates, J.M.; Han, G.; Yu, X. Androgen receptor differentially regulates the proliferation of prostatic epithelial cells in vitro and in vivo. *Oncotarget* **2016**, *7*, 70404–70419. [CrossRef]
48. Chiu, C.M.; Yeh, S.H.; Chen, P.J.; Kuo, T.J.; Chang, C.J.; Chen, P.J.; Yang, W.J.; Chen, D.S. Hepatitis B virus X protein enhances androgen receptor-responsive gene expression depending on androgen level. *Proc. Natl. Acad. Sci. USA* **2007**, *104*, 2571–2578. [CrossRef]

49. Guo, P.; Zhao, K.W.; Dong, X.Y.; Sun, X.; Dong, J.T. Acetylation of KLF5 alters the assembly of p15 transcription factors in transforming growth factor-beta-mediated induction in epithelial cells. *J. Biol. Chem.* **2009**, *284*, 18184–18193. [CrossRef]
50. Li, X.; Zhang, B.; Wu, Q.; Ci, X.; Zhao, R.; Zhang, Z.; Xia, S.; Su, D.; Chen, J.; Ma, G.; et al. Interruption of KLF5 acetylation converts its function from tumor suppressor to tumor promoter in prostate cancer cells. *Int. J. Cancer* **2015**, *136*, 536–546. [CrossRef]
51. Kumekawa, M.; Fukuda, G.; Shimizu, S.; Konno, K.; Odawara, M. Inhibition of monocyte chemoattractant protein-1 by Kruppel-like factor 5 small interfering RNA in the tumor necrosis factor- alpha-activated human umbilical vein endothelial cells. *Biol. Pharm. Bull.* **2008**, *31*, 1609–1613. [CrossRef] [PubMed]
52. Sur, I.; Unden, A.B.; Toftgard, R. Human Kruppel-like factor5/KLF5: Synergy with NF-kappaB/Rel factors and expression in human skin and hair follicles. *Eur. J. Cell Biol.* **2002**, *81*, 323–334. [CrossRef] [PubMed]
53. Ma, D.; Zhang, R.N.; Wen, Y.; Yin, W.N.; Bai, D.; Zheng, G.Y.; Li, J.S.; Zheng, B.; Wen, J.K. 1,25(OH)2D3-induced interaction of vitamin D receptor with p50 subunit of NF-kappaB suppresses the interaction between KLF5 and p50, contributing to inhibition of LPS-induced macrophage proliferation. *Biochem. Biophys. Res. Commun.* **2017**, *482*, 366–374. [CrossRef] [PubMed]
54. Chanchevalap, S.; Nandan, M.O.; McConnell, B.B.; Charrier, L.; Merlin, D.; Katz, J.P.; Yang, V.W. Kruppel-like factor 5 is an important mediator for lipopolysaccharide-induced proinflammatory response in intestinal epithelial cells. *Nucleic Acids Res.* **2006**, *34*, 1216–1223. [CrossRef]
55. Chen, C.; Hyytinen, E.R.; Sun, X.; Helin, H.J.; Koivisto, P.A.; Frierson, H.F.; Vessella, R.L.; Dong, J.T. Deletion, mutation, and loss of expression of KLF6 in human prostate cancer. *Am. J. Pathol.* **2003**, *162*, 1349–1354. [CrossRef]
56. Thalmann, G.N.; Sikes, R.A.; Wu, T.T.; Degeorges, A.; Chang, S.M.; Ozen, M.; Pathak, S.; Chung, L.W. LNCaP progression model of human prostate cancer: Androgen-independence and osseous metastasis. *Prostate* **2000**, *44*, 91–103. [CrossRef]
57. Zhang, B.; Zhang, Z.; Xia, S.; Xing, C.; Ci, X.; Li, X.; Zhao, R.; Tian, S.; Ma, G.; Zhu, Z.; et al. KLF5 activates microRNA 200 transcription to maintain epithelial characteristics and prevent induced epithelial-mesenchymal transition in epithelial cells. *Mol. Cell. Biol.* **2013**, *33*, 4919–4935. [CrossRef]
58. Zhu, S.; Zhao, D.; Yan, L.; Jiang, W.; Kim, J.S.; Gu, B.; Liu, Q.; Wang, R.; Xia, B.; Zhao, J.C.; et al. BMI1 regulates androgen receptor in prostate cancer independently of the polycomb repressive complex 1. *Nat. Commun.* **2018**, *9*, 500. [CrossRef]

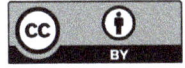

© 2020 by the authors. Licensee MDPI, Basel, Switzerland. This article is an open access article distributed under the terms and conditions of the Creative Commons Attribution (CC BY) license (http://creativecommons.org/licenses/by/4.0/).

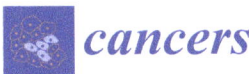

Article

The Impact of Whole Genome Data on Therapeutic Decision-Making in Metastatic Prostate Cancer: A Retrospective Analysis

Megan Crumbaker [1,2,3,†], Eva K. F. Chan [1,2,†], Tingting Gong [1,4], Niall Corcoran [5,6,7], Weerachai Jaratlerdsiri [1], Ruth J. Lyons [1], Anne-Maree Haynes [1], Anna A. Kulidjian [8,9], Anton M. F. Kalsbeek [1], Desiree C. Petersen [10], Phillip D. Stricker [11], Christina A. M. Jamieson [12], Peter I. Croucher [1,13], Christopher M. Hovens [5,6,*], Anthony M. Joshua [1,2,3,*] and Vanessa M. Hayes [1,2,4,*]

1. Garvan Institute of Medical Research, Darlinghurst, NSW 2010, Australia; m.crumbaker@garvan.org.au (M.C.); e.chan@garvan.org.au (E.K.F.C.); t.gong@garvan.org.au (T.G.); w.Jaratlerdsiri@garvan.org.au (W.J.); R.Lyons@garvan.org.au (R.J.L.); a.Haynes@garvan.org.au (A.-M.H.); amfkalsbeek@gmail.com (A.M.F.K.); p.croucher@garvan.org.au (P.I.C.)
2. St. Vincent's Clinical School, University of New South Wales, Sydney, Randwick, NSW 2031, Australia
3. Kinghorn Cancer Centre, Department of Medical Oncology, St. Vincent's Hospital, Darlinghurst, NSW 2010, Australia
4. Central Clinical School, University of Sydney, Sydney, Camperdown, NSW 2050, Australia
5. Australian Prostate Cancer Research Centre Epworth, Richmond, VIC 3121, Australia; niallmcorcoran@gmail.com
6. Department of Surgery, University of Melbourne, Melbourne, VIC 3010, Australia
7. Division of Urology, Royal Melbourne Hospital, Melbourne, VIC 3050, Australia
8. Department of Orthopedic Surgery, Scripps Clinic, La Jolla, CA 92037, USA.; Kulidjian.Anna@scrippshealth.org
9. Orthopedic Oncology Program, Scripps MD Anderson Cancer Center, La Jolla, CA 92037, USA
10. The Centre for Proteomic and Genomic Research, Cape Town 7925, South Africa; desiree.petersen@cpgr.org.za
11. Department of Urology, St. Vincent's Hospital, Darlinghurst, NSW 2010, Australia; phillip@stricker.com.au
12. Department of Urology, Moores Cancer Center, University of California, San Diego, La Jolla, CA 92037, USA; camjamieson@health.ucsd.edu
13. School of Biotechnology and Biomolecular Sciences, University of New South Wales, Sydney, Randwick, NSW 2031, Australia
* Correspondence: cbhovens@gmail.com (C.M.H.); anthony.joshua@svha.org.au (A.M.J.); v.hayes@garvan.org.au (V.M.H)
† These authors contributed equally to this work.

Received: 18 March 2020; Accepted: 28 April 2020; Published: 7 May 2020

Abstract: *Background*: While critical insights have been gained from evaluating the genomic landscape of metastatic prostate cancer, utilizing this information to inform personalized treatment is in its infancy. We performed a retrospective pilot study to assess the current impact of precision medicine for locally advanced and metastatic prostate adenocarcinoma and evaluate how genomic data could be harnessed to individualize treatment. *Methods*: Deep whole genome-sequencing was performed on 16 tumour-blood pairs from 13 prostate cancer patients; whole genome optical mapping was performed in a subset of 9 patients to further identify large structural variants. Tumour samples were derived from prostate, lymph nodes, bone and brain. *Results*: Most samples had acquired genomic alterations in multiple therapeutically relevant pathways, including DNA damage response (11/13 cases), PI3K (7/13), MAPK (10/13) and Wnt (9/13). Five patients had somatic copy number losses in genes that may indicate sensitivity to immunotherapy (*LRP1B*, *CDK12*, *MLH1*) and one patient had germline and somatic *BRCA2* alterations. *Conclusions*: Most cases, whether primary or metastatic, harboured therapeutically relevant alterations, including those associated with PARP inhibitor sensitivity, immunotherapy sensitivity and resistance to androgen pathway targeting agents. The observed intra-patient heterogeneity and presence of genomic alterations in multiple growth pathways in individual cases suggests that a precision medicine model in prostate cancer needs to simultaneously incorporate multiple pathway-targeting agents. Our whole genome approach allowed for structural variant assessment in addition to the ability to rapidly reassess an individual's molecular landscape as knowledge of relevant biomarkers evolve. This retrospective oncological assessment highlights the genomic complexity of prostate cancer and the potential impact of assessing genomic data for an individual at any stage of the disease.

Keywords: prostate cancer; precision medicine; whole genome sequencing; optical mapping; therapy

1. Introduction

Worldwide, prostate cancer (PCa) is the most commonly diagnosed non-cutaneous cancer in men and a leading cause of cancer-related male deaths [1]. Treatment strategies range from observation alone to multi-modal treatment and vary based on clinical and pathological factors such as tumour stage (T Stage), prostate specific antigen (PSA) level, Gleason or International Society of Urological Pathology (ISUP) score and life expectancy. PCa is a heterogeneous disease, and these clinical factors alone cannot predict outcomes accurately. Early disease is potentially curable whereas eventual treatment resistance is an intractable problem in metastatic disease. In both early and advanced disease, escalation of treatment including combination therapies, such as androgen deprivation therapy (ADT) administered with docetaxel with or without radiotherapy to the primary has resulted in improved outcomes [2–5]. However, the escalated treatment comes at the cost of increased toxicity and only a subset of men garner benefit. As such, predictive biomarkers for optimal treatment selection are needed at all stages of the disease.

PCa progression is driven by genomic alterations and, as such, large sequencing efforts have focused on elucidating the succession of events driving its pathogenesis and progression. These sequencing efforts aim to establish new prognostic and therapeutic targets [6–11]. Thus far, these studies have focused on primary tumours from localized cancers and/or heavily pre-treated disease that has become resistant to ADT, termed castrate-resistant prostate cancer (CRPC). It has been established that intra- and inter-patient heterogeneity is high [12–16], though certain critical events may occur early in some patients and propagate. In general, genomic changes are thought to accumulate in response to treatment as the disease progresses and the importance of structural variants (SVs) in advanced prostate cancer is an evolving area of research [10,11].

A goal of previous studies is to advance "precision medicine" in PCa. Robinson et al. found that 89% of CRPC samples harboured a clinically actionable genomic alteration [6]. However, clinical trials utilizing the precision medicine paradigm of selecting a targeted drug based on molecular criteria have yielded mixed results. For example, though phosphoinositide 3-kinase (PI3K)/Protein Kinase B (Akt) pathway activating alterations are commonly reported in PCa, PI3K inhibitors have demonstrated limited efficacy to date [17,18]. However, a randomized phase II study of abiraterone +/−ipatasertib, an Akt inhibitor, in metastatic CRPC did find improved antitumoral activity in the combination arm, particularly in men with *PTEN* loss [19]. Similarly, poly ADP ribose polymerase (PARP) inhibitors have shown promise in selected men with CRPC and homologous recombination deficiency [20–23] but not all mutations in the homologous recombination pathway predict a response [21].

Although these large genomic studies have expanded the knowledge of molecular drivers of treatment-naïve primary and metastatic CRPC, they have generally viewed the data as a cohort without looking at cumulative alterations and their potential therapeutic impact within the individuals. Likewise, hormone sensitive (HSPC) metastatic disease has also been largely neglected. In this study, we performed whole genome sequencing (WGS) on men with confirmed PCa in order to assess the collective genomic events in individual cases and their impact on real-world therapeutic decisions. Recognizing the importance of SVs in prostate cancer and the limitations of WGS in detecting large genomic rearrangements, we also performed whole genome optical mapping (WGM) on a subset of the samples.

2. Results

2.1. Shared Genomic Landscape

In this study, we retrospectively analysed 13 PCa cases that had micro- or macro-metastatic disease at the time of sampling for genomic interrogation. Patient clinical and pathological characteristics are summarized in Table 1. Sixteen tumour samples comprised of nine primary and seven metastatic biopsies and the sites of concurrent or subsequent metastases included: bone (seven cases), lymph nodes (four cases), and brain (one case), while a single case had biochemically relapsed without evidence of macro-metastatic disease on conventional imaging. Figure 1 summarizes the commonalities and differences in the genomic landscape between our primary and metastatic samples, while placing our cases in context with the current knowledge based on large PCa WGS efforts. For the latter, we focused on the study published by Wedge et al. in 2018 for 112 patients (92 primary and 20 metastatic) with the metastases evenly distributed between HSPC and CRPC and biased towards lymph node metastasis (15/20) [8].

Common predisposing germline variants (Table S1) in our samples include the *EHBP1* rs721048 (c.1185 + 30064G > A) intronic variant in five (38%) and *FGFR4* rs35185519011 (c.1162G > A, p.Gly388Arg) in ten (77%) cases. Reported in 9% of the healthy population [24], the *EHBP1* rs721048 A-allele has been associated with a more aggressive PCa [25]. The functional variant in *FGFR4*, although present in 30% of the healthy population, may predispose PCa patients to an accelerated disease course [26]. Ten patients had one of two SNPs (rs1859962, rs8072254) in non-coding regions of the 17q24.3 locus previously associated with PCa susceptibility [27].

Common somatic alterations include *ETS* fusions (seven cases) and *TP53* alterations (six cases). Tumour mutational burden (TMB) was generally low, ranging from 0.73 to 5.79 mutations/Megabase (mut/Mb) (IQR 1.30–2.09), and did not correlate with disease stage at sampling (Figure 1, Table S2). Percent genome altered (PGA) ranged from 2.2% to 63.9% (IQR 2.79–19.4%) (Table S2).

We observed a prevalence (11/13 cases) of somatic copy number alterations (SCNA) affecting at least one DNA damage response (DDR) pathway gene (Table S4). Losses in *FANCA*, which helps recruit DNA repair proteins to areas of DNA damage [28], were present in five (38%) cases, while one case harboured germline and somatic *BRCA2* alterations. With variation depending on the gene sets tested for and stage of disease, DDR gene alterations occur in approximately 20% of PCas with *BRCA2* alterations reported for 3% of prostatic and 12% of metastatic samples [6,7,29]. Aside from DDR, the most commonly impacted pathways were Phosphoinositide 3-kinase (PI3K, 7/13 (54%) cases), Mitogen-activated protein kinase (MAPK, 10 (77%) cases) and Wnt (9 (69%) cases) (Table 2). PI3K and MAPK are intracellular and extracellular signalling pathways, respectively, that are key to the regulation of the cell cycle and, like certain DDR pathways, are therapeutically targetable (manipulable) with inhibitory drugs [30,31]. The Wnt signalling pathway is a cellular pathway involved in cell growth, embryogenesis and cell cycle progression, the activation of which has been implicated in progression to CRPC and treatment resistance [32]. Previous studies have found that approximately 25% of primary PCas harbour PI3K or MAPK pathway alterations while nearly 50% of metastatic CRPC samples have PI3K alterations [6,7] and 32% MAPK amplifications [30]. In our study, 6 of the 7 samples with somatic alterations impacting PI3K were in the primary tissue, and MAPK alterations were seen in 4/7 (57%) of the metastases and 6/8 (75%) of the primaries.

Overall, SCNAs and SVs, rather than single nucleotide variants (SNVs) and small insertions and deletions (sequences of no more than 50 nucleotides in length, indels), were more commonly acquired in PCa relevant genes (Tables S1–S6). The addition of WGM identified 120 SVs not identified by WGS alone, several of which overlapped with oncogenic and/or tumour suppresser genes (Table 3, Table S6).

In particular, large insertions and duplications were typically missed by our short-read WGS approach. However, no recurrent WGM-derived SVs were observed across the cases.

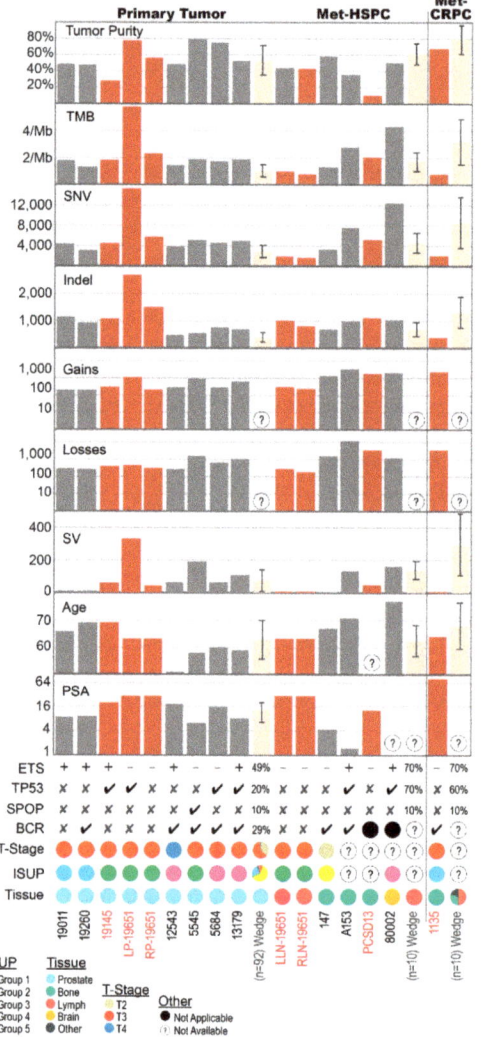

Figure 1. Summary of genomic landscape relevant to tumour purity and related to clinical and pathological features for 16 samples from 13 patients, and further compared to the Wedge et al. data. Met-HSPC: metastatic hormone sensitive PCa; met-CRPC: metastatic castration-resistant PCa; TMB: Tumour mutational burden; SNV: single nucleotide variants; Indel: small insertion or deletion; Gains and Losses: somatic copy number alterations (SCNA); SV: Structural variation including large insertions or deletions, inversions, translocations and duplications; PSA: prostate-specific antigen (ug/L); ETS: presence of ETS fusion event; TP53: presence of *TP53* alteration including SNV, SCNA or SV; SPOP: presence of *SPOP* SNV; BCR: biochemical recurrence; ISUP: International Society of Urological Pathologists cancer grade (correlates to Gleason scores). Error bars for Wedge et al. data reflect +/− one standard deviation of the sub-group totals. Sample identifiers in red, with matching red bar plots, are indicative of patients pre-treated with ADT.

Recurrent non-coding events in key PCa-associated genes have been reported [8,11,33–37], including transcription factor (TF) binding sites. Alterations at key non-coding sites within our cases are summarised in Table 4. Common to CRPC, SCNAs or SVs upstream of the androgen receptor (AR) gene were not seen in our cases, which is unsurprising given the hormone sensitive status of most of our patients. All but two of our samples contained non-coding AR binding site mutations (Table 4). Overall, 20% of the somatic SNVs or indels affected at least one TF binding cluster. However, no sample was significantly enriched for mutations within TF binding clusters and no TFs were enriched for mutations. Notably, 0.3% of the 10.5 million TF binding clusters analysed correspond to *JUN*, an average of 1.2% (0.5–1.5%) of somatic SNV in *JUN* binding clusters. JUN is a transcription factor that antagonizes AR signalling [38].

Excluding COSMIC Mutational Signature 1 common to all cancers, we observed a predominance of Mutational Signatures 3 and/or 8 (Figure 2A) that generally reduced in proportion from the clonal to subclonal stages of tumour evolution (Figure 2B). Known to be associated with DDR gene alterations [39–41], Signature 8 was particularly common in the primary 8/9 (89%) versus metastatic 3/7 (43%) samples, with notable loss in both of case 19651's lymph node metastases. In contrast, Signature 5, which is seen in most cancer types, particularly in smokers [39], and Signature 16, most often associated with liver cancer, both increased in the subclonal stage of tumour evolution.

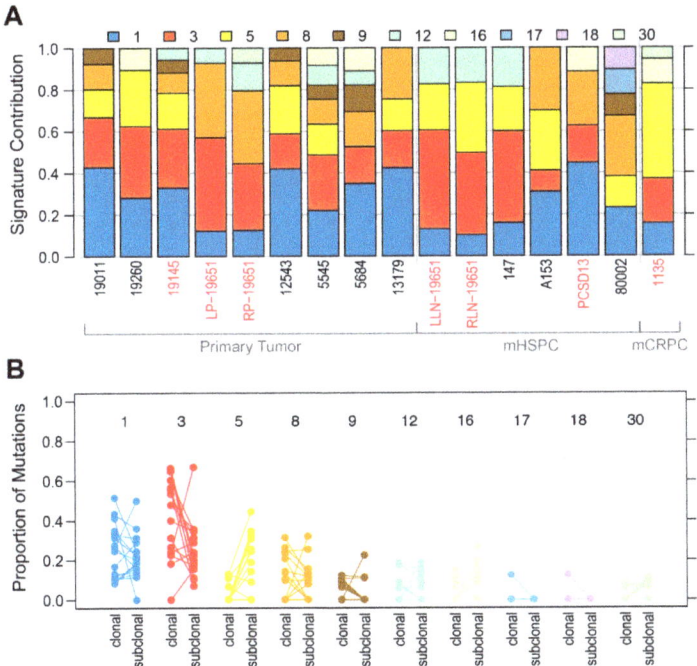

Figure 2. COSMIC Mutational Signatures (**A**) Proportion of signatures in each sample, for Signatures with >5% contribution; (**B**) Clonal vs. subclonal signature exposures. mHSPC: metastatic hormone-sensitive prostate cancer; mCRPC: metastatic castration-resistant prostate cancer.

When viewed in detail, each patient had unique features with potential therapeutic implications. This highlights the relevance of genomic information for guiding therapeutic decisions, including data derived from primary tumour tissue. Here, we discuss how the course of treatment for each patient may have been influenced by the availability of their genomic data.

Table 1. Clinical and pathological characteristics.

	Diagnosis					Time of Sample Collection for Genomic Interrogation							Relapse and Outcomes		
Patient ID	Age	Stage	Initial Treatment	ISUP	Clinical State	PSA	ECOG	Symptoms	Sample Site	ADT Prior	CRPC?	Time to BCR (mos)	Rx for BCR	Time to Mets (mos)	Duration Follow-Up (mos)
1135	64	T3N0	RP	3	Rl	80.7	1	Yes	Bone	Yes	Yes	33	ADT	68	68
19651	63	T3N1	ADT, RP, aRT	4	Dx	28	0	No	Prostate, nodes	Yes (6wks)	No	NR	NA	NR	20
147	67	T2N0	RP	2	Rl	4.4	0	Yes	Bone	No	No	84	Nil	107	135
19260	69	T3N1	RP	3	Dx	9.2	0	No	Prostate	No	No	16	sRT	NR	27
5545	58	T3N0	RP	4	Dx	6.3	0	No	Prostate	No	No	6	sRT	24	72
5684	60	T3N0	RP	5	Dx	15.7	0	No	Prostate	No	No	36	ADT	120	132
19145	69	T3N1	RP, aRT	4	Dx	20	0	No	Prostate	Yes (4wks)	No	NR	NR	NA	33
19011	66	T3N1	RP, aRT	5	Dx	8.9	0	No	Prostate	No	No	NR	NA	NA	35
12543	51	T4N0	RP, aRT	5	Dx	18.6	0	No	Prostate	No	No	72	ADT	NA	120
13179	59	T3N0	RP, aRT, ADT	5	Dx	8.4	0	No	Prostate	No	No	51	ADT	51	51
PCSD13	69	TxNxM1	ADT	-	Dx	12.8	2	Yes	Bone	Yes (8wks)	No	NA	NA	NA	9
A153	71	T2N0	RP	3	Rl	1.5	0	Yes	Bone	No	No	93	Nil	105	120
80002	77	TxNxM1	Resection, ADT	5	Dx	-	1	Yes	Brain	No	No	NA	NA	NA	1

Dx = Diagnosis; Sample = time of tissue biopsy for genomic interrogation; ADT = Androgen deprivation therapy; RP = radical prostatectomy; aRT = adjuvant radiotherapy; sRT = salvage radiotherapy; Rl = Relapse; BCR = Biochemical relapse; mos = months; NR = Not relapsed; NA = Not applicable.

Table 2. Genomic alterations affecting key genes in the PI3K, MAPK and WNT signaling pathways.

PI3K Pathway			MAPK Pathway			WNT Pathway		
Gene	Cases	Event	Gene	Cases	Event	Gene	Cases	Event
PTEN	5545 12543, 1914519145	SNVSCNASV	BRAF	1926019651LP, 13179, 1135, 147, A153, 8000219145,19651LP+RP, 80002	SNVSCNASV	APC	19651LP, 5545, A15319651LP+RP, 12543, 5545, A153	SCNASV
PIK3CA	19651LP, 13179	SCNA	EGFR	13179, 80002	SCNA	CTNNB1	19651LP, 13179	SCNA
PIK3CB	13179	SCNA	KRAS	19145, 5545, 5684	SCNA	RNF43	80002, 14780002, 147	SCNASV
PIK3R1	5684, 13179	SCNA	MAP3K1	5684, 13179,A153, 19651RP+LP	SCNASV	WNT5A	19651LP, 13179, 8000219260	SCNASV
AKT1	PCSD13	SNV, SCNA	RAF1	19651LP, 13179, 147, 80002	SCNA	MED12	19011	Germline SNV

Table 3. Structural variants identified by optical mapping as compared to whole genome sequencing. INS: Insertion; DEL: deletion; DUP: duplication; INV: inversion; Intra-Chr: intrachromosomal translocation; Inter-Chr: interchromosomal translocation.

Disease State of Sample	Sample ID	SVs from Whole Genome Optical Mapping							% Missed by Whole Genome Sequencing					
		Total	INS	DEL	DUP	INV	Intra-Chr	Inter-Chr	Total	INS	DEL	DUP	INV	Intra-Chr	Inter-Chr
Primary Tumor	5545	39	0	27	3	0	7	2	36	-	37	67	-	29	0
	13179	2	0	2	0	0	0	0	100	-	100	-	-	-	-
	5684	5	3	2	0	0	0	0	100	100	100	-	-	-	-
	12543	10	1	5	0	0	1	3	60	0	40	-	-	100	67
	19651LP	91	5	33	3	1	19	30	29	60	39	0	0	11	27
Met HSPC	A153	8	6	1	1	0	0	0	100	100	100	100	-	-	-
	147	5	4	0	1	0	0	0	100	100	-	100	-	-	-
	19651LLN	10	0	10	0	0	0	0	100	-	100	-	-	-	-
	80002	70	2	25	13	1	9	20	54	50	52	100	100	56	25
MetCRPC	1135	6	2	4	0	0	0	0	100	100	100	-	-	-	-

Table 4. Sites of recurrent non-coding alterations reported in the literature with potential clinical relevance.

Nearby Gene	Variant Positions	Data from Literature	Reference	Patient IDs
NEAT1	Chr11:65,190,268-65,213,009	13/112 cases, 6/20 mets all with previous ADT. NEAT1 produces a long non-coding RNA that regulates several growth pathways and overexpression is associated with PCa progression	Wedge [8]	5545
FOXA1	Promoter, Chr14:37587200-37597201	14 coding and 6 non-coding mutations; regulates AR signalling	Wedge	5684
FOXA1	Chr14:37886261-37888565, 37903630-37906634, 38035667-38036817, 38053354-38056060, 38056084-38059097, 38127358-38128083	FOXA1 is a co-factor for AR. These are cis-regulatory elements	Zhou [34]	5684
AR	Upstream promoter	Tandem duplications, 70–87% mCRPC vs. <2% primary PCa	Viswanathan [11]	Nil
AR	ChrX: 66117800-66128800 (66.10–66.20 bin)	1 peak, long range enhancer of AR, only 1/54 primary samples (Viswanathan); Copy number gain results in proliferation in low androgen condition and enzalutamide resistance	Takeda [35], Viswanathan	Nil
AR	Transcription Factor Binding Sites	Recurrently altered in primary PCa	Morova [33]	1135, 5545, 5684, 12543, 13179, 19011, 19145, 19260, 80002, 19651 (LP, RP, RLN), A153, PCSD13
MYC	Chr8: 128.14–128.28, 128.47–128.54, 128.54–128.62	8q24 risk loci PCa, associated with MYC enhancer activity	Ahmadiyeh [37], Yeager [36]	19651LP, 12543, A153

2.2. Primary Prostate Samples with Synchronous Lymph Node Metastases: 19011, 19260, 19145 and 19651

These cases each presented with elevated PSA levels and prostate adenocarcinomas confirmed on biopsy. Only 19651 had evidence of nodal metastases on conventional imaging preoperatively. However, at radical prostatectomy with lymph node dissection, all had pathologically involved nodes. Genomic alterations of potential relevance are summarized in Figure 3 (19011, 19260, 19145) and Figure 4 (19651). Though nodal involvement at presentation is associated with a high PCa mortality rate [42], the optimal management strategy for these men has not been established. Retrospective data suggest that adjuvant ADT with radiotherapy compared to ADT or observation is beneficial for men with lymph node metastases identified at radical prostatectomy [43]. Based on their ISUP grade group or Gleason score and tumour (T) stage, 19011, 19145 and 19651 also meet eligibility criteria for the STAMPEDE trial arms C and G that have shown benefit for adding docetaxel or abiraterone respectively to ADT [3,44,45]. Though some studies of men with high-risk localized PCa treated with neoadjuvant and/or adjuvant docetaxel demonstrate improved outcomes, these improvements occur in a small proportion, with significant toxicity to many [4,46,47]. These studies have all been based on clinical risk factors, thus, there is an urgent need for biomarkers that better select men likely to benefit, thereby avoiding over- and undertreatment.

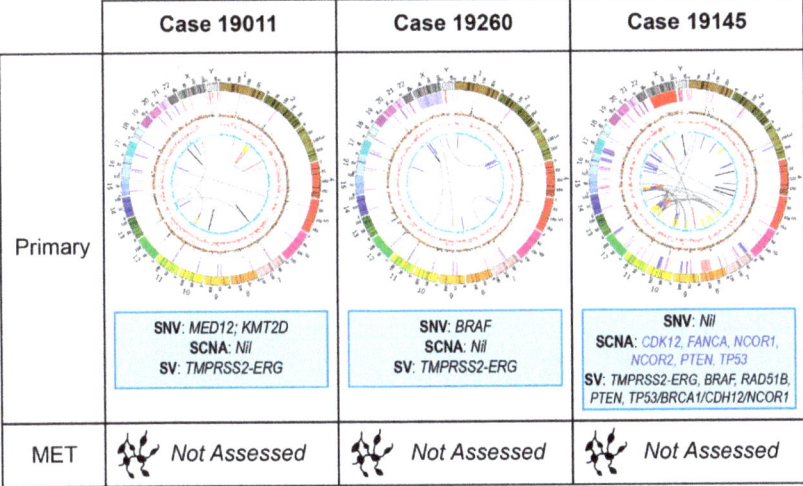

Figure 3. Summary of genomic alterations in primary prostate samples with synchronous lymph node metastases (Cases 19011, 19260 and 19145). Relevant somatic variants by type listed with SCNAs: blue indicates loss. Circos plots depict mutational load in each tumour sample. The outermost (first) track: autosome (chromosomes 1 to Y) ideograms with centromeres shown in red and the pter-qter orientation in a clockwise direction (length in Mbp); second track: somatic copy-number gains (red) and losses (blue); third track: somatic SNV allele frequencies (not corrected for tumour purity) coloured according to their mutation changes per Alexandrov et al. [39]; fourth and fifth tracks: allele frequencies (not corrected for tumour purity) of small deletions (red) and insertions (blue); innermost circle: acquired genomic rearrangements, including deletions (blue), tandem duplications (red), inversions (orange), insertions (black) and interchromosomal translocations (grey). MET: metastases.

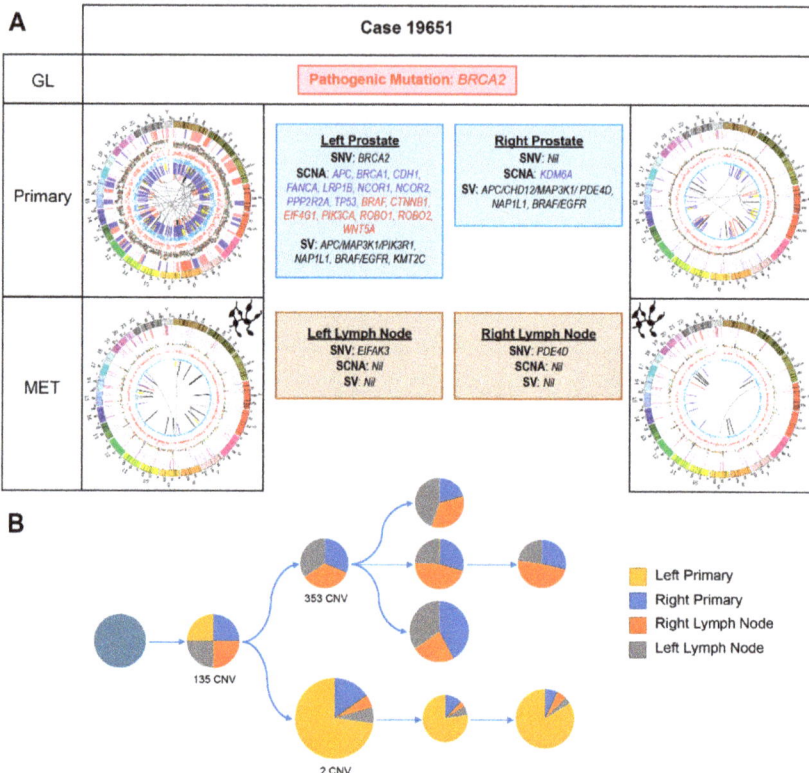

Figure 4. Case 19651. (**A**) Summary of relevant genomic alterations (germline and somatic); Circos plots as per Figure 3. GL: germline mutations; MET: metastases; (**B**) Phylogenetic reconstruction of cancer evolution predicted based on somatic SNV and copy number data. Each circle is a predicted tumour subclone, from the leftmost ancestral clone, with pie charts representing cancer cell fractions (proportion of the four samples harbouring the corresponding clone). Sizes of the circles are proportionate to the number of additional small somatic mutations acquired. Number of SCNAs acquired are indicated.

2.2.1. Case 19011: Left Prostate Tumour Core Biopsy

This *TMPRSS2-ERG* positive case had a somatic missense mutation in *MED12* (c.3670C > G; p.Leu1224Val), that is potentially pathogenic in many cancers, including prostate [48], via its upregulation of Wnt/β-catenin signalling [49]. A non-coding somatic SNV upstream of *CTNNB1* that is within the binding region of 188 TFs, may indicate misregulation of this gene involved in Wnt/β-catenin signalling [50]. No therapeutically relevant SCNA or SV was identified. PGA was low (2.7%).

Although no targetable alteration is seen in this case, the lack of mutations and low PGA may still be valuable in guiding decision-making. This patient is unlikely to respond to targeted therapies, like PARP inhibitors, but also to non-targeted agents that rely upon high mutational loads, such as immune checkpoint inhibition. The lack of poor prognostic markers, such as *TP53* loss, could mean this low volume, locally advanced PCa may respond well to aggressive local therapy without escalation to systemic therapy (e.g., addition of docetaxel). A low PGA is associated with a lower risk of BCR following definitive local therapy [51]. Despite meeting criteria for perioperative therapy trials, his genomic profile suggests aggressive local therapy will be sufficient. However, should he relapse however, the alterations in Wnt pathway-associated regions could confer resistance to AR targeting agents [32].

2.2.2. Case 19260: Right Prostate Tumour Core Biopsy

Patient 19260 was also treatment-naïve at the time of his prostatectomy and sampling for WGS. He biochemically relapsed 16 months postoperatively at which time he had salvage radiotherapy with a good PSA response.

TMPRSS2-ERG fusion positive with a low PGA (2.4%), this case presented with a pathogenic somatic missense mutation in *BRAF* (c1406G > T; p.Gly469Val). Known to confer increased kinase activity [48], this mutation may sensitise the patient to BRAF +/− MEK inhibitor therapy. Of interest in CRPC [30], with a report of response to targeted therapy in a *BRAF* mutant patient [52], clinical trials of MEK inhibitors are currently underway (NCT02881242). Though not relevant to this patient's upfront treatment, it could prove useful in the event of relapse.

2.2.3. Case 19145: Left Prostate Tumour Core Biopsy

This *TMPRSS2-ERG* positive tumour had a high PGA (10.2%), but lacked any known deleterious somatic mutation. SCNAs/SVs of note include heterozygous losses in *PTEN, FANCA, CDK12, TP53, NCOR1* and *NCOR2*, an inter-chromosomal translocation with breakpoints overlapping *RAD51B* and *PTEN* and a large heterozygous deletion overlapping with *TP53* and *NCOR1*.

Responses to PARP inhibition have been seen in patients with *FANCA* alterations [23,53] and preclinical data suggest that *PTEN* loss sensitises cancers to PARP inhibitors, with reported cases of exceptional responses to olaparib [54,55]. However, resistance to single agent PARP inhibition has been described in Pten/p53 deficient mouse models, though a synergistic response was seen upon PARP inhibition in combination with PI3K inhibition. [56]. *NCOR1* and *NCOR2* are transcriptional corepressors that negatively regulate androgen receptor (AR) signalling and androgen-induced cell proliferation [57–59]; losses in these genes increase with disease progression and are associated with anti-androgen and ADT resistance [60,61]. *TP53* loss may also predict inferior responses to novel androgen signalling inhibitors (ASIs), such as enzalutamide and abiraterone, in CRPC [62]. *CDK12* loss may predict sensitivity to immune checkpoint inhibiting therapies [63].

Many of the observed alterations in this case have therapeutic potential but are still the subject of early phase clinical trials. The presence of the *NCOR1/2* losses, however, may indicate a vulnerability in this patient for early development of CRPC. His four week course of ADT preoperatively may have induced treatment resistant clones even at this early stage. These losses together with *TP53* loss and high PGA indicate this patient may develop early resistance to ADT and, given his high-risk disease at presentation, he would be an ideal candidate for escalation of his initial treatment with chemotherapy.

2.2.4. Case 19651: Bilateral Prostate and Internal Iliac Node Tumour Core Biopsies

Reporting a family history of PCa, via his father, and breast cancer in his mother and sister, it was not surprising that this patient carries a pathogenic germline *BRCA2* stop-gain mutation (rs80359031; c.7988A > T; p.Glu2663Val) confirmed to predispose carriers to BRCA-associated cancers.

The somatic heterogeneity across the four tumour samples is striking (Figures 1 and 4A). Of the 78 overlapping SNVs (out of 24,195) present across all four samples, none had notable therapeutic relevance. Phylogenetic reconstruction of this cancer's evolution reveals distinct differences between the left primary and the other three samples (Figure 4B). Notably, the left prostatic primary acquired a somatic pathogenic *BRCA2* stop-gain mutation ((c.6308C > G; p.Ser2103Ter), variant allele frequency (VAF; 26%). Additionally, genes associated with several different growth signalling pathways, including MAPK/ERK, TGF-β, PI3K and WNT, are impacted by SCNAs in the left primary but there are few events in the other samples. No relevant SVs within the left lymph node were noted on WGM. As expected with the combined germline and somatic *BRCA2* mutations, there was a high rate of large deletions in the left primary [10], including a 3Mb deletion overlapping multiple tumour suppressor genes (TSGs) including *BTG* and *DCN*.

Inter- and intra-patient heterogeneity have been well-described in PCa [13] and most recently in multi-focal primary tumours [64], with significant therapeutic implications. The germline mutation not only informs screening for secondary cancers and testing in relatives, BRCA2 mutations may also be associated with a worse prognosis [65–69] and confer sensitivity to platinum-based chemotherapy [70] and PARP-inhibitors [23,53]. However, there is increasing evidence that responses are markedly improved with biallelic loss and many of the PARP inhibitor clinical trials have refined their inclusion criteria to include only patients with biallelic alterations. Acquiring a somatic BRCA2 mutation in a single primary tumour could result in a differential response to targeted therapies that would not be predicted based on the typical single site sampling performed in clinical practice.

Aside from the germline BRCA2 mutation, there is no unifying therapeutically relevant event across all four samples. Having had short-term ADT preoperatively, losses in NCOR1 and NCOR2 as well as other SCNAs associated with CRPC within the left primary raise the possibility that early ADT resistance is developing after minimal treatment.

In practice, knowledge of this patient's genomic landscape at baseline may have prompted his treating clinician to escalate his treatment with combination systemic therapy such as the rucaparib arm of the STAMPEDE trial. The loss of NCOR1 and NCOR2 and the poorer prognosis conferred by his TP53 and BRCA2 status represent potential indications for early chemohormonal therapy (ADT with docetaxel chemotherapy) despite him having low-volume, node only metastases [3,4,46,71]. BRCA2 alterations may also sensitize this patient to radiotherapy due to impaired DDR. Therefore, had his genomic data been available early, an upfront strategy with radiotherapy to his primary in combination with ADT and docetaxel may have been used. At progression, he may be considered for a clinical trial with a PARP inhibitor, potentially in combination with another agent given his somatic BRCA2 discordance. A metastatic biopsy at a site of progression could prove useful in determining whether new sites of disease harbour the somatic BRCA2 alteration.

2.3. Primary Prostate Samples with Relapse Post Radical Prostatectomy: 12543, 5545, 5684, and 13179

At the time of surgery, none of these cases had evidence of metastatic disease on staging scans. All men subsequently relapsed with incurable disease, including bone metastases (5545, 5684 and 13179) and persistent BCR with eventual CRPC (12543). While TMBs were similar (range 1.4–1.9), there was more marked variability in their PGAs (range 3.1–26%). Genomic alterations with patient-specific relevance are summarized in Figure 5.

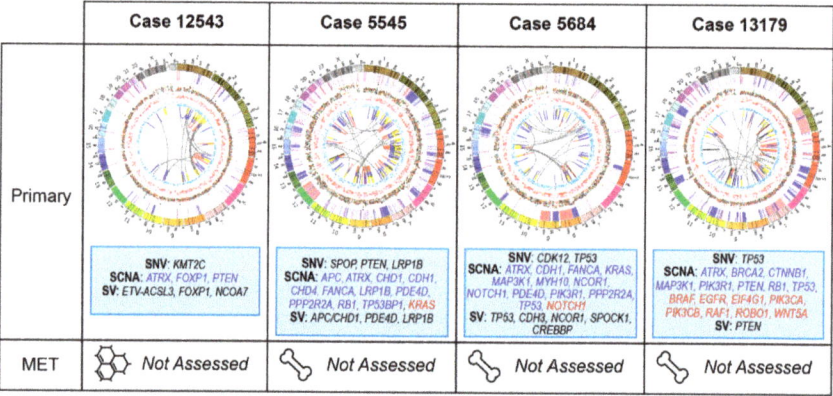

Figure 5. Summary of relevant genomic alterations for cases with subsequent metastatic relapse post radical prostatectomy (cases 12543, 5545, 5684, 13179); Circos plots as per Figure 3, with red text indicating SCNA loss.

2.3.1. Case 12543: Left Prostate Tumour Core Biopsy

This patient's tumour is characterized by *KMT2C* mutation, copy number losses (supported by large deletion) in *PTEN* and *FOXP1* and an *ETV1-ACSL3* fusion. *ETV1-ACSL3* fusion may account for this patient's prolonged ADT sensitivity (no evidence of metastatic disease following 10 years on ADT for BCR). *ACSL3* is an androgen responsive gene and thus, this fusion may lead to a strong reliance on androgen signalling [72]. Despite *PTEN* loss, loss of *FOXP1* may restore androgen receptor signalling, further enhancing this patient's response to ADT despite the *PTEN* loss [73]. At development of CRPC, this reliance on AR signalling may be exploited further with the addition of a novel ASI to his ADT, rather than docetaxel.

2.3.2. Case 5545: Left Prostate Tumour Core Biopsy

This case is characterized by a deleterious somatic *SPOP* missense variant (rs193921065, c.399C > G; p.Phe133Leu; VAF 44%) [7] and a large hemizygous deletion encompassing *CHD1*. We also predict the *LRB1B* mutation (c.3178A > G; p.Cys1060Arg) to be deleterious. Notable copy number losses include *TP53BP1* and the TSG *RB1* and the DDR genes *FANCA* and *PPP2R2A*, while a deletion overlapped *LRP1B*. Unique to WGM, we identified a large deletion involving *FILIP1L*, a gene commonly hypermethylated in PCa [74].

Point mutations in *SPOP* occur in approximately 11% of primary PCas [7] and are commonly associated with *CHD1* loss [75]. This combination of alterations is associated with increased abiraterone sensitivity in CRPC [76]. These tumours are also characterized by increased genomic instability due to error-prone double-strand DNA break repair, which results in more SVs, as seen in this case, and potential vulnerability to DNA damaging treatment such as irradiation, PARP inhibition and platinum chemotherapy [77]. Loss of *FANCA*, a gene involved in homologous recombination, may also sensitise this cancer to PARP inhibition. A recent retrospective study found that *LRP1B* alterations may predict for sensitivity to pembrolizumab [78].

SPOP/CHD1 co-altered clones persist across the disease spectrum in studies of serial patient samples [76]. Therefore, knowledge of this case's genomic data from radical prostatectomy would lead to a preference for abiraterone over docetaxel at development of CRPC. These alterations may also increase his responsiveness to PARP inhibition, though evidence is limited and preclinical models have shown that this vulnerability is reliant on elevated 53BP1 protein levels [77] and so the copy number loss in *TP53BP1* may counteract this vulnerability. This combination of alterations highlights the importance of understanding the entire genomic landscape in an individual.

2.3.3. Case 5684: Right Prostate Tumour Core Biopsy

This case harbours a small frameshift deletion in *TP53* between exons 11 and 12, in addition to heterozygous copy number loss and a deletion on SV analysis. He also presented with SCNA in *CDH1* and alterations in other DDR genes including: an SNV in *CDK12* and SCNAs in *PPP2R2A* and *FANCA*. Losses in genes affecting proliferative pathways include those in *PIK3R1*, the loss of which activates the PI3K pathway [79] and *MAP3K1*, which is associated with MEK signalling [80]. The inclusion of WGM for 5684 revealed a large insertion overlapping *SPOCK1*, which encodes a protein found to promote tumorigenesis and metastases in PCa [81]. WGM also identified an insertion in *CREBBP*, a coactivator of AR that is usually overexpressed in CRPC and the upregulation of which is associated with ADT resistance [82].

TP53 loss confers a worse prognosis and improved outcomes with chemotherapy compared to novel ASI agents [62]. Knowledge of his primary tumour *TP53* status may have guided ordering of therapies with a preference for chemotherapy, particularly upon progression to CRPC. A study of co-targeting PARP and Wee1 kinase with olaparib and AZD1775 is currently underway for *TP53* mutated solid tumours (NCT02576444). The losses in *PIK3R1* and *MAP3K1* may confer sensitivity to PI3K and MEK inhibitors respectively though these agents would only be used on a suitable clinical trial.

2.3.4. Case 13179: Right Prostate Tumour Core Biopsy

This *TMPRSS2-ERG* positive tumour is characterised by a high PGA at 26%, pathogenic somatic SNV in *TP53* (rs28934575, c.733G > A; p.Gly245Ser), as well as copy number loss of *PTEN*. Additional losses in *MAP3K1*, *PIK3R1* and *TP53* were observed, along with somatic alterations in the MAPK and PI3K pathways (Figure 5).

Co-loss of *TP53* and *PTEN* is associated with more aggressive disease, which is consistent with this patient's clinical course. Knowledge of these molecular features may have triggered more aggressive treatment upfront. Within current treatment paradigms, this may have included radiotherapy with ADT and docetaxel [5,71]. Additionally, the number of alterations in multiple targetable pathways, particularly PI3K (PI3K/AKT inhibitors) and MAPK/ERK (BRAF/MEK inhibitors), highlights the need to contextualise genomic events rather than viewing them in isolation. It is likely that this patient's treatment regimen would need to involve a tailored combination strategy if a targeted, precision-medicine approach was to be considered.

2.4. Bone Metastatic Samples: 147, A153, PCSD13 and 1135

Sampling for genomic analyses occurred at bone biopsy. Patients 147 and A153 had not yet had systemic therapy, while 1135 had CRPC, having commenced intermittent ADT for BCR 3 years postoperatively. PCSD13 presented with de novo metastatic disease manifesting as hip pain. Investigations revealed multiple bone metastases and an elevated PSA. Selected genomic events are summarized in Figure 6.

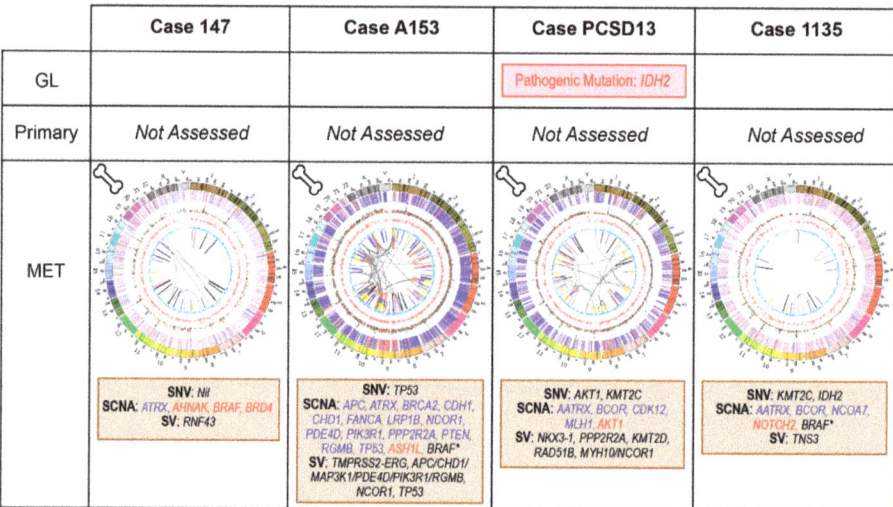

Figure 6. Summary of relevant genomic alterations for cases with metastatic disease at the time of sampling (cases 147, A153, PCSD13, 1135); Circos plots as per Figure 3.

2.4.1. Case 147: Biopsy Left Pubic Bone Corresponding to Sclerotic Region on Imaging

This case did not have any relevant somatic SNVs or WGS-identified SVs. SCNAs included gains in *BRAF*, *AHNAK* and *BRD4*.

It is unknown, yet unlikely, whether the copy number gain in *BRAF* would be sufficient to sensitize the patient to BRAF inhibition. The low level of relevant alterations in this case may explain his less aggressive disease course with a late clinical relapse (10 years post prostatectomy). The gains in *BRD4* and *AHNAK* may have contributed to metastasis formation: BRD4, part of the Bromodomain and Extraterminal (BET) protein family, regulates tumour cell migration and invasion through transcription of *AHNAK* [83]. Small molecule BRD4-selective degraders inhibit metastatic potential in PCa cell lines and a Phase I clinical trial of birabresib which included CRPC patients has been completed [84]. BRD4 is also involved in the non-homologous end joining (NHEJ) DDR pathway and higher protein levels from pre-treatment biopsies are associated with poor outcomes following radical radiotherapy in localized disease [85].

2.4.2. Case A153: Biopsy Right Iliac Crest Corresponding to Metastatic Deposit on Imaging

This *TMPRSS2-ERG* positive metastatic tumour harboured a pathogenic *TP53* mutation (rs121912656, c.734G > T; p.Gly245Val) and a high PGA (25.5%). SCNAs include losses in *APC*, *PTEN, CHD1, BRCA2, FANCA, PIK3R1* and *LRP1B*. A complex SV on chromosome 5 encompassing *PPAP2A, PDE4D, MAP3K1* and *IL6ST*, was previously associated with a worse prognosis [8].

TP53 loss is associated with a worse prognosis and decreased response to abiraterone in CRPC. *APC* loss, through its activation of Wnt signalling, may promote ASI resistance [32,62]. These two features would make docetaxel a better option than an ASI in the first instance for this patient at metastatic relapse. *BRCA2* and *FANCA* alterations were predictive for sensitivity to olaparib in the TOPARP studies [23,53] and, as previously discussed, *PTEN* and *CDH1* losses may sensitize this patient to PARP inhibition [54,77].

2.4.3. Case PCSD13: Biopsy Left Femur during Total Hip Replacement for Pathological Fracture

PCSD13 presented with a pathogenic germline *IDH2* mutation (rs121913502, c.419G > A; p.Arg140Gln). Reported to have an allele frequency of 0.00003 in The Genome Aggregation Database (gnomAD) [86], while associated with several other cancers, this mutation has not yet been reported in PCa [87]. In addition to an SNV in *AKT1*, there is a copy number gain in this gene. There are losses in the DDR genes *CDK12* and *MLH1*, and SVs also overlap multiple DDR genes. The COSMIC Mutational Signatures in this case show a subclonal increase in the proportion of Signature 3, whereas the majority of the other samples showed a decrease in this signature, which is associated with failure of double-strand DNA repair (Figure 2B).

The *AKT1* alterations may have contributed to his early ADT resistance (within 3 months of starting ADT) and confer sensitivity to AKT inhibitors [19]. These alterations could influence decisions on escalating ADT treatment with the addition of abiraterone, an androgen targeting drug, or docetaxel. However, the crosstalk between AR and PI3K/AKT signalling is well-established, [88,89] and additional pressure on the androgen axis in the context of an *AKT1* amplification may only drive further growth via the PI3K pathway. In the absence of a clinical trial with an AKT inhibitor, the addition of docetaxel rather than an AR targeting agent may have been more prudent. Immune checkpoint inhibition may have been another treatment option for this patient with his *CDK12* and *MLH1* SCNAs. This patient succumbed to his cancer shortly after developing CRPC.

2.4.4. Case 1135: Biopsy Right Posterior Iliac Crest Corresponding to Metastatic Deposit on Imaging

Despite having CRPC at the time of biopsy, case 1135 had very few alterations of interest with a TMB of 0.73 and PGA of 3.1%. This tumour contained SNVs in *KMT2C* and *IDH2* (rs121913502, c.419G > A; p.Arg140Gln) and SCNAs in *BCOR, NCOA7*, and *NOTCH2*. No significant SVs were identified with WGS but a homozygous deletion overlapping *TNS3* was identified using WGM.

The somatic SNV in *IDH2* is the same as the germline alteration seen in PCSD13 that has not been reported in PCa. It is unclear whether this mutation would drive the progression of this patient's cancer and if IDH inhibitor therapy, used to treat IDH-mutant AML, would be relevant. Based on preclinical studies, *KMT2C* alterations may confer sensitivity to PARP inhibition via its effects on the epigenetic status and expression of DDR genes. However, alterations in *KMT2C* are frequent in PCa [7] and responses to PARP inhibition only occur in a small proportion of patients [23]; therefore, it is unlikely this SNV alone will be enough to predict sensitivity to PARP monotherapy. ATRX is a DDR pathway gene while BCOR, NCOA7 and NOTCH2 are involved in androgen signalling. However, these alterations do not yet have any targeted therapeutic strategies for CRPC. While the impact of the deletion in TNS3 is again unclear, it is noted that Tensins are a family of scaffolding proteins that regulate cell motility and growth and TNS3 in involved in MET signalling [90], a target of the tyrosine kinase inhibiting drug, cabozantinib. Overall, though this case's alterations do not yet have any therapeutic relevance, the knowledge of molecular features in PCa is rapidly evolving and future findings may bring useful drugs to light.

2.5. Case 80002: Core Biopsy at Resection of Brain Metastasis

Patient 80002 presented with a solitary brain metastasis that was surgically resected. His PSA was elevated and morphology of the tumour specimen was consistent with an adenocarcinoma of prostatic origin; immunohistochemistry (IHC) markers for neuroendocrine differentiation were negative.

The relevant genomic features of this TMPRSS2-ERG fusion positive case are summarized in Figure 7 and include: TP53 mutation (rs1057519999, c.716A > C; p.Asn239Thr) and SCNAs in CDK12, RAD51C, RNF43, TP53, and BRAF. This tumour presented with a high rate of SVs, including a large deletion overlapping TP53, a partial deletion of LRP1B, and an interchromosomal translocation involving CTNNA1, the downregulation of which is associated with a worse prognosis in PCa [91]. Using our WGM approach, we identified additional large heterozygous deletions. Two overlap TSGs including TP53 and KCTD11, and another overlaps with TBX3 [92] and NRF2. NRF2 has been shown to suppress PCa cell mitosis and migration [93,94]. Another large deletion on chromosome 2 overlapped HOXD10 and HOXD3. Decreased HOXD10 expression promotes an aggressive phenotype in PCa in knockdown mice, as well on retrospective review of clinical outcomes [95] and HOXD3 methylation predicts earlier BCR [96].

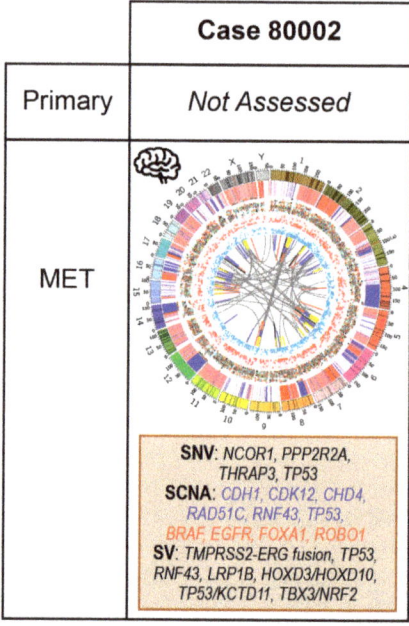

Figure 7. Summary of relevant genomic alterations for case 80002 with a brain metastasis at the time of sampling (80002) and Circos plots as per Figure 3.

Although COSMIC Mutational Signatures 1, 5, 8 and 9 are present, Signatures 17 and 18 contribute >5% each. Signature 18 may be associated with failure of base excision repair [97] and enriched in metastatic PCa [8]. Signature 17, predominantly found in gastric and oesophageal cancers, has been shown to co-occur with Signature 18 in mouse models of these cancers and this signature may be a by-product of oxidative damage [98,99].

Brain metastases are uncommon in prostate adenocarcinoma and tend to occur in cases with neuroendocrine differentiation [100]. However, gains in *FOXA1*, as seen in this case, are thought to protect against neuroendocrine trans-differentiation [101] and the *TMPRSS2-ERG* fusion supports the prostatic origin. This patient has a number of targets impacting androgen signalling, DDR and MAPK pathways. His clinical presentation would already support aggressive therapy with combination therapy and his genomic data include several poor prognostic features. The partial *LRP1B* deletion may produce sensitivity to pembrolizumab but the evidence for this is limited so this should only be considered as part of a clinical trial potentially upfront with docetaxel or later in his clinical course at development of CRPC. *KCTD11* is a negative regulator of hedgehog pathway signalling [102] and therefore its loss, identified using WGM, may increase signalling and imply this tumour would be sensitive to pathway inhibitors.

3. Materials and Methods

Included cases had adenocarcinoma of prostatic origin and were selected based on availability of tissue and matched blood specimens and micro- or overt metastatic disease either at the time of sampling or subsequent to radical prostatectomy. Patients sampled at the time of radical prostatectomy (primary tissue) had either pathologically confirmed lymph node metastases (19011, 19145, 19260, 19651) at diagnosis or subsequent metastatic relapse post-surgery (5545, 5684, 12543, 13179). Patients recruited at presentation of distant metastases had bone (1135, 147, A153, PCSD13) or brain (80002) tissue sampled.

All samples were obtained with written informed consent, as per the study approval granted from the St. Vincent's Human Research Ethics Committee (HREC), SVH/12/231 and HREC/12/SVH/323, Melbourne Health Human Research Ethics Committee HREC/12/MH/272 and Epworth Health 55512, or University of California Institute Review Board (IRB) approval 090401. Samples were shipped to the Garvan Institute of Medical Research in accordance with institutional Material Transfer Agreements (MTAs), and genomic screening and analysis were performed in accordance with approval granted by St. Vincent's Hospital HREC SVH/15/227 and governance review authorisation granted for human research at the Garvan Institute of Medical Research GHRP1522.

Primary tumour samples were collected at the time of radical prostatectomy and two core biopsies were taken from the prostate regions with cancer on preoperative biopsy. Lymph node tissue was collected at the time of radical prostatectomy from nodal masses with palpable tumour. Metastatic samples were obtained by image guided biopsy or at surgical resection (80002, PCSD13). All tissue samples were snap frozen. The presence of prostate cancer and its location within the samples was confirmed by a pathologist prior to dissection for DNA extraction. DNA was extracted from tissue and buffy coat or whole blood using one of two commercially available kits: the DNeasy blood and tissue kit protocol (Qiagen, Maryland), or for high molecular weight (HMW) DNA, the Bionano Prep Frozen Human Blood and Animal Tissue DNA isolation protocols (Bionano Genomics, San Diego document #30246 and #30077).

Demographic, clinical and pathological data were collected for each patient and are summarised in Figure 1 and Table 1. The median patient age at the time of PCa diagnosis was 65 years (range 51–77). The median time to biochemical recurrence (BCR) for those that underwent definitive first-line treatment and subsequently relapsed ($n = 8$) was 43.5 months (range 6–93); six of these patients relapsed with metastatic disease detectable on standard imaging at a median time of 86.5 months from initial diagnosis (range 24–120).

3.1. Whole Genome Sequencing (WGS)

DNA from tumour and matched blood underwent 2 × 150 bp sequencing on an Illumina HiSeq X Ten instrument (Kinghorn Centre for Clinical Genomics, Garvan Institute of Medical Research) averaging over 80× and 40× coverage, respectively. Read adapters were trimmed using Illumina's Bcl2fastq Conversion software (Illumina) and filtered to remove low quality bases (<Q15), short reads (<70 bp) and missing read pairs using cutadapt v1.9 [103]. Remaining reads were aligned to GRCh38 reference using bwa-mem v0.7.15 [104], with the ALT-aware mode. Alignment statistics were calculated using QualiMap v2.1.3 [105] and stromal contamination was calculated using Sequenza [106]. Sequencing statistics are summarized in Table S2. The sequencing data for the tumor and blood samples are available in the NCBI BioSample database under the following range of accessions: SAMN14209964–SAMN14209992.

3.2. WGS Variant Calling

The GATK pipeline version 3.5-0 was used for small variant calling [107]. We defined small variants as single nucleotide variants (SNVs) and insertions or deletions (indels) ≤ 50 bases and structural variants (SVs) as events ≥ 50 bases. Analysis-ready alignment per sample was called for SNVs and indels (GVCF mode) using GATK HaplotypeCaller (GVCF mode; [107]). Per-sample GVCFs were used for joint genotyping across genomes (GATK GenotypeGVCFs). Joint-called SNVs and indels were filtered via machine learning variant quality score recalibration and passed loci were kept. High-confidence somatic variants were called for each tumour-blood pair using MuTect2 [108]. A combination of GRIDSS and LUMPY was used for the detection of germline and somatic SVs [109,110]; potentially relevant SVs were manually inspected using Integrative Genomics Viewer (IGV) [111]. For somatic copy number alterations (SCNAs), binned copy number and segmentation profiles were determined using the copy number calling pipeline in the CNVkit package; gains (CN > 2) and losses (CN < 2) were assessed on calls adjusted for tumour purity [112].

3.3. WGS Variant Annotation

Germline and somatic SNVs and indels were annotated using Annovar [113] and pathogenic variants were manually inspected using IGV [111]. Missense mutations were further classified as potential oncogenic drivers using CanDrA [114] with PCa-specific databases.

The 30 SNV-derived Catalogue Of Somatic Mutations In Cancer (COSMIC) Mutational Signatures were annotated using the SomaticSignatures package in R [115]. Estimation of clonality and clonal segregation of somatic mutations were computed using PhyloWGS [116] and TITAN program [117].

3.4. Tumour Mutational Burden and Percentage Genome Alteration

TMB was calculated by counting the total number of small somatic mutations and dividing by genome size (3088 megabases (Mb)). PGA was calculated based on the cumulative number of base pairs altered for each gain or loss in the autosome (Chromosomes 1–22) per patient divided by the reference autosomal genome size (2875 Mb).

3.5. Whole Genome Optical Mapping

HMW DNA were fluorescently-labelled using either nicking enzyme Nt.BspQI (New England Biolabs) or non-nicking enzyme DLE-1 (BNG, Part #20351), according to the Bionano Prep Labeling NLRS Protocol (Document #30024) or Direct Label & Stain protocol (Document #30206), respectively. Samples prepared with BspQI (1135, 147, A153) were imaged using the Bionano Genomics (BNG) Irys system (San Diego, CA), while those prepared with DLE-1 (80002, 19651, 12543, 13179, 5545, 5684) were imaged using the BNG Saphyr system, to generate single molecule optical maps.

De novo assembly of single molecules into consensus genome maps was performed with the Bionano Solve (≥v3.2) software with aligner RefAligner (≥7437) [118–120]. Custom sets of parameters were used for this purpose and are included as File S1.

3.6. WGM Derived Genomic Rearrangements

SVs were identified relative to the human reference genome, GRCh38, whose genome maps were bioinformatically deduced based on predicted Nt.BspQI (GCTCTTCN) or DLE-1 (CTTAAG) motif sites. SV detection was performed as part of the Bionano Solve pipeline. Details of the underlying algorithm are described in the software's accompanying documentation (Document # 30110B).

3.7. WGM Derived Data Filtering

Filtering steps were performed on the resulting SVs. First, SVs that did not pass the Bionano recommended confidence level for the corresponding SV type were excluded; that is, all SVs other than inversion must have confidence > 0.1 and both breakpoints of an inversion event must have confidence > 0.01. Second, only rare SVs were included, defined as being observed in < 10% of a cohort of ~150 "normal" samples provided by Bionano [121]. Finally, "somatic" SVs were identified as those supported by a minimum of y_t molecules in the tumour sample but not observed in more than y_n molecules in the matching-normal sample, where $y = -0.3 + 0.13 * x$ and x being the effective coverage of the corresponding sample. This formula is recommended by Bionano as detailed in their Variant Annotation Pipeline v1.0 (BNG document # 30190). The minimum coverage cut-offs for somatic SV calling are summarized in Table S8. The WGM data are available at the following Doi: 10.25833/7wqs-gb12 [122].

3.8. Generation of a Prostate Cancer-Related Gene List

In addition to identifying annotated pathogenic and likely pathogenic alterations as well as the top genes affected by SCNAs, we reviewed alterations involving potential PCa driver genes and non-coding events associated with prostate cancer. A list of 159 PCa-associated genes was compiled from recent studies that identified recurrently mutated genes in primary and metastatic samples (Table S7) [6–9]. The list included commonly altered genes with potential functional relevance from The Cancer Genome Atlas (TCGA) primary PCa data [7,123], potential driver genes identified in primary and metastatic samples by Wedge et al. [8] and genes recurrently mutated in metastatic disease as identified by Robinson et al. [6] and Armenia et al. [9]. A list of non-coding events was compiled from recent published data (Table 4).

3.9. Other Analyses

The full list of binding clusters of 340 TFs compiled by the ENCODE project was obtained from the University of California Santa Cruz data repository (encRegTfbsClistered table; last updated 16 May 2019) and examined for somatic variants using a custom R script. Somatic variants within AR binding sites were evaluated against published putative binding sites observed in the LNCaP prostate cancer cell line (NCBI Gene Expression Omnibus accession GSE83860; [33]). The Circos plots in Figures 3–7 were generated using the CIRCOS software (v0.69-6) [124] based on SNV/indel data from MUTECT, copy number data from CNVkit, and SV data from GRIDSS. Phylogenetic reconstruction of tumour evolution for patient 19651 was performed using phyloWGS [116] based on SNV/indel data from MUTECT and copy number data from TITAN. Analyses of COSMIC Mutational Signature [125] clonal evolution was performed using the R package Palimpsest v1 [126] which utilized SNV data from MUTECT for estimates of mutation signature and SNV allele frequency data from MUTECT along with copy number segmentation data from Sequenza [106] for estimates of clonality.

4. Discussion

These real-world clinical cases demonstrate that clinically relevant mutations occur even in treatment-naïve patients across the spectrum of disease from high-risk primaries to metastatic cases. While the pathways impacted in these cases align with those identified in larger scale genomic studies, the coexistence of multiple alterations has not been explored. These findings raise several points.

Firstly, studies of neoadjuvant or adjuvant docetaxel in men with high-risk localized disease undertaking radical prostatectomy or definitive radiotherapy with ADT have had conflicting results [4,46,71] but a subgroup of men appear to benefit. Poor prognostic genomic findings, such as *TP53* deletions or deleterious *BRCA2* alterations at baseline may be useful in selecting men for additional treatment. Similarly, not all men require escalated treatment beyond ADT for HSPC but biomarkers to guide treatment selection remain limited. The findings of *TP53* and/or Wnt pathway activating alterations in 5/8 (63%) of our primary samples highlight a potential biomarker for selecting men that should be considered for escalated therapy, preferably with docetaxel rather than a novel ASI [32,62,127]. Though speculative in the hormone sensitive setting, there is mounting evidence these alterations could be useful in guiding treatment selection in CRPC. Secondly, we observed events in minimally treated patients, such as *NCOR1* and *NCOR2* losses, that may be associated with ADT resistance. These alterations again may identify patients at risk for early development of CRPC who may need escalated therapy upfront. Thirdly, pathway mutations typically enriched in metastatic CRPC, particularly PI3K and MAPK pathway SCNAs, were frequently seen in our patients and represent potential targets for neoadjuvant intervention in high risk localized and/or de novo metastatic HSPC clinical trials.

The addition of WGM in our study did not identify a current therapeutic target but it did identify SVs impacting oncogenic and tumour suppressing genes that were not identified by using WGS alone. Though we did identify non-coding events affecting the promoters, enhancers and TF binding sites of relevant genes, their therapeutic relevance has yet to be elucidated. However, as WGS and WGM data accumulate and annotations improve, we may find new relevant mutations and begin to understand how they may be integrated into clinical practice. Additionally, the use of complementary genomic technologies such as RNA-sequencing and chromatin immunoprecipitation sequencing may improve our ability to translate genomic data into real-world clinical decision-making.

In this retrospective study, we assess the current status of genome profiling, specifically WGS and WGM, to inform decision-making for 13 patients presenting with metastatic PCa. Our findings suggest that, despite being a cancer associated with a low TMB, individual PCas can harbour complex series of mutations affecting multiple growth pathways. Therefore, the precision medicine model of identifying one target to treat is unlikely to succeed. Given its heterogeneity and despite comprising only a very small fraction of the I-PREDICT study cohort [128], PCa may be the ideal cancer to test the paradigm of using genomics to identify and treat multiple targets simultaneously.

5. Conclusions

Our analyses demonstrate that whole genomic interrogation of PCas may provide invaluable information at any stage of the disease. Most of our cases had alterations affecting multiple signalling pathways highlighting the utility of a comprehensive molecular assessment in tailoring treatment strategies to an individual. Moreover, WGM identified SVs disrupting prostate cancer relevant genes that were not apparent on our WGS analyses. Many non-coding and WGM events were identified but their therapeutic relevance is yet to be established. Though these data add to our current knowledge, further research is needed, potentially integrating additional genomic technologies, to identify new treatment targets and predictive biomarkers. While several potential biomarkers that may influence treatment decisions were found in these patients, most have yet to be validated in prospective clinical trials.

Supplementary Materials: The following are available online at http://www.mdpi.com/2072-6694/12/5/1178/s1: Table S1: Potentially deleterious germline SNVs annotated by ANNOVAR, Table S2: Sequencing and mapping data including TMB and PGA, Table S3: SNVs affecting selected driver genes as annotated by ANNOVAR, Table S4: SCNAs identified by CNVKit affecting selected driver genes, Table S5: SVs affecting selected driver genes, Table S6: SVs identified by WGM, Table S7: Selected driver genes, Table S8: WGM SV calling cut-offs. File S1: Custom WGM SV calling parameters.

Author Contributions: Conceptualization, V.M.H., E.K.F.C., M.C., A.M.J., C.A.M.J., A.A.K, C.M.H. and P.I.C..; methodology, V.M.H., M.C., E.K.F.C., W.J., T.G., R.J.L., and D.C.P.; formal analysis, V.M.H., M.C, E.K.F.C., W.J., T.G.; resources, V.M.H., M.C., C.A.M.J., P.D.S., N.C., R.J.L., A.M.F.K., C.A.M.J., A.-M.H., C.M.H., A.A.K.; data curation, M.C., E.K.F.C.; writing—original draft preparation, M.C.; writing—review and editing, V.M.H., M.C., E.K.F.C., A.M.J., A.M.F.K., W.J., T.G., C.M.H., R.J.L.; visualization, E.K.F.C., M.C., V.M.H.; supervision, V.M.H.; project administration, V.M.H.; funding acquisition, V.M.H., A.M.J, C.A.M.J., P.D.S., P.I.C., N.C., C.M.H. All authors have read and agreed to the published version of the manuscript.

Funding: This work was funded by the Movember Australia and the Prostate Cancer Foundation Australia (PCFA) as part of the Movember Revolutionary Team Award (MRTA) to the Garvan Institute of Medical Research on prostate cancer bone metastasis (ProMis led by P.I.C. with team leads V.M.H., N.C. and C.M.H.), and an Ian Potter Foundation infrastructure award to V.M.H.. M.C. and T.G. was funded by an Australian Government Research Training Program Scholarship, E.K.F.C. and D.C. by MRTA-ProMis, W.J. by the Australian Prostate Cancer Research Centre NSW (APCRC-NSW), and V.M.H. by the University of Sydney Foundation and Petre Foundation, Australia.

Acknowledgments: This work is supported by the HPC resources generously provided by the National Computational Infrastructure (Raijin/Gadi), the Garvan Institute of Medical Research (Wolfpack) and the University of Sydney (Artemis). We would like to acknowledge the Bionano team for generation of Case 19651's WGM data and additional support. We also thank the patients for their participation and the Garvan Institute Biobank and its staff for access to the tumor samples.

Conflicts of Interest: The authors declare no conflict of interest. The funders had no role in the design of the study; in the collection, analyses, or interpretation of data; in the writing of the manuscript, or in the decision to publish the results.

References

1. Global Burden of Disease Cancer Collaboration; Fitzmaurice, C.; Allen, C.; Barber, R.M.; Barregard, L.; Bhutta, Z.A.; Brenner, H.; Dicker, D.J.; Chimed-Orchir, O.; Dandona, R.; et al. Global, Regional, and National Cancer Incidence, Mortality, Years of Life Lost, Years Lived With Disability, and Disability-Adjusted Life-Years for 32 Cancer Groups, 1990 to 2015: A Systematic Analysis for the Global Burden of Disease Study. *JAMA Oncol.* **2017**, *3*, 524–548. [CrossRef]
2. Sweeney, C.J.; Chen, Y.-H.; Carducci, M.; Liu, G.; Jarrard, D.F.; Eisenberger, M.; Wong, Y.-N.; Hahn, N.; Kohli, M.; Cooney, M.M.; et al. Chemohormonal Therapy in Metastatic Hormone-Sensitive Prostate Cancer. *N. Engl. J. Med.* **2015**, *373*, 737–746. [CrossRef]
3. James, N.D.; Sydes, M.R.; Clarke, N.W.; Mason, M.D.; Dearnaley, D.P.; Spears, M.R.; Ritchie, A.W.S.; Parker, C.C.; Russell, J.M.; Attard, G.; et al. Addition of docetaxel, zoledronic acid, or both to first-line hormone therapy in prostate cancer (STAMPEDE): survival results from an adaptive, multiarm, multistage, platform randomised controlled trial. *Lancet* **2016**, *387*, 1163–1177. [CrossRef]
4. Rosenthal, S.A.; Hu, C.; Sartor, O.; Gomella, L.G.; Amin, M.B.; Purdy, J.; Michalski, J.M.; Garzotto, M.G.; Pervez, N.; Balogh, A.G.; et al. Effect of Chemotherapy With Docetaxel With Androgen Suppression and Radiotherapy for Localized High-Risk Prostate Cancer: The Randomized Phase III NRG Oncology RTOG 0521 Trial. *J. Clin. Oncol.* **2019**, *37*, 1159–1168. [CrossRef] [PubMed]
5. Parker, C.C.; James, N.D.; Brawley, C.D.; Clarke, N.W.; Hoyle, A.P.; Ali, A.; Ritchie, A.W.S.; Attard, G.; Chowdhury, S.; Cross, W.; et al. Systemic Therapy for Advanced or Metastatic Prostate cancer: Evaluation of Drug Efficacy (STAMPEDE) investigators Radiotherapy to the primary tumour for newly diagnosed, metastatic prostate cancer (STAMPEDE): A randomised controlled phase 3 trial. *Lancet* **2018**, *392*, 2353–2366. [CrossRef]
6. Robinson, D.; Van Allen, E.M.; Wu, Y.-M.; Schultz, N.; Lonigro, R.J.; Mosquera, J.-M.; Montgomery, B.; Taplin, M.-E.; Pritchard, C.C.; Attard, G.; et al. Integrative clinical genomics of advanced prostate cancer. *Cell* **2015**, *161*, 1215–1228. [CrossRef] [PubMed]
7. Cancer Genome Atlas Research Network. The molecular taxonomy of primary prostate cancer. *Cell* **2015**, *163*, 1011–1025. [CrossRef]

8. Wedge, D.C.; Gundem, G.; Mitchell, T.; Woodcock, D.J.; Martincorena, I.; Ghori, M.; Zamora, J.; Butler, A.; Whitaker, H.; Kote-Jarai, Z.; et al. Sequencing of prostate cancers identifies new cancer genes, routes of progression and drug targets. *Nat. Genet.* **2018**, *50*, 682–692. [CrossRef]
9. Armenia, J.; Wankowicz, S.A.M.; Liu, D.; Gao, J.; Kundra, R.; Reznik, E.; Chatila, W.K.; Chakravarty, D.; Han, G.C.; Coleman, I.; et al. The long tail of oncogenic drivers in prostate cancer. *Nat. Genet.* **2018**, *50*, 645–651. [CrossRef]
10. Quigley, D.A.; Dang, H.X.; Zhao, S.G.; Lloyd, P.; Aggarwal, R.; Alumkal, J.J.; Foye, A.; Kothari, V.; Perry, M.D.; Bailey, A.M.; et al. Genomic hallmarks and structural variation in metastatic prostate cancer. *Cell* **2018**, *174*, 758–769. [CrossRef]
11. Viswanathan, S.R.; Ha, G.; Hoff, A.M.; Wala, J.A.; Carrot-Zhang, J.; Whelan, C.W.; Haradhvala, N.J.; Freeman, S.S.; Reed, S.C.; Rhoades, J.; et al. Structural Alterations Driving Castration-Resistant Prostate Cancer Revealed by Linked-Read Genome Sequencing. *Cell* **2018**, *174*, 433–447. [CrossRef] [PubMed]
12. Gerlinger, M.; Rowan, A.J.; Horswell, S.; Math, M.; Larkin, J.; Endesfelder, D.; Gronroos, E.; Martinez, P.; Matthews, N.; Stewart, A.; et al. Intratumor heterogeneity and branched evolution revealed by multiregion sequencing. *N. Engl. J. Med.* **2012**, *366*, 883–892. [CrossRef]
13. Boutros, P.C.; Fraser, M.; Harding, N.J.; de Borja, R.; Trudel, D.; Lalonde, E.; Meng, A.; Hennings-Yeomans, P.H.; McPherson, A.; Sabelnykova, V.Y.; et al. Spatial genomic heterogeneity within localized, multifocal prostate cancer. *Nat. Genet.* **2015**, *47*, 736–745. [CrossRef] [PubMed]
14. Ciccarese, C.; Massari, F.; Iacovelli, R.; Fiorentino, M.; Montironi, R.; Di Nunno, V.; Giunchi, F.; Brunelli, M.; Tortora, G. Prostate cancer heterogeneity: Discovering novel molecular targets for therapy. *Cancer Treat. Rev.* **2017**, *54*, 68–73. [CrossRef] [PubMed]
15. Attard, G.; Clark, J.; Ambroisine, L.; Mills, I.G.; Fisher, G.; Flohr, P.; Reid, A.; Edwards, S.; Kovacs, G.; Berney, D.; et al. Transatlantic Prostate Group Heterogeneity and clinical significance of ETV1 translocations in human prostate cancer. *Br. J. Cancer* **2008**, *99*, 314–320. [CrossRef] [PubMed]
16. Kristiansen, A.; Bergström, R.; Delahunt, B.; Samaratunga, H.; Guðjónsdóttir, J.; Grönberg, H.; Egevad, L.; Lindberg, J. Somatic alterations detected in diagnostic prostate biopsies provide an inadequate representation of multifocal prostate cancer. *Prostate* **2019**, *79*, 920–928. [CrossRef]
17. Hotte, S.J.; Joshua, A.M.; Torria, V.; Macfarlane, R.J.; Basappa, N.S.; Winquist, J.P.; Mukherjee, S.; Gregg, R.W.; Kollmannsberger, C.K.; Finch, D.L.; et al. NCIC CTG, IND-205: A phase II study of PX-866 in patients with recurrent or metastatic castration-resistant prostate cancer (CRPC). *J. Clin. Oncol.* **2013**, *31*, 5042. [CrossRef]
18. Hong, D.S.; Bowles, D.W.; Falchook, G.S.; Messersmith, W.A.; George, G.C.; O'Bryant, C.L.; Vo, A.C.H.; Klucher, K.; Herbst, R.S.; Eckhardt, S.G.; et al. A multicenter phase I trial of PX-866, an oral irreversible phosphatidylinositol 3-kinase inhibitor, in patients with advanced solid tumors. *Clin. Cancer Res.* **2012**, *18*, 4173–4182. [CrossRef]
19. de Bono, J.S.; De Giorgi, U.; Rodrigues, D.N.; Massard, C.; Bracarda, S.; Font, A.; Arranz Arija, J.A.; Shih, K.C.; Radavoi, G.D.; Xu, N.; et al. Randomized Phase II Study Evaluating Akt Blockade with Ipatasertib, in Combination with Abiraterone, in Patients with Metastatic Prostate Cancer with and without PTEN Loss. *Clin. Cancer Res.* **2019**, *25*, 928–936. [CrossRef]
20. Sandhu, S.K.; Schelman, W.R.; Wilding, G.; Moreno, V.; Baird, R.D.; Miranda, S.; Hylands, L.; Riisnaes, R.; Forster, M.; Omlin, A.; et al. The poly(ADP-ribose) polymerase inhibitor niraparib (MK4827) in BRCA mutation carriers and patients with sporadic cancer: A phase 1 dose-escalation trial. *Lancet Oncol.* **2013**, *14*, 882–892. [CrossRef]
21. Marshall, C.H.; Sokolova, A.O.; McNatty, A.L.; Cheng, H.H.; Eisenberger, M.A.; Bryce, A.H.; Schweizer, M.T.; Antonarakis, E.S. Differential Response to Olaparib Treatment Among Men with Metastatic Castration-resistant Prostate Cancer Harboring BRCA1 or BRCA2 Versus ATM Mutations. *Eur. Urol.* **2019**, *76*, 452–458. [CrossRef] [PubMed]
22. Sandhu, S.K.; Omlin, A.; Hylands, L.; Miranda, S.; Barber, L.J.; Riisnaes, R.; Reid, A.H.; Attard, G.; Chen, L.; Kozarewa, I.; et al. Poly(ADP-ribose) polymerase (PARP) inhibitors for the treatment of advanced germline BRCA2 mutant prostate cancer. *Ann. Oncol.* **2013**, *24*, 1416–1418. [CrossRef] [PubMed]
23. Mateo, J.; Carreira, S.; Sandhu, S.; Miranda, S.; Mossop, H.; Perez-Lopez, R.; Nava Rodrigues, D.; Robinson, D.; Omlin, A.; Tunariu, N.; et al. DNA-Repair Defects and Olaparib in Metastatic Prostate Cancer. *N. Engl. J. Med.* **2015**, *373*, 1697–1708. [CrossRef] [PubMed]

24. 1000 Genomes Project Consortium; Auton, A.; Brooks, L.D.; Durbin, R.M.; Garrison, E.P.; Kang, H.M.; Korbel, J.O.; Marchini, J.L.; McCarthy, S.; McVean, G.A.; et al. A global reference for human genetic variation. *Nature* **2015**, *526*, 68–74. [CrossRef] [PubMed]
25. Gudmundsson, J.; Sulem, P.; Rafnar, T.; Bergthorsson, J.T.; Manolescu, A.; Gudbjartsson, D.; Agnarsson, B.A.; Sigurdsson, A.; Benediktsdottir, K.R.; Blondal, T.; et al. Common sequence variants on 2p15 and Xp11.22 confer susceptibility to prostate cancer. *Nat. Genet.* **2008**, *40*, 281–283. [CrossRef]
26. Bange, J.; Prechtl, D.; Cheburkin, Y.; Specht, K.; Harbeck, N.; Schmitt, M.; Knyazeva, T.; Müller, S.; Gärtner, S.; Sures, I.; et al. Cancer progression and tumor cell motility are associated with the FGFR4 Arg(388) allele. *Cancer Res.* **2002**, *62*, 840–847.
27. Zhang, X.; Cowper-Sal lari, R.; Bailey, S.D.; Moore, J.H.; Lupien, M. Integrative functional genomics identifies an enhancer looping to the SOX9 gene disrupted by the 17q24.3 prostate cancer risk locus. *Genome Res.* **2012**, *22*, 1437–1446. [CrossRef]
28. Wang, W. Emergence of a DNA-damage response network consisting of Fanconi anaemia and BRCA proteins. *Nat. Rev. Genet.* **2007**, *8*, 735–748. [CrossRef]
29. Lang, S.H.; Swift, S.L.; White, H.; Misso, K.; Kleijnen, J.; Quek, R.G.W. A systematic review of the prevalence of DNA damage response gene mutations in prostate cancer. *Int. J. Oncol.* **2019**, *55*, 597–616. [CrossRef]
30. Nickols, N.G.; Nazarian, R.; Zhao, S.G.; Tan, V.; Uzunangelov, V.; Xia, Z.; Baertsch, R.; Neeman, E.; Gao, A.C.; Thomas, G.V.; et al. MEK-ERK signaling is a therapeutic target in metastatic castration resistant prostate cancer. *Prostate Cancer Prostatic Dis.* **2019**, *22*, 531–538. [CrossRef]
31. Crumbaker, M.; Khoja, L.; Joshua, A.M. AR signaling and the PI3K pathway in prostate cancer. *Cancers* **2017**, *9*, 34. [CrossRef] [PubMed]
32. Isaacsson Velho, P.; Fu, W.; Wang, H.; Mirkheshti, N.; Qazi, F.; Lima, F.A.S.; Shaukat, F.; Carducci, M.A.; Denmeade, S.R.; Paller, C.J.; et al. Wnt-pathway Activating Mutations Are Associated with Resistance to First-line Abiraterone and Enzalutamide in Castration-resistant Prostate Cancer. *Eur. Urol.* **2020**, *77*, 14–21. [CrossRef] [PubMed]
33. Morova, T.; McNeill, D.R.; Lallous, N.; Gönen, M.; Dalal, K.; Wilson, D.M.; Gürsoy, A.; Keskin, Ö.; Lack, N.A. Androgen receptor-binding sites are highly mutated in prostate cancer. *Nat. Commun.* **2020**, *11*, 1–10. [CrossRef] [PubMed]
34. Zhou, S.; Hawley, J.R.; Soares, F.; Grillo, G.; Teng, M.; Madani Tonekaboni, S.A.; Hua, J.T.; Kron, K.J.; Mazrooei, P.; Ahmed, M.; et al. Noncoding mutations target cis-regulatory elements of the FOXA1 plexus in prostate cancer. *Nat. Commun.* **2020**, *11*, 441. [CrossRef] [PubMed]
35. Takeda, D.Y.; Spisák, S.; Seo, J.-H.; Bell, C.; O'Connor, E.; Korthauer, K.; Ribli, D.; Csabai, I.; Solymosi, N.; Szállási, Z.; et al. A somatically acquired enhancer of the androgen receptor is a noncoding driver in advanced prostate cancer. *Cell* **2018**, *174*, 422–432. [CrossRef] [PubMed]
36. Yeager, M.; Orr, N.; Hayes, R.B.; Jacobs, K.B.; Kraft, P.; Wacholder, S.; Minichiello, M.J.; Fearnhead, P.; Yu, K.; Chatterjee, N.; et al. Genome-wide association study of prostate cancer identifies a second risk locus at 8q24. *Nat. Genet.* **2007**, *39*, 645–649. [CrossRef]
37. Ahmadiyeh, N.; Pomerantz, M.M.; Grisanzio, C.; Herman, P.; Jia, L.; Almendro, V.; He, H.H.; Brown, M.; Liu, X.S.; Davis, M.; et al. 8q24 prostate, breast, and colon cancer risk loci show tissue-specific long-range interaction with MYC. *Proc. Natl. Acad. Sci. USA* **2010**, *107*, 9742–9746. [CrossRef] [PubMed]
38. Hsu, C.-C.; Hu, C.-D. Transcriptional activity of c-Jun is critical for the suppression of AR function. *Mol. Cell. Endocrinol.* **2013**, *372*, 12–22. [CrossRef]
39. Alexandrov, L.B.; Nik-Zainal, S.; Wedge, D.C.; Aparicio, S.A.J.R.; Behjati, S.; Biankin, A.V.; Bignell, G.R.; Bolli, N.; Borg, A.; Børresen-Dale, A.-L.; et al. Signatures of mutational processes in human cancer. *Nature* **2013**, *500*, 415–421. [CrossRef]
40. Ma, J.; Setton, J.; Lee, N.Y.; Riaz, N.; Powell, S.N. The therapeutic significance of mutational signatures from DNA repair deficiency in cancer. *Nat. Commun.* **2018**, *9*, 1–12. [CrossRef]
41. Nik-Zainal, S.; Davies, H.; Staaf, J.; Ramakrishna, M.; Glodzik, D.; Zou, X.; Martincorena, I.; Alexandrov, L.B.; Martin, S.; Wedge, D.C.; et al. Landscape of somatic mutations in 560 breast cancer whole-genome sequences. *Nature* **2016**, *534*, 47–54. [CrossRef]
42. Eggener, S.E.; Scardino, P.T.; Walsh, P.C.; Han, M.; Partin, A.W.; Trock, B.J.; Feng, Z.; Wood, D.P.; Eastham, J.A.; Yossepowitch, O.; et al. Predicting 15-year prostate cancer specific mortality after radical prostatectomy. *J. Urol.* **2011**, *185*, 869–875. [CrossRef]

43. Touijer, K.A.; Karnes, R.J.; Passoni, N.; Sjoberg, D.D.; Assel, M.; Fossati, N.; Gandaglia, G.; Eastham, J.A.; Scardino, P.T.; Vickers, A.; et al. Survival Outcomes of Men with Lymph Node-positive Prostate Cancer After Radical Prostatectomy: A Comparative Analysis of Different Postoperative Management Strategies. *Eur. Urol.* **2018**, *73*, 890–896. [CrossRef]
44. James, N.D.; de Bono, J.S.; Spears, M.R.; Clarke, N.W.; Mason, M.D.; Dearnaley, D.P.; Ritchie, A.W.S.; Amos, C.L.; Gilson, C.; Jones, R.J.; et al. STAMPEDE Investigators Abiraterone for Prostate Cancer Not Previously Treated with Hormone Therapy. *N. Engl. J. Med.* **2017**, *377*, 338–351. [CrossRef]
45. James, N.; Woods, B.; Sideris, E.; Spears, M.R.; Dearnaley, D.P.; Mason, M.; Clarke, N.; Parmar, M.K.B.; Sydes, M.R.; Sculpher, M. STAMPEDE Investigators Addition of docetaxel to first-line long-term hormone therapy in prostate cancer (STAMPEDE): Long-term survival, quality-adjusted survival, and cost-effectiveness analysis. *J. Clin. Oncol.* **2018**, *36*, 162. [CrossRef]
46. Hurwitz, M.D.; Harris, J.; Sartor, O.; Xiao, Y.; Shayegan, B.; Sperduto, P.W.; Badiozamani, K.R.; Lawton, C.A.F.; Horwitz, E.M.; Michalski, J.M.; et al. Adjuvant radiation therapy, androgen deprivation, and docetaxel for high-risk prostate cancer postprostatectomy: Results of NRG Oncology/RTOG study 0621. *Cancer* **2017**, *123*, 2489–2496. [CrossRef]
47. Eastham, J.A.; Heller, G.; Halabi, S.; Monk, P.; Clinton, S.K.; Szmulewitz, R.Z.; Coleman, J.; Gleave, M.; Evans, C.P.; Hillman, D.W.; et al. CALGB 90203 (Alliance): Radical prostatectomy (RP) with or without neoadjuvant chemohormonal therapy (CHT) in men with clinically localized, high-risk prostate cancer (CLHRPC). *J. Clin. Oncol.* **2019**, *37*, 5079. [CrossRef]
48. Chang, M.T.; Asthana, S.; Gao, S.P.; Lee, B.H.; Chapman, J.S.; Kandoth, C.; Gao, J.; Socci, N.D.; Solit, D.B.; Olshen, A.B.; et al. Identifying recurrent mutations in cancer reveals widespread lineage diversity and mutational specificity. *Nat. Biotechnol.* **2016**, *34*, 155–163. [CrossRef] [PubMed]
49. Kim, S.; Xu, X.; Hecht, A.; Boyer, T.G. Mediator is a transducer of Wnt/beta-catenin signaling. *J. Biol. Chem.* **2006**, *281*, 14066–14075. [CrossRef] [PubMed]
50. Linch, M.; Goh, G.; Hiley, C.; Shanmugabavan, Y.; McGranahan, N.; Rowan, A.; Wong, Y.N.S.; King, H.; Furness, A.; Freeman, A.; et al. Intratumoural evolutionary landscape of high-risk prostate cancer: The PROGENY study of genomic and immune parameters. *Ann. Oncol.* **2017**, *28*, 2472–2480. [CrossRef]
51. Lalonde, E.; Ishkanian, A.S.; Sykes, J.; Fraser, M.; Ross-Adams, H.; Erho, N.; Dunning, M.J.; Halim, S.; Lamb, A.D.; Moon, N.C.; et al. Tumour genomic and microenvironmental heterogeneity for integrated prediction of 5-year biochemical recurrence of prostate cancer: A retrospective cohort study. *Lancet Oncol.* **2014**, *15*, 1521–1532. [CrossRef]
52. Prophet, M.; Xiao, K.; Gourdin, T.S.; Nagy, R.J.; Kiedrowski, L.A.; Ledet, E.; Sonpavde, G.; Sartor, A.O.; Lilly, M.B. Detection of actionable *BRAF* missense mutations by ctDNA-based genomic analysis in prostate cancer. *J. Clin. Oncol.* **2018**, *36*, 306. [CrossRef]
53. Mateo, J.; Porta, N.; Bianchini, D.; McGovern, U.; Elliott, T.; Jones, R.; Syndikus, I.; Ralph, C.; Jain, S.; Varughese, M.; et al. Olaparib in patients with metastatic castration-resistant prostate cancer with DNA repair gene aberrations (TOPARP-B): A multicentre, open-label, randomised, phase 2 trial. *Lancet Oncol.* **2020**, *21*, 162–174. [CrossRef]
54. Forster, M.D.; Dedes, K.J.; Sandhu, S.; Frentzas, S.; Kristeleit, R.; Ashworth, A.; Poole, C.J.; Weigelt, B.; Kaye, S.B.; Molife, L.R. Treatment with olaparib in a patient with PTEN-deficient endometrioid endometrial cancer. *Nat. Rev. Clin. Oncol.* **2011**, *8*, 302–306. [CrossRef]
55. Wang, J. Complete pathological remission after treatment with olaparib in a patient with PTEN-deficient sarcomatoid prostate cancer. *J. Mol. Cancer* **2018**, *1*, 17–19.
56. González-Billalabeitia, E.; Seitzer, N.; Song, S.J.; Song, M.S.; Patnaik, A.; Liu, X.-S.; Epping, M.T.; Papa, A.; Hobbs, R.M.; Chen, M.; et al. Vulnerabilities of PTEN-TP53-deficient prostate cancers to compound PARP-PI3K inhibition. *Cancer Discov.* **2014**, *4*, 896–904. [CrossRef] [PubMed]
57. Hodgson, M.C.; Astapova, I.; Cheng, S.; Lee, L.J.; Verhoeven, M.C.; Choi, E.; Balk, S.P.; Hollenberg, A.N. The androgen receptor recruits nuclear receptor CoRepressor (N-CoR) in the presence of mifepristone via its N and C termini revealing a novel molecular mechanism for androgen receptor antagonists. *J. Biol. Chem.* **2005**, *280*, 6511–6519. [CrossRef]
58. Cui, J.; Yang, Y.; Zhang, C.; Hu, P.; Kan, W.; Bai, X.; Liu, X.; Song, H. FBI-1 functions as a novel AR co-repressor in prostate cancer cells. *Cell Mol. Life Sci.* **2011**, *68*, 1091–1103. [CrossRef]

59. Wong, M.M.; Guo, C.; Zhang, J. Nuclear receptor corepressor complexes in cancer: Mechanism, function and regulation. *Am. J. Clin. Exp. Urol.* **2014**, *2*, 169–187.
60. Lopez, S.M.; Agoulnik, A.I.; Zhang, M.; Peterson, L.E.; Suarez, E.; Gandarillas, G.A.; Frolov, A.; Li, R.; Rajapakshe, K.; Coarfa, C.; et al. Nuclear Receptor Corepressor 1 Expression and Output Declines with Prostate Cancer Progression. *Clin. Cancer Res.* **2016**, *22*, 3937–3949. [CrossRef]
61. Lorenzin, F.; Demichelis, F. Evolution of the prostate cancer genome towards resistance. *JTGG J. Transl. Genet. Genom.* **2019**, *3*, 1–12. [CrossRef]
62. Maughan, B.L.; Guedes, L.B.; Boucher, K.; Rajoria, G.; Liu, Z.; Klimek, S.; Zoino, R.; Antonarakis, E.S.; Lotan, T.L. p53 status in the primary tumor predicts efficacy of subsequent abiraterone and enzalutamide in castration-resistant prostate cancer. *Prostate Cancer Prostatic Dis.* **2018**, *21*, 260–268. [CrossRef] [PubMed]
63. Wu, Y.-M.; Cieślik, M.; Lonigro, R.J.; Vats, P.; Reimers, M.A.; Cao, X.; Ning, Y.; Wang, L.; Kunju, L.P.; de Sarkar, N.; et al. Inactivation of CDK12 delineates a distinct immunogenic class of advanced prostate cancer. *Cell* **2018**, *173*, 1770–1782. [CrossRef] [PubMed]
64. Løvf, M.; Zhao, S.; Axcrona, U.; Johannessen, B.; Bakken, A.C.; Carm, K.T.; Hoff, A.M.; Myklebost, O.; Meza-Zepeda, L.A.; Lie, A.K.; et al. Multifocal primary prostate cancer exhibits high degree of genomic heterogeneity. *Eur. Urol.* **2019**, *75*, 498–505. [CrossRef] [PubMed]
65. Edwards, S.M.; Evans, D.G.R.; Hope, Q.; Norman, A.R.; Barbachano, Y.; Bullock, S.; Kote-Jarai, Z.; Meitz, J.; Falconer, A.; Osin, P.; et al. UK Genetic Prostate Cancer Study Collaborators and BAUS Section of Oncology Prostate cancer in BRCA2 germline mutation carriers is associated with poorer prognosis. *Br. J. Cancer* **2010**, *103*, 918–924. [CrossRef] [PubMed]
66. Castro, E.; Goh, C.; Leongamornlert, D.; Saunders, E.; Tymrakiewicz, M.; Dadaev, T.; Govindasami, K.; Guy, M.; Ellis, S.; Frost, D.; et al. Effect of BRCA Mutations on Metastatic Relapse and Cause-specific Survival After Radical Treatment for Localised Prostate Cancer. *Eur. Urol.* **2015**, *68*, 186–193. [CrossRef]
67. Na, R.; Zheng, S.L.; Han, M.; Yu, H.; Jiang, D.; Shah, S.; Ewing, C.M.; Zhang, L.; Novakovic, K.; Petkewicz, J.; et al. Germline Mutations in ATM and BRCA1/2 Distinguish Risk for Lethal and Indolent Prostate Cancer and are Associated with Early Age at Death. *Eur. Urol.* **2017**, *71*, 740–747. [CrossRef]
68. Castro, E.; Goh, C.; Olmos, D.; Saunders, E.; Leongamornlert, D.; Tymrakiewicz, M.; Mahmud, N.; Dadaev, T.; Govindasami, K.; Guy, M.; et al. Germline BRCA mutations are associated with higher risk of nodal involvement, distant metastasis, and poor survival outcomes in prostate cancer. *J. Clin. Oncol.* **2013**, *31*, 1748–1757. [CrossRef]
69. Annala, M.; Struss, W.J.; Warner, E.W.; Beja, K.; Vandekerkhove, G.; Wong, A.; Khalaf, D.; Seppälä, I.-L.; So, A.; Lo, G.; et al. Treatment Outcomes and Tumor Loss of Heterozygosity in Germline DNA Repair-deficient Prostate Cancer. *Eur. Urol.* **2017**, *72*, 34–42. [CrossRef]
70. Pomerantz, M.M.; Spisák, S.; Jia, L.; Cronin, A.M.; Csabai, I.; Ledet, E.; Sartor, A.O.; Rainville, I.; O'Connor, E.P.; Herbert, Z.T.; et al. The association between germline BRCA2 variants and sensitivity to platinum-based chemotherapy among men with metastatic prostate cancer. *Cancer* **2017**, *123*, 3532–3539. [CrossRef]
71. Oudard, S.; Latorzeff, I.; Caty, A.; Miglianico, L.; Sevin, E.; Hardy-Bessard, A.C.; Delva, R.; Rolland, F.; Mouret, L.; Priou, F.; et al. Effect of Adding Docetaxel to Androgen-Deprivation Therapy in Patients With High-Risk Prostate Cancer With Rising Prostate-Specific Antigen Levels After Primary Local Therapy: A Randomized Clinical Trial. *JAMA Oncol.* **2019**, *5*, 623–632. [CrossRef]
72. Migita, T.; Takayama, K.-I.; Urano, T.; Obinata, D.; Ikeda, K.; Soga, T.; Takahashi, S.; Inoue, S. ACSL3 promotes intratumoral steroidogenesis in prostate cancer cells. *Cancer Sci.* **2017**, *108*, 2011–2021. [CrossRef] [PubMed]
73. Hieronymus, H.; Iaquinta, P.J.; Wongvipat, J.; Gopalan, A.; Murali, R.; Mao, N.; Carver, B.S.; Sawyers, C.L. Deletion of 3p13-14 locus spanning FOXP1 to SHQ1 cooperates with PTEN loss in prostate oncogenesis. *Nat. Commun.* **2017**, *8*, 1–10. [CrossRef] [PubMed]
74. Desotelle, J.; Truong, M.; Ewald, J.; Weeratunga, P.; Yang, B.; Huang, W.; Jarrard, D. CpG island hypermethylation frequently silences FILIP1L isoform 2 expression in prostate cancer. *J. Urol.* **2013**, *189*, 329–335. [CrossRef] [PubMed]
75. Barbieri, C.E.; Baca, S.C.; Lawrence, M.S.; Demichelis, F.; Blattner, M.; Theurillat, J.-P.; White, T.A.; Stojanov, P.; Van Allen, E.; Stransky, N.; et al. Exome sequencing identifies recurrent SPOP, FOXA1 and MED12 mutations in prostate cancer. *Nat. Genet.* **2012**, *44*, 685–689. [CrossRef]

76. Boysen, G.; Rodrigues, D.N.; Rescigno, P.; Seed, G.; Dolling, D.; Riisnaes, R.; Crespo, M.; Zafeiriou, Z.; Sumanasuriya, S.; Bianchini, D.; et al. SPOP-Mutated/CHD1-Deleted Lethal Prostate Cancer and Abiraterone Sensitivity. *Clin. Cancer Res.* **2018**, *24*, 5585–5593. [CrossRef]
77. Shenoy, T.R.; Boysen, G.; Wang, M.Y.; Xu, Q.Z.; Guo, W.; Koh, F.M.; Wang, C.; Zhang, L.Z.; Wang, Y.; Gil, V.; et al. CHD1 loss sensitizes prostate cancer to DNA damaging therapy by promoting error-prone double-strand break repair. *Ann. Oncol.* **2017**, *28*, 1495–1507. [CrossRef]
78. Tucker, M.D.; Zhu, J.; Marin, D.; Gupta, R.T.; Gupta, S.; Berry, W.R.; Ramalingam, S.; Zhang, T.; Harrison, M.; Wu, Y.; et al. Pembrolizumab in men with heavily treated metastatic castrate-resistant prostate cancer. *Cancer Med.* **2019**, *8*, 4644–4655. [CrossRef]
79. Yu, J.; Zhang, Y.; McIlroy, J.; Rordorf-Nikolic, T.; Orr, G.A.; Backer, J.M. Regulation of the p85/p110 phosphatidylinositol 3′-kinase: Stabilization and inhibition of the p110alpha catalytic subunit by the p85 regulatory subunit. *Mol. Cell. Biol.* **1998**, *18*, 1379–1387. [CrossRef]
80. Xue, Z.; Vis, D.J.; Bruna, A.; Sustic, T.; van Wageningen, S.; Batra, A.S.; Rueda, O.M.; Bosdriesz, E.; Caldas, C.; Wessels, L.F.A.; et al. MAP3K1 and MAP2K4 mutations are associated with sensitivity to MEK inhibitors in multiple cancer models. *Cell Res.* **2018**, *28*, 719–729. [CrossRef]
81. Chen, Q.; Yao, Y.-T.; Xu, H.; Chen, Y.-B.; Gu, M.; Cai, Z.-K.; Wang, Z. SPOCK1 promotes tumor growth and metastasis in human prostate cancer. *Drug Des. Dev. Ther.* **2016**, *10*, 2311–2321. [PubMed]
82. Comuzzi, B.; Nemes, C.; Schmidt, S.; Jasarevic, Z.; Lodde, M.; Pycha, A.; Bartsch, G.; Offner, F.; Culig, Z.; Hobisch, A. The androgen receptor co-activator CBP is up-regulated following androgen withdrawal and is highly expressed in advanced prostate cancer. *J. Pathol.* **2004**, *204*, 159–166. [CrossRef] [PubMed]
83. Shafran, J.S.; Andrieu, G.P.; Györffy, B.; Denis, G.V. BRD4 Regulates Metastatic Potential of Castration-Resistant Prostate Cancer through AHNAK. *Mol. Cancer Res.* **2019**, *17*, 1627–1638. [CrossRef]
84. Lewin, J.; Soria, J.-C.; Stathis, A.; Delord, J.-P.; Peters, S.; Awada, A.; Aftimos, P.G.; Bekradda, M.; Rezai, K.; Zeng, Z.; et al. Phase Ib Trial With Birabresib, a Small-Molecule Inhibitor of Bromodomain and Extraterminal Proteins, in Patients With Selected Advanced Solid Tumors. *J. Clin. Oncol.* **2018**, *36*, 3007–3014. [CrossRef]
85. Li, X.; Baek, G.; Ramanand, S.G.; Sharp, A.; Gao, Y.; Yuan, W.; Welti, J.; Rodrigues, D.N.; Dolling, D.; Figueiredo, I.; et al. BRD4 Promotes DNA Repair and Mediates the Formation of TMPRSS2-ERG Gene Rearrangements in Prostate Cancer. *Cell Rep.* **2018**, *22*, 796–808. [CrossRef]
86. Karczewski, K.J.; Francioli, L.C.; Tiao, G.; Cummings, B.B.; Alföldi, J.; Wang, Q.; Collins, R.L.; Laricchia, K.M.; Ganna, A.; Birnbaum, D.P.; et al. Variation across 141,456 human exomes and genomes reveals the spectrum of loss-of-function intolerance across human protein-coding genes. *BioRxiv* **2019**.
87. Kotredes, K.P.; Razmpour, R.; Lutton, E.; Alfonso-Prieto, M.; Ramirez, S.H.; Gamero, A.M. Characterization of cancer-associated IDH2 mutations that differ in tumorigenicity, chemosensitivity and 2-hydroxyglutarate production. *Oncotarget* **2019**, *10*, 2675–2692. [CrossRef]
88. Mulholland, D.J.; Tran, L.M.; Li, Y.; Cai, H.; Morim, A.; Wang, S.; Plaisier, S.; Garraway, I.P.; Huang, J.; Graeber, T.G.; et al. Cell autonomous role of PTEN in regulating castration-resistant prostate cancer growth. *Cancer Cell* **2011**, *19*, 792–804. [CrossRef]
89. Carver, B.S.; Chapinski, C.; Wongvipat, J.; Hieronymus, H.; Chen, Y.; Chandarlapaty, S.; Arora, V.K.; Le, C.; Koutcher, J.; Scher, H.; et al. Reciprocal feedback regulation of PI3K and androgen receptor signaling in PTEN-deficient prostate cancer. *Cancer Cell* **2011**, *19*, 575–586. [CrossRef]
90. Qian, X.; Li, G.; Vass, W.C.; Papageorge, A.; Walker, R.C.; Asnaghi, L.; Steinbach, P.J.; Tosato, G.; Hunter, K.; Lowy, D.R. The Tensin-3 protein, including its SH2 domain, is phosphorylated by Src and contributes to tumorigenesis and metastasis. *Cancer Cell* **2009**, *16*, 246–258. [CrossRef]
91. Jiang, T.; Jiang, H.; Su, X.-M.; Zheng, L.; Li, Q.-L.; Zhang, Z.-W.; Li, X.-C. Expressions of E-cadherin and alpha-catenin in benign, malignant and metastatic prostate tumors. *Zhonghua Nan Ke Xue* **2012**, *18*, 499–503. [PubMed]
92. Chang, F.; Xing, P.; Song, F.; Du, X.; Wang, G.; Chen, K.; Yang, J. The role of T-box genes in the tumorigenesis and progression of cancer. *Oncol. Lett.* **2016**, *12*, 4305–4311. [CrossRef] [PubMed]
93. Xue, D.; Zhou, C.; Shi, Y.; Lu, H.; Xu, R.; He, X. Nuclear transcription factor Nrf2 suppresses prostate cancer cells growth and migration through upregulating ferroportin. *Oncotarget* **2016**, *7*, 78804–78812. [CrossRef] [PubMed]
94. Frohlich, D.A.; McCabe, M.T.; Arnold, R.S.; Day, M.L. The role of Nrf2 in increased reactive oxygen species and DNA damage in prostate tumorigenesis. *Oncogene* **2008**, *27*, 4353–4362. [CrossRef]

95. Mo, R.J.; Lu, J.M.; Wan, Y.P.; Hua, W.; Liang, Y.X.; Zhuo, Y.J.; Kuang, Q.W.; Liu, Y.L.; He, H.C.; Zhong, W.D. Decreased hoxd10 expression promotes a proliferative and aggressive phenotype in prostate cancer. *Curr. Mol. Med.* **2017**, *17*, 70–78. [CrossRef]
96. Kron, K.J.; Liu, L.; Pethe, V.V.; Demetrashvili, N.; Nesbitt, M.E.; Trachtenberg, J.; Ozcelik, H.; Fleshner, N.E.; Briollais, L.; van der Kwast, T.H.; et al. DNA methylation of HOXD3 as a marker of prostate cancer progression. *Lab. Investig.* **2010**, *90*, 1060–1067. [CrossRef]
97. Pilati, C.; Shinde, J.; Alexandrov, L.B.; Assié, G.; André, T.; Hélias-Rodzewicz, Z.; Ducoudray, R.; Le Corre, D.; Zucman-Rossi, J.; Emile, J.-F.; et al. Mutational signature analysis identifies MUTYH deficiency in colorectal cancers and adrenocortical carcinomas. *J. Pathol.* **2017**, *242*, 10–15. [CrossRef]
98. Tomkova, M.; Tomek, J.; Kriaucionis, S.; Schuster-Böckler, B. Mutational signature distribution varies with DNA replication timing and strand asymmetry. *Genome Biol.* **2018**, *19*, 1–12. [CrossRef]
99. Tomkova, M.; Renard, C.; Urban, L.; Kolli, S.; Ardin, M.; Pandey, M.; Zhivagui, M.; Huskova, H.; Olivier, M.; Marusawa, H.; et al. Abstract 4661: Deciphering the causes of the COSMIC mutational signature 17 by combining pan-cancer data with experimental mouse models. In *Tumor Biology*; American Association for Cancer Research: Amherst, MA, USA, 2019; p. 4661.
100. Hatzoglou, V.; Patel, G.V.; Morris, M.J.; Curtis, K.; Zhang, Z.; Shi, W.; Huse, J.; Rosenblum, M.; Holodny, A.I.; Young, R.J. Brain metastases from prostate cancer: An 11-year analysis in the MRI era with emphasis on imaging characteristics, incidence, and prognosis. *J. Neuroimag.* **2014**, *24*, 161–166. [CrossRef]
101. Kim, J.; Jin, H.; Zhao, J.C.; Yang, Y.A.; Li, Y.; Yang, X.; Dong, X.; Yu, J. FOXA1 inhibits prostate cancer neuroendocrine differentiation. *Oncogene* **2017**, *36*, 4072–4080. [CrossRef]
102. Zazzeroni, F.; Nicosia, D.; Tessitore, A.; Gallo, R.; Verzella, D.; Fischietti, M.; Vecchiotti, D.; Ventura, L.; Capece, D.; Gulino, A.; et al. KCTD11 tumor suppressor gene expression is reduced in prostate adenocarcinoma. *Biomed Res. Int.* **2014**, *2014*, 380398. [CrossRef] [PubMed]
103. Martin, M. Cutadapt removes adapter sequences from high-throughput sequencing reads. *EMBnet J.* **2011**, *17*, 10–12. [CrossRef]
104. Li, H.; Durbin, R. Fast and accurate short read alignment with Burrows-Wheeler transform. *Bioinformatics* **2009**, *25*, 1754–1760. [CrossRef] [PubMed]
105. Okonechnikov, K.; Conesa, A.; García-Alcalde, F. Qualimap 2: Advanced multi-sample quality control for high-throughput sequencing data. *Bioinformatics* **2016**, *32*, 292–294. [CrossRef] [PubMed]
106. Favero, F.; Joshi, T.; Marquard, A.M.; Birkbak, N.J.; Krzystanek, M.; Li, Q.; Szallasi, Z.; Eklund, A.C. Sequenza: Allele-specific copy number and mutation profiles from tumor sequencing data. *Ann. Oncol.* **2015**, *26*, 64–70. [CrossRef] [PubMed]
107. Van der Auwera, G.A.; Carneiro, M.O.; Hartl, C.; Poplin, R.; Del Angel, G.; Levy-Moonshine, A.; Jordan, T.; Shakir, K.; Roazen, D.; Thibault, J.; et al. From FastQ data to high confidence variant calls: The Genome Analysis Toolkit best practices pipeline. *Curr. Protoc. Bioinform.* **2013**, *43*, 1–11.
108. Cibulskis, K.; Lawrence, M.S.; Carter, S.L.; Sivachenko, A.; Jaffe, D.; Sougnez, C.; Gabriel, S.; Meyerson, M.; Lander, E.S.; Getz, G. Sensitive detection of somatic point mutations in impure and heterogeneous cancer samples. *Nat. Biotechnol.* **2013**, *31*, 213–219. [CrossRef]
109. Cameron, D.L.; Schröder, J.; Penington, J.S.; Do, H.; Molania, R.; Dobrovic, A.; Speed, T.P.; Papenfuss, A.T. GRIDSS: Sensitive and specific genomic rearrangement detection using positional de Bruijn graph assembly. *Genome Res.* **2017**, *27*, 2050–2060. [CrossRef]
110. Layer, R.M.; Chiang, C.; Quinlan, A.R.; Hall, I.M. LUMPY: A probabilistic framework for structural variant discovery. *Genome Biol.* **2014**, *15*, R84. [CrossRef]
111. Thorvaldsdóttir, H.; Robinson, J.T.; Mesirov, J.P. Integrative Genomics Viewer (IGV): High-performance genomics data visualization and exploration. *Brief. Bioinform.* **2013**, *14*, 178–192. [CrossRef]
112. Talevich, E.; Shain, A.H.; Botton, T.; Bastian, B.C. CNVkit: Genome-Wide Copy Number Detection and Visualization from Targeted DNA Sequencing. *PLoS Comput. Biol.* **2016**, *12*, e1004873. [CrossRef] [PubMed]
113. Wang, K.; Li, M.; Hakonarson, H. ANNOVAR: Functional annotation of genetic variants from high-throughput sequencing data. *Nucleic Acids Res.* **2010**, *38*, e164. [CrossRef] [PubMed]
114. Mao, Y.; Chen, H.; Liang, H.; Meric-Bernstam, F.; Mills, G.B.; Chen, K. CanDrA: Cancer-specific driver missense mutation annotation with optimized features. *PLoS ONE* **2013**, *8*, e77945. [CrossRef] [PubMed]
115. Gehring, J.S.; Fischer, B.; Lawrence, M.; Huber, W. SomaticSignatures: Inferring mutational signatures from single-nucleotide variants. *Bioinformatics* **2015**, *31*, 3673–3675. [CrossRef] [PubMed]

116. Deshwar, A.G.; Vembu, S.; Yung, C.K.; Jang, G.H.; Stein, L.; Morris, Q. PhyloWGS: Reconstructing subclonal composition and evolution from whole-genome sequencing of tumors. *Genome Biol.* **2015**, *16*, 1–29. [CrossRef]
117. Ha, G.; Roth, A.; Khattra, J.; Ho, J.; Yap, D.; Prentice, L.M.; Melnyk, N.; McPherson, A.; Bashashati, A.; Laks, E.; et al. TITAN: Inference of copy number architectures in clonal cell populations from tumor whole-genome sequence data. *Genome Res.* **2014**, *24*, 1881–1893. [CrossRef]
118. Lam, E.T.; Hastie, A.; Lin, C.; Ehrlich, D.; Das, S.K.; Austin, M.D.; Deshpande, P.; Cao, H.; Nagarajan, N.; Xiao, M.; et al. Genome mapping on nanochannel arrays for structural variation analysis and sequence assembly. *Nat. Biotechnol.* **2012**, *30*, 771–776. [CrossRef]
119. Hastie, A.R.; Dong, L.; Smith, A.; Finklestein, J.; Lam, E.T.; Huo, N.; Cao, H.; Kwok, P.-Y.; Deal, K.R.; Dvorak, J.; et al. Rapid genome mapping in nanochannel arrays for highly complete and accurate de novo sequence assembly of the complex Aegilops tauschii genome. *PLoS ONE* **2013**, *8*, e55864. [CrossRef]
120. Hastie, A.R.; Lam, E.T.; Pang, A.W.C.; Zhang, X.; Andrews, W.; Lee, J.; Liang, T.Y.; Wang, J.; Zhou, X.; Zhu, Z.; et al. Rapid Automated Large Structural Variation Detection in a Diploid Genome by NanoChannel Based Next-Generation Mapping. *BioRxiv* **2017**.
121. Levy-Sakin, M.; Pastor, S.; Mostovoy, Y.; Li, L.; Leung, A.K.Y.; McCaffrey, J.; Young, E.; Lam, E.T.; Hastie, A.R.; Wong, K.H.Y.; et al. Genome maps across 26 human populations reveal population-specific patterns of structural variation. *Nat. Commun.* **2019**, *10*, 1–14. [CrossRef]
122. Bionano Data. Available online: https://protect-au.mimecast.com/s/QtA0COMK24uZZWrtEuAv2?domain=dx.doi.org (accessed on 2 March 2020).
123. Gonzalez-Perez, A.; Perez-Llamas, C.; Deu-Pons, J.; Tamborero, D.; Schroeder, M.P.; Jene-Sanz, A.; Santos, A.; Lopez-Bigas, N. IntOGen-mutations identifies cancer drivers across tumor types. *Nat. Methods* **2013**, *10*, 1081–1082. [CrossRef]
124. Krzywinski, M.; Schein, J.; Birol, I.; Connors, J.; Gascoyne, R.; Horsman, D.; Jones, S.J.; Marra, M.A. Circos: An information aesthetic for comparative genomics. *Genome Res.* **2009**, *19*, 1639–1645. [CrossRef] [PubMed]
125. Alexandrov, L.; Kim, J.; Haradhvala, N.J.; Huang, M.N.; Ng, A.W.T.; Boot, A.; Covington, K.R.; Gordenin, D.A.; Bergstrom, E.; Lopez-Bigas, N.; et al. The repertoire of mutational signatures in human cancer. *Nature.* **2020**, *578*, 94–101. [CrossRef] [PubMed]
126. Shinde, J.; Bayard, Q.; Imbeaud, S.; Hirsch, T.Z.; Liu, F.; Renault, V.; Zucman-Rossi, J.; Letouzé, E. Palimpsest: An R package for studying mutational and structural variant signatures along clonal evolution in cancer. *Bioinformatics* **2018**, *34*, 3380–3381. [CrossRef] [PubMed]
127. De Laere, B.; Oeyen, S.; Mayrhofer, M.; Whitington, T.; van Dam, P.-J.; Van Oyen, P.; Ghysel, C.; Ampe, J.; Ost, P.; Demey, W.; et al. TP53 Outperforms Other Androgen Receptor Biomarkers to Predict Abiraterone or Enzalutamide Outcome in Metastatic Castration-Resistant Prostate Cancer. *Clin. Cancer Res.* **2019**, *25*, 1766–1773. [CrossRef] [PubMed]
128. Sicklick, J.K.; Kato, S.; Okamura, R.; Schwaederle, M.; Hahn, M.E.; Williams, C.B.; De, P.; Krie, A.; Piccioni, D.E.; Miller, V.A.; et al. Molecular profiling of cancer patients enables personalized combination therapy: The I-PREDICT study. *Nat. Med.* **2019**, *25*, 744–750. [CrossRef]

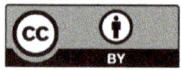

© 2020 by the authors. Licensee MDPI, Basel, Switzerland. This article is an open access article distributed under the terms and conditions of the Creative Commons Attribution (CC BY) license (http://creativecommons.org/licenses/by/4.0/).

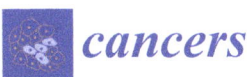

Review

Applications of Artificial Intelligence to Prostate Multiparametric MRI (mpMRI): Current and Emerging Trends

Michelle D. Bardis [1,*], Roozbeh Houshyar [1], Peter D. Chang [1], Alexander Ushinsky [2], Justin Glavis-Bloom [1], Chantal Chahine [1], Thanh-Lan Bui [1], Mark Rupasinghe [1], Christopher G. Filippi [3] and Daniel S. Chow [1]

1. Department of Radiology, University of California, Irvine, Orange, CA 92868-3201, USA; rhoushya@hs.uci.edu (R.H.); changp6@hs.uci.edu (P.D.C.); jglavisb@hs.uci.edu (J.G.-B.); cchahin1@hs.uci.edu (C.C.); thanhltb@hs.uci.edu (T.-L.B.); mrupasin@hs.uci.edu (M.R.); chowd3@hs.uci.edu (D.S.C.)
2. Mallinckrodt Institute of Radiology, Washington University Saint Louis, St. Louis, MO 63110, USA; aushinsky@wustl.edu
3. Department of Radiology, North Shore University Hospital, Manhasset, NY 11030, USA; sairaallapeikko@gmail.com
* Correspondence: mbardis@hs.uci.edu

Received: 2 April 2020; Accepted: 8 May 2020; Published: 11 May 2020

Abstract: Prostate carcinoma is one of the most prevalent cancers worldwide. Multiparametric magnetic resonance imaging (mpMRI) is a non-invasive tool that can improve prostate lesion detection, classification, and volume quantification. Machine learning (ML), a branch of artificial intelligence, can rapidly and accurately analyze mpMRI images. ML could provide better standardization and consistency in identifying prostate lesions and enhance prostate carcinoma management. This review summarizes ML applications to prostate mpMRI and focuses on prostate organ segmentation, lesion detection and segmentation, and lesion characterization. A literature search was conducted to find studies that have applied ML methods to prostate mpMRI. To date, prostate organ segmentation and volume approximation have been well executed using various ML techniques. Prostate lesion detection and segmentation are much more challenging tasks for ML and were attempted in several studies. They largely remain unsolved problems due to data scarcity and the limitations of current ML algorithms. By contrast, prostate lesion characterization has been successfully completed in several studies because of better data availability. Overall, ML is well situated to become a tool that enhances radiologists' accuracy and speed.

Keywords: prostate carcinoma; prostate mpMRI; machine learning; artificial intelligence; deep learning; neural network

1. Introduction

Prostate carcinoma (PCa) is the most common cancer and the third leading cause of cancer-related death among men in the United States [1]. A major challenge for PCa management is the lack of non-invasive tools that can differentiate aggressive versus non-aggressive cancer types [2]. This limitation can result in overdiagnosis and overtreatment, as evidenced by the fact that only one death is prevented for every 48 patients treated for PCa [3]. This overdiagnosis and overtreatment can lead to unnecessary biopsies, surgeries, radiotherapy, chemotherapy, and patient anxiety [2]. Better diagnostic methods could mitigate these unwarranted procedures. To meet this need for more effective screening, multiparametric magnetic resonance imaging (mpMRI) could be implemented to examine the entire prostate.

MpMRI of the prostate has been increasingly used for PCa screening in recent years [4]. MpMRI's current utility in screening stems from a high negative predictive value for prostate cancer. However, the full potential of mpMRI has not yet been achieved [5]. PCa overdiagnosis could be reduced with an mpMRI analysis that accomplishes better lesion detection, lesion classification (benign versus malignant), and lesion volume quantification.

Accurate prostate segmentation and volume estimation can provide invaluable information for the diagnosis and clinical management of benign prostatic hyperplasia (BPH) and PCa. This can improve BPH treatment, surgical planning, and predictions of PCa prognosis [6–8]. Prostate segmentation is necessary for magnetic resonance imaging (MRI) transrectal ultrasound (TRUS) fusion biopsy, which is increasingly used to diagnose PCa. MRI/TRUS fusion biopsy yield depends on accurate prostate segmentation on magnetic resonance images because the prostate edges form the reference frames for fusion with the ultrasound data [8]. Therefore, any inaccuracy in tracing prostate boundaries may lead to biopsy errors [9]. In addition to segmentation, prostate volume estimation is also a useful metric, especially with regard to BPH treatment, surgical planning, and PCa prognosis. BPH is one of the most common diseases that affects elderly men and reaches a prevalence of 90% by the ninth decade of life [10]. Large prostate volumes in men with BPH indicate a higher likelihood of more severe lower urinary tract symptoms and urinary retention [11–13]. Furthermore, studies have shown that patients have differential responses to BPH-targeted medications, depending on prostate size [11]. Additionally, prostate volume is considered when determining a surgical approach, with each procedure having its own risk profile [14]. In addition to guiding BPH treatment, prostate volume is used in PCa prognosis. Prostate size alone is a valuable marker for PCa prognosis; PCa is more accurately detected in prostates under 50 cm^3 than in those over 50 cm^3 [6]. Prostate volume is also used to calculate prostate-specific antigen density, a figure that helps to differentiate BPH from PCa and can also be used to predict radical prostatectomy outcomes [15–17].

Accuracy of prostate lesion detection, segmentation, and volume estimation is important at different stages of PCa management. Lesion detection identifies regions for biopsy. Accurate segmentation is crucial for improved fusion biopsy yields. Additionally, segmentation improves radiotherapy delivery. Volume estimation predicts prognosis after prostatectomy [18–20]. Prostate lesion detection is crucial because the effective treatment of PCa directly depends on identifying cancer at its earliest stage [21–23]. Even though PCa most often follows an indolent course, it can show rapid progression in some cases. In these instances, lesion recognition on mpMRI is critical because it provides a region of high suspicion and a higher yield from targeted biopsy [24]. Without mpMRI lesion detection, random 12 core TRUS biopsies are performed, which may miss small or anteriorly located PCa [25].

While early prostate lesion detection improves timely PCa treatment, accurate lesion segmentation can improve radiotherapy [26]. Prostate lesion contouring is a major source of error when administering radiation therapy. This inexact segmentation can lead to the underdosage of the tumor as well as the overdosage of normal cells [20]. Although radiotherapy is an effective cancer treatment, its use is hampered by imprecise delineation. More precise contouring of a malignant lesion can improve lesion targeting and relative radiotherapeutic dosage, which can lead to lower recurrence rates [26,27].

Pre-operative prostate lesion volume estimation is a key metric for predicting the likelihood of positive surgical margins, biochemical prostate-specific antigen (PSA) recurrence, and cancer-specific survival post-prostatectomy [28–31]. This volume is a better indicator of surgical margins than other factors such as Gleason score and extracapsular extension [28]. Lesion volume also functions as an independent variable for PSA recurrence, an early sign of recurrent disease which may require salvage radiation therapy [32]. In addition, lesion volume predicts cancer-specific survival more accurately than variables such as lymphadenopathy, seminal vesical invasion, and Gleason score [29].

After prostate lesions have been detected on mpMRI, lesion characterization is important for selecting appropriate management options. Accurate prostate lesion classification on mpMRI could preclude biopsies in men with low-grade tumors, reduce the number of biopsy cores, and decrease the rate of overdiagnosis and false-negative biopsies [33]. Reduction in unnecessary biopsies is important, as potential TRUS biopsy complications include hematuria, lower urinary tract symptoms, and temporary erectile dysfunction [34]. Additionally, the number of biopsy cores obtained correlates with increased risk of complications, including rectal bleeding, hematospermia, bleeding complications, and acute urinary retention [34]. Furthermore, the overdetection of PCa exerts a major psychological toll on quality of life and increases the risk of overtreatment [2]. Overtreatment side effects that may occur after radical prostatectomy and radiotherapy include urinary incontinence, rectal bleeding and fistulae, and erectile dysfunction [2,35–37].

Artificial intelligence (AI) is a promising tool to improve prostate lesion detection, lesion characterization, and lesion volume quantification. AI can systematically evaluate mpMRI images [38]. Machine learning (ML), a branch of AI, and its sub-discipline, deep learning (DL), have become attractive techniques in medical imaging because of their ability to interpret large amounts of data [39]. By applying ML to prostate mpMRI data, imaging-based clinical decisions could be improved. The purpose of this review is to summarize ML applications for prostate mpMRI in regards to (1) prostate organ segmentation, (2) prostate lesion detection and segmentation, and (3) prostate lesion characterization.

2. Multiparametric Magnetic Resonance Imaging

Multiparametric magnetic resonance imaging (mpMRI) of the prostate is a form of advanced non-invasive imaging that combines standard anatomical sequences with functional imaging. It consists of T1-weighted images, T2-weighted images (T2W), and the following functional sequences: diffusion-weighted images (DWI) including the apparent diffusion coefficient maps (ADC) and dynamic contrast-enhanced images (DCE). Certain protocols also incorporate proton magnetic resonance spectroscopy imaging (MRSI) [40,41]. Typically, the functional techniques used are DWI and DCE. MRSI is more demanding than DWI and DCE because it requires more acquisition time, greater technical expertise, and intensive post-processing of the data. Therefore, it is not commonly used [42].

The advantages of seeing both the anatomy and functional ability of the prostate have made mpMRI an attractive imaging technique with many applications. It can accurately identify clinically relevant cancer. The combination of T2W, DWI, and DCE has high specificity, sensitivity, and negative predictive value in detecting PCa [43–45]. The use of all three functional sequences has been found to have a positive predictive value for PCa of 98% [46]. In addition to diagnosing PCa, mpMRI is also used in the management of the disease as the functional sequences aid in predicting tumor behavior. Prostate mpMRI has been used for active surveillance, tumor localization, staging, treatment planning, and monitoring of recurrence [40,41].

While mpMRI is a powerful imaging modality, it does have limitations. Differences in image acquisition techniques and protocols across institutions lead to heterogeneity in imaging quality and make it challenging to compare images [47]. Additionally, the learning curve for reading mpMRIs is steep, and there exists inter-observer variability [48–50]. The experience of radiologists reading these scans impacts the utility of prostate mpMRI images. In addition, the prostate gland is difficult to delineate, and various benign and pre-malignant processes can mimic PCa [51]. For example, the sensitivity for the detection of PCa in the transitional zone is limited by the heterogeneous nature of this zone in the setting of BPH, which can also exhibit increased cellularity further complicating the distinction. Furthermore, patient-related factors, including body habitus, prior procedures, and unconventional anatomy, can impact imaging. Artifacts, such as field inhomogeneity from rectal gas and metal implants, can substantially impede the interpretation and reporting of prostate mpMRI. Finally, it can be difficult to discriminate between post-treatment changes and local recurrence following treatment on mpMRI.

In an effort to assist in standardizing the acquisition, interpretation, and reporting of prostate mpMRI, the Prostate Imaging Reporting and Data System (PI-RADS) was developed by the European Society of Urogenital Radiology (ESUR) in 2012 [52]. The ESUR, in collaboration with the American

College of Radiology and the AdMeTech Foundation, released updated versions PI-RADS v2 in 2015 and PI-RADS v2.1 in 2019 [53,54]. All of the PI-RADS versions offer guidance for protocols and specifications for image acquisition. The scoring systems provide frameworks to evaluate individual sequences of T2W, DWI, and DCE and to integrate these findings into an overall risk assessment category from 1 to 5. These risk categories assist in the determination of biopsies and the management of clinically significant PCa.

3. Artificial Intelligence Paradigms: Machine Learning and Deep Learning

Although the terms AI, ML, and DL are commonly used interchangeably, each term has its own specific definition. AI is the broad, umbrella term that encompasses both ML and DL, with DL being a subset of ML (Figure 1). Marvin Minsky, an early AI developer, described AI as "the science of making machines do things that would require intelligence if done by men" [55]. AI is the ability of any tool to accept inputs of prior knowledge, experience, goals, and observations and then create an output that implements an action. This definition covers a wide range of tools varying from a simple thermostat to a self-driving car. AI research often falls under the domain of computer science because AI tools perform many computations to create appropriate outputs [56].

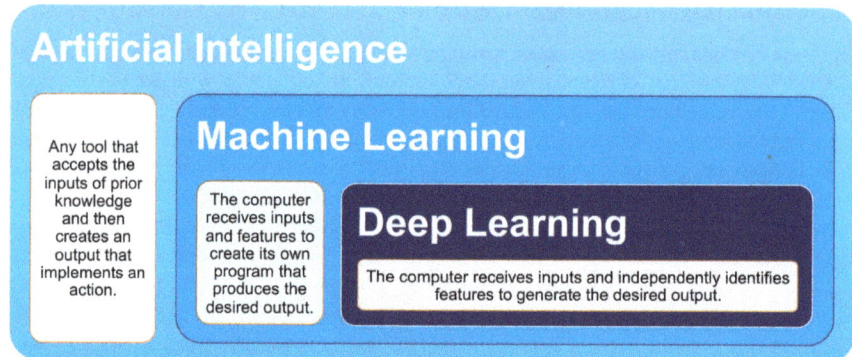

Figure 1. Relationship between artificial intelligence, machine learning, and deep learning. Artificial intelligence is an umbrella term that includes machine learning and deep learning. Deep learning is a hyponym of machine learning.

Whereas AI typically entails a fixed, rules-based computational method, ML dynamically improves upon computational methods as data is input and trained. In traditional programming, a computer receives data and a program as inputs and then produces the output in a one-to-one manner. All improvements to the results derive from alterations to the program rules. In ML, a computer receives data and labels as inputs and then creates a program to refine the outputs. The computer learns by comparing its own outputs, also known as predictions, to data that has already been defined and associated with a label. Over time, the ML algorithm will improve upon its ability to create a program that can match its own output to a label. The effectiveness of the program is highly dependent on the quality and size of data that the ML algorithm receives as input.

The data types that can be input into an ML algorithm vary widely, encompassing digitized handwriting, text from documents, DNA sequences, facial images, and more. A ML algorithm can utilize this data to train and make predictions. Two of the most common ML implementations are classification and regression [57]. In classification, ML receives data and then decides upon a category for each item in the data. For example, ML could look at images and decide whether the image is a plane, car, or boat. In regression, ML receives data and then predicts a numerical value for each item in the data. Examples include predicting tomorrow's ambient temperature or the price of a stock.

Within the ML discipline, DL has garnered significant attention because of the groundbreaking results that it achieved in the ImageNet Large Scale Visual Recognition Challenge competition, where competitors developed algorithms using a subset of a public dataset of images [58]. DL has flourished with the rise of big data and faster hardware [39]. In traditional ML, the algorithm has features that it will extract from the data before training begins [57] (Figure 2). These features are constant and are based upon established rules. For example, the algorithm can look for eyes when trying to recognize a face or search for wings when identifying an airplane. By contrast, a DL algorithm does not require feature selection before training. DL simply receives input and learns its salient features during training (Figure 2). DL architecture is also notable because it is formed by many tiered layers, which resemble a brain's neuronal network. These layers enable DL to extract features from progressively smaller sizes of input data and allow for increased feature complexity [59]. Although various DL architectures exist, convolutional neural networks (CNN) are considered well suited for medical imaging. The overall goal of these techniques is to allow the machine to determine and optimize features automatically for evaluating and classifying images.

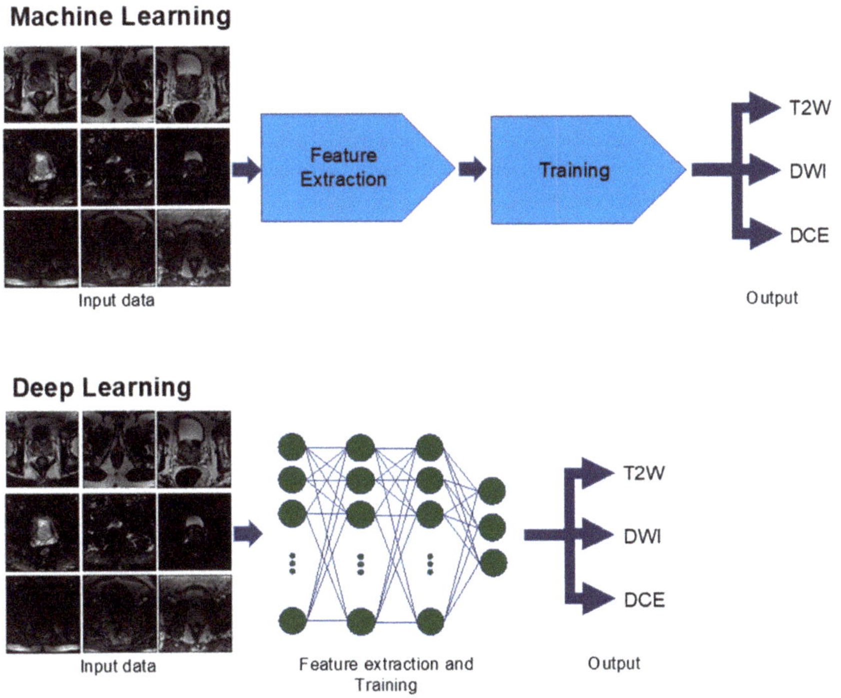

Figure 2. Machine learning versus deep learning used for multiparametric magnetic resonance imaging (mpMRI) sequence identification. In machine learning, the computer receives inputs of mpMRI images and goes through feature extraction specific to the different sequences of T2-weighted (T2W), diffusion-weighted imaging (DWI), and dynamic contrast-enhanced (DCE). Then, the computer is trained on additional images and is able to identify the correct sequence as an output. Deep learning differs from machine learning in that feature extraction and training can be done simultaneously to produce the output.

Medical imaging studies that use ML algorithms are frequently designed with three dataset types: training, validation, and test [60]. The study will first use training data as its input to develop an algorithm that produces the desired output. During this training period, the algorithm constantly uses validation data to provide correct feedback to modify itself. After the algorithm has finished development, final performance is then assessed with test data. Because test data was not used during the algorithm training, it is an objective method to assess performance.

4. Prostate Organ: Segmentation and Volume Estimation

Although prostate segmentation and volume approximation could greatly improve PCa and BPH management, existing techniques are limited. Currently, prostate segmentation is performed in a manual or semi-automated fashion and is limited by inter-observer variability [61]. According to a study by Rash et al. [62], the mean prostate organ volume among three radiation oncologists varied between 0.95 and 1.08. Currently, prostate volume is most often calculated during TRUS utilizing an ellipsoid estimate [63] or estimated during a prostate exam. Even though this volume approximation with TRUS is commonly used, it has significant intra-observer variation and is not as accurate as an approximation with mpMRI images [64,65]. Prostate volume approximation with software has been attempted with limited results. Medical students outperform the accuracy of a commercially available tool [66].

To meet this need for an automatic, accurate prostate segmentation and volume approximation tool, ML methods have been applied by various groups (Figure 3). A ML technique, fuzzy c-means clustering, categorizes data into groups via unsupervised learning and was used by Rundo et al. [67] to segment the prostate on T1-weighted and T2-weighted mpMRI images. Rundo et al. evaluated 21 patients to yield an average Dice score of 0.91 [67]. The Dice score is a standard statistic for assessing the spatial intersection between two images and ranges from 0 (no overlap) to 1 (perfect overlap) [68]. Therefore, a Dice score of 0.91 demonstrates that the technique was able to segment and estimate the volume of prostates with a high level of precision.

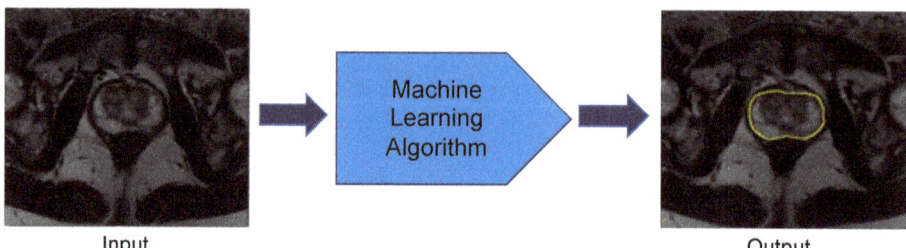

Figure 3. Prostate organ segmentation performed by machine learning methods. The computer takes multiparametric magnetic resonance imaging images as inputs and applies the developed machine learning algorithm to correctly identify the borders of the prostate.

Besides fuzzy c-means clustering, DL has been extensively used for complete prostate segmentation. In 2012, the release of the PROMISE12 challenge dataset, which contained 100 patients, prompted many studies on this topic [69,70]. Two groups led by Tian et al. [71] and Karimi et al. [70] both employed CNNs. Tian et al. [71] trained their CNN on T2-weighted mpMRI images from 140 patients and achieved a Dice score of 0.85. Karimi et al.'s [70] CNN was trained on a limited dataset of 49 T2-weighted mpMRI images supplemented by data augmentation. Their Dice score was 0.88. Both studies achieved high Dice scores and demonstrated that prostate segmentation could be achieved with commonly used technical designs.

Additionally, a uniquely designed DL network for biomedical images, U-Net, has also been proposed for complete prostate segmentation [72]. U-Net is an algorithm that successively compresses an image, derives features during these contractions, and classifies every pixel in the image [72]. Three studies used U-Net for prostate segmentation and obtained Dice scores of 0.89, 0.93, and 0.89 [73–75]. These three groups showed that U-Net could effectively segment the prostate with dataset sizes between 81 and 163 patients. The high Dice scores across multiple studies with comparable network architectures demonstrate substantial progress towards completely automated prostate segmentation and volume approximation. Table 1 lists the previously discussed studies along with several others that also segmented the prostate using various CNNs. To establish the ground truth label, which is used in establishing a Dice score, five studies used radiologists, two studies used clinicians of unstated specialties, one study used an expert, and one study used a radiologist for most of its data and an unnamed source for the rest of its data [67,70,71,73–78].

Table 1. Machine learning techniques applied to prostate organ segmentation.

Reference	Year	ML Algorithm	Patients	Dice	Modalities
Rundo et al. [67]	2017	Fuzzy C-means clustering. Features: T1 intensity, T2 intensity	21	0.91	T1W, T2W
Tian et al. [71]	2018	CNN: 7 layers	140	0.85	T2W
Karimi et al. [70]	2018	CNN: 3 layers	49	0.88	T2W
Clark et al. [73]	2017	CNN: U-Net	134	0.89	DWI
Zhu, Y. et al. [74]	2018	CNN: U-Net	163	0.93	DWI, T2W
Zhu, Q. et al. [75]	2017	CNN: U-Net	81	0.89	T2W
Milletari et al. [76]	2016	CNN: V-Net	80	0.87	T2W
Wang, B. et al. [77]	2019	CNN: 3D DSD-FCN	40	0.86	T2W
Cheng et al. [78]	2016	CNN and Active Appearance Model	120	0.93	T2W

5. Prostate Lesion: Detection, Segmentation, and Volume Estimation

Although prostate lesion detection, segmentation, and volume approximation could benefit PCa management, an effective tool that can automate these processes has not been created. For prostate lesion detection, satellite small lesions can be challenging to detect [19]. In a study by Steenbergen et al. [19], six different teams, each composed of one radiologist and one radiation oncologist, missed 66 out of 69 satellite lesions distributed across 20 patients. In addition to prostate lesion detection, segmentation is difficult because sparse tumors composed of benign glands and stroma are challenging to outline [79]. When segmentation across multiple institutions is compared, the contours reveal considerable differences [80]. As a result of inexact segmentation, volume approximation of prostate lesions is also challenging and often underestimates the histopathological volume [79]. This need for improved lesion metrics could be satisfied using ML algorithms that could learn to identify these features within mpMRI images.

For prostate lesion detection, ML approaches have been used to identify potential malignancies (Figure 4). Lay et al. [81] used a prostate computer-aided diagnosis (CAD) based on a random forest for prostate lesion detection (Table 2). This study's dataset used 224 patient cases across three sequences (T2-weighted, ADC, and DWI) for a total of 287 benign lesions and 123 lesions with a Gleason score of 6 or higher [81]. The Gleason scoring system describes PCa grades on a scale of 1 to 5 based on the pattern that the cancerous cells fall into, with 1 or 2 being low grade and 5 being high grade. It uses the combined grades of the most prominent and second most prominent patterns in a biopsy as the final score. A Gleason score of 6 or greater has malignant potential [82]. Lay et al.'s random forest technique yielded an area under the curve (AUC) score of 0.93 [81]; AUC is a measurement for binary classification and ranges from 0 to 1. Therefore, this study demonstrates that the ML model can detect lesions with high accuracy.

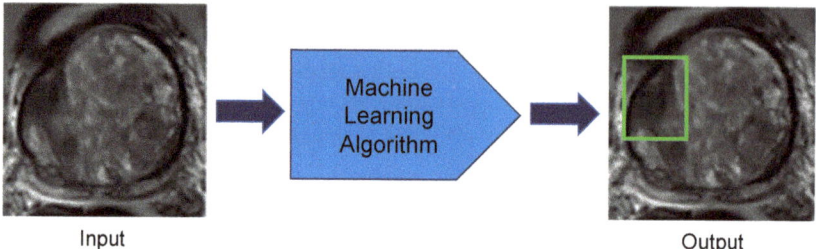

Figure 4. Prostate lesion detection using machine learning methods. The computer takes multiparametric magnetic resonance imaging images of the prostate as inputs and applies the developed machine learning algorithm to correctly localize lesions in the prostate.

Table 2. Machine learning techniques applied to prostate lesion detection.

Reference	Year	ML Algorithm	Patients	Lesions	AUC	Modalities
Lay et al. [81]	2017	Random Forest. Features: Intensity, Haralick texture	224	410	0.93	T2W, ADC, DWI
Sumathipala et al. [83]	2018	CNN: Holistically Nested Edge Detection	186	N/A	0.93	T2W, ADC, DWI
Xu et al. [84]	2019	CNN: ResNet	346	N/A	0.97	T2W, ADC, DWI
Tsehay et al. [85]	2017	CNN, 5 Layers	52	125	0.90	T2W, ADC, DWI

DL techniques have also been applied to prostate lesion detection (Table 2). Xu et al. [84] implemented a type of neural network with extensive layers, ResNet [86], to find lesions on T2-weighted, ADC, and DWI images. This study used images from the Cancer Imaging Archive data portal and included 346 patients. They achieved an AUC of 0.97 [84]. Tsehay et al. [85] also used a DL algorithm with a 5-layer CNN architecture that used an individual loss function for each layer. The CNN was trained and validated on a dataset of 39 benign lesions and 86 lesions with a Gleason 6 or higher [85]. Tsehay's group achieved an impressive AUC of 0.90 [85], which demonstrates high accuracy of prostate lesion detection. All four studies in Table 2 used radiologists for labeling the ground truth [81,83–85].

Although prostate lesion detection has been implemented with ML, automated prostate lesion segmentation and volume approximation remain largely unsolved (Figure 5). Few studies have attempted this task due to a dearth of well-curated data and its technical requirements. One obstacle for prostate lesion segmentation is a lack of guidelines across institutions for prostate lesion contours, which results in significant inter-observer variability [19,80]. Despite the lack of standardization, three studies have attempted prostate lesion segmentation (Table 3). A study by Liu et al. [87] used fuzzy Markov random fields to achieve a Dice score of 0.62 with 11 patients. Two other groups, Kohl et al. [88] and Dai et al. [89], both employed DL algorithms and used U-Net and Mask R-CNN, respectively. Kohl's group used a dataset of 152 patients and implemented U-Net combined with an adversarial network. Their architecture resulted in an average Dice score for prostate lesion segmentation of 0.41 [88]. Dai's group used a highly specialized DL algorithm, Mask R-CNN, and trained with 63 patients to achieve a prostate lesion Dice score of 0.46 [89]. To label the ground truth, Dai et al. [89] used a clinician, Kohl et al. [88] used a radiologist, and Liu et al. [87] used a pathologist. These studies' lower Dice scores demonstrate that the current techniques have limited precision. These studies show that prostate lesion segmentation and volume estimation remain challenging. A bigger dataset with more uniform labeling would permit the development of more ML models geared toward these tasks.

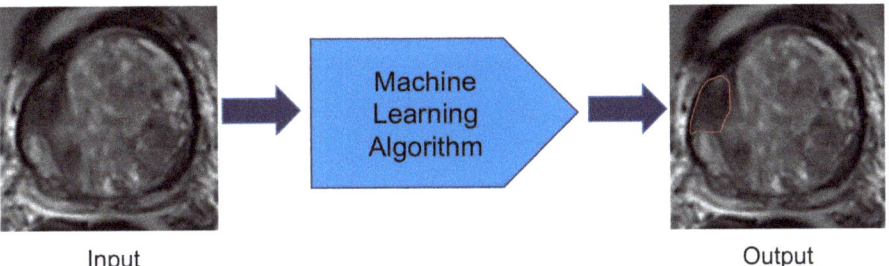

Figure 5. Prostate lesion segmentation using machine learning techniques. The computer takes multiparametric magnetic resonance imaging images of the prostate as inputs and applies the developed machine learning algorithm to correctly identify the borders of the lesion.

Table 3. Machine learning techniques applied to prostate lesion segmentation.

Reference	Year	ML Algorithm	Patients	Dice	Modalities
Dai et al. [89]	2019	CNN: Mask R-CNN	63	0.46	T2W, ADC
Kohl et al. [88]	2017	Adversarial Network and CNN: U-Net	152	0.41	T2W, ADC, DWI
Liu et al. [87]	2009	Fuzzy Markov Random Fields	11	0.62	T2W, quantitative T2, DWI, DCE

6. Prostate Lesion: Characterization

Although prostate lesions have been increasingly imaged with mpMRI since 2013 [4], their characterization has been hindered by the variability in classification conventions across different radiologists and institutions [4,47,90]. To establish better standardization, the PI-RADS scoring system was created in 2012, with an updated version PI-RADS v2 released in 2015, and the newest version PI-RADS v2.1 released in 2019 [53,54,91]. Since their conception, multiple studies have attempted to elucidate the clinical utility of PI-RADS, PI-RADS v2, and PI-RADS v2.1. Challenges to its broader acceptance include inter-reader agreement, radiologist experience, and the substantial interpretation time of images [4,47,90]. This need for more consistent lesion characterization makes ML an attractive method for accurate, quick classification.

ML algorithms can augment the PI-RADS scoring system as well as independently classify lesions (Table 4). Regarding PI-RADS, Litjens et al. [92] created a CAD system that applied a random forest for characterizing prostate lesions on a scale of suspicion for malignancy. After combining the ML generated scores and the radiologist provided PI-RADS scores on a dataset of 107 patients, the overall AUC was greater than either the ML generated scores or the PI-RADS scores [92]. Similarly, Wang, J. et al. [93], who used 54 patients in their dataset, also concluded that a support vector machine (SVM) algorithm enhanced the PI-RADS performance of radiologists. Song et al. [94] opted to use a DL algorithm based off of VGG-Net, a deep CNN, as a tool for improving PI-RADS scores assigned by radiologists. Song's group gathered data from 195 patients and also observed that their AUC improved when radiologists' decisions were combined with the VGG-Net [94].

Table 4. Machine-learning techniques applied to prostate lesion characterization.

Reference	Year	Algorithm	Patients	Lesions	AUC	Modalities
Litjens et al. [92]	2015	Random Forest. Features: Intensity, Position, Pharmacokinetic, Texture, Spatial Filter	107	141	Benign vs. Cancer; AUC increased from 0.81 to 0.88 with their ML tool Indolent vs. Aggressive; AUC increased from 0.78 to 0.88 with their ML tool	T2W, DCE, DWI
Wang, J. et al. [93]	2017	SVM. Features: Volumetric Radiomics	54	149	0.95	T2W, DWI
Song et al. [94]	2018	CNN: Deep CNN and Augmentation	195	547	0.94	T2W, ADC, DWI
Kwak et al. [95]	2015	SVM. Features: Texture	244	479	0.89	T2W, DWI
Wang, Z. et al. [96]	2018	CNN: Deep CNN	360	600	0.96	T2W, ADC
Seah et al. [97]	2017	CNN: Deep CNN	346	538	0.84	T2W, ADC, DCE
Liu et al. [98]	2017	CNN: XmasNet	341	538	0.84	T2W, ADC, DWI, Ktrans
Mehrtash et al. [99]	2017	CNN: 3D Implementation	344	538	0.80	ADC, DWI, DCE
Chen et al. [100]	2019	Two CNNs: Inception V3 and VGG-16	Training Data: 204 Test Data: N/A	538	Inception V3, 0.81 VGG-16, 0.83	T2W, DWI, DCE

In addition to bolstering lesion classification by radiologists, ML algorithms have been trained to characterize prostate lesions independently (Figure 6, Table 4). Many studies explored this task with the PROSTATEx challenge dataset that was released in 2017 [101]. The PROSTATEx dataset was gathered from 344 patients and contained segmented lesions along with their respective pathology-defined Gleason scores [101]. From this public database, Wang, Z. et al. [96] achieved an AUC of 0.96 by running two CNNs in parallel. Both Seah et al. [97] and Liu et al. [98] obtained an AUC of 0.84 by using deep layered CNNs. Mehrtash et al. [99] implemented a 3D CNN to reach an AUC of 0.80. One study by Kwak et al. [95] used its own proprietary dataset to implement an SVM that trained on T2-weighted and DWI images to characterize prostate lesions. In this study, 244 patients were used for a total of 333 benign and 146 malignant lesions [95]. The SVM method used discriminative features in training that resulted in an AUC score of 0.89 [95]. All of the studies listed in Table 4 used radiologists to determine their ground truth [77,92–95,97–100]. These studies highlight the ability of DL algorithms to predict the likelihood of a lesion's malignancy based upon Gleason scores.

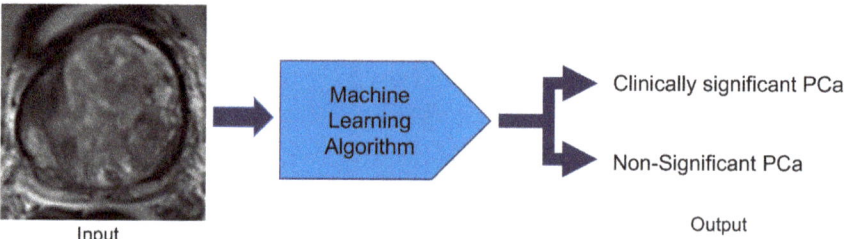

Figure 6. Prostate lesion characterization using machine-learning techniques. The computer receives multiparametric magnetic imaging images of prostate lesions and applies the developed machine learning algorithm to categorize the lesion as clinically significant prostate cancer or non-significant prostate cancer.

7. Future Work

The potential applications of ML to PCa surpass volume estimation, lesion detection, and lesion characterization. Further developments in prostate lesion classification may lead to a more practical clinical use, include training ML algorithms for tumor grade prediction. In addition to analyzing data solely from images, ML could augment the clinical management of PCa by incorporating demographic and biochemical data. ML could enable clinicians to make more assured decisions regarding the need for biopsy, medication dosing, and cancer recurrence. Biopsies that are performed for diagnosing PCa could be rendered unnecessary with a ML tool. Two studies by Hu et al. [102] and Chen et al. [103] used data such as age, digital rectal exam findings, PSA, and prostate volume for biopsy prediction. These studies made accurate PCa diagnoses and showed the potential for ML to eliminate the need for biopsy. In addition to diagnosis, ML could impact PCa medication dosing in PCa management. Radiation therapy requires accurate dosing, which is frequently operator dependent [104]. By minimizing operator dependency, ML could offer better standardization leading to more precise dosing. Nicola et al. [105] employed ML to predict prostate brachytherapy dosing by analyzing images and prior treatment plans from other patients. This study showed that ML implementation was comparable to brachytherapists and could be advanced by using a DL instead of a traditional ML algorithm. Along with diagnosis and dosing, ML could be used for predicting cancer recurrence after prostatectomy. Two studies by Wong et al. [106] and Cordon et al. [107] gathered data such as Gleason score, PSA, seminal vesical invasion, and surgical margins to predict recurrence after prostatectomy. The accuracy of these studies could be increased by adding postoperative imaging data for improved recurrence prediction.

8. Conclusions

AI applications in prostate mpMRI are promising tools for more effective and efficient image interpretation, leading to improved care. In pure image interpretation, ML has shown noteworthy progress in prostate organ segmentation and volume estimation. As better-curated data becomes available for prostate lesions, ML will likely become more successful at lesion detection, volume estimation, and characterization. As ML evolves, it will indisputably change radiologists' workflow by performing many of the simple tasks in image interpretation. However, ML will not replace the role of radiologists, who are critical to solving complex clinical problems [104]. AI is poised to enhance the decisions made by radiologists. It will enable radiologists to better care for their patients rather than supersede the need for radiologists.

Similarly, ML's ability to evaluate complex datasets across different domains suggests this technique may facilitate the bridging of advanced imaging, such as mpMRI, with emerging biomarker analysis or tumor genetics. Thus, ML may form the underpinnings of radiogenomics, allowing for the integration of imaging data, blood chemistry analysis, and pathologic evaluation in forming complex models that can predict treatment response. Enabled by larger datasets and more sophisticated mathematical techniques, ML could progress to creating completely automated tools that receive a patient's prostate mpMRI images and then delineate a range of desired features, as well as giving likelihood metrics for an array of pathologies.

Funding: This review was partially funded by the Radiological Society of North America Medical Student Research Grant RMS1902 and the Alpha Omega Alpha Carolyn L. Kuckein Student Research Fellowship.

Conflicts of Interest: Author Peter D. Chang, MD, is a co-founder and shareholder of Avicenna.ai, a medical imaging startup. Author Daniel S. Chow, MD, is a shareholder of Avicenna.ai, a medical imaging startup, and a grant recipient from Cannon Inc. The other authors declare no conflicts of interest. The funders had no role in the design of the study; in the collection, analyses, or interpretation of data; in the writing of the manuscript, or in the decision to publish the results.

References

1. Siegel, R.L.; Miller, K.D.; Jemal, A. Cancer statistics, 2017. *CA Cancer J. Clin.* **2017**, *67*, 7–30. [CrossRef] [PubMed]
2. Hugosson, J.; Carlsson, S. Overdetection in screening for prostate cancer. *Curr. Opin. Urol.* **2014**, *24*, 256–263. [CrossRef] [PubMed]
3. Schröder, F.H.; Hugosson, J.; Roobol, M.J.; Tammela, T.L.; Ciatto, S.; Nelen, V.; Kwiatkowski, M.; Lujan, M.; Lilja, H.; Zappa, M.; et al. Screening and prostate-cancer mortality in a randomized European study. *N. Engl. J. Med.* **2009**, *360*, 1320–1328. [CrossRef] [PubMed]
4. Oberlin, D.T.; Casalino, D.D.; Miller, F.H.; Meeks, J.J. Dramatic increase in the utilization of multiparametric magnetic resonance imaging for detection and management of prostate cancer. *Abdom. Radiol. (Ny)* **2017**, *42*, 1255–1258. [CrossRef] [PubMed]
5. Monni, F.; Fontanella, P.; Grasso, A.; Wiklund, P.; Ou, Y.C.; Randazzo, M.; Rocco, B.; Montanari, E.; Bianchi, G. Magnetic resonance imaging in prostate cancer detection and management: A systematic review. *Minerva. Urol. Nefrol.* **2017**, *69*, 567–578. [CrossRef] [PubMed]
6. Uzzo, R.G.; Wei, J.T.; Waldbaum, R.S.; Perlmutter, A.P.; Byrne, J.C.; Vaughan, D., Jr. The influence of prostate size on cancer detection. *Urology* **1995**, *46*, 831–836. [CrossRef]
7. Boyle, P.; Gould, A.L.; Roehrborn, C.G. Prostate volume predicts outcome of treatment of benign prostatic hyperplasia with finasteride: Meta-analysis of randomized clinical trials. *Urology* **1996**, *48*, 398–405. [CrossRef]
8. Sparks, R.; Bloch, B.N.; Feleppa, E.; Barratt, D.; Madabhushi, A. Fully automated prostate magnetic resonance imaging and transrectal ultrasound fusion via a probabilistic registration metric. *Proc. SPIE Int. Soc. Opt. Eng.* **2013**, *8671*. [CrossRef]
9. Tay, K.J.; Gupta, R.T.; Rastinehad, A.R.; Tsivian, E.; Freedland, S.J.; Moul, J.W.; Polascik, T.J. Navigating MRI-TRUS fusion biopsy: Optimizing the process and avoiding technical pitfalls. *Expert Rev. Anticancer Ther.* **2016**, *16*, 303–311. [CrossRef]
10. Lim, K.B. Epidemiology of clinical benign prostatic hyperplasia. *Asian J. Urol.* **2017**, *4*, 148–151. [CrossRef]
11. Garvey, B.; Türkbey, B.; Truong, H.; Bernardo, M.; Periaswamy, S.; Choyke, P.L. Clinical value of prostate segmentation and volume determination on MRI in benign prostatic hyperplasia. *Diagn. Interv. Radiol.* **2014**, *20*, 229. [CrossRef] [PubMed]
12. Kolman, C.; Girman, C.J.; Jacobsen, S.J.; Lieber, M.M. Distribution of post-void residual urine volume in randomly selected men. *J. Urol.* **1999**, *161*, 122–127. [CrossRef]
13. Girman, C.J.; Jacobsen, S.J.; Guess, H.A.; Oesterling, J.E.; Chute, C.G.; Panser, L.A.; Lieber, M.M. Natural history of prostatism: Relationship among symptoms, prostate volume and peak urinary flow rate. *J. Urol.* **1995**, *153*, 1510–1515. [CrossRef]
14. Oelke, M.; Bachmann, A.; Descazeaud, A.; Emberton, M.; Gravas, S.; Michel, M.C.; N'dow, J.; Nordling, J.; Jean, J. EAU guidelines on the treatment and follow-up of non-neurogenic male lower urinary tract symptoms including benign prostatic obstruction. *Eur. Urol.* **2013**, *64*, 118–140. [CrossRef] [PubMed]
15. Bretton, P.R.; Evans, W.P.; Borden, J.D.; Castellanos, R.D. The use of prostate specific antigen density to improve the sensitivity of prostate specific antigen in detecting prostate carcinoma. *Cancer Interdiscip. Int. J. Am. Cancer Soc.* **1994**, *74*, 2991–2995. [CrossRef]
16. Benson, M.C.; Seong Whang, I.; Pantuck, A.; Ring, K.; Kaplan, S.A.; Olsson, C.A.; Cooner, W.H. Prostate specific antigen density: A means of distinguishing benign prostatic hypertrophy and prostate cancer. *J. Urol.* **1992**, *147*, 815–816. [CrossRef]
17. Sfoungaristos, S.; Perimenis, P. PSA density is superior than PSA and Gleason score for adverse pathologic features prediction in patients with clinically localized prostate cancer. *Can. Urol. Assoc. J.* **2012**, *6*, 46. [CrossRef]
18. May, M.; Siegsmund, M.; Hammermann, F.; Loy, V.; Gunia, S. Visual estimation of the tumor volume in prostate cancer: A useful means for predicting biochemical-free survival after radical prostatectomy? *Prostate Cancer Prostatic Dis.* **2007**, *10*, 66. [CrossRef]
19. Steenbergen, P.; Haustermans, K.; Lerut, E.; Oyen, R.; De Wever, L.; Van den Bergh, L.; Kerkmeijer, L.G.; Pameijer, F.A.; Veldhuis, W.B.; Pos, F.J. Prostate tumor delineation using multiparametric magnetic resonance imaging: Inter-observer variability and pathology validation. *Radiother. Oncol.* **2015**, *115*, 186–190. [CrossRef]

20. Njeh, C. Tumor delineation: The weakest link in the search for accuracy in radiotherapy. *J. Med. Phys./Assoc. Med. Phys. India* **2008**, *33*, 136. [CrossRef]
21. Denis, L.J.; Murphy, G.P.; Schroder, F.H. Report of the consensus workshop on screening and global strategy for prostate cancer. *Cancer* **1995**, *75*, 1187–1207. [CrossRef]
22. Edwards, B.K.; Ward, E.; Kohler, B.A.; Eheman, C.; Zauber, A.G.; Anderson, R.N.; Jemal, A.; Schymura, M.J.; Lansdorp-Vogelaar, I.; Seeff, L.C.; et al. Annual report to the nation on the status of cancer, 1975-2006, featuring colorectal cancer trends and impact of interventions (risk factors, screening, and treatment) to reduce future rates. *Cancer* **2010**, *116*, 544–573. [CrossRef] [PubMed]
23. Etzioni, R.; Tsodikov, A.; Mariotto, A.; Szabo, A.; Falcon, S.; Wegelin, J.; DiTommaso, D.; Karnofski, K.; Gulati, R.; Penson, D.F.; et al. Quantifying the role of PSA screening in the US prostate cancer mortality decline. *Cancer Causes Control.* **2008**, *19*, 175–181. [CrossRef] [PubMed]
24. Lahdensuo, K.; Erickson, A.; Saarinen, I.; Seikkula, H.; Lundin, J.; Lundin, M.; Nordling, S.; Bützow, A.; Vasarainen, H.; Bostrom, P.J.; et al. Loss of PTEN expression in ERG-negative prostate cancer predicts secondary therapies and leads to shorter disease-specific survival time after radical prostatectomy. *Mod. Pathol.* **2016**, *29*, 1565–1574. [CrossRef]
25. Rothwax, J.T.; George, A.K.; Wood, B.J.; Pinto, P.A. Multiparametric MRI in biopsy guidance for prostate cancer: Fusion-guided. *Biomed. Res. Int.* **2014**, *2014*, 439171. [CrossRef]
26. Lips, I.M.; van der Heide, U.A.; Haustermans, K.; van Lin, E.N.; Pos, F.; Franken, S.P.; Kotte, A.N.; van Gils, C.H.; van Vulpen, M. Single blind randomized phase III trial to investigate the benefit of a focal lesion ablative microboost in prostate cancer (FLAME-trial): Study protocol for a randomized controlled trial. *Trials* **2011**, *12*, 255. [CrossRef]
27. Cellini, N.; Morganti, A.G.; Mattiucci, G.C.; Valentini, V.; Leone, M.; Luzi, S.; Manfredi, R.; Dinapoli, N.; Digesu', C.; Smaniotto, D. Analysis of intraprostatic failures in patients treated with hormonal therapy and radiotherapy: Implications for conformal therapy planning. *Int. J. Radiat. Oncol. Biol. Phys.* **2002**, *53*, 595–599. [CrossRef]
28. Chun, F.K.-H.; Briganti, A.; Jeldres, C.; Gallina, A.; Erbersdobler, A.; Schlomm, T.; Walz, J.; Eichelberg, C.; Salomon, G.; Haese, A. Tumour volume and high grade tumour volume are the best predictors of pathologic stage and biochemical recurrence after radical prostatectomy. *Eur. J. Cancer* **2007**, *43*, 536–543. [CrossRef]
29. Chung, B.I.; Tarin, T.V.; Ferrari, M.; Brooks, J.D. Comparison of prostate cancer tumor volume and percent cancer in prediction of biochemical recurrence and cancer specific survival. *Urol. Oncol.* **2011**, *29*, 314–318. [CrossRef]
30. Nelson, B.A.; Shappell, S.B.; Chang, S.S.; Wells, N.; Farnham, S.B.; Smith, J.A., Jr.; Cookson, M.S. Tumour volume is an independent predictor of prostate-specific antigen recurrence in patients undergoing radical prostatectomy for clinically localized prostate cancer. *BJU Int.* **2006**, *97*, 1169–1172. [CrossRef]
31. Fukuhara, H.; Kume, H.; Suzuki, M.; Fujimura, T.; Enomoto, Y.; Nishimatsu, H.; Ishikawa, A.; Homma, Y. Maximum tumor diameter: A simple independent predictor for biochemical recurrence after radical prostatectomy. *Prostate Cancer Prostatic Dis.* **2010**, *13*, 244. [CrossRef] [PubMed]
32. Stephenson, A.J.; Scardino, P.T.; Kattan, M.W.; Pisansky, T.M.; Slawin, K.M.; Klein, E.A.; Anscher, M.S.; Michalski, J.M.; Sandler, H.M.; Lin, D.W. Predicting the outcome of salvage radiation therapy for recurrent prostate cancer after radical prostatectomy. *J. Clin. Oncol. Off. J. Am. Soc. Clin. Oncol.* **2007**, *25*, 2035. [CrossRef] [PubMed]
33. Bjurlin, M.A.; Taneja, S.S. Standards for prostate biopsy. *Curr. Opin. Urol.* **2014**, *24*, 155–161. [CrossRef] [PubMed]
34. Borghesi, M.; Ahmed, H.; Nam, R.; Schaeffer, E.; Schiavina, R.; Taneja, S.; Weidner, W.; Loeb, S. Complications After Systematic, Random, and Image-guided Prostate Biopsy. *Eur. Urol.* **2017**, *71*, 353–365. [CrossRef] [PubMed]
35. Walsh, P.C.; Marschke, P.; Ricker, D.; Burnett, A.L. Patient-reported urinary continence and sexual function after anatomic radical prostatectomy. *Urology* **2000**, *55*, 58–61. [CrossRef]
36. Hu, K.; Wallner, K. Clinical course of rectal bleeding following I-125 prostate brachytherapy. *Int. J. Radiat. Oncol. Biol. Phys.* **1998**, *41*, 263–265. [CrossRef]
37. Theodorescu, D.; Gillenwater, J.Y.; Koutrouvelis, P.G. Prostatourethral-rectal fistula after prostate brachytherapy: Incidence and risk factors. *Cancer Interdiscip. Int. J. Am. Cancer Soc.* **2000**, *89*, 2085–2091. [CrossRef]

38. Shaver, M.M.; Kohanteb, P.A.; Chiou, C.; Bardis, M.D.; Chantaduly, C.; Bota, D.; Filippi, C.G.; Weinberg, B.; Grinband, J.; Chow, D.S. Optimizing neuro-oncology imaging: A review of deep learning approaches for glioma imaging. *Cancers* **2019**, *11*, 829. [CrossRef]
39. Jordan, M.I.; Mitchell, T.M. Machine learning: Trends, perspectives, and prospects. *Science* **2015**, *349*, 255–260. [CrossRef]
40. Johnson, L.M.; Turkbey, B.; Figg, W.D.; Choyke, P.L. Multiparametric MRI in prostate cancer management. *Nat. Rev. Clin. Oncol.* **2014**, *11*, 346–353. [CrossRef]
41. Stabile, A.; Giganti, F.; Rosenkrantz, A.B.; Taneja, S.S.; Villeirs, G.; Gill, I.S.; Allen, C.; Emberton, M.; Moore, C.M.; Kasivisvanathan, V. Multiparametric MRI for prostate cancer diagnosis: Current status and future directions. *Nat. Rev. Urol.* **2020**, *17*, 41–61. [CrossRef] [PubMed]
42. Dickinson, L.; Ahmed, H.U.; Allen, C.; Barentsz, J.O.; Carey, B.; Futterer, J.J.; Heijmink, S.W.; Hoskin, P.J.; Kirkham, A.; Padhani, A.R.; et al. Magnetic resonance imaging for the detection, localisation, and characterisation of prostate cancer: Recommendations from a European consensus meeting. *Eur. Urol.* **2011**, *59*, 477–494. [CrossRef] [PubMed]
43. De Rooij, M.; Hamoen, E.H.; Futterer, J.J.; Barentsz, J.O.; Rovers, M.M. Accuracy of multiparametric MRI for prostate cancer detection: A meta-analysis. *AJR Am. J. Roentgenol.* **2014**, *202*, 343–351. [CrossRef] [PubMed]
44. Fütterer, J.J.; Briganti, A.; De Visschere, P.; Emberton, M.; Giannarini, G.; Kirkham, A.; Taneja, S.S.; Thoeny, H.; Villeirs, G.; Villers, A. Can clinically significant prostate cancer be detected with multiparametric magnetic resonance imaging? A systematic review of the literature. *Eur. Urol.* **2015**, *68*, 1045–1053. [CrossRef] [PubMed]
45. Daun, M.; Fardin, S.; Ushinsky, A.; Batra, S.; Nguyentat, M.; Lee, T.; Uchio, E.; Lall, C.; Houshyar, R. PI-RADS version 2 is an excellent screening tool for clinically significant prostate cancer as designated by the validated international society of urological pathology criteria: A retrospective analysis. *Curr. Probl. Diagn. Radiol.* **2019**. [CrossRef]
46. Turkbey, B.; Mani, H.; Shah, V.; Rastinehad, A.R.; Bernardo, M.; Pohida, T.; Pang, Y.; Daar, D.; Benjamin, C.; McKinney, Y.L.; et al. Multiparametric 3T prostate magnetic resonance imaging to detect cancer: Histopathological correlation using prostatectomy specimens processed in customized magnetic resonance imaging based molds. *J. Urol.* **2011**, *186*, 1818–1824. [CrossRef]
47. Leake, J.L.; Hardman, R.; Ojili, V.; Thompson, I.; Shanbhogue, A.; Hernandez, J.; Barentsz, J. Prostate MRI: Access to and current practice of prostate MRI in the United States. *J. Am. Coll. Radiol.* **2014**, *11*, 156–160. [CrossRef]
48. Latchamsetty, K.C.; Borden, L.S., Jr.; Porter, C.R.; Lacrampe, M.; Vaughan, M.; Lin, E.; Conti, N.; Wright, J.L.; Corman, J.M. Experience improves staging accuracy of endorectal magnetic resonance imaging in prostate cancer: What is the learning curve? *Can. J. Urol.* **2007**, *14*, 3429–3434.
49. Gaziev, G.; Wadhwa, K.; Barrett, T.; Koo, B.C.; Gallagher, F.A.; Serrao, E.; Frey, J.; Seidenader, J.; Carmona, L.; Warren, A.; et al. Defining the learning curve for multiparametric magnetic resonance imaging (MRI) of the prostate using MRI-transrectal ultrasonography (TRUS) fusion-guided transperineal prostate biopsies as a validation tool. *BJU Int.* **2016**, *117*, 80–86. [CrossRef]
50. Rosenkrantz, A.B.; Babb, J.S.; Taneja, S.S.; Ream, J.M. Proposed adjustments to PI-RADS Version 2 decision rules: Impact on prostate cancer detection. *Radiology* **2017**, *283*, 119–129. [CrossRef]
51. De Visschere, P.J.; Vral, A.; Perletti, G.; Pattyn, E.; Praet, M.; Magri, V.; Villeirs, G.M. Multiparametric magnetic resonance imaging characteristics of normal, benign and malignant conditions in the prostate. *Eur. Radiol.* **2017**, *27*, 2095–2109. [CrossRef] [PubMed]
52. Barentsz, J.O.; Richenberg, J.; Clements, R.; Choyke, P.; Verma, S.; Villeirs, G.; Rouviere, O.; Logager, V.; Futterer, J.J.; European Society of Urogenital, R. ESUR prostate MR guidelines 2012. *Eur. Radiol.* **2012**, *22*, 746–757. [CrossRef] [PubMed]
53. Weinreb, J.C.; Barentsz, J.O.; Choyke, P.L.; Cornud, F.; Haider, M.A.; Macura, K.J.; Margolis, D.; Schnall, M.D.; Shtern, F.; Tempany, C.M.; et al. PI-RADS Prostate imaging—Reporting and data system: 2015, version 2. *Eur. Urol.* **2016**, *69*, 16–40. [CrossRef] [PubMed]
54. Turkbey, B.; Rosenkrantz, A.B.; Haider, M.A.; Padhani, A.R.; Villeirs, G.; Macura, K.J.; Tempany, C.M.; Choyke, P.L.; Cornud, F.; Margolis, D.J.; et al. Prostate imaging reporting and data system version 2.1: 2019 update of prostate imaging reporting and data system version 2. *Eur. Urol.* **2019**, *76*, 340–351. [CrossRef] [PubMed]

55. Stonier, T. The evolution of machine intelligence. In *Beyond Information: The Natural History of Intelligence*; Springer: London, UK, 1992; pp. 107–133. [CrossRef]
56. Poole, D.; Mackworth, A.; Goebel, R. *Computational Intelligence*; Oxford University Press: Oxford, UK, 1998; Volume 1.
57. Goodfellow, I.; Bengio, Y.; Courville, A. *Deep Learning*; MIT Press: Cambridge, MA, USA, 2016.
58. Krizhevsky, A.; Sutskever, I.; Hinton, G.E. Imagenet classification with deep convolutional neural networks. In Proceedings of the Advances in Neural information Processing Systems, Lake Tahoe, NV, USA, 3–6 December 2012; pp. 1097–1105.
59. LeCun, Y.; Bengio, Y.; Hinton, G. Deep learning. *Nature* **2015**, *521*, 436. [CrossRef] [PubMed]
60. Ueda, D.; Shimazaki, A.; Miki, Y. Technical and clinical overview of deep learning in radiology. *Jpn. J. Radiol.* **2019**, *37*, 15–33. [CrossRef] [PubMed]
61. Ghose, S.; Oliver, A.; Martí, R.; Lladó, X.; Vilanova, J.C.; Freixenet, J.; Mitra, J.; Sidibé, D.; Meriaudeau, F. A survey of prostate segmentation methodologies in ultrasound, magnetic resonance and computed tomography images. *Comput. Methods Prog. Biomed.* **2012**, *108*, 262–287. [CrossRef] [PubMed]
62. Rasch, C.; Barillot, I.; Remeijer, P.; Touw, A.; van Herk, M.; Lebesque, J.V. Definition of the prostate in CT and MRI: A multi-observer study. *Int. J. Radiat. Oncol. Biol. Phys.* **1999**, *43*, 57–66. [CrossRef]
63. Kachouie, N.N.; Fieguth, P.; Rahnamayan, S. An elliptical level set method for automatic TRUS prostate image segmentation. In Proceedings of the 2006 IEEE International Symposium on Signal Processing and Information Technology, Vancouver, BC, Canada, 27–30 August 2006; pp. 191–196.
64. Ko, J.S.; Landis, P.; Carter, H.B.; Partin, A.W. Effect of intra-observer variation in prostate volume measurement on prostate-specific antigen density calculations among prostate cancer active surveillance participants. *BJU Int.* **2011**, *108*, 1739–1742. [CrossRef]
65. Dianat, S.S.; Ruiz, R.M.R.; Bonekamp, D.; Carter, H.B.; Macura, K.J. Prostate volumetric assessment by magnetic resonance imaging and transrectal ultrasound: Impact of variation in calculated prostate-specific antigen density on patient eligibility for active surveillance program. *J. Comput. Assist. Tomogr.* **2013**, *37*, 589–595. [CrossRef]
66. Bezinque, A.; Moriarity, A.; Farrell, C.; Peabody, H.; Noyes, S.L.; Lane, B.R. Determination of prostate volume: A comparison of contemporary methods. *Acad. Radiol.* **2018**, *25*, 1582–1587. [CrossRef] [PubMed]
67. Rundo, L.; Militello, C.; Russo, G.; Garufi, A.; Vitabile, S.; Gilardi, M.C.; Mauri, G. Automated prostate gland segmentation based on an unsupervised fuzzy C-means clustering technique using multispectral T1w and T2w MR imaging. *Information* **2017**, *8*, 49. [CrossRef]
68. Zou, K.H.; Warfield, S.K.; Bharatha, A.; Tempany, C.M.; Kaus, M.R.; Haker, S.J.; Wells III, W.M.; Jolesz, F.A.; Kikinis, R. Statistical validation of image segmentation quality based on a spatial overlap index1: Scientific reports. *Acad. Radiol.* **2004**, *11*, 178–189. [CrossRef]
69. Litjens, G.; Toth, R.; van de Ven, W.; Hoeks, C.; Kerkstra, S.; van Ginneken, B.; Vincent, G.; Guillard, G.; Birbeck, N.; Zhang, J.; et al. Evaluation of prostate segmentation algorithms for MRI: The PROMISE12 challenge. *Med. Image Anal.* **2014**, *18*, 359–373. [CrossRef] [PubMed]
70. Karimi, D.; Samei, G.; Kesch, C.; Nir, G.; Salcudean, S.E. Prostate segmentation in MRI using a convolutional neural network architecture and training strategy based on statistical shape models. *Int. J. Comput. Assist. Radiol. Surg.* **2018**. [CrossRef] [PubMed]
71. Tian, Z.; Liu, L.; Zhang, Z.; Fei, B. PSNet: Prostate segmentation on MRI based on a convolutional neural network. *J. Med. Imaging* **2018**, *5*, 021208. [CrossRef]
72. Ronneberger, O.; Fischer, P.; Brox, T. U-net: Convolutional networks for biomedical image segmentation. In Proceedings of the 2015 International Conference on Medical Image Computing and Computer-Assisted Intervention, Munich, Germany, 5–9 October 2015; pp. 234–241.
73. Clark, T.; Wong, A.; Haider, M.A.; Khalvati, F. *Fully Deep Convolutional Neural Networks for Segmentation of the Prostate Gland in Diffusion-Weighted MR Images*; Springer: Cham, Switzerland, 2017; pp. 97–104.
74. Zhu, Y.; Wei, R.; Gao, G.; Ding, L.; Zhang, X.; Wang, X.; Zhang, J. Fully automatic segmentation on prostate MR images based on cascaded fully convolution network. *J. Magn. Reson. Imaging* **2018**, *49*, 1149–1156. [CrossRef]
75. Zhu, Q.; Du, B.; Turkbey, B.; Choyke, P.L.; Yan, P. Deeply-supervised CNN for prostate segmentation. In Proceedings of the 2017 International Joint Conference on Neural Networks (IJCNN), Anchorage, AK, USA, 14–19 May 2017; pp. 178–184.

76. Milletari, F.; Navab, N.; Ahmadi, S.-A. V-net: Fully convolutional neural networks for volumetric medical image segmentation. In Proceedings of the 2016 Fourth International Conference on 3D Vision (3DV), Stanford, CA, USA, 25–28 October 2016; pp. 565–571.
77. Wang, B.; Lei, Y.; Tian, S.; Wang, T.; Liu, Y.; Patel, P.; Jani, A.B.; Mao, H.; Curran, W.J.; Liu, T.; et al. Deeply supervised 3D fully convolutional networks with group dilated convolution for automatic MRI prostate segmentation. *Med. Phys.* **2019**, *46*, 1707–1718. [CrossRef]
78. Cheng, R.; Roth, H.R.; Lu, L.; Wang, S.; Turkbey, B.; Gandler, W.; McCreedy, E.S.; Agarwal, H.K.; Choyke, P.; Summers, R.M. Active appearance model and deep learning for more accurate prostate segmentation on MRI. In Proceedings of the Medical Imaging 2016: Image Processing, San Diego, CA, USA, 27 February–3 March 2016; p. 97842I.
79. Le Nobin, J.; Orczyk, C.; Deng, F.M.; Melamed, J.; Rusinek, H.; Taneja, S.S.; Rosenkrantz, A.B. Prostate tumour volumes: Evaluation of the agreement between magnetic resonance imaging and histology using novel co-registration software. *BJU Int.* **2014**, *114*, E105–E112. [CrossRef]
80. Van Schie, M.A.; Dinh, C.V.; van Houdt, P.J.; Pos, F.J.; Heijmink, S.W.; Kerkmeijer, L.G.; Kotte, A.N.; Oyen, R.; Haustermans, K.; van der Heide, U.A. Contouring of prostate tumors on multiparametric MRI: Evaluation of clinical delineations in a multicenter radiotherapy trial. *Radiother. Oncol.* **2018**, *128*, 321–326. [CrossRef]
81. Lay, N.; Tsehay, Y.; Greer, M.D.; Turkbey, B.; Kwak, J.T.; Choyke, P.L.; Pinto, P.; Wood, B.J.; Summers, R.M. Detection of prostate cancer in multiparametric MRI using random forest with instance weighting. *J. Med. Imaging (Bellingham)* **2017**, *4*, 024506. [CrossRef] [PubMed]
82. Epstein, J.I.; Zelefsky, M.J.; Sjoberg, D.D.; Nelson, J.B.; Egevad, L.; Magi-Galluzzi, C.; Vickers, A.J.; Parwani, A.V.; Reuter, V.E.; Fine, S.W. A contemporary prostate cancer grading system: A validated alternative to the Gleason score. *Eur. Urol.* **2016**, *69*, 428–435. [CrossRef] [PubMed]
83. Sumathipala, Y.; Lay, N.; Turkbey, B.; Smith, C.; Choyke, P.L.; Summers, R.M. Prostate cancer detection from multi-institution multiparametric MRIs using deep convolutional neural networks. *J. Med. Imaging* **2018**, *5*, 044507. [CrossRef] [PubMed]
84. Xu, H.; Baxter, J.S.; Akin, O.; Cantor-Rivera, D. Prostate cancer detection using residual networks. *Int. J. Comput. Assist. Radiol. Surg.* **2019**, *14*, 1647–1650. [CrossRef]
85. Tsehay, Y.K.; Lay, N.S.; Roth, H.R.; Wang, X.; Kwak, J.T.; Turkbey, B.I.; Pinto, P.A.; Wood, B.J.; Summers, R.M. Convolutional neural network based deep-learning architecture for prostate cancer detection on multiparametric magnetic resonance images. In *Medical Imaging 2017: Computer-Aided Diagnosis*; SPIE: Bellingham, WA, USA, 2017; p. 1013405. [CrossRef]
86. He, K.; Zhang, X.; Ren, S.; Sun, J. Deep residual learning for image recognition. In Proceedings of the 2016 IEEE Conference on Computer Vision and Pattern Recognition, Las vegas, NV, USA, 26 June–1 July 2016; pp. 770–778.
87. Liu, X.; Langer, D.L.; Haider, M.A.; Yang, Y.; Wernick, M.N.; Yetik, I.S. Prostate cancer segmentation with simultaneous estimation of Markov random field parameters and class. *IEEE Trans. Med. Imaging* **2009**, *28*, 906–915. [CrossRef]
88. Kohl, S.; Bonekamp, D.; Schlemmer, H.-P.; Yaqubi, K.; Hohenfellner, M.; Hadaschik, B.; Radtke, J.-P.; Maier-Hein, K. Adversarial networks for the detection of aggressive prostate cancer. *ArXiv* **2017**, arXiv:1702.08014.
89. Dai, Z.; Carver, E.; Liu, C.; Lee, J.; Feldman, A.; Zong, W.; Pantelic, M.; Elshaikh, M.; Wen, N. Segmentation of the Prostatic Gland and the Intraprostatic Lesions on Multiparametic MRI Using Mask-RCNN. *ArXiv* **2019**, arXiv:1904.02575.
90. Dickinson, L.; Ahmed, H.U.; Allen, C.; Barentsz, J.O.; Carey, B.; Futterer, J.J.; Heijmink, S.W.; Hoskin, P.; Kirkham, A.P.; Padhani, A.R. Scoring systems used for the interpretation and reporting of multiparametric MRI for prostate cancer detection, localization, and characterization: Could standardization lead to improved utilization of imaging within the diagnostic pathway? *J. Magn. Reson. Imaging* **2013**, *37*, 48–58. [CrossRef]
91. Nguyentat, M.; Ushinsky, A.; Miranda-Aguirre, A.; Uchio, E.; Lall, C.; Shirkhoda, L.; Lee, T.; Green, C.; Houshyar, R. Validation of Prostate Imaging-Reporting and Data System Version 2: A Retrospective Analysis. *Curr. Probl. Diagn. Radiol.* **2018**, *47*, 404–409. [CrossRef]
92. Litjens, G.J.; Barentsz, J.O.; Karssemeijer, N.; Huisman, H.J. Clinical evaluation of a computer-aided diagnosis system for determining cancer aggressiveness in prostate MRI. *Eur. Radiol.* **2015**, *25*, 3187–3199. [CrossRef]

93. Wang, J.; Wu, C.-J.; Bao, M.-L.; Zhang, J.; Wang, X.-N.; Zhang, Y.-D. Machine learning-based analysis of MR radiomics can help to improve the diagnostic performance of PI-RADS v2 in clinically relevant prostate cancer. *Eur. Radiol.* **2017**, *27*, 4082–4090. [CrossRef] [PubMed]
94. Song, Y.; Zhang, Y.D.; Yan, X.; Liu, H.; Zhou, M.; Hu, B.; Yang, G. Computer-aided diagnosis of prostate cancer using a deep convolutional neural network from multiparametric MRI. *J. Magn. Reson. Imaging* **2018**, *48*, 1570–1577. [CrossRef] [PubMed]
95. Kwak, J.T.; Xu, S.; Wood, B.J.; Turkbey, B.; Choyke, P.L.; Pinto, P.A.; Wang, S.; Summers, R.M. Automated prostate cancer detection using T2-weighted and high-b-value diffusion-weighted magnetic resonance imaging. *Med. Phys.* **2015**, *42*, 2368–2378. [CrossRef] [PubMed]
96. Wang, Z.; Liu, C.; Cheng, D.; Wang, L.; Yang, X.; Cheng, K.-T. Automated detection of clinically significant prostate cancer in mp-MRI images based on an end-to-end deep neural network. *IEEE Trans. Med. Imaging* **2018**, *37*, 1127–1139. [CrossRef]
97. Seah, J.C.; Tang, J.S.; Kitchen, A. Detection of prostate cancer on multiparametric MRI. In Proceedings of the Medical Imaging 2017: Computer-Aided Diagnosis, Orlando, FL, USA, 13–16 February 2017; p. 1013429.
98. Liu, S.; Zheng, H.; Feng, Y.; Li, W. Prostate cancer diagnosis using deep learning with 3D multiparametric MRI. In Proceedings of the Medical Imaging 2017: Computer-Aided Diagnosis, Orlando, FL, USA, 13–16 February 2017; p. 1013428.
99. Mehrtash, A.; Sedghi, A.; Ghafoorian, M.; Taghipour, M.; Tempany, C.M.; Wells, W.M., III; Kapur, T.; Mousavi, P.; Abolmaesumi, P.; Fedorov, A. Classification of clinical significance of MRI prostate findings using 3D convolutional neural networks. *Proc. Spie Int. Soc. Opt. Eng.* **2017**, *10134*. [CrossRef]
100. Chen, Q.; Hu, S.; Long, P.; Lu, F.; Shi, Y.; Li, Y. A transfer learning approach for malignant prostate lesion detection on multiparametric MRI. *Technol. Cancer Res. Treat.* **2019**, *18*. [CrossRef]
101. Armato, S.G.; Huisman, H.; Drukker, K.; Hadjiiski, L.; Kirby, J.S.; Petrick, N.; Redmond, G.; Giger, M.L.; Cha, K.; Mamonov, A. PROSTATEx Challenges for computerized classification of prostate lesions from multiparametric magnetic resonance images. *J. Med. Imaging* **2018**, *5*, 044501. [CrossRef]
102. Hu, X.; Cammann, H.; Meyer, H.-A.; Miller, K.; Jung, K.; Stephan, C. Artificial neural networks and prostate cancer—Tools for diagnosis and management. *Nat. Rev. Urol.* **2013**, *10*, 174. [CrossRef]
103. Chen, T.; Li, M.; Gu, Y.; Zhang, Y.; Yang, S.; Wei, C.; Wu, J.; Li, X.; Zhao, W.; Shen, J. Prostate cancer differentiation and aggressiveness: Assessment with a radiomic-based model vs. PI-RADS v2. *J. Magn. Reson. Imaging* **2019**, *49*, 875–884. [CrossRef]
104. European Society of Radiology. What the radiologist should know about artificial intelligence—An ESR white paper. *Insights Imaging* **2019**, *10*, 44. [CrossRef]
105. Nicolae, A.; Morton, G.; Chung, H.; Loblaw, A.; Jain, S.; Mitchell, D.; Lu, L.; Helou, J.; Al-Hanaqta, M.; Heath, E.; et al. Evaluation of a machine-learning algorithm for treatment planning in prostate low-dose-rate brachytherapy. *Int. J. Radiat. Oncol. Biol. Phys.* **2017**, *97*, 822–829. [CrossRef]
106. Wong, N.C.; Lam, C.; Patterson, L.; Shayegan, B. Use of machine learning to predict early biochemical recurrence after robot-assisted prostatectomy. *BJU Int.* **2019**, *123*, 51–57. [CrossRef] [PubMed]
107. Cordon-Cardo, C.; Kotsianti, A.; Verbel, D.A.; Teverovskiy, M.; Capodieci, P.; Hamann, S.; Jeffers, Y.; Clayton, M.; Elkhettabi, F.; Khan, F.M.; et al. Improved prediction of prostate cancer recurrence through systems pathology. *J. Clin. Invest.* **2007**, *117*, 1876–1883. [CrossRef] [PubMed]

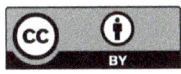

© 2020 by the authors. Licensee MDPI, Basel, Switzerland. This article is an open access article distributed under the terms and conditions of the Creative Commons Attribution (CC BY) license (http://creativecommons.org/licenses/by/4.0/).

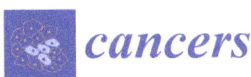

Review

Angiogenesis Inhibition in Prostate Cancer: An Update

Chandrani Sarkar [1,2], Sandeep Goswami [1], Sujit Basu [1,2,3] and Debanjan Chakroborty [1,*]

1. Department of Pathology, Ohio State University, Columbus, OH 43210, USA; Chandrani.Sarkar@osumc.edu (C.S.); Sandeep.Goswami@osumc.edu (S.G.); Sujit.Basu@osumc.edu (S.B.)
2. Comprehensive Cancer Center, Ohio State University, Columbus, OH 43210, USA
3. Department of Medical Oncology, Ohio State University, Columbus, OH 43210, USA
* Correspondence: Debanjan.Chakroborty@osumc.edu; Tel.: +1-614-247-6361

Received: 23 July 2020; Accepted: 21 August 2020; Published: 23 August 2020

Abstract: Prostate cancer (PCa), like all other solid tumors, relies on angiogenesis for growth, progression, and the dissemination of tumor cells to other parts of the body. Despite data from in vitro and in vivo preclinical studies, as well as human specimen studies indicating the crucial role played by angiogenesis in PCa, angiogenesis inhibition in clinical settings has not shown significant benefits to patients, thus challenging the inclusion and usefulness of antiangiogenic agents for the treatment of PCa. However, one of the apparent reasons why these antiangiogenic agents failed to meet expectations in PCa can be due to the choice of the antiangiogenic agents, because the majority of these drugs target vascular endothelial growth factor-A (VEGFA) and its receptors. The other relevant causes might be inappropriate drug combinations, the duration of treatment, and the method of endpoint determination. In this review, we will first discuss the role of angiogenesis in PCa growth and progression. We will then summarize the different angiogenic growth factors that influence PCa growth dynamics and review the outcomes of clinical trials conducted with antiangiogenic agents in PCa patients and, finally, critically assess the current status and fate of antiangiogenic therapy in this disease.

Keywords: prostate cancer; angiogenesis; angiogenic growth factors; antiangiogenic therapy

---

1. Introduction

Prostate cancer (PCa) is the most commonly diagnosed non-skin cancer in the United States and the second major cause of cancer-related death in men [1]. Although nearly 80% of cases are diagnosed as localized diseases that can be cured by radiotherapy or surgery, there is relapse of the disease in 30–60% of patients [2,3]. Androgen deprivation therapy (ADT) is commonly used in PCa treatment to block the androgens required for cancer growth [4–6]. However, aggressive disease relapse frequently occurs following ADT, and the disease becomes castration-resistant prostate cancer (CRPC) [4–8]. Treatment and management thus pose a real challenge at this stage of the disease [7,8]. Advancement of clinical research over the last two decades, along with the approval of several targeted and immunomodulatory agents, together with chemotherapeutic agents such as docetaxel, prednisone, and mitoxantrone, have substantially changed the treatment landscape of metastatic CRPC (mCRPC). Although these agents have shown significant benefits to a percentage of patients, these benefits are short-lived [9–13]. Accordingly, there is a constant need to identify newer and better treatments that can be used alone or in combination with currently available therapies for better disease management and outcomes.

Angiogenesis, the sprouting of new blood vessels from pre-existing vessels, is essential for tumor growth and metastasis [14–17]. Inhibiting angiogenesis has emerged as an effective strategy for the treatment of many solid tumors [18–20]. Unlike other angiogenic solid tumors, the inhibition of angiogenesis in PCa did not meet the clinical expectations, thereby igniting concerns about its relevance in PCa progression [21–25]. However, several preclinical observations as well as studies involving patient samples and cell lines support and reinforce the importance of angiogenesis in PCa [21,23–25]. Based on our current knowledge and relevant reports in literature, we will here discuss the importance of angiogenesis in PCa and the relevance of antiangiogenic strategies for the management of this disease.

2. Angiogenesis and Tumor Progression

Angiogenesis, a multistep process tightly regulated by several stimulatory and inhibitory growth factors, is essential not only for normal physiological processes but also for abnormal conditions, such as tumor growth [14,15,22,26]. Tumor growth often depends on its ability to sustain adequate blood supply by newly formed blood vessels (neovessels), thus making angiogenesis a rate-limiting step [14–16,26,27]. Vascular endothelial growth factors (VEGFs) are the most prominent and well-studied proangiogenic factors associated with tumor growth, including PCa [15,22,25]. Other angiogenic factors, such as fibroblast growth factors (FGFs), angiopoietins (Ang), hepatocyte growth factor (HGF), epidermal growth factor (EGF), platelet-derived growth factor (PDGF), placental growth factor (PlGF), insulin-like growth factors (IGFs), tumor necrosis factor (TNF), interleukin-6 (IL-6), and lysophosphatidic acid (LPA), have also been mentioned in the literature [22,28]. The antiangiogenic factors include angiostatin, endostatin, platelet factor-4 (PF4), tissue inhibitors of metalloproteinases (TIMPs), interleukins (ILs), and interferons (IFs) [22,25]. The neovessels formed during tumorigenesis differ from normal vasculature both in structure and in function, as they lack hierarchy, are chaotic in their arrangement, and the blood flow in them is sluggish [25,27,29,30].

Dr. Folkman, in his pioneer study, first described the essential role of angiogenesis in tumor growth in 1971, which led to the idea that targeting this process might be a promising therapeutic strategy to combat the growth and metastatic spread of cancer. Accordingly, antiangiogenic agents have been developed and tested in clinics, and many have been approved for the treatment of different cancer types [31].

3. Angiogenesis and Prostate Cancer

Preclinical animal experiments and studies with clinical samples have indicated significant angiogenic activity within malignant prostate tumor tissues often measured as microvessel density (MVD), a well-established marker of angiogenesis, which correlated well with the tumor growth, Gleason score, and metastasis in PCa [23,25,32]. Thus, MVD in PCa has been designated as a valuable prognostic indicator that may predict the clinical and biochemical recurrence of the disease [23,25,32–35]. In addition, several reports have demonstrated the importance of angiogenic factors such as VEGFs, FGFs, ILs, transforming growth factor β (TGFβ), and different metalloproteinases which support the role of angiogenesis in PCa progression. However, the presently approved antiangiogenic agents could not meet acceptable outcomes in PCa patients, as was expected from the results of preclinical studies [23–25,36]. Although, in some cases, the response rate and progression-free survival were significantly improved, the overall survival (OS) did not increase following treatment [25]. Because there are discrepancies between these results and the reports from the preclinical animal studies and histopathology studies using PCa samples, it would be therefore prudent to discuss and analyze the possible reasons for these apparent differences.

3.1. Angiogenic Growth Factors in Prostate Cancer

Vascular Endothelial Growth factors (VEGFs): VEGFs are part of the platelet-derived growth factor family and have been most extensively studied and described among all the angiogenic growth factors. VEGFs (VEGFA, VEGFB, VEGFC, and VEGFD) along with their cognate cell surface receptors (VEGFR1, VEGFR2, VEGFR3) play critical roles in PCa starting from cell growth to motility and cellular dissemination to other parts of the body [14,21,22]. Vascular endothelial growth factor

–A (VEGFA), which is a 45 KDa heparin-binding protein, is the most predominant growth factor among all the VEGFs [14,22,37]. VEGFA has long been identified to influence every aspect of endothelial cell (EC) behavior and the maintenance of vascular integrity, and therefore plays a crucial role during tumor growth [14,17,22,37] and is overexpressed in PCa [37,38]. Both human PCa and PCa tissues of animal origin, including prostate tumors isolated from TRansgenic Adenocarcinoma Mouse Prostate (TRAMP)models, show an increased expression of VEGFA in comparison to normal prostate tissues [21,22,37–41]. Along with prostatic glandular epithelial cells, non-vascular cells of the tumor microenvironment, such as macrophages, fibroblasts, and mast cells, also secrete VEGFA [42,43]. The role of VEGFA in PCa progression is further evident from studies that correlate the increased VEGFA expression in PCa tissues to angiogenesis, advanced disease stages, increased recurrence, and decreased survival among patients [41,44,45]. Increased amounts of VEGFA are also present in the urine samples of PCa patients, which has been reported to serve as a prognostic indicator of hormone-refractory PCa progression and survivability of these patients [46,47]. In addition, the results from several preclinical studies indicate that VEGFA inhibition or treatment with anti-VEGFA antibodies blocks the growth of human prostate tumors through suppression of angiogenesis [21,22,48], further supporting the role of VEGFA-mediated angiogenesis in PCa growth and progression. Reports also show the efficacy of anti-VEGFA treatment in combination with other therapeutic agents in preclinical mouse PCa models [49,50]. Interestingly, a dose-dependent regulation in the expression of VEGFA and its receptor FLT1 (FMS-like tyrosine kinase receptor domain 1) or VEGFR1 by androgen during PCa progression has been reported [51]. The expression of VEGFR1 has been further correlated with higher MVD, advanced pathologic state, and poor outcome in PCa [51]. Moreover, patients with advanced PCa receiving ADT show genetic polymorphisms in the androgen receptor (AR) binding site of FLT1 [52,53]. These reports, therefore, indicate that the expression of VEGFA and its receptors in PCa are subjected to androgen regulation, which together regulates the process of angiogenesis.

Fibroblast growth factors (FGFs): In addition to the VEGF family, the FGF family of growth factors is another major cytokine family that plays diverse roles during PCa progression [54,55]. FGFs are potent mitogens to many cell types, including ECs, and are expressed in many tissues, where they play significant roles in both physiological and pathological processes [54,55]. FGFs, particularly FGF2, FGF7, and FGF10, play vital roles in normal prostatic development, such as organogenesis, tissue homeostasis, and the acquisition of androgen dependency [54–56]. Both PCa cells and stromal cells in the PCa microenvironment secrete FGFs and express FGF receptors (FGFRs) [54,56,57]. FGF1 and FGF2 were among the first identified angiogenic factors which promote angiogenesis during tumor growth [57]. FGF/FGFR signaling regulates PCa angiogenesis both in a VEGFA-dependent and -independent manner [54–59]. Enhanced FGF levels and FGFR expressions such as type 1 FGFR (FGFR1), together with aberrant FGFR signaling and the loss of the intrinsic FGF7/FGF10-type 2 FGFR (FGFR2), are associated with enhanced PCa growth and angiogenesis [54,57,58]. The serum basic FGF (bFGF) level has also been shown to increase in PCa patients [59]. Furthermore, the correlation between FGF8 expression and VEGFA has been reported to be associated with advanced disease stage, higher serum PSA values, and poor survival [60]. These studies on the FGF/FGFR signaling cascade form the basis of FGF/VEGFR dual inhibition as a therapeutic strategy in PCa [61]. The prognostic implication of FGF, however, is controversial, as some studies have failed to find any relation between the FGF expression and PCa disease stage [62,63]. The specific role of FGF thus needs to be studied in more details.

Matrix metalloproteinases (MMPs): MMPs, together with TIMPs, form a classic regulatory unit that drives angiogenic processes both positively and negatively [64,65]. Metalloproteinases are zinc-containing calcium-dependent endopeptidases belonging to the metzincin superfamily [64,65]. Although MMPs are better known for their roles in tumor invasion and metastasis, as they help in breaking down the connective tissue barrier and thus help cancer cells to metastasize, they also play a crucial role in regulating angiogenesis by controlling EC attachment /detachment to the extracellular matrix, therefore helping in EC migration and invasion [64–66]. The expression of TIMPs controls the

MMP activities in the tissue environment, and an imbalance in the expression of MMPs and TIMPs has been shown in PCa angiogenesis [64]. Studies reveal a higher MMPs to TIMPs ratio in advanced PCa tumors (Gleason score of 8 and above) compared to tumors with a favorable prognosis (Gleason score of less than 6) [67]. Knowledge about the involvement of MMPs in PCa progression is mostly derived from knockdown and overexpression studies using animal models of PCa due to the lack of availability of specific MMP inhibitors [68]. Among different members of the metalloproteinase family, the roles of MMP-2, -7, -9, and MT1-MMP are well documented in PCa. MMP-2, MMP-7, and MMP-9 have been shown to stimulate PCa angiogenesis, as conditional knockouts of these MMPs in mice resulted in PCa that showed reduced vascularity and angiogenesis [68]. While MMP-2 deficiency is associated with a reduction in the number of immature blood vessels along with reduced tumor burden, MMP-9 primarily plays a role in vascular remodeling [68]. Studies have further shown that knocking down of MMP-9 in PCa cells has a negative effect on the expression of proangiogenic molecules, such as VEGFA and intercellular adhesion molecule1 (ICAM-1). It helps in the upregulation of the expression of angiostatin and other endogenous inhibitors of angiogenesis in PCa [64,69–71]. Furthermore, not only in primary tumors, MMPs, specifically MMP-9, derived from osteoclasts directly affect angiogenesis in the prostate tumor-bone microenvironment [72]. However, controversies exist regarding the roles of MMPs in PCa progression, particularly that of MMP-9, as some studies correlate the increased expression of MMP-9 with a high Gleason score, disease progression, and poorer clinical outcomes [68,73]. On the contrary, others fail to demonstrate MMP-9 expression in PCa and describe the increased perivascular invasion of PCa cells in mice lacking MMP9 [68,73].

Transforming growth factor (TGF) β: TGFβ, a pleiotropic molecule comprised of three isoforms, exhibits potent tumor suppressor properties in the early stages of tumor development [74,75], while harboring a tumor-promoting effect during the later stages of tumor progression [75,76]. This paradoxical nature of TGFβ in PCa is mostly due to its capability to differentially activate the ERK/MAP kinase pathway in benign and malignant PCa cells [76]. Although no unanimous opinion exists regarding the time point when TGFβ switches from being a tumor suppressor to a tumor promoter, studies mostly report that it acts in the interphase of stromal -epithelial interaction and exerts its effect through three different TGFβ receptors—TGFβ1, TGFβ2, and TGFβ3on tumor cells, as well as on nonmalignant stromal cells such as fibroblasts and ECs [76]. Increased TGFβ1 in PCa tissues and high levels of TGFβ1 in the urinary and serum samples of PCa patients have been reported to be associated with enhanced angiogenesis, metastasis, and poor clinical outcomes [76,77]. TGFβ indirectly affects PCa angiogenesis via the upregulation of VEGFA through the activation of SMAD-mediated transcriptional regulation and activation of the Src/Focal Adhesion Kinase (FAK)/Protein kinase B (PKB or AKT) signaling pathways [78]. TGFβ also regulates PCa angiogenesis by promoting the differentiation of cancer-associated fibroblasts (CAFs), which in turn promote tumor angiogenesis through increased VEGFA production [79]. Besides this, VEGFA also influences TGFβ expression through a positive feedback mechanism [78]. However, some studies also report the negative association between TGFβ and VEGFA expression, especially in ECs [79]. Among the TGFβ receptors, TGFβ1 expression is associated with higher clinical tumor stages and a lower 5-year survival rate. Furthermore, apigenin, a natural flavone compound, and an inhibitor for TGFβ have been shown to inhibit angiogenesis in PCa through the suppression of VEGFA, which further proves the role of TGFβ in PCa angiogenesis [78].

Cyclooxygenases: Cyclooxygenases are enzymes that form prostaglandins and thromboxanes from arachidonic acids and are mainly associated with inflammatory responses [80,81]. Fatty acids and inflammation and their role in genitourinary cancer is an actively growing area of research [80,81]. Although clinical data at this point does not strongly support the effect of nonsteroidal anti-inflammatory drugs (NSAIDs) in inhibiting or preventing PCa progression in patients, the results from several preclinical studies are encouraging [80–82]. Cyclooxygenases and their eicosanoids products, prostaglandins and thromboxanes, play multiple roles in the regulation of EC biology [82]. There are two different forms of cyclooxygenase: cyclooxygenase 1 (COX1), which is expressed constitutively, and cyclooxygenase 2 (COX2), which expresses under the influence of various growth factors and cytokines [80,81]. The increased expression of COX2 has been reported in different cell types of the tumor microenvironment, and it promotes angiogenesis through enhanced VEGFA production, EC mobilization, vascular sprouting, and increased EC survival [82]. COX2 has been reported to overexpress in PCa tissues compared to the normal prostate, which shows low to no expression [83–85]. Increased COX2 expression is associated with increased MVDs in PCa tissues [84,85]. The inhibition of COX2 with its specific inhibitor, NS398, inhibits the growth of PC3 human prostate tumors in athymic mice through the suppression of neovessel formation in these tumors [85]. The inhibition of COX2 induces apoptosis in ECs via the suppression of AKT phosphorylation in PCa [86]. Importantly, epidemiologic studies show a lower risk of PCa in men taking aspirin and other NSAIDs, which has been attributed to COX2 inhibition that leads to the inhibition of subsequent angiogenesis [80,81]. However, specific patient data showing the grade-specific upregulation of COX2 in PCa is still lacking and is needed in order to ascertain the role of COX2 in PCa in a more definitive way.

Interleukins (ILs): ILs, which are cytokines primarily secreted by leukocytes, play a major role in shaping the tumor microenvironment during tumor progression primarily through their immune regulatory properties [87,88]. In addition to lymphocytes, monocytes, and macrophages, ECs in the tumor microenvironment are regarded as major contributors of ILs [88]. To date, 50 different ILs have been identified [89]. ILs play diverse roles in PCa, such as being molecular determinants of progression from androgen-dependent to androgen-independent stages, or acting as tumor suppressors [90]. They regulate EC properties and angiogenesis in PCa either positively or negatively [91,92]. While some ILs, such as IL8, have been linked to increased PCa angiogenesis, others such as IL27 and IL10 have been linked to angiogenesis suppression in PCa [93–95]. IL8 expression in PCa has been shown to correlate with intra-tumoral MVD [93]. In addition, PCa cells transfected with IL8 have been shown to grow faster in mice with increased tumor vascularity compared to non-transfected cells [93]. As a result, targeting IL8 in PCa has emerged as a novel strategy for PCa treatment [93]. Other ILs such as IL27 and IL10, however, negatively regulate the process of angiogenesis during PCa progression. Rather than directly affecting ECs, the antiangiogenic properties of IL27 are mediated through the downregulation of proangiogenic-related genes such as FLT1, prostaglandin G/H synthase 1/cyclooxygenase-1 (PTGS1/COX-1), and FGFR3s and the upregulation of antiangiogenic genes such as CXCL10 and TIMP3 [94]. In addition to IL27, IL10 also negatively affects proangiogenic cells in the tumor microenvironment, such as activated macrophages, by inhibiting proangiogenic MMP2 and upregulating TIMP 1 and thereby suppressing the process of angiogenesis during PCa progression [95].

Other factors: In addition to the above factors, in recent years, there have been reports that other novel factors, such as microRNAs (miRNAs), which are short segments (21- to 25-nucleotides) of non-coding RNAs; long noncoding RNAs (lncRNAs), which are RNA transcripts longer than 200 nucleotides that do not encode proteins; and extracellular vesicles (EVs), which are small cell-derived membranous structures containing proteins, lipids, and genetic material, either directly or indirectly affect the angiogenic response in PCa [96–102]. In the past decades, these factors have attracted attention, as they play important roles in the progression of the disease. Increasing evidence indicates that cancer cells communicate among themselves as well as with cells of the surrounding microenvironment via the secretion and transfer of these factors. We will discuss some of these recent findings.

miRNAs can modulate the functions of ECs via non-cell-autonomous as well as cell-autonomous mechanisms, and thus regulate angiogenesis [103]. They regulate the expressions of both pro- or anti-angiogenic growth factors, and target the growth factor receptors and signaling molecules required in the process. Both the upregulation and downregulation of miRNAs have impact on PCa progression and angiogenesis. While miRNAs such as miR-296, miR-30d, miR-323, miR-21, and miR-182 are upregulated in PCa [104–109], the decreased expressions of miR-195, miR-218, and miR-146a are also shown to be associated with increased angiogenesis in PCa [97,110–112]. The upregulation of miR-30d [104] and miR-323 [105] were reported to enhance VEGF synthesis and secretion by PCa cells and therefore promote VEGF-mediated angiogenesis in PCa. miR-296, which is frequently upregulated in PCa, regulates the levels of VEGF and PDGF receptors in angiogenic ECs [108,109]. miR-21 and miR-182 regulate the expression of HIF1α and thereby HIF 1α-mediated angiogenesis [106,107]. The decreased expression of miR-146a was reported in CRPC, where it regulates the expression of epidermal growth factor receptor (EGFR) and MMP2 in PCa tissues [112]. On the other hand, the decreased expression of miR-195 in PCa results in the upregulation of ribosomal protein S6 kinase B1 (RPS6KB1), which leads to increased expressions of MMP-9 and VEGF proteins, which regulate angiogenesis [110]. miR-218, which inhibits angiogenesis through targeting the rapamycin-insensitive companion of mTOR (RICTOR)/VEGFA axis, is also downregulated during PCa progression [97]. In addition, the reduced expression of miR-130b in PCa tissues correlates with poor prognosis and increased angiogenesis, as the miR-130b/TNF-α/NF-κB/VEGFA loop inhibits PCa angiogenesis [113].

Among the lncRNAs, prostate cancer antigens (PCAs) and prostate cancer-associated transcripts (PCAT) are of immense interest, as they regulate several aspects of PCa progression. PCA3, a prostate-specific RNA which is overexpressed in more than 95% of PCa patients' urine samples, has been reported to regulate the expression of genes involved in angiogenesis, in addition to genes controlling signal transduction and apoptosis [114,115]. The knockdown of lncRNAs, PCAT3, and PCAT9 in PCa cells leads to the suppression of VEGF synthesis and angiogenesis via the modulation of the miR-203/SNAI2 axis [116]. RBMS3-AS3, which poorly expresses in PCa, can suppress PCa angiogenesis and cell proliferation by upregulating the expression of an intrinsic angiogenesis inhibitor, vasohibin1 (VASH1), through the RBMS3-AS3/miR-4534/VASH1 axis [117].

EVs, including apoptotic bodies, microvesicles, and exosomes, play vital roles in vascular development, growth, and maturation [118]. EVs can act both in a positive and negative way to modulate the process of tumor growth and angiogenesis, therefore they are considered as promising targets for therapeutic intervention [102,119,120]. While exosomes secreted from PCa cells, cells in the PCa microenvironment, and also from PCa stem cells mostly promote angiogenesis, exosomes derived from other cell types and tissues have been reported to negatively affect the process and thereby PCa growth, suggesting a crucial role of EVs in tumor angiogenesis, which largely depends on their origin [102,120,121]. Cancer-derived EVs bestow aggressive phenotypes to cancer cells by affecting ECs within the tumor microenvironment and promoting angiogenesis. The exosomes in bodily fluids, secreted during hypoxia or acidocis, cause increased angiogenesis [122]. EVs contain miRNAs, mRNAs, and proteins that mediate the communication between various cell types and ECs and induce either pro- or antiangiogenic signaling. Sphingomyelin transferred into ECs by EVs secreted by PCa cells promotes the migration and proangiogenic activity of these cells [123]. Exosomes from PCa cell lines contain TGFβ1, which stimulates the differentiation of fibroblasts to highly aggressive myofibroblasts [124,125], an important source of matrix-remodeling proteins within the tumor microenvironment, via the activation of TGFβ/SMAD3 signaling, and thereby support PCa angiogenesis [124,125]. PCa cell-derived exosomes promote the differentiation of mesenchymal stem cells (MSCs) to proangiogenic myofibroblasts that support angiogenesis during PCa progression [126]. Furthermore, PCa-associated exosomes contain c-Src, IGF-1R, and FAK proteins that promote angiogenesis and PCa development [127]. Prostate-specific membrane antigen (PSMA), which is an important tumor marker for PCa progression, including angiogenesis and metastasis, is enriched in exosomes derived from PCa cells [128].

A schematic diagram representing the role of angiogenic growth factors in PCa is presented in Figure 1.

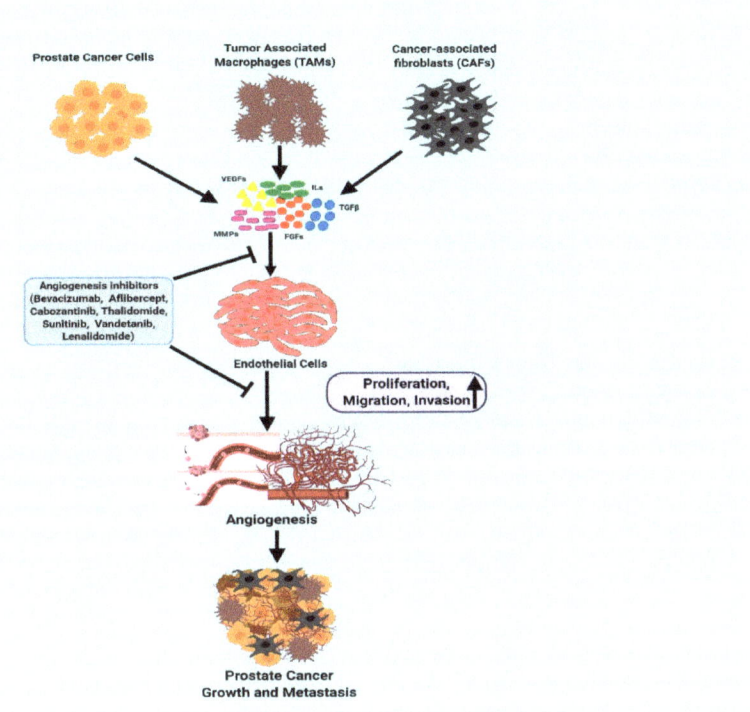

Figure 1. Schematic diagram of the role of angiogenic growth factors in prostate cancer (created with BioRender.com https://biorender.com/). VEGFs = Vascular endothelial growth factors; ILs = Interleukins; MMPs = Matrix metalloproteinases; FGFs = Fibroblast growth factors; TGFβ = Transforming growth factor beta.

3.2. Current Antiangiogenic Treatment Strategies for Prostate Cancer

Several mechanisms, such as inhibiting the activity of the proangiogenic factors directly, blocking the receptors of these proangiogenic factors, or elevating the levels of endogenous antiangiogenic factors, can be employed to inhibit angiogenesis [24,25]. In PCa, strategies were mainly designed to inhibit the proangiogenic factors or target downstream signaling effector pathways using monoclonal antibodies or small molecule inhibitors or using agents that are capable of immune modulation. Due to the multitude of factors regulating the process of angiogenesis, monotherapy, as well as combination therapy with different chemotherapeutic agents or antiangiogenic agents, have been tested for optimal therapeutic effects. Since VEGFA is a critical growth factor associated with PCa, it has been extensively studied [25,41,44,45]. As the overexpression of VEGFA correlates with poor prognosis and metastasis, the main antiangiogenic strategies in PCa at present were designed to mainly inhibit the VEGF pathway by targeting VEGFA or its receptors [25,41,44,45]. In this section, we will discuss some of these prominent antiangiogenic strategies that were developed for the treatment of PCa.

Bevacizumab is a humanized anti-VEGF monoclonal IgG1 antibody (molecular weight, 149 kDa) that selectively binds to and neutralizes VEGF, thereby preventing it from binding to its cell surface VEGFRs, leading to reduced MVD in tumors, thus limiting the blood supply to tumor tissues and lowering interstitial tissue pressure and vascular permeability [25]. A Phase II trial with bevacizumab in combination with ADT consisting of 102 recurrent hormone-sensitive PCa patients reported a significant improvement in relapse-free survival (RFS). Hypertension was the most commonly observed adverse effect in these patients [129]. Other Phase II studies with CRPC patients where bevacizumab was combined with docetaxel, thalidomide, and prednisone [130] or where bevacizumab was combined with estramustine and docetaxel for the treatment of HRPC or CRPC patients [131,132] have all demonstrated that the combination with bevacizumab was tolerated and led to encouraging antitumor activity, median survival and OS. On the contrary, the Phase III Cancer and Leukemia Group B (CALGB)trial that followed with 1050 metastatic PCa patients demonstrated some improvement in progression-free survival (PFS) with the combination therapy; there was no significant increase in OS. Bevacizumab also showed other adverse events (AE), which included cardiovascular and neutropenic complications [133]. Furthermore, in a very recent Phase I/II trial in patients with mCRPC, bevacizumab when used in combination with temsirolimus showed limited clinical activity, and only a transient decrease in the circulating tumor cells (CTC) level was observed, which was associated with significant AE [134]. These studies thus indicate that the addition of bevacizumab to standard therapy does not result in any significant clinical benefit in CRPC.

Sunitinib is a novel oral small-molecule tyrosine kinase inhibitor that targets VEGFR1 and VEGFR2. [135]. Not many clinical studies have been conducted using sunitinib in PCa. In a randomized, placebo-controlled, Phase III trial conducted with 873 progressive mCRPC patients who either received prednisone in combination with sunitinib or prednisone alone, sunitinib did not improve OS and severe AE was reported, which led to the discontinuation of the study [136].

Vandetanib is an oral multi-tyrosine kinase inhibitor that targets VEGFR2, epidermal growth factor receptor (EGFR), and RET (rearranged during transfection) pathways in cancer [25]. In a randomized, double-blinded, placebo-controlled Phase II trial of vandetanib in combination with docetaxel/prednisolone in 86 hormone-refractory PCa patients, the combination with vandetanib did not demonstrate any benefit [137]. Additionally, in another randomized Phase II trial with mCRPC patients, a combination of vandetanib with bicalutamide did not exhibit superior efficacy compared to the treatment with bicalutamide alone. These approaches were also associated with considerable toxicity [138].

Aflibercept (VEGF Trap) is a recombinant human fusion protein comprised of extracellular domains of human VEGFR1 and 2 fused to the constant region (Fc) of human immunoglobulin G1 (IgG1), which has a very high VEGF binding affinity and binds to all isomers of the VEGFA and B family and PlGF [25]. In a Phase III double-blinded randomized trial, where men with mCRPC received aflibercept with docetaxel and prednisone as first-line chemotherapy, no improvement in OS was reported. Furthermore, a high incidence of severe AE and treatment-related fatal events were reported in the aflibercept group compared to the placebo group [139].

Thalidomide is an oral agent that inhibits the activity of angiogenic factors such as VEGF, bFGF, and IL-6. In CRPC patients who have failed multiple therapies, thalidomide monotherapy showed some clinical activity [140]. Results from an open-label Phase II trial of thalidomide in patients with androgen-independent PCa [141] indicated thalidomide to be an option for patients who do not respond to other forms of therapy. Upon combination with docetaxel in a randomized Phase II trial, more than half (53%) of the CRPC patients had a PSA decrease of at least 50%, as compared to 35% of the patients in the docetaxel-alone treatment arm [142].

Lenalidomide is a thalidomide derivative that inhibits VEGF-mediated phosphatidylinositol-3,4,5-trisphosphate (PI3K)-Akt signaling pathway. The results of an open-label, Phase II clinical trial with 63 CRPC patients where lenalidomide was combined with docetaxel, bevacizumab, and prednisone showed that combining different angiogenesis inhibitors was safe with appropriate supportive measures and could potentially provide clinical benefit to patients [143]. In a Phase I/II double-blinded, randomized study with 60 non-metastatic PCa patients, treatment with lenalidomide showed an acceptable toxicity, with disease stabilization and reduction in PSA [144]. However, in a randomized, double-blind, placebo-controlled, Phase III study with 1059 chemotherapy-naive mCRPC patients, a combination of lenalidomide with docetaxel and prednisone resulted in a significantly worse OS with increased AE such as hematological side effects, diarrhea, pulmonary embolism, and asthenia [145].

Cabozantinib is an orally available small-molecule inhibitor of kinases, including VEGFR2. Preclinical studies show that cabozantinib can effectively inhibit PCa growth and metastasis by suppressing angiogenesis [146]. Clinical studies conducted so far with cabozantinib have demonstrated positive effects mostly in context to bone metastasis inhibition, bone lesion resolution, and improvement in patient CTC counts [25]. In a Phase II randomized trial of cabozantinib with patients with advanced solid tumors, randomization was halted, and the patients were unblinded because the drug showed efficacy and the largest PFS improvement in CRPC patients [147]. Furthermore, cabozantinib treatment also reduced soft tissue and bone lesions, bone turnover markers, pain, and narcotic use [148]. However, in a Phase III study with previously treated mCRPC patients, cabozantinib did not improve the OS, disease progression, or PSA response [149].

From the results of the clinical studies that have been summarized in Table 1, it can be concluded that the antiangiogenic approach in PCa has only been moderately successful. Treatment-related toxicities, often grade 3 or greater, were observed with these agents, which also resulted in treatment-related deaths. The main AE reported were hypertension, gastrointestinal perforation, proteinuria, hemorrhage, thrombosis, fistula formation, cardiac toxicity, endocrine dysfunction, and reversible posterior leukoencephalopathy [25,150].

Table 1. Summary of clinical studies of antiangiogenic drugs in the treatment of prostate cancer.

Drug	Mechanism of Action	Phase	Drugs in Combination Treatment	Outcomes	Adverse Events	Reference
Bevacizumab (Avastin®; Genentech, Inc.)	Recombinant humanized monoclonal antibody against VEGF-A	I/II	Temsirolimus	Transient decrease in circulating tumor cell levels in metastatic CRPC patients	• Anorexia • Fatigue • Mucositis • Lymphopenia • Thrombocytopenia	[134]
			ADT	Significant improvement in relapse-free survival in recurrent hormone-sensitive PCa patients	• Hypertension • Musculoskeletal pain • Infection • Headache	[129]
		II	Docetaxel, Thalidomide, and Prednisone	Improved median survival in CRPC patients	• Neutropenia • Anemia • Thrombocytopenia • Constipation	[130]
			Estramustine and Docetaxel	Improved overall survival in CRPC patients	• Leukopenia • Neutropenia • Fatigue • Pulmonary embolism • Deep venous thrombosis • Epistaxis • Hypertension	[132]
		III	Docetaxel and Prednisone	No improvement in overall survival in metastatic CRPC patients	• Neutropenia • Fatigue • Leucopenia • Hypertension • GI hemorrhage and perforation • Mucositis	[133]

Table 1. Cont.

Drug	Mechanism of Action	Phase	Drugs in Combination Treatment	Outcomes	Adverse Events	Reference
Sunitinib malate (Sutent®, Pfizer)	Novel oral small-molecule tyrosine kinase inhibitor that targets VEGFR1 and VEGFR2	III	Prednisone	No improvement in overall survival in metastatic CRPC patients	• Diarrhea • Nausea • Vomiting • Fatigue • Hand/Foot Syndrome • Hypertension • Mucosal inflammation • Asthenia	[136]
Vandetanib (Caprelsa, AstraZeneca & Sanofi)	Oral multi-tyrosine kinase inhibitor that targets VEGFR2, epidermal growth factor receptor (EGFR), and RET pathways in cancer	II	Docetaxel and Prednisolone	No efficacy benefit in HRPC patients	• Fatigue • Diarrhea • Nausea • Erythematous and exfoliative rash	[137]
			Bicalutamide	No efficacy benefit in metastatic CRPC patients	• Hypertension • Fatigue • Diarrhea • Dyspnea • Skin rash • Hand/Foot syndrome • Anorexia • Prolonged QTc interval	[138]
Aflibercept/VEGF Trap (Eylea and Zaltrap, Regeneron Pharmaceuticals)	Recombinant human fusion protein that has high VEGF binding affinity and binds to all isomers of the VEGFA and B family and placental growth factor (PGF)	III	Docetaxel and Prednisone	No improvement in overall survival in metastatic CRPC patients	• Hypertension • Vascular Disorder • GI hemorrhage • Epistaxis • Perforation • Stomatitis • Ulceration	[139]
Thalidomide (Thalomid, Celgene)	Oral agent that inhibits VEGF, bFGF, and IL-6	II	Docetaxel	PSA decrease in CRPC patients	• Thrombocytopenia • Anemia • Venous thromboembolism	[142]

Table 1. Cont.

Drug	Mechanism of Action	Phase	Drugs in Combination Treatment	Outcomes	Adverse Events	Reference
Lenalidomide (Revlimid, Celgene)	Thalidomide derivative that inhibits VEGF-mediated phosphatidylinositol-3,4,5-trisphosphate (PI3K)-Akt signaling pathway	I/II		Disease stabilization and reduction of PSA in non-metastatic PCa patients	• Neutropenia • Venous thromboembolism • Fatigue • Hyperglycemia • Constipation • Anemia	[144]
		II	Docetaxel, Bevacizumab, and Prednisone	PSA decline and partial responses in CRPC patients	• Neutropenia • Anemia • Thrombocytopenia • Diarrhea • Fatigue	[143]
		III	Docetaxel and Prednisone	Significantly worse overall survival in chemotherapy-naïve metastatic CRPC patients	• Hematological side effects • Diarrhea • Pulmonary embolism • Asthenia • Pneumonia	[145]
Cabozantinib (Cometriq™ and Cabometyx™, Exelixis Inc.)	Orally available small-molecule inhibitor of kinases, including VEGFR2	II		Proliferation-free survival improvement in CRPC patients	• Fatigue • Diarrhea • Hypertension • Muscle spasms • Asthenia	[147]
		III		No improvement in overall survival, disease progression, or PSA response in previously treated metastatic CRPC patients. Some improvement in bone scan response, radiographic progression-free survival, symptomatic skeletal events, circulating tumor cell conversion, and bone biomarkers	• Nausea • Diarrhea • Fatigue • Asthenia • Weight loss • Constipation • Anemia • Hypertension • Bone pain	[149]

4. Conclusions and Future Direction

In summary, there is substantial evidence regarding the critical role of angiogenesis in the progression of PCa, with studies reporting correlations between expressions of angiogenic markers, Gleason scores, metastatic disease progression, and clinical outcomes [23,25,32–35]. Several studies have also demonstrated the efficacies of antiangiogenic agents in preclinical PCa models [23,25]. However, despite these promising results, antiangiogenic treatment has only been moderately successful in some hormone-sensitive PCa patients [96]. On the contrary, in mCRPC, which to date has limited treatment options, antiangiogenic treatment has failed to show any significant effects in terms of improvement in OS or improvement in the quality of life of patients in the clinics [21,25].

Reviews on PCa and angiogenesis have discussed many factors that may be responsible for the moderate effectiveness of antiangiogenic agents in PCa [22,151,152]. Importantly, the failure of these agents may be attributed to several factors, such as differences in the design of clinical trials from preclinical studies, choosing appropriate angiogenic agents or combination of agents, the determination of treatment response and endpoints, and lastly the side effects encountered by the patients [23,25].

Treatment response measured as a decrease in the PSA level, improvement in PFS, or OS may not also be sufficient and appropriate for antiangiogenic agents, as the PSA level may not always accurately indicate the clinical status and disease progression, and these drugs often increase the PSA level despite a positive disease response [22,23,25]. The measurement of alternative biomarkers such as CTC counts in the peripheral blood samples isolated from patients can be an indicator of drug efficacy as CTC counts can predict OS better than PSA levels at all time points [153,154]. OS as an endpoint may not be the best evaluator of survival benefit from an antiangiogenic agent, considering the long survival rate of PCa patients normally, and PFS is not an ideal endpoint to determine the efficacy of a drug, as it may or may not necessarily translate into an OS improvement [23]. Therefore, new biomarkers of disease progression and the establishment of clinical endpoints following the administration of antiangiogenic agents may help in the determination of the efficacy of these drugs. Furthermore, at present there are no established markers to assess the angiogenic activity in PCa. MVD, which is considered as a potent surrogate marker, may not be an independent prognostic factor in untreated tumors, and studies have not yet established a strong correlation between MVD and the effectiveness of antiangiogenic agents in PCa [155]. The determination of vascularization in two-dimensional histological slides may not also be the most appropriate method for evaluating the efficacy of antiangiogenic agents [155–157]. With improved imaging techniques and other noninvasive techniques such as Doppler, it will be prudent to assess the whole vascular architecture within the tumors. Moreover, the study of the functional aspects of angiogenesis, such as the detection of vascular permeability and blood flow in tumors, will help to provide previously unavailable information and also help in decision-making [29,156,157].

Finally, although several growth factors regulate angiogenesis in PCa, most of the preclinical studies and clinical trials have been undertaken with anti-VEGFA or anti-VEGFR agents, which demonstrated modest clinical response and severe AE in patients. Therefore, it will be necessary to investigate the roles of other novel proangiogenic growth factors in PCa, which will identify newer, effective, and safe antiangiogenic agents for the treatment of PCa. Resistance, both intrinsic and acquired, to the currently used antiangiogenic agents is another possible reason for the suboptimal performance of these agents in the clinics. A number of growth factors can activate different signaling pathways during the process of angiogenesis in PCa. Recent findings indicate the probable regulatory roles of miRNAs, lncRNAs, and EVs in PCa angiogenesis. Therefore, targeting the angiogenic process using agents that are capable of inhibiting multiple pathways or by combining agents that can target different pathways may help to overcome drug resistance and result in better clinical outcomes. Combination therapy with antiangiogenic agents have actually shown promising results in clinics [143,151]. Furthermore, to find out more effective drug combinations and minimize toxicity, detailed studies determining the effective dose of each drug in a combination and monitoring the pharmacodynamic endpoints is required. Importantly, a deeper understanding of the process of angiogenesis and signaling pathways regulating the process is needed in order to design novel targeted antiangiogenic therapies in PCa.

Author Contributions: Conceptualization, C.S. and D.C.; Writing—original draft preparation, C.S., S.G., and D.C.; Writing—review and editing, C.S., S.B., and D.C. All authors have read and agreed to the published version of the manuscript.

Funding: This work was supported by the US Department of Defense Grant W81XWH-07-1-0051 (to S.B.).

Conflicts of Interest: The authors declare no conflict of interest.

References

1. Siegel, R.L.; Miller, K.D.; Jemal, A. Cancer statistics, 2020. *CA Cancer J. Clin.* **2020**, *70*, 7–30. [CrossRef] [PubMed]
2. Merino, M.; Pinto, A.; González, R.; Espinosa, E. Antiangiogenic agents and endothelin antagonists in advanced castration resistant prostate cancer. *Eur. J. Cancer* **2011**, *47*, 1846–1851. [CrossRef]
3. Shipley, W.U.; Seiferheld, W.; Lukka, H.R.; Major, P.P.; Heney, N.M.; Grignon, D.J.; Sartor, O.; Patel, M.P.; Bahary, J.P.; Zietman, A.L.; et al. NRG Oncology RTOG Radiation with or without Antiandrogen Therapy in Recurrent Prostate Cancer. *N. Engl. J. Med.* **2017**, *376*, 417–428. [CrossRef] [PubMed]
4. Cannata, D.H.; Kirschenbaum, A.; Levine, A.C. Androgen deprivation therapy as primary treatment for prostate cancer. *J. Clin. Endocrinol. Metab.* **2012**, *97*, 360–365. [CrossRef] [PubMed]
5. Schmidt, L.J.; Tindall, D.J. Androgen receptor: Past, present and future. *Curr. Drug Targets.* **2013**, *14*, 401–407. [CrossRef]
6. Yap, T.A.; Smith, A.D.; Ferraldeschi, R.; Al-Lazikani, B.; Workman, P.; de Bono, J.S. Drug discovery in advanced prostate cancer: Translating biology into therapy. *Nat. Rev. Drug Discov.* **2016**, *15*, 699–718. [CrossRef]
7. Katsogiannou, M.; Ziouziou, H.; Karaki, S.; Andrieu, C.; Henry de Villeneuve, M.; Rocchi, P. The hallmarks of castration-resistant prostate cancers. *Cancer Treat. Rev.* **2015**, *41*, 588–597. [CrossRef]
8. Craft, N.; Chhor, C.; Tran, C.; Belldegrun, A.; DeKernion, J.; Witte, O.N.; Said, J.; Reiter, R.E.; Sawyers, C.L. Evidence for clonal outgrowth of androgen-independent prostate cancer cells from androgen-dependent tumors through a two-step process. *Cancer Res.* **1999**, *59*, 5030–5036.
9. Pham, T.; Sadowski, M.C.; Li, H.; Richard, D.J.; d'Emden, M.C.; Richard, K. Advances in hormonal therapies for hormone naïve and castration-resistant prostate cancers with or without previous chemotherapy. *Exp. Hematol. Oncol.* **2016**, *22*, 5. [CrossRef]
10. Donkena, K.V.; Yuan, H.; Young, C.Y. Recent advances in understanding hormonal therapy resistant prostate cancer. *Curr. Cancer Drug Targets* **2010**, *10*, 402–410. [CrossRef]
11. Janiczek, M.; Szylberg, Ł.; Kasperska, A.; Kowalewski, A.; Parol, M.; Antosik, P.; Radecka, B.; Marszałek, A. Immunotherapy as a Promising Treatment for Prostate Cancer: A Systematic Review. *J. Immunol. Res.* **2017**, *2017*, 4861570. [CrossRef]
12. Nevedomskaya, E.; Baumgart, S.J.; Haendler, B. Recent Advances in Prostate Cancer Treatment and Drug Discovery. *Int. J. Mol. Sci.* **2018**, *19*, 1359. [CrossRef] [PubMed]
13. Sumanasuriya, S.; De Bono, J. Treatment of Advanced Prostate Cancer-A Review of Current Therapies and Future Promise. *Cold Spring Harb. Perspect. Med.* **2018**, *8*, a030635. [CrossRef] [PubMed]
14. Carmeliet, P.; Jain, R.K. Angiogenesis in cancer and other diseases. *Nature* **2000**, *407*, 249–257. [CrossRef]
15. Basu, S.; Nagy, J.A.; Pal, S.; Vasile, E.; Eckelhoefer, I.A.; Bliss, V.S.; Manseau, E.J.; Dasgupta, P.S.; Dvorak, H.F.; Mukhopadhyay, D. The neurotransmitter dopamine inhibits angiogenesis induced by vascular permeability factor/vascular endothelial growth factor. *Nat. Med.* **2001**, *5*, 569–574. [CrossRef]
16. Bielenberg, D.R.; Zetter, B.R. The Contribution of Angiogenesis to the Process of Metastasis. *Cancer J.* **2015**, *21*, 267–273. [CrossRef] [PubMed]
17. Chakroborty, D.; Sarkar, C.; Basu, B.; Dasgupta, P.S.; Basu, S. Catecholamines regulate tumor angiogenesis. *Cancer Res.* **2009**, *69*, 3727–3730. [CrossRef]
18. Chakroborty, D.; Sarkar, C.; Mitra, R.B.; Banerjee, S.; Dasgupta, P.S.; Basu, S. Depleted dopamine in gastric cancer tissues: Dopamine treatment retards growth of gastric cancer by inhibiting angiogenesis. *Clin. Cancer Res.* **2004**, *10*, 4349–4356. [CrossRef]

19. Sarkar, C.; Chakroborty, D.; Dasgupta, P.S.; Basu, S. Dopamine is a safe antiangiogenic drug which can also prevent 5-fluorouracil induced neutropenia. *Int. J. Cancer* **2015**, *137*, 744–749. [CrossRef]
20. Schmidt, T.; Carmeliet, P. Angiogenesis: A target in solid tumors, also in leukemia? *Hematol. Am. Soc. Hematol. Educ. Program* **2011**, *2011*, 1–8. [CrossRef]
21. Guo, Y.; Wang, S.; Hoot, D.R.; Clinton, S.K. Suppression of VEGF-mediated autocrine and paracrine interactions between prostate cancer cells and vascular endothelial cells by soy isoflavones. *J. Nutr. Biochem.* **2007**, *18*, 408–417. [CrossRef] [PubMed]
22. Hwang, C.; Heath, E.I. Angiogenesis inhibitors in the treatment of prostate cancer. *J. Hematol. Oncol.* **2010**, *3*, 26. [CrossRef] [PubMed]
23. Bilusic, M.; Wong, Y.N. Anti-angiogenesis in prostate cancer: Knocked down but not out. *Asian J. Androl.* **2014**, *16*, 372–377. [CrossRef]
24. Aragon-Ching, J.B.; Jain, L.; Gulley, J.L.; Arlen, P.M.; Wright, J.J.; Steinberg, S.M.; Draper, D.; Venitz, J.; Jones, E.; Chen, C.C.; et al. Final analysis of a phase II trial using sorafenib for metastatic castration-resistant prostate cancer. *BJU Int.* **2009**, *103*, 1636–1640. [CrossRef]
25. Mukherji, D.; Temraz, S.; Wehbe, D.; Shamseddine, A. Angiogenesis and antiangiogenic therapy in prostate cancer. *Crit. Rev. Oncol. Hematol.* **2013**, *87*, 122–131. [CrossRef]
26. Carmeliet, P. Angiogenesis in health and disease. *Nat. Med.* **2003**, *9*, 653–660. [CrossRef]
27. Hanahan, D.; Folkman, J. Patterns and emerging mechanisms of the angiogenic switch during tumorigenesis. *Cell* **1996**, *86*, 353–364. [CrossRef]
28. Rivera-Lopez, C.M.; Tucker, A.L.; Lynch, K.R. Lysophosphatidic acid (LPA) and angiogenesis. *Angiogenesis* **2008**, *11*, 301–310. [CrossRef]
29. Chakroborty, D.; Sarkar, C.; Yu, H.; Wang, J.; Liu, Z.; Dasgupta, P.S.; Basu, S. Dopamine stabilizes tumor blood vessels by upregulating angiopoietin 1 expression in pericytes and Kruppel-like factor-2 expression in tumor endothelial cells. *Proc. Natl. Acad. Sci. USA* **2011**, *108*, 20730–20735. [CrossRef]
30. Winkler, F.; Kozin, S.V.; Tong, R.T.; Chae, S.S.; Booth, M.F.; Garkavtsev, I.; Xu, L.; Hicklin, D.J.; Fukumura, D.; di Tomaso, E.; et al. Kinetics of vascular normalization by VEGFR2 blockade governs brain tumor response to radiation: Role of oxygenation, angiopoietin-1, and matrix metalloproteinases. *Cancer Cell.* **2004**, *6*, 553–563. [CrossRef]
31. Folkman, J. Tumor angiogenesis: Therapeutic implications. *N. Engl. J. Med.* **1971**, *21*, 1182–1186. [CrossRef]
32. Gettman, M.T.; Pacelli, A.; Slezak, J.; Bergstralh, E.J.; Zincke, H.; Bostwick, D.G. Role of microvessel density inpredicting recurrence in pathologic Stage T3 prostatic adenocarcinoma. *Urology* **1999**, *54*, 479–485. [CrossRef]
33. Weidner, N.; Carroll, P.R.; Flax, J.; Blumenfeld, W.; Folkman, J. Tumor angiogenesis correlates with metastasis in invasive prostate carcinoma. *Am. J. Pathol.* **1993**, *143*, 401–409. [PubMed]
34. Siegal, J.A.; Yu, E.; Brawer, M.K. Topography of neovascularity in human prostate carcinoma. *Cancer* **1995**, *75*, 2545–2551. [CrossRef]
35. Brawer, M.K.; Deering, R.E.; Brown, M.; Preston, S.D.; Bigler, S.A. Predictors of pathologic stage in prostatic carcinoma. The role of neovascularity. *Cancer* **1994**, *73*, 678–687. [CrossRef]
36. Chi, K.N.; Ellard, S.L.; Hotte, S.J.; Czaykowski, P.; Moore, M.; Ruether, J.D.; Schell, A.J.; Taylor, S.; Hansen, C.; Gauthier, I.; et al. A phase II study of sorafenib in patients with chemo-naive castration-resistant prostate cancer. *Ann. Oncol.* **2008**, *19*, 746–751. [CrossRef]
37. Dvorak, H.F. Vascular permeability factor/vascular endothelial growth factor: A critical cytokine in tumor angiogenesis and a potential target for diagnosis and therapy. *J. Clin. Oncol.* **2002**, *20*, 4368–4380. [CrossRef]
38. Roberts, E.; Cossigny, D.A.; Quan, G.M. The role of vascular endothelial growth factor in metastatic prostate cancer to the skeleton. *Prostate Cancer* **2013**, *418340*. [CrossRef]
39. Jackson, M.W.; Roberts, J.S.; Heckford, S.E.; Ricciardelli, C.; Stahl, J.; Choong, C.; Horsfall, D.J.; Tilley, W.D. A potential autocrine role for vascular endothelial growth factor in prostate cancer. *Cancer Res.* **2002**, *62*, 854–859.
40. Huss, W.J.; Hanrahan, C.F.; Barrios, R.J.; Simons, J.W.; Greenberg, N.M. Angiogenesis and prostate cancer: Identification of a molecular progression switch. *Cancer Res.* **2001**, *61*, 2736–2743.
41. Strohmeyer, D.; Rössing, C.; Bauerfeind, A.; Kaufmann, O.; Schlechte, H.; Bartsch, G.; Loening, S. Vascular endothelial growth factor and its Fargoncorrelation with angiogenesis and p53 expression in prostate cancer. *Prostate* **2000**, *45*, 216–224. [CrossRef]

42. Chen, P.C.; Cheng, H.C.; Wang, J.; Wang, J.; Wang, S.W.; Tai, H.C.; Lin, C.W.; Tang, C.H. Prostate cancer-derived CCN3 induces M2 macrophage infiltration and contributes to angiogenesis in prostate cancer microenvironment. *Oncotarget* **2014**, *5*, 1595–1608. [CrossRef] [PubMed]
43. Taverna, G.; Giusti, G.; Seveso, M.; Hurle, R.; Colombo, P.; Stifter, S.; Grizzi, F. Mast cells as a potential prognostic marker in prostate cancer. *Dis. Markers* **2013**, *35*, 711–720. [CrossRef] [PubMed]
44. Aragon-Ching, J.B.; Dahut, W.L. VEGF inhibitors and prostate cancer therapy. *Curr. Mol. Pharmacol.* **2009**, *2*, 161–168. [CrossRef] [PubMed]
45. Borre, M.; Nerstrøm, B.; Overgaard, J. Association between immunohistochemical expression of vascular endothelial growth factor (VEGF), VEGF-expressing neuroendocrine-differentiated tumor cells, and outcome in prostate cancer patients subjected to watchful waiting. *Clin. Cancer Res.* **2000**, *6*, 1882–1890.
46. Jamaspishvili, T.; Kral, M.; Khomeriki, I.; Student, V.; Kolar, Z.; Bouchal, J. Urine markers in monitoring for prostate cancer. *Prostate Cancer Prostatic Dis.* **2010**, *13*, 12–19. [CrossRef]
47. George, D.J.; Halabi, S.; Shepard, T.F.; Vogelzang, N.J.; Hayes, D.F.; Small, E.J.; Kantoff, P.W. Prognostic significance of plasma vascular endothelial growth factor levels in patients with hormone-refractory prostate cancer treated on Cancer and Leukemia Group B 9480. *Clin. Cancer Res.* **2001**, *7*, 1932–1936.
48. Mateus, P.A.M.; Kido, L.A.; Silva, R.S.; Cagnon, V.H.A.; Montico, F. Association of anti-inflammatory and antiangiogenic therapies negatively influences prostate cancer progression in TRAMP mice. *Prostate* **2019**, *79*, 515–535. [CrossRef]
49. Zurita, A.J.; George, D.J.; Shore, N.D.; Liu., G.; Wilding, G.; Hutson, T.E.; Kozloff, M.; Mathew, P.; Harmon, C.S.; Wang, S.L.; et al. Sunitinib in combination with docetaxel and prednisone in chemotherapy-naive patients with metastatic, castration-resistant prostate cancer: A phase 1/2 clinical trial. *Ann. Oncol.* **2012**, *23*, 688–694. [CrossRef]
50. Antonarakis, E.S.; Armstrong, A.J. Emerging therapeutic approaches in the management of metastatic castration-resistant prostate cancer. *Prostate Cancer Prostatic Dis.* **2011**, *14*, 206–218. [CrossRef]
51. Sieveking, D.P.; Lim, P.; Chow, R.W.; Dunn, L.L.; Bao, S.; McGrath, K.C.; Heather, A.K.; Handels, D.J.; Celermajer, D.S.; Ng, M.K. A sex-specific role for androgens in angiogenesis. *J. Exp. Med.* **2010**, *207*, 345–352. [CrossRef] [PubMed]
52. Pallares, J.; Rojo, F.; Iriarte, J.; Morote, J.; Armadans, L.I.; de Torres, I. Study of microvessel density and the expression of the angiogenic factors VEGF, bFGF and the receptors Flt-1 and FLK-1 in benign, premalignant and malignant prostate tissues. *Histol. Histopathol.* **2006**, *21*, 857–865. [CrossRef] [PubMed]
53. Huang, C.N.; Huang, S.P.; Pao, J.B.; Hour, T.C.; Chang, T.Y.; Lan, Y.H.; Lu, T.-L.; Lee, H.-Z.; Juang, S.-H.; Huang, C.Y.; et al. Genetic polymorphisms in androgen receptor-binding sites predict survival in prostate cancer patients receiving androgen-deprivation therapy. *Ann. Oncol.* **2012**, *23*, 707–713. [CrossRef] [PubMed]
54. Huss, W.J.; Barrios, R.J.; Foster, B.A.; Greenberg, N.M. Differential expression of specific FGF ligand and receptor isoforms during angiogenesis associated with prostate cancer progression. *Prostate* **2003**, *54*, 8–16. [CrossRef] [PubMed]
55. Doll, J.A.; Reiher, F.K.; Crawford, S.E.; Pins, M.R.; Campbell, S.C.; Bouck, N.P. Thrombospondin-1, vascular endothelial growth factor and fibroblast growth factor-2 are key functional regulators of angiogenesis in the prostate. *Prostate* **2001**, *49*, 293–305. [CrossRef] [PubMed]
56. Thomson, A.A. Role of androgens and fibroblast growth factors in prostatic development. *Reproduction* **2001**, *121*, 187–195. [CrossRef]
57. Kwabi-Addo, B.; Ozen, M.; Ittmann, M. The role of fibroblast growth factors and their receptors in prostate cancer. *Endocr. Relat. Cancer* **2004**, *11*, 709–724. [CrossRef]
58. Wang, C.; Liu, Z.; Ke, Y.; Wang, F. Intrinsic FGFR2 and Ectopic FGFR1 Signaling in the Prostate and Prostate Cancer. *Front. Genet.* **2019**, *10*, 12. [CrossRef]
59. Meyer, G.E.; Yu, E.; Siegal, J.A.; Petteway, J.C.; Blumenstein, B.A.; Brawer, M.K. Serum basic fibroblast growth factor in men with and without prostate carcinoma. *Cancer* **1995**, *76*, 2304–2311. [CrossRef]
60. West, A.F.; O'Donnell, M.; Charlton, R.G.; Neal, D.E.; Leung, H.Y. Correlation of vascular endothelial growth factor expression with fibroblast growth factor-8 expression and clinico-pathologic parameters in human prostate cancer. *Br. J. Cancer* **2001**, *85*, 576–583. [CrossRef]

61. Bok, R.A.; Halabi, S.; Fei, D.T.; Rodriquez, C.R.; Hayes, D.F.; Vogelzang, N.J.; Kantoff, P.; Shuman, M.A.; Small, E.J. Vascular endothelial growth factor and basic fibroblast growth factor urine levels as predictors of outcome in hormone-refractory prostate cancer patients: A cancer and leukemia group B study. *Cancer Res.* **2001**, *61*, 2533–2536. [PubMed]
62. Dorkin, T.J.; Robinson, M.C.; Marsh, C.; Bjartell, A.; Neal, D.E.; Leung, H.Y. FGF8 over-expression in prostate cancer is associated with decreased patient survival and persists in androgen independent disease. *Oncogene* **1999**, *18*, 2755–2761. [CrossRef] [PubMed]
63. Casanovas, O.; Hicklin, D.J.; Bergers, G.; Hanahan, D. Drug resistance by evasion of antiangiogenic targeting of VEGF signaling in late-stage pancreatic islet tumors. *Cancer Cell.* **2005**, *8*, 299–309. [CrossRef]
64. Gong, Y.; Chippada-Venkata, U.D.; Oh, W.K. Roles of matrix metalloproteinases and their natural inhibitors in prostate cancer progression. *Cancers* **2014**, *6*, 1298–1327. [CrossRef] [PubMed]
65. Kessenbrock, K.; Plaks, V.; Werb, Z. Matrix metalloproteinases: Regulators of the tumor microenvironment. *Cell* **2010**, *141*, 52–67. [CrossRef] [PubMed]
66. Gialeli, C.; Theocharis, A.D.; Karamanos, N.K. Roles of matrix metalloproteinases in cancer progression and their pharmacological targeting. *FEBS J.* **2011**, *278*, 16–27. [CrossRef] [PubMed]
67. Wood, M.; Fudge, K.; Mohler, J.L.; Frost, A.R.; Garcia, F.; Wang, M.; Stearns, M.E. In situ hybridization studies of metallo-proteinases 2 and 9 and TIMP-1 and TIMP-2 expression in human prostate cancer. *Clin. Exp. Metastasis* **1997**, *15*, 246–258. [CrossRef]
68. Littlepage, L.E.; Sternlicht, M.D.; Rougier, N.; Phillips, J.; Gallo, E.; Yu, Y.; Williams, K.; Brenot, A.; Gordon, J.I.; Werb, Z. Matrix metalloproteinases contribute distinct roles in neuroendocrine prostate carcinogenesis, metastasis, and angiogenesis progression. *Cancer Res.* **2010**, *70*, 2224–2234. [CrossRef]
69. Aalinkeel, R.; Nair, M.P.; Sufrin, G.; Mahajan, S.D.; Chadha, K.C.; Chawda, R.P.; Schwartz, S.A. Gene expression of angiogenic factors correlates with metastatic potential of prostate cancer cells. *Cancer Res.* **2004**, *64*, 5311–5321. [CrossRef]
70. Aalinkeel, R.; Nair, B.B.; Reynolds, J.L.; Sykes, D.E.; Mahajan, S.D.; Chadha, K.C.; Schwartz, S.A. Overexpression of MMP-9 contributes to invasiveness of prostate cancer cell line LNCaP. *Immunol. Investig.* **2011**, *40*, 447–464. [CrossRef]
71. Gupta, A.; Zhou, C.Q.; Chellaiah, M.A. Osteopontin and MMP9: Associations with VEGF Expression/Secretion and Angiogenesis in PC3 Prostate Cancer Cells. *Cancers* **2013**, *5*, 617–638. [CrossRef] [PubMed]
72. Bruni-Cardoso, A.; Johnson, L.C.; Vessella, R.L.; Peterson, T.E.; Lynch, C.C. Osteoclast-derived matrix metalloproteinase-9 directly affects angiogenesis in the prostate tumor-bone microenvironment. *Mol. Cancer Res.* **2010**, *8*, 459–470. [CrossRef] [PubMed]
73. Trudel, D.; Fradet, Y.; Meyer, F.; Têtu, B. Matrix metalloproteinase 9 is associated with Gleason score in prostate cancer but not with prognosis. *Hum. Pathol.* **2010**, *41*, 1694–1701. [CrossRef] [PubMed]
74. Akhurst, R.J.; Derynck, R. TGF-beta signaling in cancer–a double-edged sword. *Trends Cell Biol.* **2001**, *11*, S44–S51. [CrossRef] [PubMed]
75. Inman, G.J. Switching TGFβ from a tumor suppressor to a tumor promoter. *Curr. Opin. Genet. Dev.* **2011**, *21*, 93–99. [CrossRef] [PubMed]
76. Principe, D.R.; Doll, J.A.; Bauer, J.; Jung, B.; Munshi, H.G.; Bartholin, L.; Pasche, B.; Lee, C.; Grippo, P.J. TGF-β: Duality of function between tumor prevention and carcinogenesis. *J. Natl. Cancer Inst.* **2014**, *106*, djt369. [CrossRef]
77. Lu, S.; Lee, J.; Revelo, M.; Wang, X.; Lu, S.; Dong, Z. Smad3 is overexpressed in advanced human prostate cancer and necessary for progressive growth of prostate cancer cells in nude mice. *Clin. Cancer Res.* **2007**, *13*, 5692–5702. [CrossRef]
78. Mirzoeva, S.; Franzen, C.A.; Pelling, J.C. Apigenin inhibits TGF-β-induced VEGF expression in human prostate carcinoma cells via a Smad2/3- and Src-dependent mechanism. *Mol. Carcinog.* **2014**, *53*, 598–609. [CrossRef]
79. Ji, H.; Li, Y.; Jiang, F.; Wang, X.; Zhang, J.; Shen, J.; Yanget, X. Inhibition of transforming growth factor beta/SMAD signal by MiR-155 is involved in arsenic trioxide-induced anti-angiogenesis in prostate cancer. *Cancer Sci.* **2014**, *105*, 1541–1549. [CrossRef]
80. Mahmud, S.; Franco, E.; Aprikian, A. Prostate cancer and use of nonsteroidal anti-inflammatory drugs: Systematic review and meta-analysis. *Br. J. Cancer* **2004**, *90*, 93–99. [CrossRef]

81. Cai, T.; Santi, R.; Tamanini, I.; Galli, I.C.; Perletti, G.; Bjerklund Johansen, T.E.; Nesi, G. Current Knowledge of the Potential Links between Inflammation and Prostate Cancer. *Int. J. Mol. Sci.* **2019**, *20*, 3833. [CrossRef] [PubMed]
82. Masferrer, J.L.; Leahy, K.M.; Koki, A.T.; Zweifel, B.S.; Settle, S.L.; Woerner, B.M.; Edwaeds, D.A.; Flickinger, A.G.; More, R.J.; Seibert, K. Antiangiogenic and antitumor activities of cyclooxygenase-2 inhibitors. *Cancer Res.* **2000**, *60*, 1306–1311. [PubMed]
83. Khor, L.Y.; Bae, K.; Pollack, A.; Hammond, M.E.; Grignon, D.J.; Venkatesan, V.M.; Rosenthal, S.A.; Ritter, M.A.; Sandler, H.M.; Hanks, G.E.; et al. COX-2 expression predicts prostate-cancer outcome: Analysis of data from the RTOG 92-02 trial. *Lancet Oncol.* **2007**, *8*, 912–920. [CrossRef]
84. Dandekar, D.S.; Lokeshwar, B.L. Inhibition of cyclooxygenase (COX)-2 expression by Tet-inducible COX-2 antisense cDNA in hormone-refractory prostate cancer significantly slows tumor growth and improves efficacy of chemotherapeutic drugs. *Clin. Cancer Res.* **2004**, *10*, 8037–8047. [CrossRef]
85. Liu, X.H.; Kirschenbaum, A.; Yao, S.; Lee, R.; Holland, J.F.; Levine, A.C. Inhibition of cyclooxygenase-2 suppresses angiogenesis and the growth of prostate cancer in vivo. *J. Urol.* **2000**, *164*, 820–825. [CrossRef]
86. Gately, S. The contributions of cyclooxygenase-2 to tumor angiogenesis. *Cancer Metastasis Rev.* **2000**, *19*, 19–27. [CrossRef]
87. Setrerrahmane, S.; Xu, H. Tumor-related interleukins: Old validated targets for new anti-cancer drug development. *Mol. Cancer* **2017**, *16*, 153. [CrossRef]
88. Anestakis, D.; Petanidis, S.; Kalyvas, S.; Nday, C.M.; Tsave, O.; Kioseoglou, E.; Salifoglou, A. Mechanisms and applications of interleukins in cancer immunotherapy. *Int. J. Mol. Sci.* **2015**, *16*, 1691–1710. [CrossRef]
89. Jiang, X.; Wang, J.; Deng, X.; Xiong, F.; Ge, J.; Xiang, B.; Wu, X.; Ma, J.; Zhou, M.; Li, X.; et al. Role of the tumor microenvironment in PD-L1/PD-1-mediated tumor immune escape. *Mol. Cancer* **2019**, *18*, 10. [CrossRef]
90. Araki, S.; Omori, Y.; Lyn, D.; Lyn, D.; Singh, R.K.; Meinbach, D.M.; Sandman, Y.; Lokeshwar, V.B.; Lokeshwar, B.L. Interleukin-8 is a molecular determinant of androgen independence and progression in prostate cancer. *Cancer Res.* **2007**, *67*, 6854–6862. [CrossRef]
91. Inoue, K.; Slaton, J.W.; Eve, B.Y.; Kim, S.J.; Perrotte, P.; Balbay, M.D.; Yano, S.; Bar-Eli, M.; Radinsky, R.; Pettaway, C.A.; et al. Interleukin 8 expression regulates tumorigenicity and metastases in androgen-independent prostate cancer. *Clin. Cancer Res.* **2000**, *6*, 2104–2119. [PubMed]
92. Middleton, K.; Jones, J.; Lwin, Z.; Coward, J.I. Interleukin-6: An angiogenic target in solid tumours. *Crit. Rev. Oncol. Hematol.* **2014**, *89*, 129–139. [CrossRef] [PubMed]
93. Roumeguère, T.; Legrand, F.; Rassy, E.E.; Kaitouni, M.; Albisinni, S.; Rousseau, A.; Vanhaeverbeek, M.; Rorive, S.; Decaestecker, C.; Debeir, O.; et al. A prospective clinical study of the implications of IL-8 in the diagnosis, aggressiveness and prognosis of prostate cancer. *Future Sci. OA* **2017**, *4*, FSO266. [CrossRef] [PubMed]
94. Di Carlo, E.; Sorrentino, C.; Zorzoli, A.; Di Meo, S.; Tupone, M.G.; Ognio, E.; Mincione, G.; Airoldi, I. The antitumor potential of Interleukin-27 in prostate cancer. *Oncotarget* **2014**, *5*, 10332–10341. [CrossRef]
95. Stearns, M.E.; Wang, M.; Hu, Y.; Garcia, F.U.; Rhim, J. Interleukin 10 blocks matrix metalloproteinase-2 and membrane type 1-matrix metalloproteinase synthesis in primary human prostate tumor lines. *Clin. Cancer Res.* **2003**, *3*, 1191–1199.
96. Vanacore, D.; Boccellino, M.; Rossetti, S.; Cavaliere, C.; D'Aniello, C.; Di Franco, R.; Romano, F.J.; Montanari, M.; Mantia, E.L.; Piscitelli, R.; et al. Micrornas in prostate cancer: An overview. *Oncotarget* **2017**, *8*, 50240–50251. [CrossRef]
97. Guan, B.; Wu, K.; Zeng, J.; Xu, S.; Mu, L.; Gao, Y.; Wang, K.; Ma, Z.; Tian, J.; Shi, Q.; et al. Tumor-suppressive microRNA-218 inhibits tumor angiogenesis via targeting the mTOR component RICTOR in prostate cancer. *Oncotarget* **2017**, *8*, 8162–8172. [CrossRef]
98. Misawa, A.; Takayama, K.I.; Inoue, S. Long non-coding RNAs and prostate cancer. *Cancer Sci.* **2017**, *108*, 2107–2114. [CrossRef]
99. Takayama, K.I.; Misawa, A.; Inoue, S. Significance of microRNAs in Androgen Signaling and Prostate Cancer Progression. *Cancers* **2017**, *9*, 102. [CrossRef]
100. Saber, S.H.; Ali, H.E.A.; Gaballa, R.; Gaballah, M.; Ali, H.I.; Zerfaoui, M.; Elmageed, Z.Y.A. Exosomes are the Driving Force in Preparing the Soil for the Metastatic Seeds: Lessons from the Prostate Cancer. *Cells* **2020**, *9*, 564. [CrossRef]

101. Liu, C.M.; Hsieh, C.L.; Shen, C.N.; Lin, C.C.; Shigemura, K.; Sung, S.Y. Exosomes from the tumor microenvironment as reciprocal regulators that enhance prostate cancer progression. *Int. J. Urol.* **2016**, *23*, 734–744. [CrossRef] [PubMed]
102. Vlaeminck-Guillem, V. Extracellular Vesicles in Prostate Cancer Carcinogenesis, Diagnosis, and Management. *Front. Oncol.* **2018**, *8*, 222. [CrossRef] [PubMed]
103. Wang, Y.; Wang, L.; Chen, C.; Chu, X. New insights into the regulatory role of microRNA in tumor angiogenesis and clinical implications. *Mol. Cancer* **2018**, *17*, 22. [CrossRef] [PubMed]
104. Lin, Z.Y.; Chen, G.; Zhang, Y.Q.; He, H.C.; Liang, Y.X.; Ye, J.H.; Liang, Y.K.; Mo, R.J.; Lu, J.M.; Zhou, Y.J.; et al. MicroRNA-30d promotes angiogenesis and tumor growth via MYPT1/c-JUN/VEGFA pathway and predicts aggressive outcome in prostate cancer [published correction appears in prostate cancer. *Mol. Cancer* **2019**, *18*, 122]. *Mol. Cancer* **2017**, *16*, 48. [CrossRef] [PubMed]
105. Gao, Q.; Yao, X.; Zheng, J. MiR-323 Inhibits Prostate Cancer Vascularization Through Adiponectin Receptor. *Cell Physiol. Biochem.* **2015**, *36*, 1491–1498. [CrossRef]
106. Li, Y.; Zhang, D.; Wang, X.; Yao, X.; Ye, C.; Zhang, S.; Wang, H.; Chang, C.; Xia, H.; Wang, Y.; et al. Hypoxia-inducible miR-182 enhances HIF1α signaling via targeting PHD2 and FIH1 in prostate cancer. *Sci. Rep.* **2015**, *5*, 12495. [CrossRef]
107. Liu, L.Z.; Li, C.; Chen, Q.; Jing, Y.; Carpenter, R.; Jiang, Y.; Kung, H.F.; Lai, L.; Jiang, B.H. MiR-21 induced angiogenesis through AKT and ERK activation and HIF-1α expression. *PLoS ONE.* **2011**, *6*, e19139. [CrossRef]
108. Würdinger, T.; Tannous, B.A.; Saydam, O.; Skog, J.; Grau, S.; Soutschek, J.; Weissleder, R.; Breakefield, X.O.; Krichevsky, A.M. miR-296 regulates growth factor receptor overexpression in angiogenic endothelial cells. *Cancer Cell.* **2008**, *14*, 382–393. [CrossRef]
109. Lou, W.; Liu, J.; Gao, Y.; Lou, W.; Liu, J.; Gao, Y.; Zhong, G.; Chen, D.; Shen, J.; Ding, B.; et al. MicroRNAs in cancer metastasis and angiogenesis. *Oncotarget* **2017**, *8*, 115787–115802. [CrossRef]
110. Cai, C.; Chen, Q.B.; Han, Z.D.; Zhang, Y.Q.; He, H.C.; Chen, J.H.; Chen, Y.R.; Yang, S.B.; Wu, Y.D.; Qin, G.Q.; et al. miR-195 Inhibits Tumor Progression by Targeting RPS6KB1 in Human Prostate Cancer. *Clin. Cancer Res.* **2015**, *21*, 4922–4934. [CrossRef]
111. Cai, C.; He, H.; Duan, X.; Wu, W.; Mai, Z.; Zhang, T.; Fan, J.; Deng, T.; Zhong, W.; Liu, Y.; et al. miR-195 inhibits cell proliferation and angiogenesis in human prostate cancer by downregulating PRR11 expression. *Oncol. Rep.* **2018**, *39*, 1658–1670. [CrossRef]
112. Xu, B.; Wang, N.; Wang, X.; Tong, N.; Shao, N.; Tao, J.; Li, P.; Niu, X.; Feng, N.; Zhang, L.; et al. MiR-146a suppresses tumor growth and progression by targeting EGFR pathway and in a p-ERK-dependent manner in castration-resistant prostate cancer. *Prostate* **2012**, *72*, 1171–1178. [CrossRef]
113. Mu, H.Q.; He, Y.H.; Wang, S.B.; Yang, S.; Wang, Y.J.; Nan, C.J.; Bao, Y.F.; Xie, Q.P.; Chen, Y.H. MiR-130b/TNF-α/NF-κB/VEGFA loop inhibits prostate cancer angiogenesis. *Clin. Transl. Oncol.* **2020**, *22*, 111–121. [CrossRef] [PubMed]
114. De Oliveira, J.C.; Oliveira, L.C.; Mathias, C.; Pedroso, G.A.; Lemos, D.S.; Salviano-Silva, A.; Gradia, D.F.; Jucoski, T.S.; Lobo-Alves, S.C.; Zamalde, E.P.; et al. Long non-coding RNAs in cancer: Another layer of complexity. *J. Gene Med.* **2019**, *21*, e3065. [CrossRef]
115. Salameh, A.; Lee, A.K.; Cardó-Vila, M.; Nunes, D.; Efstathiou, E.; Staquicini, F.; Dobroff, A.S.; Machio, S.; Navone, N.; Hpsoya, H.; et al. PRUNE2 is a human prostate cancer suppressor regulated by the intronic long noncoding RNA PCA3. *Proc. Natl. Acad. Sci. USA* **2015**, *112*, 8403–8408. [CrossRef] [PubMed]
116. Tao, F.; Tian, X.; Zhang, Z. The PCAT3/PCAT9-miR-203-SNAI2 axis functions as a key mediator for prostate tumor growth and progression. *Oncotarget* **2018**, *9*, 12212–12225. [CrossRef] [PubMed]
117. Jiang, Z.; Zhang, Y.; Chen, X.; Wu, P.; Chen, D. Long noncoding RNA RBMS3-AS3 acts as a microRNA-4534 sponge to inhibit the progression of prostate cancer by upregulating VASH1. *Gene Ther.* **2020**, *27*, 143–156. [CrossRef]
118. Naito, Y.; Yoshioka, Y.; Yamamoto, Y.; Ochiya, T. How cancer cells dictate their microenvironment: Present roles of extracellular vesicles. *Cell Mol. Life Sci.* **2017**, *74*, 697–713. [CrossRef] [PubMed]
119. Ciardiello, C.; Leone, A.; Budillon, A. The Crosstalk between Cancer Stem Cells and Microenvironment Is Critical for Solid Tumor Progression: The Significant Contribution of Extracellular Vesicles. *Stem Cells Int.* **2018**, 6392198. [CrossRef]

120. Alcayaga-Miranda, F.; González, P.L.; Lopez-Verrilli, A.; Varas-Godoy, M.; Aguila-Díaz, C.; Contreras, L.; Khoury, M. Prostate tumor-induced angiogenesis is blocked by exosomes derived from menstrual stem cells through the inhibition of reactive oxygen species. *Oncotarget* **2016**, *7*, 44462–44477. [CrossRef]
121. Lorenc, T.; Klimczyk, K.; Michalczewska, I.; Słomka, M.; Kubiak-Tomasze wska, G.; Olejarz, W. Exosomes in Prostate Cancer Diagnosis, Prognosis and Therapy. *Int. J. Mol. Sci.* **2020**, *21*, 2118. [CrossRef] [PubMed]
122. Mashouri, L.; Yousefi, H.; Aref, A.R.; Ahadi, A.M.; Molaei, F.; Alahari, S.K. Exosomes: Composition, biogenesis, and mechanisms in cancer metastasis and drug resistance. *Mol. Cancer* **2019**, *18*, 75. [CrossRef] [PubMed]
123. Kim, C.W.; Lee, H.M.; Lee, T.H.; Kang, C.; Kleinman, H.K.; Gho, Y.S. Extracellular membrane vesicles from tumor cells promote angiogenesis via sphingomyelin. *Cancer Res.* **2002**, *62*, 6312–6317.
124. Webber, J.; Steadman, R.; Mason, M.D.; Tabi, Z.; Clayton, A. Cancer exosomes trigger fibroblast to myofibroblast differentiation. *Cancer Res.* **2010**, *70*, 9621–9630. [CrossRef]
125. Webber, J.P.; Spary, L.K.; Sanders, A.J.; Chowdhury, R.; Jiang, W.G.; Steadman, R.; Wymant, J.; Jones, A.T.; Kynastion, H.; Tabi, Z.; et al. Differentiation of tumour-promoting stromal myofibroblasts by cancer exosomes. *Oncogene* **2015**, *34*, 290–302. [CrossRef]
126. Chowdhury, R.; Webber, J.P.; Gurney, M.; Mason, M.D.; Tabi, Z.; Clayton, A. Cancer exosomes trigger mesenchymal stem cell differentiation into pro-angiogenic and pro-invasive myofibroblasts. *Oncotarget* **2015**, *6*, 715–731. [CrossRef]
127. DeRita, R.M.; Zerlanko, B.; Singh, A.; Lu, H.; Iozzo, R.V.; Benovic, J.L.; Languino, L.R. c-Src, Insulin-Like Growth Factor I Receptor, G-Protein-Coupled Receptor Kinases and Focal Adhesion Kinase are Enriched Into Prostate Cancer Cell Exosomes. *J. Cell. Biochem.* **2017**, *118*, 66–73. [CrossRef]
128. Liu, T.; Mendes, D.E.; Berkman, C.E. Functional prostate-specific membrane antigen is enriched in exosomes from prostate cancer cells. *Int. J. Oncol.* **2014**, *44*, 918–922. [CrossRef]
129. McKay, R.R.; Zurita, A.J.; Werner, L.; Bruce, J.Y.; Carducci, M.A.; Stein, M.N.; Heath, E.I.; Hussain, A.; Tran, T.H.; Sweeney, C.J.; et al. A Randomized Phase II Trial of Short-Course Androgen Deprivation Therapy With or Without Bevacizumab for Patients With Recurrent Prostate Cancer After Definitive Local Therapy. *J. Clin. Oncol.* **2016**, *34*, 1913–1920. [CrossRef]
130. Ning, Y.M.; Gulley, J.L.; Arlen., P.M.; Woo, S.; Steinberg, S.M.; Wright, J.J.; Parnes, H.L.; Trepel, J.B.; Lee, M.; Kim, Y.S.; et al. Phase II trial of bevacizumab, thalidomide, docetaxel, and prednisone in patients with metastatic castration-resistant prostate cancer. *J. Clin. Oncol.* **2010**, *28*, 2070–2076. [CrossRef]
131. Picus, J.; Halabi, S.; Rini, B.; Vogelzang, N.; Whang, Y.; Kaplan, E.; Kelly, W.; Small, E. The use of bevacizumab (B) with docetaxel (D) and estramustine (E) in hormone refractory prostate cancer (HRPC): Initial results of CALGB 90006 (abstract 1578). *Proc. Am. Soc. Oncol.* **2003**, *22*, 393.
132. Picus, J.; Halabi, S.; Kelly, W.K.; Vogelzang, N.J.; Whang, Y.E.; Kaplan, E.B.; Stadler, W.M.; Small, E.J.; The Cancer and Leukemia Group B. A phase 2 study of estramustine, docetaxel, and bevacizumab in men with castrate-resistant prostate cancer: Results from Cancer and Leukemia Group B Study 90006. *Cancer* **2011**, *117*, 526–533. [CrossRef] [PubMed]
133. Kelly, W.K.; Halabi, S.; Carducci, M.; George, D.; Mahoney, J.F.; Stadler, W.M.; Morris, M.; Kantoff, P.; Monk, J.P.; Kaplan, E.; et al. Randomized, double-blind, placebo-controlled phase III trial comparing docetaxel and prednisone with or without bevacizumab in men with metastatic castration-resistant prostate cancer: CALGB 90401. *J. Clin. Oncol.* **2012**, *30*, 1534–1540. [CrossRef] [PubMed]
134. Barata, P.C.; Cooney, M.; Mendiratta, P.; Gupta, R.; Dreicer, R.; Garcia, J.A. Phase I/II study evaluating the safety and clinical efficacy of temsirolimus and bevacizumab in patients with chemotherapy refractory metastatic castration-resistant prostate cancer. *Investig. New Drugs* **2019**, *37*, 331–337. [CrossRef] [PubMed]
135. Mendel, D.B.; Laird, A.D.; Xin, X.; Louie, S.G.; Christensen, J.G.; Li, G.; Schreck, R.E.; Abrams, T.J.; Ngai, T.J.; Lee, L.B.; et al. In vivo antitumor activity of SU11248, a novel tyrosine kinase inhibitor targeting vascular endothelial growth factor and platelet-derived growth factor receptors: Determination of a pharmacokinetic/pharmacodynamic relationship. *Clin. Cancer Res.* **2003**, *9*, 327–337. [PubMed]
136. Michaelson, M.D.; Oudard, S.; Ou, Y.C.; Sengeløv, L.; Saad, F.; Houede, N.; Ostler, P.; Stenzl, A.; Daugaard, G.; Jones, R.; et al. Randomized, placebo-controlled, phase III trial of sunitinib plus prednisone versus prednisone alone in progressive, metastatic, castration-resistant prostate cancer. *J. Clin. Oncol.* **2014**, *32*, 76–82. [CrossRef] [PubMed]

137. Horti, J.; Widmark, A.; Stenzl, A.; Federico, M.H.; Abratt, R.P.; Sanders, N.; Pover, G.M.; Bodrogi, I. A randomized, double-blind, placebo-controlled phase II study of vandetanib plus docetaxel/prednisolone in patients with hormone-refractory prostate cancer. *Cancer Biother. Radiopharm.* **2009**, *24*, 175–180. [CrossRef]
138. Azad, A.A.; Beardsley, E.K.; Hotte, S.J.; Ellard, S.L.; Klotz, L.; Chin, J.; Kollmannsberger, C.; Mukherjee, S.D.; Chi, K.N. A randomized phase II efficacy and safety study of vandetanib (ZD6474) in combination with bicalutamide versus bicalutamide alone in patients with chemotherapy naïve castration-resistant prostate cancer. *Investig. New Drugs* **2014**, *32*, 746–752. [CrossRef]
139. Tannock, I.F.; Fizazi, K.; Ivanov, S.; Karlsson, C.T.; Fléchon, A.; Skoneczna, I.; Orlandi, F.; Gravis, G.; Matveev, V.; Bavbek, S.; et al. Aflibercept versus placebo in combination with docetaxel and prednisone for treatment of men with metastatic castration-resistant prostate cancer (VENICE): A phase 3, double-blind randomised trial. *Lancet Oncol.* **2013**, *14*, 760–768. [CrossRef]
140. Figg, W.D.; Dahut, W.; Duray, P.; Hamilton, M.; Tompkins, A.; Steinberg, S.M.; Jones, E.; Premkumar, A.; MarstonLinehan, W.; KayFloeter, M.; et al. A randomized phase II trial of thalidomide, an angiogenesis inhibitor, in patients with androgen-independent prostate cancer. *Clin. Cancer Res.* **2001**, *7*, 1888–1893.
141. Drake, M.J.; Robson, W.; Mehta, P.; Schofield, I.; Neal, D.E.; Leung, H.Y. An open-label phase II study of low-dose thalidomide in androgen-independent prostate cancer. *Br. J. Cancer* **2003**, *88*, 822–827. [CrossRef] [PubMed]
142. Figg, W.D.; Arlen, P.; Gulley, J.; Fernandez, P.; Noone, M.; Fedenko, K.; Hamilton, M.; Parker, C.; Kruger, E.A.; Pluda, J.; et al. A randomized phase II trial of docetaxel (taxotere) plus thalidomide in androgen-independent prostate cancer. *Semin. Oncol.* **2001**, *28*, 62–66. [CrossRef]
143. Madan, R.A.; Karzai, F.H.; Ning, Y.M.; Adesunloye, B.A.; Huang, X.; Harold, N.; Couvillon, A.; Chun, G.; Cordes, L.; Sissung, T.; et al. Phase II trial of docetaxel, bevacizumab, lenalidomide and prednisone in patients with metastatic castration-resistant prostate cancer. *BJU Int.* **2016**, *11*, 590–597. [CrossRef] [PubMed]
144. Keizman, D.; Zahurak, M.; Sinibaldi, V.; Carducci, M.; Denmeade, S.; Drake, C.; Pili, R.; Antonarakis, E.S.; Hudock, S.; Eisenberger, M. Lenalidomide in non-metastatic biochemically relapsed prostate cancer: Results of a phase I/II double-blinded, randomized study. *Clin. Cancer Res.* **2010**, *16*, 5269–5276. [CrossRef]
145. Petrylak, D.P.; Vogelzang, N.J.; Budnik, N.; Jan Wiechno, P.; Sternberg, C.N.; Doner, K.; Bellmunt, J.; Burke, J.M.; de Olza, M.O.; Choudhury, A.; et al. Docetaxel and prednisone with or without lenalidomide in chemotherapy-naive patients with metastatic castration-resistant prostate cancer (MAINSAIL): A randomised, double-blind, placebo-controlled phase 3 trial. *Lancet Oncol.* **2015**, *16*, 417–425. [CrossRef]
146. Yakes, F.M.; Chen, J.; Tan, J.; Yamaguchi, K.; Shi, Y.; Yu, P.; Qian, F.; Chu, F.; Bentzien, F.; Cancilla, B.; et al. Cabozantinib (XL184), a novel MET and VEGFR2 inhibitor, simultaneously suppresses metastasis, angiogenesis, and tumor growth. *Mol. Cancer Ther.* **2011**, *12*, 2298–2308. [CrossRef]
147. Schöffski, P.; Gordon, M.; Smith, D.C.; Kurzrock, R.; Daud, A.; Vogelzang, N.J.; Lee, Y.; Scheffold, C.; Shapiro, G.I. Phase II randomised discontinuation trial of cabozantinib in patients with advanced solid tumours. *Eur. J. Cancer* **2017**, *86*, 296–304. [CrossRef]
148. Smith, D.C.; Smith., M.R.; Sweeney, C.; Elfiky, A.A.; Logothetis, C.; Corn, P.G.; Vogelzang, N.J.; Small, E.J.; Harzstark, A.L.; Gordonet, M.S.; et al. Cabozantinib in patients with advanced prostate cancer: Results of a phase II randomized discontinuation trial. *J. Clin. Oncol.* **2013**, *31*, 412–419. [CrossRef]
149. Smith, M.; De Bono, J.; Sternberg, C.; Oudard, S.; De Giorgi, U.; Krainer, M.; Bergman, A.; Hoelzer, W.; De Wit, R.; Bögemann, M.; et al. Phase III Study of Cabozantinib in Previously Treated Metastatic Castration-Resistant Prostate Cancer: COMET-1. *J. Clin. Oncol.* **2016**, *34*, 3005–3013. [CrossRef]
150. Kluetz, P.G.; Figg, W.D.; Dahut, W.L. Angiogenesis inhibitors in the treatment of prostate cancer. *Expert Opin. Pharmacother.* **2010**, *11*, 233–247. [CrossRef]
151. Melegh, Z.; Oltean, S. Targeting Angiogenesis in Prostate Cancer. *Int. J. Mol. Sci.* **2019**, *20*, 2676. [CrossRef] [PubMed]
152. Adesunloye, B.A.; Karzai, F.H.; Dahut, W.L. Angiogenesis inhibitors in the treatment of prostate cancer. *Chem. Immunol. Allergy* **2014**, *99*, 197–215. [CrossRef] [PubMed]
153. Yu, E.M.; Jain, M.; Aragon-Ching, J.B. Angiogenesis inhibitors in prostate cancer therapy. *Discov. Med.* **2010**, *10*, 521–530. [PubMed]
154. De Bono, J.S.; Scher, H.I.; Montgomery, R.B.; Parker, C.; Miller, M.C.; Tissing, H.; Doyle, G.V.; Terstappen, L.W.; Pienta, K.J.; Raghavan, D.; et al. Circulating tumor cells predict survival benefit from treatment in metastatic castration-resistant prostate cancer. *Clin. Cancer Res.* **2008**, *14*, 6302–6309. [CrossRef] [PubMed]

155. Hlatky, L.; Hahnfeldt, P.; Folkman, J. Clinical application of antiangiogenic therapy: Microvessel density, what it does and doesn't tell us. *J. Natl. Cancer Inst.* **2002**, *94*, 883–893. [CrossRef]
156. Jain, R.K.; Schlenger, K.; Höckel, M.; Yuan, F. Quantitative angiogenesis assays: Progress and problems. *Nat. Med.* **1997**, *3*, 1203–1208. [CrossRef]
157. Jiang, J.; Chen, Y.; Zhu, Y.; Yao, X.; Qi, J. Contrast-enhanced ultrasonography for the detection and characterization of prostate cancer: Correlation with microvessel density and Gleason score. *Clin. Radiol.* **2011**, *66*, 732–737. [CrossRef]

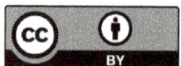

© 2020 by the authors. Licensee MDPI, Basel, Switzerland. This article is an open access article distributed under the terms and conditions of the Creative Commons Attribution (CC BY) license (http://creativecommons.org/licenses/by/4.0/).

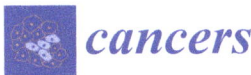

Perspective

Repurposing of α1-Adrenoceptor Antagonists: Impact in Renal Cancer

Meredith Mihalopoulos [1], Zachary Dovey [1], Maddison Archer [1,2], Talia G. Korn [1], Kennedy E. Okhawere [1], William Nkemdirim [1], Hassan Funchess [1], Ami Rambhia [1], Nihal Mohamed [1], Steven A. Kaplan [1], Reza Mehrazin [1], Dara Lundon [1], Che-Kai Tsao [3], Ketan K. Badani [1] and Natasha Kyprianou [1,2,4,*]

1. Department of Urology, Tisch Cancer Institute, Icahn School of Medicine at Mount Sinai, New York, NY 10029, USA; meredith.mihalopoulos@icahn.mssm.edu (M.M.); zachary.dovey@mountsinai.org (Z.D.); Maddison.Archer@mountsinai.org (M.A.); Talia.korn@mountsinai.org (T.G.K.); Kennedy.Okhawere@mountsinai.org (K.E.O.); wn442@nyu.edu (W.N.); hf1031@nyu.edu (H.F.); ar6326@nyu.edu (A.R.); nihal.mohamed@mountsinai.org (N.M.); steven.kaplan@mountsinai.org (S.A.K.); reza.mehrazin@mountsinai.org (R.M.); Dara.Lundon@mountsinai.org (D.L.); ketan.badani@mountsinai.org (K.K.B.)
2. Department of Oncological Sciences, Icahn School of Medicine at Mount Sinai, New York, NY 10029, USA
3. Department of Medicine/Division of Hematology-Oncology, Icahn School of Medicine at Mount Sinai, New York, NY 10029, USA; che-kai.tsao@mssm.edu
4. Department of Pathology and Laboratory Medicine, Icahn School of Medicine at Mount Sinai, New York, NY 10029, USA
* Correspondence: natasha.kyprianou@mountsinai.org

Received: 20 July 2020; Accepted: 24 August 2020; Published: 28 August 2020

Abstract: Renal cancer ranks twelfth in incidence among cancers worldwide. Despite improving outcomes due to better therapeutic options and strategies, prognosis for those with metastatic disease remains poor. Current systemic therapeutic approaches include inhibiting pathways of angiogenesis, immune checkpoint blockade, and mTOR inhibition, but inevitably resistance develops for those with metastatic disease, and novel treatment strategies are urgently needed. Emerging molecular and epidemiological evidence suggests that quinazoline-based α1-adrenoceptor-antagonists may have both chemopreventive and direct therapeutic actions in the treatment of urological cancers, including renal cancer. In human renal cancer cell models, quinazoline-based α1-adrenoceptor antagonists were shown to significantly reduce the invasion and metastatic potential of renal tumors by targeting focal adhesion survival signaling to induce anoikis. Mechanistically these drugs overcome anoikis resistance in tumor cells by targeting cell survival regulators AKT and FAK, disrupting integrin adhesion (α5β1 and α2β1) and engaging extracellular matrix (ECM)-associated tumor suppressors. In this review, we discuss the current evidence for the use of quinazoline-based α1-adrenoceptor antagonists as novel therapies for renal cell carcinoma (RCC) and highlight their potential therapeutic action through overcoming anoikis resistance of tumor epithelial and endothelial cells in metastatic RCC. These findings provide a platform for future studies that will retrospectively and prospectively test repurposing of quinazoline-based α1-adrenoceptor-antagonists for the treatment of advanced RCC and the prevention of metastasis in neoadjuvant, adjuvant, salvage and metastatic settings.

Keywords: renal tumors; prevention; α1-adrenoceptor antagonists; anoikis; vascularity

---

1. Introduction: The Therapeutic Challenge

Renal cancer ranks twelfth in incidence among cancers worldwide and has a lifetime risk of 1 to 63 for a given individual, with numbers estimated to be increasing at a rate of 2.4% per year [1,2].

Globally, 6 in 100,000 males and 3 in 100,000 females are diagnosed annually with renal cancer, with the incidence estimated to be increasing at a rate of 2.4% per year [1,2] with limited therapeutic management options [3–5]. In the United States alone, over 60,000 individuals were diagnosed with renal cell carcinoma (RCC) in 2018, with an estimated 14,970 deaths resulting from the illness [6]. Despite the introduction of systemic targeted therapies, five-year survival rates for locally advanced and metastatic disease remain at 70% and 12%, respectively in the year 2020 [7].

The most common genetic abnormality for clear cell RCC (ccRCC) is the chromosome 3p deletion and inactivation of the von Hippel Lindau (VHL) tumor suppressor gene, present in almost all familial and up to 60% of sporadic RCCs [8,9]. Loss of the VHL gene leads to the upregulation of hypoxia-inducible factor (HIF) and activation of vascular endothelial growth factor receptors (VEGFR) and other signaling pathways, leading to tumorigenesis with an aggressive angiogenic phenotype [8,9]. Current treatment of RCC is based on the tumor stage at diagnosis. Localized disease, with or without evidence of regional spread, is typically managed surgically alone. For those with more advanced localized or loco-regional disease after nephrectomy, treatment with adjuvant VEGFR TKI sunitinib has been approved by the Federal Drug Administration, although the modest clinical benefit and concern for the potential side effects has largely limited its clinical application to data [10].

For metastatic ccRCC, a number of approaches combining immune checkpoint inhibitors or with VEGFR-TKIs have now become the standard of care after demonstrating a definitive survival benefit in the first-line setting [11], compared to sunitinib alone [2]. However, the optimal first-line and sequence of subsequent therapies are not well defined. The current systemic therapeutic approaches include: targeting pathways of angiogenesis, immune checkpoint blockade, and mTOR inhibition. Inevitably, treatment resistance is either intrinsic or eventually develops. New mechanistic approaches are urgently needed to improve survival outcomes in this patient population.

Investigative efforts from our group and others have focused on the role of quinazoline-derived α1-adrenoreceptor antagonists in the treatment of renal cancer. By inducing smooth muscle relaxation and vasodilation, these drugs are currently used in the treatment of hypertension (HTN) and renal and ureteric stones [12,13], as well as of benign prostatic hyperplasia (BPH) [13]. More recently the potential efficacy of these drugs in the treatment of prostate cancer has been proposed, due to the ability to induce apoptosis and overcome anoikis resistance in tumor cells [14–18]. Reassuringly, in earlier clinical trials assessing their use for the treatment of BPH, they were well tolerated with only reversible adverse effects in a minority of patients, including postural hypotension (4%), asthenia or light-headedness (10%), somnolence (3%) and retrograde ejaculation (8%) [19,20].

Expression and distribution of α1-adrenoreceptors has been found in the cortex, pelvis, calyces, blood vessels and tubules of the kidney, suggesting potential effects of α1 adrenoceptor antagonists in renal pathophysiology [21–25]. Evidence at the cellular level suggests that the antitumor effect of α1-adrenoreceptor antagonists in renal tumors proceeds via reducing vascularity and impairing growth within the tumor microenvironment (via apoptosis and overcoming anoikis resistance). In this review, we outline the mechanism of α1-adrenoreceptor antagonists in targeting renal cancer epithelial and endothelial cells and the potential therapeutic efficacy of using these clinically used FDA-approved drugs for the treatment of advanced RCC.

2. Mechanism of Action of α-Adrenoreceptor Antagonists in Human Disease

Adrenergic receptors (adrenoreceptors) are G-Protein coupled-receptors that are distributed throughout the body. They serve as receptors for catecholamines (noradrenaline and epinephrine) secreted from the autonomic sympathetic nervous system and play an important role in the regulation of a wide range of physiological systems in the body [23,24]. Alpha (α) receptors mediate smooth muscle contraction and vasoconstriction, while beta (β) receptors mediate vasodilation, smooth muscle relaxation, bronchodilation, and excitatory cardiac function [17,21]. The α-adrenoceptors are divided into two classes: α1 and α2, both of which are present in the renal vasculature and mediate vasoconstriction of exogenous and endogenous noradrenaline [22,24]. The α1-adrenoceptors are further sub-divided into α1A, α1B, α1D, with α1A subtype of therapeutic interest because of its location in the prostate, vas deferens, and urethra in humans [21,23–25].

Quinazoline-derived compounds blocking α1-adrenoreceptors have been found to reduce prostatic smooth muscle tone and relieve overall obstruction, as seen by their success in treating BPH [19]. This mechanism of action is also utilized in the treatment of renal and ureteric stones, as α1 blockers reduce intra-ureteral pressure and increase fluid passage [12,26–28]. Remarkably in human prostatic disease, these compounds not only target the alpha1-adrenergic-receptor mediated smooth muscle contraction [29], but they can also effectively induce apoptosis of tumor epithelial and endothelial cells [17,30,31]. It is important to note that the quinazoline-derived compounds can induce apoptosis among benign prostate epithelial cells, as well as in both androgen-dependent and castration-resistant prostate cancer cells, via α1-adrenoceptor –independent mechanisms [30–35]. This supports a strong cellular basis for their pharmacologic use in other cancer types.

The signaling mechanisms driving the intracellular antitumor action by quinazoline-based α1-adrenoceptor antagonists against prostate cancer epithelial and endothelial cells are summarized on Figure 1. (1) Smad activation of transforming growth factor (TGF)-β1 signaling, which controls cellular proliferation, differentiation, and apoptosis in human cancers cell including prostate cancer cells [3,30–32]; (2) Engaging the death receptor Fas-associated death domain (FADD)-mediated caspase-8 activation and apoptosis induction [3,32,33]; (3) Inhibition of the VEGF-mediated angiogenesis and Akt survival mechanisms navigating tumor vascularity [3,33,34]; and (4) α1-adrenoceptor antagonists have the ability to block cellular adhesion and invasion by targeting cell-cell interaction and impairing cell tight junctions (and also between epithelial and endothelial cells with the extracellular matrix; ECM), consequentially impacting epithelial–mesenchymal-transition (EMT) to mesenchymal–epithelial-transition (MET) phenotypic interconversions and increasing cellular vulnerability to anoikis (Figure 1) [3,35,36].

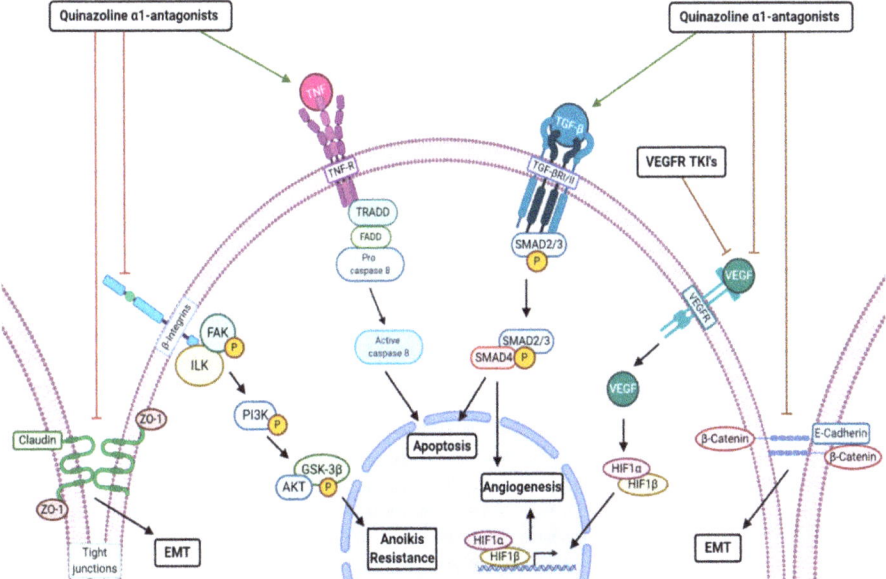

Figure 1. Biological Mechanisms of Anti-tumor Action of Quinazoline α1-Adrenoceptor Antagonists. Schematic diagram demonstrating the signaling mechanisms potentially targeted by quinazolne α1-andrenoceptor antagonists in attenuating renal tumor initiation and progression to metastasis. Quinazoline based α1-adrenoceptor antagonists influence the interconversion of epithelial– mesenchymal-transition (EMT) to mesenchymal–epithelial-transition (MET) phenotypes by targeting

tight junctions and E-cadherin-mediates cell adherence. Tumor cells succumb to anoikis by disruption of integrin-mediated cell survival via integrin-linked kinase (ILK). Quinazoline based α1-andrenoceptor antagonists induce apoptosis by either tumor necrosis factor (TNF)-mediated Fas-associated death domain (FADD)/caspase 8 activity and DNA fragmentation and/or Smad4 activation and apoptotic gene induction by transforming growth factor (TGF)-β. Angiogenesis is inhibited by vascular endothelial growth factor receptor (VEGFR)–tyrosine kinase inhibitors and quinazoline based α1-andrenoceptor antagonists can also target tumor vascularity by disruption of VEGF-mediated HIF1 transcriptional expression and potentially TGF-β signaling.

Moreover we previously established that integrin-linked kinase (ILK), a serine and threonine protein kinase, plays a key role in anoikis resistance by interacting with the cytoplasmic domains of β1-integrin and β3-integrin, which are pivotal in regulating cell adhesion, fibronectin–ECM assembly, and anchorage-dependent cell growth [34–37]. Within the tumor microenvironment (TME), ILK is activated in its phosphorylated form by focal adhesion kinase (FAK) and phosphatidylinositol 3-kinase (PI3-kinase)/Akt pathways [33,38–40]. By inhibiting ILK, quinazoline-derived α1-adrenoceptor antagonists can disrupt these cell-survival signals towards anoikis induction [3,41,42]. Considering that resistance to anoikis (and evasion of apoptosis in detached cells) is a primary contributor to cancer metastasis [43,44] and ultimately lethal disease, the ability to overcome this resistance points to a unique therapeutic value of quinazoline-derived α1-adrenoceptor antagonists.

3. Antitumor Effects of α1-Adrenoceptor Antagonists

Table 1 summarizes the updated evidence from clinical, translational and epidemiological studies, suggesting the antitumor action of α1-adrenoceptor antagonists in human malignancies. The published work from our group and other investigators makes a strong case in support of the repurposing of the α1-adrenoceptor antagonists (with a good safety profile) and advance our current understanding of the clinical value of these therapeutic modalities for the treatment of GU-cancers including renal cancer

Table 1. Therapeutic Impact of α1-Adrenoreceptor Antagonists Use against Human Cancers.

Drug	Neoplasm	Effect		Cellular Mechanism
Naftopidil, Prazosin [14,45]	Bladder Cancer	Inhibit cell growth and viability in vitro in ACHN human cell lines	-	Induce apoptosis via caspase activity
Doxazosin [46]	Colorectal Cancer	Decrease tumor numbers and size in vitro in RKO human cell lines and in vivo in mouse models	-	Induce apoptosis via caspase activity
Doxazosin, Naftopidil, Prozasin, Terozasin, DZ-50 [14,17,32,35,45]	Prostate Cancer	Reduce cell viability and tumor vascularity in vitro and in vivo, including in castration-resistant prostate cancer	-	G2 checkpoint arrest Inhibit cell growth Decrease microvessel density Induce apoptosis via caspase activity, Smad activation of TGF-β1 signaling (Doxazosin) Induce anoikis by disrupting integrin-mediated cell survival pathways (DZ-50)
Doxazosin, Naftodipil, DZ-50 [3,45]	RCC	Inhibit cell proliferation and reduce vascularity in vitro and in vivo in lines with and without VHL mutation	-	Induce apoptosis by disabling FADD inhibitors, Smad activation of TGF-β1 signaling (Dozazosin) G1 cell cycle induction arrested in tumor and vascular epithelial cells (Naftopidil) Induce anoikis by disrupting integrin-mediated cell survival pathways (DZ-50)
Terazosin [46]	TCC	Reduce tumor vascularity and cell growth in vivo	-	Induce apoptosis and decrease microvessel density

3.1. Prostate Cancer

Based on these pharmacological mechanisms of actions, α1-adrenoceptor antagonists have been shown to have efficacy in the treatment of several genitourinary cancers. There is mounting evidence of the effectiveness of quinazoline-derived α1 blockers in the clinical treatment patients with BPH and prostate tumors. Studies have shown that α1-adrenoceptor antagonists like prozasin and naftopidil inhibit cell growth, arrest cell cycling, decrease microvessel density, and induce apoptosis in human prostate cancer cells [34,35,45]. Doxazosin, a clinically used quinazoline-based α1-adrenoreceptor antagonist, reduced endothelial cell viability and suppressed tumor vascularity in prostate cancer xenografts. The drug additionally exhibited significant antitumor efficacy against models of metastatic castration-resistant prostate cancer (CRPC) [17,30]. In a retrospective observational cohort study at the VA Medical Center in Kentucky, Harris et al. (2007) found that in over a 5-year period in this clinical setting, exposure to quinazoline-based α1-adrenoreceptors antagonists, such as doxazosin and terazosin, significantly decreased the incidence of prostate cancer from 2.4% to 1.65%, corroborating the results of previous investigations [15,45]. While a case-control study of 23,320 men in the Finnish Cancer Registry and national prescription database found tamsulosin and alfuzosin did not improve the odds of developing prostate cancer, the study did discover the drugs significantly decreased the incidence of high-grade tumors in the cohort [47].

More recently, Hart et al. (2020) studied 303 prostate cancer patients to retrospectively determine if α1-blockers influenced response to radiotherapy for localized prostate cancer. The authors found that those treated with prazosin had a 3.9 lower relative risk of biochemical relapse. While not statistically significant, both tamsulosin and prazosin extended survival without recurrence by 13.15 and 9.21 months, respectively [48]. Furthermore, drug optimization efforts led to the development of the quinazoline-derived drug DZ-50. This novel α1 blocker has exerted chemoprotective qualities in vivo in BPH and prostate cancer cells through decreasing angiogenesis and increasing anoikis via inhibition of the TGF-β1 and insulin-like growth factor (IGF) pro-growth pathways [34,35].

3.2. Bladder Cancer

When evaluating antitumor activity of α1 blockers in terms of cell viability, cell cycle progression, competition, and apoptotic signaling in bladder cancer, Nakagawa et al. (2016) showed that naftopidil was one of the strongest antitumor α1-adrenoceptor antagonists [45]. Significantly enough, oral administration of naftopidil reduced tumor volume in a xenograft model in a concentration (10–100 µmol/L)-dependent manner, suggesting promising outcomes of α1 blockers in bladder cancer treatment [16]. To a lesser extent, prazosin has been shown to reduce survival of human bladder cancer cells at concentrations more than 30 µmol/L [14]. Terazosin, proven to induce apoptosis in prostate cancer cells, reduced tumor vascularity and induced apoptosis in transitional cell carcinoma (TCC) of the bladder in a retrospective case-control study using a pathological examination of specimens from patients undergoing radical cystectomy (Table 1) [49]. An independent retrospective observational study of 27,183 men confirmed these results and found that those treated with the quinazoline based adrenoceptor antagonists terazosin and doxazosin had a 43% lower relative risk of developing bladder cancer than unexposed men [50].

3.3. Colorectal Cancer

Epidemiological evidence from case-control studies enabled promising insights into the use of doxazosin as therapeutic and a chemopreventive strategy in treating colorectal cancer. An in vitro case-control study found that the α1 adrenoceptor antagonist, doxazosin significantly suppressed the proliferation of RKO colon cancer cell lines within human colorectal cancer cell assays. Recent pre-clinical studies demonstrated in vivo treatment of mice harboring colon cancer xenografts with doxazosin resulted in a significant decrease in tumor numbers and size compared to control untreated mice [46]. While limited, these results support the ongoing pursuit of the use of α1-adrenoreceptors antagonists in cancer treatment.

3.4. Adrenal Cancer

While not directly related to the genitourinary system as the other malignancies we have discussed, it is important to address the recent discoveries of the effect of α1-adrenoreceptors antagonists on adrenal cancer, specifically pheochromocytoma. While limited, there are promising preliminary results in the anti-adrenergic effects of α1-blockade in managing unchecked catecholamine production in pheochromocytoma. High circulating catecholamine levels stimulate alpha receptors on blood vessels, thereby causing vasoconstriction and increased total peripheral resistance. Thus, α-adrenergic blockade helps control blood pressure and prevent hypertensive crisis in the preoperative setting of surgical resection for metastatic pheochromocytomas [51]. While randomized controlled trials are lacking, a literature review has shown the effectiveness of doxazosin and phenoxybenzamine in the preoperative treatment of pheochromocytomas; however, further research is needed in better understanding the use of these drugs, especially in combination with β-blockers for preoperative treatment [51,52].

4. Potential Therapeutic Value in Renal Cancer

Original studies by our group provided initial translational insights into the therapeutic effects of α1-adrenoceptor antagonists in RCC preclinical models [3]. Doxazosin induces apoptosis in cancer cells through similar α1-adrenoceptor-independent mechanisms as found in human prostate cancer cell models [3]. Molecular assays have demonstrated this quanizoline-based α1-adrenoceptor antagonist induces apoptosis in prostate cancer cells expressing C-Flip, an endogenous inhibitor of FADD-mediated activation, and subsequently cleaving caspase-8 [3]. As illustrated on Figure 1, doxazosin also induces apoptosis in renal cancer cells through activation of TGF-β1 signaling via Smad effector phosphorylation and targeting Akt survival mechanisms [31–34].

Additional cell-based evidence suggests that α1-blockers impair cancer progression to metastasis via anoikis induction at pharmacologically relevant doses, proceeding via an α1-adrenoreceptor-independent mechanism. Structural optimization studies led to the generation of a quinazoline-based derivative, of α1-adrenoreceptors antagonist, DZ-50, that was shown to overcome anoikis resistance in human renal cancer cells by disrupting integrin/FAK-mediated cell survival pathways in vitro and in vivo [3]. Doxazosin and DZ-50 were both found to exert potent antitumor action against human renal cancer cell lines 786-0 (harboring a VHL tumor-suppressor gene mutation and a highly angiogenic phenotype) and Caki cells (without a VHL mutation) [3].

DZ-50 has the chemoprotective potential to suppress angiogenesis and reverse the hypoxic nature of cancer through disrupting the tumor microenvironment [30]. The process of EMT, directed by TGF-β within the tumor microenvironment phenotypic landscape, confers acquisition of an invasive phenotype via resistance to anoikis, promoting angiogenesis, metastatic progression, and treatment failure. We first reported the ability of the novel quinazoline-derivative, DZ-50 to disrupt the ILK-1/integrin β1 complex and reduce phosphorylation of its downstream targets, AKT and GSK-3β [3]. As mentioned, this is an important mechanism in inducing anoikis in cancer cells because ILK regulates several integrin-mediated cellular processes, including cell adhesion, fibronectin-ECM assembly and anchorage-dependent cell growth [35,39]. By inhibiting ILK, DZ-50 is then able to kill tumor cells via blocking AKT and FAK phosphorylation and subsequent cell survival, disrupting integrin adhesion (α5β1 and α2β1), and engaging ECM associated tumor suppressors [3,30]. Through anoikis induction, DZ-50 has been found to significantly impair RCC metastasis in in vitro and in vivo models [3,17]. In vitro metastasis assays found that DZ-50 significantly decreased the adhesion potential of RCC to fibronectin and laminin in a time-dependent manner and subsequently suppressed the cells' migratory and invasive capabilities. Mechanistic analysis of anoikis induction (determined by Annexin V-based flow cytometry) revealed that this novel agent inactivates critical cellular survival pathways through inhibition of FAK phosphorylation, inactivation of AKT and GSK-β in the focal adhesion complex signaling cascade, and disruption of integrin-mediated focal adhesion complexes, such as FAK, ILK-1 and paxillin [3]. By interfering with this survival signaling, DZ-50 successfully reverses anoikis resistance and induces cancer cell death [3,17]. By sensitizing cells to anoikis through disruption of integrin β1-mediated focal adhesion complexes, the novel quinazoline-derived agent acquires a high therapeutic value by effectively reversing anoikis resistance in metastatic RCC tumors [3]. Temporal analysis of cell death in response to DZ-50, established that anoikis occurred prior to apoptosis [3]. Furthermore, DZ-50 exerted a more potent inhibitor effect than doxazosin on ILK-1, FAK, and paxillin binding to integrin-β1 in vivo in human renal cancer 786-0 and Caki cells [3,17,18]. In both RCC cell lines, DZ-50 led to significantly greater inhibition of tumor cell adhesion, migration and invasion than doxasozin did at pharmacologically relevant doses [3]. These findings support that the structural optimization of this particular quinazoline-based α1-adrenoreceptor antagonist has furthered a promising effect in inducing anoikis and impairing renal tumor vascularity to impair metastasis. Naftopidil has also been investigated in this context, with studies demonstrating in vitro suppression of proliferation in ACHN and Caki-2 RCC cell lines [13,53]. Fluorescence-activated cell sorting (FACS) analysis revealed that renal cancer cells treated with naftopidil underwent G_1-cell cycle arrest in vitro; the drug also decreased tumor weight and vascularity in RCC xenograft models in naftopidiol-treated excised human RCC [53]. Therefore, naftopidil provides another putative systemic therapy for the treatment and prevention of RCC that, based on this evidence, warrants further investigation.

5. The Repurposing of α1-Blockade in the Management of RCC

Drug repurposing refers to the development of new applications and uses for existing drugs. The advantage of this method is that the drugs under investigation have already been "de-risked," have been approved by the FDA, have an established safety/toxicity profile and their subsequent development timelines and costs are significantly reduced. Historically, the concept of drug repurposing has been based on incidental discoveries, but a more formal approach has been proposed internationally to realize the potential in reusing currently available drugs. Emerging recommendations for integrative platforms of data analysis to systematically synthesize results from industry drug trials for more efficient discovery of new therapeutic uses and effects of novel compounds, advance combinatorial approaches for efficacy and treatment optimization. Drug repurposing has also been accelerated by the removal of patency and regulatory barriers that may prevent clinical use and the increasing funding opportunities for drug repurposing initiatives, particularly for less common diseases [54].

Quinazoline-based α1-adrenoceptor-antagonists represent an important category of drug repurposing, having already been FDA approved, with an established safety profile and extensively prescribed for the treatment of HTN and BPH for the last 30 years. Moreover, RCC patients, who have an average age at diagnosis of 65 years, commonly suffer from comorbidities including HTN and BPH (if male), notwithstanding the common association of HTN with RCC as a paraneoplastic syndrome secondary to renin and adrenocorticotropic hormone (ACTH) secretion, parenchymal or ureteral compression, and polycythaemia or an arterio-venous fistula. This would lend itself to the use of quinazoline-α1-adrenoceptor-antagonists as a logical choice in RCC patients with HTN for a potential bimodal treatment effect. Clinicians treating patients with RCC have a strong advantage to further explore such treatment and impact patient survival.

Analogous to the observational cohort study in prostate cancer discussed earlier, epidemiology studies retrospectively exploring the use of quinazoline-based α1-adrenoceptor-antagonists for the treatment of HTN or BPH for patients who were subsequently diagnosed with RCC would allow comparisons of cumulative incidence with populations of RCC patients who were unexposed, thus providing insight into the chemopreventive effects of the drug [17,46]. In a surgical setting, retrospective analyses of patient cohorts who underwent nephrectomy for renal masses with and without extensive exposure to α1-adrenoceptors for the treatment of HTN or BPH pre-operatively, as well as patients who continued α1 blockade for a period of time post-surgery, would allow an assessment of the efficacy of neoadjuvant or adjuvant quinazoline-based α1-adrenoceptor-antagonists on long-term RCC oncological outcomes. Moreover, immunohistochemical profiling of renal tumors may establish a novel anoikis signature that could correlate with the effects of α1 blockade on clinical outcome and survival in patients with high-risk RCC, potentially contributing to risk stratification and treatment decisions. Finally, applying translational research to further investigate the mechanisms of quinazoline-induced anoikis in RCC and its influence on both the tumor microenvironment and EMT may reveal additional actions on alternative signaling pathways and guide the development of combination regimes with other emerging targeted therapies.

6. Conclusions and Future Directions

In summary, this review accomplishes the aim of the study to investigate the effectiveness of quinazoline-based α1-adrenoceptor antagonists in the treatment of RCC by demonstrating the translational value of quinazoline-based α1-adrenoceptor-antagonists as anti-tumor-modalities with potential efficacy at all stages of the RCC patients' journey (neoadjuvant, adjuvant, salvage and metastatic). Retrospective epidemiological studies are underway to assess the impact of quinazoline-derived α1 adrenoceptor antagonists as chemopreventive agents, and prospective clinical trials designed to investigate their efficacy in pre-surgical, post-surgical, and in-patient settings of metastatic disease. There is high translational significance in the repurposing of the α1-adrenoceptor antagonists (FDA-approved drugs) to establish their therapeutic benefit as effective treatment modalities for patients with metastatic renal cell carcinoma (RCC). Our current research efforts pursue this drug repurposing at three levels: (a) the mechanistic level, by interrogating the functional exchanges between anoikis signaling and phenotypic EMT within the kidney TME to define novel mechanisms of action; (b) the translational level by directly examining precision combination therapies in pre-clinical models of RCC with and without VHL mutations; and (c). at the clinical setting by undertaking retrospective epidemiological studies to determine the impact of the use of quinazoline-derived α1 adrenoceptor antagonists as chemopreventive agents in RCC cancan also by prospective clinical trials designed to investigate their efficacy in pre-surgical, post-surgical, and in-patient settings of RCC patients with metastatic disease [54]. If such investigative efforts demonstrate clear efficacy, RCC patients with advanced disease can therapeutically benefit from their clinical use in the near future. With the international initiatives in place encouraging the use of repurposed drugs, the introduction of new, effective RCC treatment modalities based on α1-blockade can rapidly be integrated into clinical use and markedly improve oncological outcomes of RCC patients.

Author Contributions: Conceptualization, M.M., Z.D., K.K.B. and N.K.; methodology, M.M., Z.D., M.A., T.G.K.; software, M.A., K.E.O., W.N., H.F.; validation, M.M., A.R., N.M., and N.K.; formal analysis, M.M., Z.D., T.G.K., S.A.K., R.M., D.L., C.-K.T., K.K.B.; investigation, M.M., Z.D., K.E.O., R.M., K.K.B., N.K.; resources, S.A.K., C.-K.T., K.K.B., N.K.; data curation, Z.D., N.M., D.L., N.K.; writing—original draft preparation, M.M., Z.D., S.A.K., R.M., K.K.B., N.K.; writing—review and editing, M.M., Z.D., N.K.; visualization, M.M., M.A., T.G.K.; supervision, N.K.; project administration, K.K.B., N.K.; funding acquisition, N.K. All authors have read and agreed to the published version of the manuscript.

Funding: This research received support from an NIH/NCI R01 grant CA232574 (NK).

Acknowledgments: The authors wish to acknowledge the support of the Department of Urology and the Kidney Cancer Center of Excellence at the Icahn School of Medicine at Mount Sinai for the completion of this work.

Conflicts of Interest: The authors declare no conflict of interest.

Abbreviations

ACTH	Adrenocorticotropic Hormone
ASCO	American Society of Clinical Oncology
BPH	Benign Prostatic Hyperplasia
CRPC	Castration-Resistant Prostate Cancer
ECM	Extracellular Matrix
EMT	Epithelial–Mesenchymal Transition
MET	Mesennchymal–Epithelial-Transition
FACS	Fluorescence-activated cell sorting
FADD	Fas-Associated Death Domain
FAK	Focal Adhesion Kinase

FDA	Food and Drug Administration
HIF-α	Hypoxia-Inducible Factor-α
HTN	Hypertension
IGF	Insulin-Like Growth Factor
ILK	Integrin-Linked Kinase
PI3-K	Phosphatidylinositol 3-Kinase
RCC	Renal Cell Carcinoma
TCC	Transitional Cell Carcinoma (of the bladder)
TGF-β	Transforming Growth Factor-β
TKI	Tyrosine Kinase Inhibitors
TME	Tumor Microenvironment
TNF	Tumor Necrosis Factor
VHL	von Hippel-Lindau
VEGF	Vascular Endothelial Growth Factor
VEGFR	Vascular Endothelial Growth Factor Receptor

References

1. Saad, A.M.; Gad, M.M.; Al-Husseini, M.J.; Ruhban, I.A.; Sonbol, M.B.; Ho, T.H. Trends in Renal-Cell Carcinoma Incidence and Mortality in the United States in the Last 2 Decades: A SEER-Based Study. *Clin. Genitourin Cancer* **2019**, *17*, 46–57.e45. [CrossRef] [PubMed]
2. Ljungberg, B.; Albiges, L.; Bensalah, K.; Bex, A.; Giles, G.H.; Hora, M.; Kuczyk, M.A.; Lam, T.; Marconi, L.; Merseburger, A.S.; et al. EAU Guidelines: Renal Cell Carcinoma. Available online: http://uroweb.org/guidelines/compilations-of-all-guidelines/ (accessed on 15 June 2020).
3. Sakamoto, S.; Schwarze, S.; Kyprianou, N. Anoikis disruption of focal adhesion-Akt signaling impairs renal cell carcinoma. *Eur. Urol.* **2011**, *59*, 734–744. [CrossRef] [PubMed]
4. Gangadaran, S.G.D. Current Management Options in Metastatic Renal Cell Cancer. *Oncol. Rev.* **2017**, *11*, 339. [CrossRef] [PubMed]
5. Gandaglia, G.; Ravi, P.; Abdollah, F.; Abd-El-Barr, A.E.; Becker, A.; Popa, I.; Briganti, A.; Karakiewicz, P.I.; Trinh, Q.D.; Jewett, M.A.; et al. Contemporary incidence and mortality rates of kidney cancer in the United States. *Can. Urol. Assoc. J.* **2014**, *8*, 247–252. [CrossRef] [PubMed]
6. Siegel, R.L.; Miller, K.D.; Jemal, A. Cancer statistics, 2018. *CA Cancer J. Clin.* **2018**, *68*, 7–30. [CrossRef]
7. A.S.O.C. Kidney Cancer: Statistics. Available online: https://www.cancer.net/cancer-types/kidney-cancer/statistics (accessed on 15 June 2020).
8. Cairns, P. Renal cell carcinoma. *Cancer Biomark.* **2010**, *9*, 461–473. [CrossRef] [PubMed]
9. Chappell, J.C.; Payne, L.B.; Rathmell, W.K. Hypoxia, angiogenesis, and metabolism in the hereditary kidney cancers. *J. Clin. Investig.* **2019**, *129*, 442–451. [CrossRef]
10. Ravaud, A.; Motzer, R.J.; Pandha, H.S.; George, D.J.; Pantuck, A.J.; Patel, A.; Chang, Y.H.; Escudier, B.; Donskov, F.; Magheli, A.; et al. Adjuvant Sunitinib in High-Risk Renal-Cell Carcinoma after Nephrectomy. *N. Engl. J. Med.* **2016**, *375*, 2246–2254. [CrossRef]
11. Zhang, T.; Hwang, J.K.; George, D.J.; Pal, S.K. The landscape of contemporary clinical trials for untreated metastatic clear cell renal cell carcinoma. *Cancer Treat. Res. Commun.* **2020**, *24*, 100183. [CrossRef]
12. Campschroer, T.; Zhu, Y.; Duijvesz, D.; Grobbee, D.E.; Lock, M.T. Alpha-blockers as medical expulsive therapy for ureteral stones. *Cochrane Database Syst. Rev.* **2014**. [CrossRef]
13. Lepor, H. Landmark studies impacting the medical management of benign prostatic hyperplasia. *Rev. Urol.* **2003**, *5*, S34–S41. [PubMed]
14. Batty, M.; Pugh, R.; Rathinam, I.; Simmonds, J.; Walker, E.; Forbes, A.; Anoopkumar-Dukie, S.; McDermott, C.M.; Spencer, B.; Christie, D.; et al. The Role of α1-Adrenoceptor Antagonists in the Treatment of Prostate and Other Cancers. *Int. J. Mol. Sci.* **2016**, *17*, 1339. [CrossRef] [PubMed]
15. Harris, A.M.; Warner, B.W.; Wilson, J.M.; Becker, A.; Rowland, R.G.; Conner, W.; Lane, M.; Kimbler, K.; Durbin, E.B.; Baron, A.T.; et al. Effect of alpha1-adrenoceptor antagonist exposure on prostate cancer incidence: An observational cohort study. *J. Urol.* **2007**, *178*, 2176–2180. [CrossRef] [PubMed]
16. Gotoh, A.; Nagaya, H.; Kanno, T.; Nishizaki, T. Antitumor action of α(1)-adrenoceptor blockers on human bladder, prostate and renal cancer cells. *Pharmacology* **2012**, *90*, 242–246. [CrossRef] [PubMed]
17. Wade, C.A.; Goodwin, J.; Preston, D.; Kyprianou, N. Impact of α-adrenoceptor antagonists on prostate cancer development, progression and prevention. *Am. J. Clin. Exp. Urol.* **2019**, *7*, 46–60.
18. Bilbro, J.; Mart, M.; Kyprianou, N. Therapeutic value of quinazoline-based compounds in prostate cancer. *Anticancer Res.* **2013**, *33*, 4695–4700.

19. Lepor, H. Alpha blockers for the treatment of benign prostatic hyperplasia. *Rev. Urol.* **2007**, *9*, 181–190. [CrossRef]
20. Karabacak, O.R.; Sener, N.C.; Yilmazer, D.; Karabacak, Y.; Goktug, H.N.; Yigitbasi, O.; Alper, M. Alpha adrenergic receptors in renal pelvis and calyces: Can rat models be used? *Int. Braz. J. Urol.* **2014**, *40*, 683–689. [CrossRef]
21. Minamisawa, K.; Umemura, S.; Hirawa, N.; Hayashi, S.; Toya, Y.; Ishikawa, Y.; Yasuda, G.; Ishii, M. Characteristic localization of alpha 1- and alpha 2-adrenoceptors in the human kidney. *Clin. Exp. Pharmacol. Physiol.* **1993**, *20*, 523–526. [CrossRef]
22. Uhlén, S.; Lindblom, J.; Kindlundh, A.; Mugisha, P.; Nyberg, F. Nandrolone treatment decreases the level of rat kidney alpha(1B)-adrenoceptors. *Naunyn. Schmiedebergs Arch. Pharmacol.* **2003**, *368*, 91–98. [CrossRef]
23. Bylund, D.B. Adrenergic Receptors. In *The Adrenergic Receptors: In the 21st Century*; Perez, D.M., Ed.; Humana Press: Totowa, NJ, USA, 2006; pp. 3–21. [CrossRef]
24. Civantos Calzada, B.; Aleixandre de Artiñano, A. Alpha-adrenoceptor subtypes. *Pharmacol. Res.* **2001**, *44*, 195–208. [CrossRef] [PubMed]
25. Hesse, I.F.; Johns, E.J. An in vivo study of the alpha-adrenoreceptor subtypes on the renal vasculature of the anaesthetized rabbit. *J. Auton Pharmacol.* **1984**, *4*, 145–152. [CrossRef] [PubMed]
26. Kobayashi, S.; Tang, R.; Shapiro, E.; Lepor, H. Characterization and localization of prostatic alpha 1 adrenoceptors using radioligand receptor binding on slide-mounted tissue section. *J. Urol.* **1993**, *150*, 2002–2006. [CrossRef]
27. Marshall, I.; Burt, R.P.; Chapple, C.R. Noradrenaline contractions of human prostate mediated by alpha 1A-(alpha 1c-) adrenoceptor subtype. *Br. J. Pharmacol.* **1995**, *115*, 781–786. [CrossRef]
28. Taniguchi, N.; Ukai, Y.; Tanaka, T.; Yano, J.; Kimura, K.; Moriyama, N.; Kawabe, K. Identification of alpha1-adrenoceptor subtypes in the human prostatic urethra. *Naunyn Schmiedeberg's Arch. Pharmacol.* **1997**, *355*, 412–416. [CrossRef]
29. Forray, C.; Bard, J.A.; Wetzel, J.M.; Chiu, G.; Shapiro, E.; Tang, R.; Lepor, H.; Hartig, P.R.; Weinshank, R.L.; Branchek, T.A.; et al. The alpha 1-adrenergic receptor that mediates smooth muscle contraction in human prostate has the pharmacological properties of the cloned human alpha 1c subtype. *Mol. Pharmacol.* **1994**, *45*, 703–708.
30. Kyprianou, N.; Benning, C.M. Suppression of human prostate cancer cell growth by alpha1-adrenoceptor antagonists doxazosin and terazosin via induction of apoptosis. *Cancer Res.* **2000**, *60*, 4550–4555.
31. Anglin, I.E.; Glassman, D.T.; Kyprianou, N. Induction of prostate apoptosis by alpha1-adrenoceptor antagonists: Mechanistic significance of the quinazoline component. *Prostate Cancer Prostatic Dis.* **2002**, *5*, 88–95. [CrossRef]
32. Benning, C.M.; Kyprianou, N. Quinazoline-derived alpha1-adrenoceptor antagonists induce prostate cancer cell apoptosis via an alpha1-adrenoceptor-independent action. *Cancer Res.* **2002**, *62*, 597–602.
33. Garrison, J.B.; Kyprianou, N. Novel targeting of apoptosis pathways for prostate cancer therapy. *Curr. Cancer Drug Targets* **2004**, *4*, 85–95. [CrossRef]
34. Partin, J.V.; Anglin, I.E.; Kyprianou, N. Quinazoline-based alpha 1-adrenoceptor antagonists induce prostate cancer cell apoptosis via TGF-beta signalling and I kappa B alpha induction. *Br. J. Cancer* **2003**, *88*, 1615–1621. [CrossRef] [PubMed]
35. Keledjian, K.; Garrison, J.B.; Kyprianou, N. Doxazosin inhibits human vascular endothelial cell adhesion, migration, and invasion. *J. Cell Biochem.* **2005**, *94*, 374–388. [CrossRef] [PubMed]
36. Hannigan, G.E.; Leung-Hagesteijn, C.; Fitz-Gibbon, L.; Coppolino, M.G.; Radeva, G.; Filmus, J.; Bell, J.C.; Dedhar, S. Regulation of cell adhesion and anchorage-dependent growth by a new beta 1-integrin-linked protein kinase. *Nature* **1996**, *379*, 91–96. [CrossRef] [PubMed]
37. Li, F.; Liu, J.; Mayne, R.; Wu, C. Identification and characterization of a mouse protein kinase that is highly homologous to human integrin-linked kinase. *Biochim. Biophys. Acta* **1997**, *1358*, 215–220. [CrossRef]
38. Wu, C.; Dedhar, S. Integrin-linked kinase (ILK) and its interactors: A new paradigm for the coupling of extracellular matrix to actin cytoskeleton and signaling complexes. *J. Cell Biol.* **2001**, *155*, 505–510. [CrossRef] [PubMed]
39. Radeva, G.; Petrocelli, T.; Behrend, E.; Leung-Hagesteijn, C.; Filmus, J.; Slingerland, J.; Dedhar, S. Overexpression of the integrin-linked kinase promotes anchorage-independent cell cycle progression. *J. Biol. Chem.* **1997**, *272*, 13937–13944. [CrossRef]

40. Cieslik, K.; Zembowicz, A.; Tang, J.L.; Wu, K.K. Transcriptional regulation of endothelial nitric-oxide synthase by lysophosphatidylcholine. *J. Biol. Chem.* **1998**, *273*, 14885–14890. [CrossRef]
41. Attwell, S.; Roskelley, C.; Dedhar, S. The integrin-linked kinase (ILK) suppresses anoikis. *Oncogene* **2000**, *19*, 3811–3815. [CrossRef]
42. Fukuda, T.; Chen, K.; Shi, X.; Wu, C. PINCH-1 is an obligate partner of integrin-linked kinase (ILK) functioning in cell shape modulation, motility, and survival. *J. Biol. Chem.* **2003**, *278*, 51324–51333. [CrossRef]
43. Frisch, S.M.; Francis, H. Disruption of epithelial cell-matrix interactions induces apoptosis. *J. Cell Biol.* **1994**, *124*, 619–626. [CrossRef]
44. Frisch, S.M.; Screaton, R.A. Anoikis mechanisms. *Curr. Opin. Cell Biol.* **2001**, *13*, 555–562. [CrossRef]
45. Nakagawa, Y.U.; Nagaya, H.; Miyata, T.; Wada, Y.; Oyama, T.; Gotoh, A. Piperazine-based Alpha-1 AR Blocker, Naftopidil, Selectively Suppresses Malignant Human Bladder Cells via Induction of Apoptosis. *Anticancer Res.* **2016**, *36*, 1563–1570. [PubMed]
46. Suzuki, N.; Niikura, R.; Ihara, S.; Hikiba, Y.; Kinoshita, H.; Higashishima, N.; Hayakawa, Y.; Yamada, A.; Hirata, Y.; Nakata, R.; et al. Alpha-Blockers As Colorectal Cancer Chemopreventive: Findings from a Case-Control Study, Human Cell Cultures, and In Vivo Preclinical Testing. *Cancer Prev. Res.* **2019**, *12*, 185–194. [CrossRef] [PubMed]
47. Murtola, T.J.; Tammela, T.L.; Määttänen, L.; Ala-Opas, M.; Stenman, U.H.; Auvinen, A. Prostate cancer incidence among finasteride and alpha-blocker users in the Finnish Prostate Cancer Screening Trial. *Br. J. Cancer* **2009**, *101*, 843–848. [CrossRef] [PubMed]
48. Hart, J.; Spencer, B.; McDermott, C.M.; Chess-Williams, R.; Sellers, D.; Christie, D.; Anoopkumar-Dukie, S. A Pilot retrospective analysis of alpha-blockers on recurrence in men with localised prostate cancer treated with radiotherapy. *Sci. Rep.* **2020**, *10*, 8191. [CrossRef]
49. Tahmatzopoulos, A.; Lagrange, C.A.; Zeng, L.; Mitchell, B.L.; Conner, W.T.; Kyprianou, N. Effect of terazosin on tissue vascularity and apoptosis in transitional cell carcinoma of bladder. *Urology* **2005**, *65*, 1019–1023. [CrossRef]
50. Martin, F.M.; Harris, A.M.; Rowland, R.G.; Conner, W.; Lane, M.; Durbin, E.; Baron, A.T.; Kyprianou, N. Decreased risk of bladder cancer in men treated with quinazoline-based α1-adrenoceptor antagonists. *Gene Ther. Mol. Biol.* **2008**, *12*, 253–258.
51. Blake, M.; Sweeney, A.T.; Griffing, G. Pheochromocytoma. Available online: https://emedicine.medscape.com/article/124059-overview (accessed on 18 August 2020).
52. Van der Zee, P.; de Boer, A. Pheochromocytoma: A review on preoperative treatment with phenoxybenzamine or doxazosin. *Neth. J. Med.* **2014**, *72*, 190–201.
53. Iwamoto, Y.; Ishii, K.; Sasaki, T.; Kato, M.; Kanda, H.; Yamada, Y.; Arima, K.; Shiraishi, T.; Sugimura, Y. Oral naftopidil suppresses human renal-cell carcinoma by inducing G(1) cell-cycle arrest in tumor and vascular endothelial cells. *Cancer Prev. Res.* **2013**, *6*, 1000–1006. [CrossRef]
54. Pushpakom, S.; Iorio, F.; Eyers, P.A.; Escott, K.J.; Hopper, S.; Wells, A.; Doig, A.; Guilliams, T.; Latimer, J.; McNamee, C.; et al. Drug repurposing: Progress, challenges and recommendations. *Nat. Rev. Drug Discov.* **2019**, *18*, 41–58. [CrossRef]

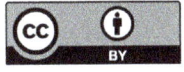

© 2020 by the authors. Licensee MDPI, Basel, Switzerland. This article is an open access article distributed under the terms and conditions of the Creative Commons Attribution (CC BY) license (http://creativecommons.org/licenses/by/4.0/).

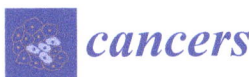

Review

Cellular and Molecular Progression of Prostate Cancer: Models for Basic and Preclinical Research

Sirin Saranyutanon [1,2], Sachin Kumar Deshmukh [1,2], Santanu Dasgupta [1,2], Sachin Pai [3], Seema Singh [1,2,4] and Ajay Pratap Singh [1,2,4,*]

1. Cancer Biology Program, Mitchell Cancer Institute, University of South Alabama, Mobile, AL 36604, USA; ss1830@jagmail.southalabama.edu (S.S.); skdeshmukh@health.southalabama.edu (S.K.D.); dasgupta@southalabama.edu (S.D.); seemasingh@health.southalabama.edu (S.S.)
2. Department of Pathology, College of Medicine, University of South Alabama, Mobile, AL 36617, USA
3. Department of Medical Oncology, Mitchell Cancer Institute, University of South Alabama, Mobile, AL 36604, USA; spai@health.southalabama.edu
4. Department of Biochemistry and Molecular Biology, University of South Alabama, Mobile, AL 36688, USA
* Correspondence: asingh@health.southalabama.edu; Tel.: +1-251-445-9843; Fax: +1-251-460-6994

Received: 26 August 2020; Accepted: 11 September 2020; Published: 17 September 2020

Simple Summary: The molecular progression of prostate cancer is complex and elusive. Biological research relies heavily on in vitro and in vivo models that can be used to examine gene functions and responses to the external agents in laboratory and preclinical settings. Over the years, several models have been developed and found to be very helpful in understanding the biology of prostate cancer. Here we describe these models in the context of available information on the cellular and molecular progression of prostate cancer to suggest their potential utility in basic and preclinical prostate cancer research. The information discussed herein should serve as a hands-on resource for scholars engaged in prostate cancer research or to those who are making a transition to explore the complex biology of prostate cancer.

Abstract: We have witnessed noteworthy progress in our understanding of prostate cancer over the past decades. This basic knowledge has been translated into efficient diagnostic and treatment approaches leading to the improvement in patient survival. However, the molecular pathogenesis of prostate cancer appears to be complex, and histological findings often do not provide an accurate assessment of disease aggressiveness and future course. Moreover, we also witness tremendous racial disparity in prostate cancer incidence and clinical outcomes necessitating a deeper understanding of molecular and mechanistic bases of prostate cancer. Biological research heavily relies on model systems that can be easily manipulated and tested under a controlled experimental environment. Over the years, several cancer cell lines have been developed representing diverse molecular subtypes of prostate cancer. In addition, several animal models have been developed to demonstrate the etiological molecular basis of the prostate cancer. In recent years, patient-derived xenograft and 3-D culture models have also been created and utilized in preclinical research. This review is an attempt to succinctly discuss existing information on the cellular and molecular progression of prostate cancer. We also discuss available model systems and their tested and potential utility in basic and preclinical prostate cancer research.

Keywords: prostate cancer; research model; oncogenes; tumor suppressor genes

1. Introduction

Prostate cancer (PCa) is the most commonly diagnosed malignancy and the second leading cause of cancer-related death in men in the United States. It is estimated that PCa will afflict approximately

191,930 men and cause nearly 33,330 deaths this year in the United States alone [1]. Notably, PCa incidence and associated mortality are nearly two-thirds and over two times higher, respectively, in African-American (AA) men compared to their Caucasian-American (CA) counterparts [2,3]. PCa follows a defined pattern of cellular progression but exhibits diverse molecular pathobiology making it one of most highly heterogeneous cancers [4,5]. The prostate-specific antigen (PSA) test is the primary detection tool for PCa screening. However, due to the lack of accuracy and specificity, the usefulness of PSA for PCa diagnosis has been questioned [6–8]. Most PCa patients are generally subjected to localized radical prostatectomy, radiation therapy, proton beam therapy, and cryosurgery after the initial diagnosis [9–11]. However, for patients with metastatic disease or recurrent cancer with locoregional and distant metastases, androgen-deprivation therapy (ADT) or castration therapy is considered the primary line of treatment [12]. Unfortunately, despite the initial outstanding therapeutic response, most PCa patients treated with ADT eventually have the relapse of PCa in a highly aggressive and therapy-resistant form leading to poor clinical outcomes [13,14].

To meet the challenges associated with prostate cancer clinical management, research labs across the world have been working tirelessly to understand underlying molecular diversity and biology of PCa. These efforts have resulted in novel therapies that are currently in clinics, while researchers continue to gather more insights to address new hurdles and failures faced in clinical settings. These advances have been possible through the development of several in vitro and in vivo research models, while new models continue to be developed to address the genetic and biological complexities associated with the PCa. In this review, we discuss the cellular and molecular progression of PCa as well as the available in vitro and in vivo models for PCa research. We believe that the information presented herein will be helpful to the researchers, especially those who are new to the field, in understanding the molecular pathobiology of PCa and guide them in choosing the correct model(s) for their laboratory and preclinical research.

2. Cellular and Molecular Progression of Prostate Cancer

The human prostate is a walnut-size glandular organ that develops from the embryonic urogenital sinus [15]. Its primary function is to produce seminal fluid containing zinc, citric acid, and various enzymes, including a protease named prostate-specific antigen (PSA). Histologically, the prostate can be divided into central, peripheral, and transition zones comprised of a secretory ductal-acinar structure located within a fibromuscular stroma [16,17]. The ductal-acinar structure is formed of tall columnar secretory luminal cells, a flattened basal epithelium attached to the basement membrane, and scattered neuroendocrine cells (Figure 1). Luminal epithelial cells express cytokeratins (CK) 8 and 18, NKX3.1, androgen receptor (AR), and PSA, whereas basal epithelial cells express CK5, CK14, glutathione S-transferase Pi 1 (GSTP1), p63, and low levels of AR [18,19].

The cellular origin of prostate cancer is not very clear, partly because of the lack of well-characterized prostate epithelial lineage [20–22]. PCa develops from normal prostate epithelium through a multistep histological transformation process, governed by various underlying molecular changes [23] (Figure 2). Low-grade and high-grade prostate intraepithelial neoplasia (PIN) lesions develop from normal prostate epithelium through the loss of phosphatase and the tensin homolog *(PTEN)*, NK3 Homeobox 1 *(NKX3.1)*, overexpression of *MYC* proto-oncogene, B-cell lymphoma 2 *(BCL-2)*, and the glutathione S-transferase pi 1 gene *(GSTP1)*, accompanied with Speckle Type BTB/POZ Protein *(SPOP)* mutation and Transmembrane Serine Protease 2- ETS-related gene *(TMPRSS2-ERG)* fusion [24–36]. Further loss of the retinoblastoma protein *(RB1)*, along with telomerase activation and frequent Forkhead Box A1 *(FOXA1)* mutation, leads to the development of prostate adenocarcinoma from the advanced PIN lesion [37–43]. Further molecular aberrations including the loss of SMAD Family Member 4 *(SMAD4)*, AR corepressors, mutations in AR, *FOXA1*, *BRCA1/2*, *ATM*, *ATR*, and *RAD51* accompanied with the gain of function of the AR coactivator, *CXCL12*, *CXCR4*, *RANK-RANKL*, EMT, *BAI1*, and *EZH2* lead to the development of metastatic prostate cancer [44–59].

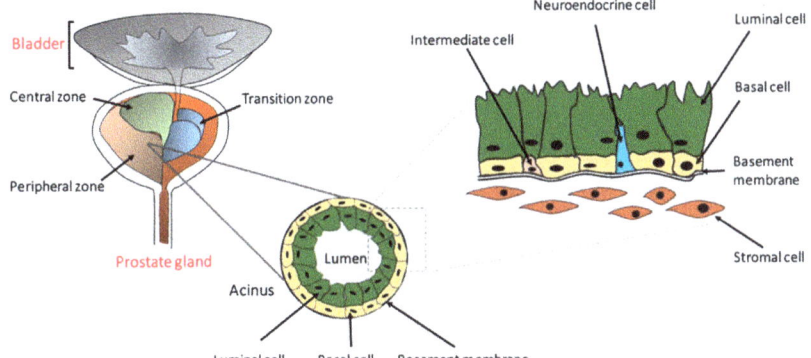

Figure 1. The location and architecture of the human prostate gland. The prostate gland is located below the bladder and consists of a central, a peripheral, and a transition zone. Histologically, it is comprised of secretary luminal, basal, and rare intermediate and neuroendocrine cells. The prostatic epithelium is separated from the stromal cells by the basement membrane as indicated. Preneoplastic or neoplastic cellular transformation can initiate from either basal or luminal cells.

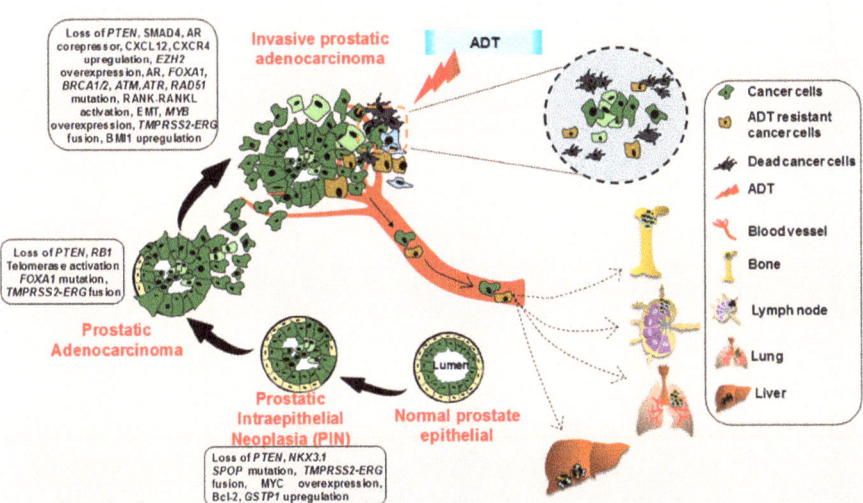

Figure 2. Histopathological and molecular progression of human prostate cancer. Metastatic prostate cancer develops via progression through prostate intraepithelial neoplasia (PIN) and invasive adenocarcinoma through the acquirement of various molecular alterations as depicted. The invasive adenocarcinoma cells and androgen-deprivation therapy resistant cancer cells metastasize to the bone, lymph node, lung, and liver.

As evident from the PCa progression model (Figure 2), inactivation of *PTEN* appears to be a critical event in PCa carcinogenesis and associated with aggressive disease manifestation. *PTEN* alterations occur in various ways in prostate cancer, such as genomic deletion and rearrangement, intragenic breakage, or translocation. The loss of *PTEN* is linked with an upregulation of PI3K/AKT/mTOR signaling that regulates cell survival, proliferation, and energy metabolism [60,61]. Another critical determinant of PCa tumorigenesis is *SMAD4*, a tumor suppressor gene (18q21.1), which mediates the transforming growth factor β (TGF-β) signaling pathway and suppresses epithelial cell growth.

Transcriptome analysis revealed significantly lower levels of *SMAD4* in PCa tissues compared to adjacent non-cancerous tissues [46]. Of note, in a mouse model, prostate specific ablation of *Smad4* and *Pten* leads to the development of an invasive and metastatic potential of PCa (discussed below) [45].

In the PCa initiation and progression cascade, tumor suppressor *NKX3.1* (8p21) plays a pivotal role and found to be frequently lost due to the loss of heterozygosity (LOH) [62,63]. Of note, LOH at 8p21 appears to be an early event in PCa tumorigenesis [63–65]. Thus, it is likely that the genes that reside within these frequently deleted regions are associated with PCa initiation. Under the normal condition, *NKX3.1* drives growth-suppressing and differentiating effects on the prostatic epithelium [66]. *Nkx3.1* heterozygous mice develop abnormal prostate morphology with the dysplastic epithelium [67,68]. Importantly, *Nkx3.1*-null mice show changes in prostate epithelial morphology with severe dysplasia [67]. Kim et al. demonstrated that the loss of function of *Pten* and *Nkx3.1* in mice cooperated in PCa development. Importantly, *Pten;Nkx3.1* compound mutant mice showed a higher incidence of High-grade prostatic intraepithelial neoplasia (HGPIN) [69]. In addition to the critical tumor suppressor genes described above, the *MYC* proto-oncogene is also amplified in PCa [70–72]. *MYC* encodes a transcription factor that regulates the expression of several genes involved in cell proliferation, metabolism, mitochondrial function, and stem cell renewal [73–75]. Several studies suggest that *MYC* is activated through overexpression, amplification, rearrangement, Wnt/β-catenin pathway activation, germline *MYC* promotor variation, and loss of *FOXP3* in PCa [76–79], and is a critical oncogenic event driving PCa initiation and progression [71,80].

Other than *MYC*, *TMPRSS2:ERG* gene fusion, resulting from the chromosomal rearrangement, is also reported in approximately 45% of PCa. This alteration leads to the expression of the truncated *ERG* protein under the control androgen-responsive gene promoter of *TMPRSS2* [81–85]. *ERG* belongs to the *ETS* family of transcription factors (*ERG*, *ETV1*, and *ETV4*), and its activation is associated with PCa progression in both early- and late-stages [82,83,86]. *MYB*, another gene encoding a transcription factor, is also reported to be amplified in PCa and exhibits an increased amplification frequency in castration resistant PCa (CRPC) [87]. Research from our laboratory has shown that *MYB* plays a vital role in PCa growth, malignant behavior, and androgen-depletion resistance [56].

3. Prostate Cancer Research Models

As discussed above, we have made appreciable progress in our understanding of PCa pathobiology over the past several years. These insights resulted from the efforts at multiple levels: (i) recording of clinicopathological data and histopathological examination of tumor sections at the microscopic levels, (ii) molecular profiling of clinical specimens to identify molecular aberrations associated with defined histopathological characteristics, and (iii) conducting laboratory assays to define the functional significance of identified molecular aberrations. The development of PCa research models by scientists played a significant role in these laboratory and preclinical efforts. Prostate cell lines (cancer and non-cancer) established from patients have been instrumental as research models to gain functional and mechanistic insight. A comprehensive list of cell lines used in PCa research is given in Table 1. Moreover, quite a few mouse models have also been developed that not only provide direct evidence for the oncogenic function of a gene or gene-set but also serve as models for furthering basic and translational cancer research. Recently, 3-D in vitro cultures and patient-derived tumor xenografts (PDXs) have been developed as well, which are mostly used for translational research. Below we describe some of these models and discuss their characteristics and potential significance.

Table 1. Prostate cancer cell line models and their characteristics.

Cell Line	Origin	Doubling Time	AR	PSA	Markers	Cyto-Keratin	Source	Refs.
Non-cancerous prostate epithelial cell lines								
RWPE-1	NPEC in peripheral zone	120 h	+	+	p53, Rb	8, 18	ATCC	[88,89]
BPH-1	Primary prostatic tissue	35 h	−	−	p53, BAX, PTEN, p21	8, 18, 19	ACCEGEN, Creative Bioarray, DSMZ	[90]
pRNS-1-1	radical prostatectomy	72 h	−	−	PTEN	5, 8	NCI and Stanford University	[91]
RC77N/E	Non-malignant tissue of a PCa patient	No report	+	−	NKX3.1, p16	8	Tuskegee University	[92]
HprEpC	Normal human prostate	No report	+	+	Cytokeratin 18	14, 18, 19	Cell applications, iXcells Biotechnologies, EZ biosystem	[93]
Hormone sensitive								
LNCaP	lymph node metastatic	28–60 h	+	+	WT p53, PTEN loss, vimentin, PAP, CBP, negative desmin	8, 18, 20	ATCC, Creative Bioarray, ACCEGEN, SIGMA	[94]
LAPC-4	lymph node metastatic from an androgen insensitive patient	72 h	+	+	p53 mutation	5, 8, 18	ATCC *	[95]
LAPC-9	bone metastasis from a patient with ADT	No report	+	+	Ki67, PTEN loss	5	ATCC *	[96]
VCaP	metastatic tumor	51 h	+	+	p53 mutation, Rb, PAP, PTEN	8, 18	ATCC, SIGMA, ACCEGEN	[97]
MDA-PCa 2a/2b	bone metastasis from an African-American male	82–93 h/42–73 h	+	+	WT p53, p21, Rb, Bcl-2	5, 8, 18	ATCC	[98]
LuCaP 23.1	lymph node and liver metastatic	11–21 days	+	+	5α-reductase type I, WT PTEN	No report	University of Washington	[99]
RC-77T/E	Radical prostatectomy from an African-American patient	No report	+	+	p16, NKX3.1, β-catenin, α-actinin-1, filamin-A	8	Tuskegee University	[92]
Castration resistant								
PC-3	lumbar vertebral metastasis	33 h	−	−	PTEN loss, no p53 expression, TGF-α, EGFR, transferrin receptor	7, 8, 18, 19	ATCC, SIGMA, ACCEGEN, Creative Bioarray	[100]
DU-145	Brain metastasis	34 h	−	−	TGF-α/β, EGFR, IGF-1, EGF	5, 7, 8, 18	ATCC, ACCEGEN	[101]

Table 1. Cont.

Cell Line	Origin	Doubling Time	AR	PSA	Markers	Cyto-Keratin	Source	Refs.
C4-2/ C4-2B	mouse vertebral metastasis LNCaP cell xenograft	48 h	+	+	p53, PTEN loss, marker chromosome m1	8	ATCC	[102,103]
22Rv1	CWR22R xenograft derivative	35–40 h	+	+	kallikrien-like serine protease, AR splice variant	8, 18	ATCC, SIGMA, ACCEGEN, Creative Bioarray	[104]
ARCaP	ascites fluid of a patient with advanced metastatic disease	No report	+	+	EGFR, c-erb B2/neu, c-erb B3, bombesin, serotonin	8, 18	Novicure Biotechnology	[105]

(* = Discontinued).

3.1. Cell Line Models

3.1.1. Non-Cancerous Prostate Epithelial Cell Lines

RWPE-1

This cell line model was established from the peripheral zone of a histologically normal adult human prostate from a 54-year-old man. The cells were immortalized by transduction with human papillomavirus 18 (HPV-18) to establish a stable line [88]. RWPE-1 cells exhibit the expression of AR and androgen-inducible expression of kallikrein-3 (KLK3) or PSA. These cells also express CK8 and CK18, which are the characteristic markers of the luminal prostatic epithelium [89]. Further, RWPE-1 cells exhibit heterogeneous nuclear staining for p53 and Rb proteins as well [89]. The growth of these cells is induced upon treatment with the epidermal growth factor (EGF) and fibroblast growth factor (FGF) in a dose-dependent manner, whereas TGF-β treatment inhibits their growth [89,106,107].

BPH-1

BPH-1 is an immortalized benign prostatic hyperplasia cell line model established from primary prostatic tissue obtained by transurethral resection from a 68-year-old patient [90]. Immortalization of these cells was achieved by transduction with simian virus 40 (SV40) large T antigen [90]. BPH-1 cells express wild type (WT) PTEN, WT p53 as well as CK8, CK18, and CK19 suggestive of their luminal epithelial origin [108], but are negative for AR, PSA, and prostatic acid phosphatase (PAP) [90]. Cytogenetic analysis of these cells revealed an aneuploidy karyotype with a modal chromosome number of 76 (range 71-79). EGF, TGF-β, FGF-1, and FGF-7 treatment induces the proliferation of these cells, while FGF-2, TGF-β1, and TGF-β2 are shown to have an opposite effect [90]. Due to the lack of AR expression, these cells do not respond to androgen treatment [90]. They are non-tumorigenic in nude mice [108].

pRNS-1-1

pRNS-1-1 is a human prostatic epithelial cell line model derived from a 53-year-old male who had undergone radical prostatectomy. These cells were transfected with a plasmid, pRNS-1-1, containing the SV40 genome expressing T-antigen to establish a stable line. pRNS-1-1 cells express WTPTEN, and CK5 and CK8 suggestive of their epithelial origin [91]. The pRNS-1-1 cells do not express either AR or PSA [109,110]. The growth of these cells is promoted by EGF, IGF, and bovine pituitary extract treatment, while TGF-β has an inhibitory effect. pRNS-1-1 cells do not form tumors when injected subcutaneously in nude mice [109].

RC-77N/E

The RC-77N/E prostate epithelial cell line model was derived from the non-malignant prostate tissue isolated from a 63-year-old African American (AA) man diagnosed with PCa [92]. RC-77N/E cells are immortalized by the expression of HPV-16E6/E7 and exhibit an epithelial morphology. These cells are androgen-sensitive and express CK8, AR, PSA, and p16. RC-77N/E does not form tumors in severe combined immunodeficiency (SCID) mice [92]. This line could be useful for racial disparity associated PCa studies.

HprEpC

Human prostate epithelial cells (HprEpCs) were isolated from the normal human prostate. HPrEpC model cells express both prostatic basal epithelial marker CK14 and luminal prostatic epithelium markers CK18 and CK19 suggesting that they are intermediate cells [93]. Besides their application as normal control cells for PCa research, HprEpC cells are useful tools in studying the hormonal regulation and secretory function of the prostate.

3.1.2. Prostate Cancer Cell Lines

Prostate cancer cell lines established from human patients are broadly categorized into two types (castration-sensitive and castration-resistant) depending upon their survivability under androgen-deprived conditions.

Castration-Sensitive

LNCaP

LNCaP is a widely used human PCa cell line model. This cell line was developed in 1980 from a lesion in the left supraclavicular lymph node metastasis of human prostatic adenocarcinoma from a 50-year-old Caucasian male [94]. LNCaP cells are weakly adherent and slow-growing and have a doubling time of about 60-72 h. LNCaP cells express AR and PSA and exhibit a biphasic regulation of growth following androgen treatment [111]. These cells have a point mutation in AR (T877A) and express WT p53 [112,113]. These cells also harbor one mutated and other deleted alleles of *PTEN* [114]. Additionally, these cells are CK8, CK18, CK20, and vimentin-positive [115]. LNCaP cells require androgens to sustain their growth, but several derivative androgen-depletion resistant cell lines have been developed following slow and long-term androgen-deprivation or through their selection from mouse-xenograft tumors [116,117].

LAPC-4

LAPC-4 (Los Angeles prostate cancer 4) model cell line was established from a lymph node metastasis of a hormone-refractory PCa patient through direct transfer of surgically removed tissues (2–3 mm sections) into male SCID mice. The tissue explants were subcutaneously xenografted into the mice, and later tumor cells were harvested from mouse xenografts and plated on the culture dish to generate the cell line [95]. These cells are very slow growing, with a doubling rate of around 72 h [113]. LAPC-4 cells express wild type AR and PSA [118]. The expression of both CK5 (a basal epithelial marker) and CK8 (luminal epithelium marker) is also detected in these cells suggestive of their dedifferentiation [95]. Although these cells are castration-sensitive, forced overexpression of human epidermal growth factor receptor 2 (HER-2/neu) is shown to cause ligand independence by activation of the AR pathway [119]. Further, HER2 overexpression synergizes with low levels of androgen to potentiate AR activation [119]. LAPC4 are tumorigenic and can grow subcutaneously, orthotopically, or intratibially in nude mice [120–122].

LAPC-9

The LAPC-9 (Los Angeles prostate cancer 9) cell line was derived from the bone metastasis of the prostate cancer patient that had undergone androgen-ablation therapy [96]. These cells express AR and PSA and undergo growth arrest upon androgen ablation [123]. It is shown that LAPC-9 cells can remain in a dormant state for at least six months following castration and can emerge as castration-resistant following a long period of androgen deprivation [96]. LAPC-9 cells develop tumors in nude mice upon subcutaneous injection [96,124]. They can respond rapidly to androgen replenishment and re-enter the cell cycle and resume growth [96].

RWPE-2

The RWPE-2 cell line is derived from the HPV-18 immortalized RWPE-1 cells by transformation with Ki-ras using the Kirsten murine sarcoma virus (Ki-MuSV). The overexpression of Ki-ras bestowed tumorigenicity to these cells since Ki-ras activation is implicated in prostate carcinogenesis [89]. These cells express CK8, CK18, WT p53, WT Rb, AR, and PSA and are hormone responsive. EGF and FGF promote RWPE-2 cell growth, and in contrast, TGF-β has growth inhibitory effects on these cells. RWPE-2 cells that form colonies in agar have an invasive potential [89] and form tumors when injected subcutaneously into the nude mice [125].

VCaP

The VCaP (vertebral cancer of the prostate) cell line was established in 1997 from a metastatic prostate tumor that developed in the vertebrae of a 59-year-old Caucasian patient with the hormone-refractory disease who had failed androgen deprivation therapy [97]. VCaP was passaged as xenografts in nude mice and then cultured in vitro. The VCaP cells exhibit multiple features of clinical PCa, including expression of PSA, PAP, and AR. One study has also shown the elevated expression of the AR-V7 variant in VCaP xenograft after castration by next-generation RNA-Seq [126]. Additionally, these cells express CK-8, CK-18, Rb, and p53 (with A248W mutation). As per the American Type Culture Collection, the doubling time of this cell line was about 51 h (VCaP ATCC CRL-2876TM). These cells form tumors when injected subcutaneously in SCID mice [97,127]. The presence of the *TMPRSS2:ERG* fusion gene has been shown to stimulate the growth of the VCaP orthotopic mouse model [128].

MDA-PCa 2a/2b

MDA-PCa 2a and MDA-PC 2b cell lines were established from two distinct areas of prostate tumor derived from a 63-year-old African American (AA) subject having a late-stage bone metastasis [98]. The patient was under relapse following castration therapy at the time of cell isolation. MDA-PCa 2a/2b cells express WT AR, WT p53, KLK3/PSA, WT PTEN, and p21 [129,130]. Coming from two different areas of the tumor, they have different doubling times. MDA-PCa 2a cells double in number in about 82–93 h, whereas MDA-PCa2b has a doubling time of 42–73 h [98]. These cells can form tumors in mice when injected subcutaneously [98]. Although, the MDA-PCa 2a/2b cells are derived from an androgen-independent tumor but are sensitive and responsive to androgens [98]. Among these lines, MDA-PCa 2b is androgen dependent [131]. Later, a new androgen refractory subline MDA-PCa 2b-hr was developed following 35 weeks of androgen depletion to represent clinical PCa recurrence during androgen ablation treatment [131]. These lines could also be useful for racial disparity-associated PCa studies.

LuCaP 23.1

LuCaP 23.1, Lucan 23.8, and LuCaP 23.12 cell line series were developed in 1996 from two different lymph node metastases (LNM) of a 63-year-old Caucasian PCa patient (adenocarcinoma with Gleason score 8). Cancer tissues from this subject were xenografted subcutaneously in nude mice and passaged serially to establish these xenograft lines. All three lines are AR-positive and responsive to androgen and express WT PTEN at mRNA levels [99]. Notably, androgen depletion in mice harboring these three lines prolonged tumor growth with a concomitant decrease in the PSA expression level. However, some of the tumors eventually relapsed following castration and were considered hormone-refractory. Thus, studying these models could be invaluable to unravel the sequential molecular events driving relapse and acquirement of androgen independence. Moreover, tumor progression in these models can be monitored by measuring the PSA level. The LuCaP 35 model was developed from the LNM of a 66-year-old PCa patient (Stage T4c) through subcutaneous implantation in nude mice, as described above. This line expresses PSA and AR (harbors AR amplification and C1863T mutation) and is androgen-sensitive [132]. The LuCaP 35 cells can be cultured in vitro, unlike the LuCaP 23 cells, and produce LN and pulmonary metastases when implanted orthotopically. The LuCaP 35V cells were established from recurrent LuCaP 35 cells and are androgen-independent. Collectively, these are unique in vivo and in vitro models to study the mechanism of castration resistance [133]. Later, several cell lines such as LuCaP 23.12, LuCaP 23.8, LuCaP 35, LuCaP 41, LuCaP 49, LuCaP 58, and LuCaP 73 were developed. LuCaP 23.1, LuCaP 23.12, LuCaP 23.8, LuCaP 35, LuCaP 41, LuCaP 49, LuCaP 58, and LuCaP 73 cells express AR and PSA.

RC-77T/E

The RC-77T/E cell line was developed from the radical prostatectomy specimen of a 63-year-old AA patient with a clinical-stage T3c adenocarcinoma [92]. From the same patient, anon-malignant cell line RC-77N/E was also developed (discussed above). The RC-77T/E cells express AR, PSA, NKX 3.1, CK8, and p16 [92]. RC-77T/E cells also express β-catenin, α-actinin-1, and filamin-A [134]. These cells are androgen-responsive and form tumors when injected subcutaneously in nude mice [92]. This cell line model could be useful for racial disparity-associated PCa studies.

12T-7f

12T-7f (12: 12 kb, T: Tag transgene, f: fast) is a mouse cell line developed from the probasin-large T antigen transgenic mouse (a.k.a LADY) model along with six other transgenic cell lines. These cells were split into three groups based on the stage of neoplasia and their rapid growth pattern. Inoculation of these cells in mice resulted in the development of prostate tumors. The most aggressive line from these pools was designated as 12T-7f, which could progress to late-stage adenocarcinoma [135]. Notably, tumors developed through 12T-7f xenografting regressed upon castration but progressed after androgen administration.

Castration-Resistant Cell Lines

As discussed in the earlier section, castration-resistance could develop due to AR-dependent and AR-independent mechanisms. Therefore, two types of castration-resistant cell lines (AR-positive and AR-negative) have been developed and are discussed below:

Androgen-Receptor Expressing

C4-2/C4-2B

These cell lines were derived from LNCaP mouse xenografts. C4-2 was isolated from the vertebral metastasis of the LNCaP xenograft, whereas C4-2B was derived from the bone metastasis of the C4-2 tumor-bearing mice [102,103]. Both cell lines express AR and PSA and low levels of p53 and develop tumors when subcutaneously injected in the nude mice [103].

Rv1

The 22Rv1cell line was introduced in 1999. This cell line was derived from the mouse CWR22R xenograft developed from the prostate tumor of a patient with bone metastasis [104]. The 22Rv1 cells harbor the H874Y mutation in the AR like CWR22R xenograft and express PSA and kallikrein-like serine protease [104,136]. EGF is shown to promote the growth of 22Rv1 in vitro [104]. Recently, it has been shown that 22Rv1 prostate carcinoma cells produce high-titer of the human retrovirus XMRV (xenotropic murine leukemia virus-related virus) [137].

Androgen-Receptor Non-Expressing

PC-3

The PC-3 cell line was developed from lumbar vertebral metastasis of a grade IV prostatic adenocarcinoma from a 62-year-old Caucasian man [100]. In the karyotypic analysis, these cells were found to be near triploid having 62 chromosomes. PC3 cells express CK7, CK8, CK18, and CK19 but not AR and PSA and exhibit characteristics of a poorly differentiated adenocarcinoma with a doubling time of about 33 h [138,139]. These cells respond positively to EGF while being insensitive to FGF and are tumorigenic when orthotopically injected in mice [100,140–143].

DU-145

The DU145 cell line was established from the brain metastasis of a 69-year-old prostate cancer patient [101]. These cells express CK5, CK7, CK8, CK18, and CK19 [93,144,145]. Being AR negative, DU145 cells are hormone-insensitive and do not express PSA [146]. This cell line has a doubling time of about 34 h and exhibits a growth response to EGF [147] and also a high level of EGFR expression [148]. DU-145 cells metastasize to spleen and liver when injected subcutaneously in a nude mouse [149,150].

ARCaP

ARCaP (androgen-refractory cancer of the prostate) was established from the ascites of a patient with advanced metastatic disease. Interestingly, it is shown that androgen and estrogen treatment as a dose-dependent suppressive impact on the growth of ARCaP cells [105]. ARCaP cells express low levels of AR and PSA and exhibit positive immunostaining for EGFR, HER2/neu, HER3, bombesin, serotonin, neuron-specific enolase, and the mesenchymal–epithelial transition factor (C-MET). These cells are tumorigenic and highly metastatic that preferably colonize to the lung, pancreas, liver, kidney, and bone [151–153]. These cells form ascites fluid in athymic mice [105].

3.2. Genetically Engineered Mouse Models of Prostate Cancer

The mouse models are beneficial resources to improve our understanding of the disease pathobiology and to establish the role of candidate oncogenes in the pathogenic processes. As discussed below, several genetically engineered mouse models of PCa have been developed that have provided insights into tumor initiation, progression, and metastasis and are being used in preclinical research.

3.2.1. TRAMP

The transgenic adenocarcinoma of the mouse prostate (TRAMP) mice model was generated and characterized in 1996. The chloramphenicol acetyltransferase (CAT) gene was introduced into the germ line of mice under the control of the rat probasin (PB) promoter. In TRAMP mice, expression of both the large and small SV40 T antigens (TAG) is regulated by the prostate-specific rat PB promoter [154]. The PB-SV40 T antigen (PB-Tag) transgene is spatially restricted to the dorsolateral and ventral lobes of the prostate. The gene expression is male specific and restricted to the epithelial cells of the lateral, dorsal, and ventral prostatic lobes of the murine prostate [155]. TRAMP is a very useful model for studying the pathology of PCa as the progression occurs through PIN lesions to malignant disease, like human disease, in a predictable time. Epithelial hyperplasia develops by 10 weeks of age, PIN by 18 weeks of age, and lymphatic metastases after 28 weeks of age [154,156,157].

The TRAMP model has been used for PCa prevention and treatment studies [158,159]. It is also the first genetically engineered mouse model (GEMM) that displays castration-resistant disease progression [160]. One of the limitations of the TRAMP model, however, is that these mice often develop neuroendocrine PCa [161]. A simultaneous loss of *Rb* and *p53* could be the reason for the development of neuroendocrine cancer [161,162]. Considering the higher chances of neuroendocrine disease, the TRAMP mouse model is clinically more relevant to study PCa of neuroendocrine origin.

3.2.2. LADY

The LADY PCa mouse model was developed in 1998 and is similar to the TRAMP model [163]. There are, however, a few key differences between the TRAMP and LADY. In the LADY, a larger fragment (12 kb) of the PB (a.k.a. LPB) promoter upstream of the SV40 T-antigen is used that contains additional androgen and growth factor-responsive sequences and thus allows consistently high transgene expression. Additionally, the LPB promoter is linked with a deletion mutant of the SV40 T-antigen (deleted small T-antigen) to allow the expression of large T-antigen, unlike small t-antigen in the TRAMP model. The purpose of deleting small t-antigen was to analyze the importance of neuroendocrine differences in metastatic lesions developed by LADY [164]. LADY model mice develop metastases to the liver, lymph nodes, and bones [164]. The metastases, however, primarily contain neuroendocrine cells, which is unlike the human metastasis [135,165]. Thus, the LADY mice are different from the most common type of human PCa from the perspective of rapid tumor growth and neuroendocrine tumor development. Nevertheless, the LADY model possesses the molecular changes similar to the human prostate, such as the multifocal nature of tumorigenesis, histopathologically changes from low- to high-grade dysplasia similar to PIN in humans, and the androgen-dependent growth of the primary tumors. Hence, the LADY model could be beneficial for investigating the stepwise mechanisms of PCa progression as well as therapeutic intervention [163].

3.2.3. Pten Deficient Mice

Loss of the *PTEN* tumor suppressor is a critical event in PCa initiation, as discussed above. However, homozygous knockout of *Pten* in mice embryonic stem cells through the deletion of the phosphatase domain led to embryonic lethality [166,167]. To overcome this limitation, Wang et al. generated *Pten* null mice by conditional deletion of *Pten* in the murine prostatic epithelium. They generated *Pten*$^{loxp/loxp}$: PB-Cre4 mice in order to attain the prostate-specific *Pten* biallelic deletion. They showed that *Pten* null PCa progressed with a short latency of PIN formation by 6 weeks of age compared to heterozygous *Pten* deletion mice, which developed PIN by 10 months. Moreover, homozygous *Pten* deletion mice developed invasive adenocarcinoma by 9 weeks of age and metastasis to the lymph node and lung by 12 weeks of age. The effect of hormone ablation therapy on *Pten* null mice was evaluated by performing the castration of mice at week 16. The response of *Pten* null tumors at day 3 and day 6 post-castration was analyzed. In response to androgen abolition, the AR-positive prostatic epithelium showed an increase in the apoptosis leading to the decrease of prostate volume. Hence, these homozygous *Pten* mutant mice recapitulate the PCa by mimicking the histopathological features of human disease [40]. In contrast, heterozygous mutant *(Pten*$^{+/-}$*)* mice developed neoplasia in multiple tissues, including mammary glands, lymphoid cells, small intestines, thyroid, endometrial, and adrenal glands [166,168,169], further limiting the applicability of the heterozygous mutant over *Pten* null mice.

The *Pten* knockout model has been used to demonstrate the role of the tumor microenvironment, particularly interleukin-17 (IL-17), in the growth and progression of PCa [170,171]. To test how tumor suppressor *Rb* interacts with *Pten*, Bai et al. developed mice with double mutations in both the cyclin-dependent kinase (CDK) inhibitor *p18Ink4c* and *Pten* [172]. The double mutant mice develop a broader spectrum of prostate tumors in the anterior and dorsolateral lobes at an accelerated rate [172]. Loss of function of *Nkx3.1* is crucial for PCa progression and has been associated with the development of prostatic epithelial hyperplasia, dysplasia, and PIN [30,67,173]. *Nkx3.1* and *Pten* are shown to cooperate in prostate carcinogenesis in mice. *Nkx3.1;Pten* double mutant mice demonstrated an increased incidence of HGPIN, which resembles the early stages of human PCa [69].

3.2.4. $Pten^{pc-/-}Smad4^{pc-/-}$

To examine a cooperative action of *Pten* and *Smad4* loss in PCa pathogenesis, De Pinho lab developed mice having prostate-specific genetic ablation of *Smad4* in Pten-null mice. These mice were highly aggressive and exhibited profound lymph node and pulmonary metastasis [45]. The importance of *Smad4* in PCa was further revealed by the development of metastatic and lethal PCa with 100% penetrance in *Smad4* and *Pten* double knockout mouse prostate [45]. $Pten^{pc-/-}Smad4^{pc-/-}$ has been used to analyze the efficacy of hypoxia-prodrug TH-302 and checkpoint blockade combination therapy. The combination of the hypoxia-prodrug and checkpoint blockade significantly extended the survival of $Pten^{pc-/-}Smad4^{pc-/-}$ mice [174]. Furthermore, Wang and colleagues utilized the $Pten^{pc-/-}Smad4^{pc-/-}$ mice model and identified that polymorphonuclear myeloid-derived suppressor cells (MDSCs) are one of the significant infiltrating immune cells in PCa and their depletion blocks PCa progression [175].

3.2.5. Hi/Lo-Myc

Two plasmids having a rat probasin (PB) promoter alone (PB-Mycfor lo-Myc) and PB coupled with a sequence of the ARR2 (ARR2PB for hi-Myc) were used to achieve prostate-specific overexpression of c-Myc. The ARR2PB promotor contained two additional androgen response elements that forced the development of invasive adenocarcinoma from prostatic intraepithelial neoplasia (mPIN) in about 26 weeks [27,176,177]. Hi-Myc mice also displayed a decreased expression of Nkx3.1 at both mRNA and protein levels [27]. The PB-Myc mice showed similar pathological changes, but a slower progression of 30 weeks (time to invasive PCa development from PIN lesions) [27]. The main differences between these two models are their androgen responsiveness. The Hi-Myc is androgen-responsive, while the Lo-myc model displays no such sensitivity [27]. The mice model generated by non-viral oncogene ARR2PB-Myc and PB-Myc develop invasive adenocarcinoma and offer advantages over those expressing SV40. However, they do not develop metastasis, which is a major drawback of this model. Hubbard et al. in 2016 showed that the combination of *Myc* overexpression and *Pten* loss in mice resulted in the development of lethal prostatic adenocarcinoma with distant metastases [29]. Moreover, homeobox protein Hox-B13 (HOXB13) was suggested to participate in the *MYC* activation and *Pten* loss genomic instability and aggressive prostate cancer [29,178].

3.2.6. MPAKT

The mouse prostate Akt (MPAKT) model is useful in studying the role of protein kinase B (Akt) in the transformation of prostate epithelial cells and in developing the biomarkers relevant to human PCa. This mouse model was developed by the introduction of Akt1 along with a myristoylation sequence (myr) and a hemagglutinin (HA) epitope in the form of the linearized rPb-myr-HA-Akt1. This insert was injected into the pronuclei of fertilized oocytes, and the friend leukemia virus B (FVB) mice founders were verified [179]. These mice exhibited the formation of PIN by 8 weeks. Immunohistochemistry analysis of the PIN lesions of MPAKT demonstrated numerous important findings such as Akt results in the activation of p70S6K and is associated with the development of PIN in MPAKT mice and Akt-induced PIN might be linked to neovascularization. Histological evaluation revealed that MPAKT mice had distinct phenotypic characteristics, including disorganized epithelial layers, loss of cell polarity, intraepithelial lumen formation, and nuclear atypia and apoptotic bodies. However, the MPAKT did not develop invasive carcinoma even after 78 weeks [180].

3.3. Patient Tumor-Derived Models

Patient-derived models are useful tools for translational research as they mimic human tumors. They are instrumental in studying the response of various therapies undergoing preclinical evaluation since they carry intrinsic tumor factors and microenvironmental presence involved in disease progression and therapy resistance.

3.3.1. Three-Dimensional (3-D) Organoid Cultures

The transition from monolayer PCa cultures to the three-dimensional (3-D) cultures is a remarkable breakthrough in cancer research. Although culturing cancer cell lines is cost-effective and easy to handle, established cell lines do not carry the heterogeneity and genetic makeup of tumors from which they were initially derived [181,182]. These limitations are mostly overridden by the establishment of 3-D organoid culture models from the patient-derived tumors [183]. Dong et al. established the first PCa 3-D organoid culture from the biopsy of a patient in 2014 [184]. This organoid culture maintained the molecular signature of PCa, including *TMPRSS2-ERG* fusion, *SPOP* mutation, Chromodomain Helicase DNA Binding Protein 1 (*CHD1*) loss, and serine protease inhibitor Kazal-type 1 (*SPINK1*) overexpression. Further, whole-exome sequencing revealed mutations in several other genes, as well as the loss of the p53 and RB tumor suppressor pathway function [184]. Puca and colleges developed patient-derived organoids from needle biopsies of metastatic lesions from patients with neuroendocrine CRPC. These organoids showed genomic, epigenomic, and transcriptomic association with corresponding patient tumors [185]. 3-D models are thus beneficial for drug discovery and preclinical evaluation of therapeutic drugs for efficacy under in vitro setting that mimics the complex in vivo environment.

3.3.2. Patient-Derived Xenografts (PDX)

Patient-derived xenografts (PDXs) are essential tools in cancer research as the results obtained from these resources more accurately predict clinical responses in patients (Table 2). The reason is that these models retain the genetic diversity of patient tumors and maintain a closely resembling tumor microenvironment [186]. PDX grown in immunocompromised mice carry essential histological and molecular features of the patient tumors, including gene expression programs, mutations, epigenetic regulators, and structural genomic events that ultimately drive their 3D growth [187,188]. Recent technical advancements, including the co-injection of PCa tissues with extracellular matrix (ECM) and transplantation into renal capsules, have increased the success rate of PDX establishment in mice [189–191]. The first androgen-dependent PCa xenograft model, designated as PC-82, was developed in 1977 by Schröder and colleagues at Erasmus University Rotterdam [192]. For this, the patient prostatic tumor tissue was grafted into the shoulder of nude mice. Later, two more androgen-independent in vivo models, designated as PC-133 and PC-135, were developed [192]. In 1996, seven other PDX models were established [193]. During 1991-2005, numerous other PDX models were developed that carried the *TMPRSS-ERG* rearrangement, *RB1* loss, AR amplification, *PTEN* deletion, *SPOP* mutation, *Tp53* deletion and mutation, and *BRCA2* loss [132,194,195]. The success rate of the localized PDX model has been increased in recent years due to the implantation of the chimeric graft with neonatal mouse mesenchyme. This method improved the survival rate and doubled the proliferation index of xenografted cancer cells [196]. The PDX models, however, have two significant limitations, i.e., the absence of functional human immunity and the lack of orthotopic modeling in the mice [197]. Further, the model takes a long time (about 8 months) for validation of detectable tumor growth in mice that limits its utility for the high-throughput drug screening [198].

Table 2. The advantages and limitations of patient-derived xenograft models.

Model	Advantages	Limitations	Sources
3D-organoid	<ul><li>In vivo-like complexity</li><li>Retain 3D architecture</li><li>Maintain heterogeneity</li><li>Good for high-throughput screening</li><li>Good for drug response testing</li></ul>	<ul><li>Low establishment rate with primary hormone-sensitive tumor</li><li>Success in only aggressive PCa specimens</li><li>Lack vasculature</li><li>Deficient microenvironment and immunity</li></ul>	Primary prostate cancer patient-derived tissue

Table 2. Cont.

Model	Advantages	Limitations	Sources
PDX	• Maintain heterogeneity • Retain 3D architecture • Intact endocrine system • Includes microenvironment	• Time-consuming and expensive • Established in a mouse with deficient immunity • Microenvironment is different from a human	Primary prostate cancer patient-derived tissue, CrownBio, The Jackson Laboratory

3.4. Other Models

3.4.1. Rat Models

Rat is one of the models for PCa research that was first established in the year 1937 by Moore and Melchionna after injecting the white rat prostate with benzpyrene. Following treatment, the columnar prostate epithelium underwent squamous metaplasia and also led to the induction of cancer in both the healthy and atrophic prostates [199]. These tumors spontaneously developed from a dorsal prostatic adenocarcinoma in an inbred Copenhagen rat and then were transplanted into a syngenic Copenhagen × Fischer F1 hybrid rat. These rat prostate tumors are well differentiated and slow growing [200]. The albino Lobund–Wistar (LW) rat model was first described by Pollard [201]. The LW rat developed spontaneous tumors at a mean age of 26 months. Moreover, a combination of N-methyl-N-nitrosourea (MNU) and testosterone treatments induced the development of prostate adenocarcinoma in the LW rat at a mean time of 10.5 months. The cancer of the LW rat resembles the human PCa in several aspects, including spontaneous development and progression to androgen independence and metastasis [201]. However, a major limitation of the rat models is that they have a long latency period for tumor development (2–3 years), have low tumor incidence, and lack spontaneous metastases.

3.4.2. Zebrafish Model

The zebrafish model for cancer research has been utilized by many to acquire information that is traditionally obtained by mice and cell culture systems, although there are limited studies on zebrafish in an in vivo model for PCa research. The zebrafish model is suitable for visual observation of labeled tumor cells through the imaging technique since they are transparent. Nevertheless, the limitation of orthotopic transplantation could be the hurdle owing to the anatomical difference between zebrafish and the human body such as the breast, prostate, or lung [202]. The cancer cells can be injected into a different site in the zebrafish embryos, such as the blastodisc region, the yolk sac, the hindbrain ventricle, and into the circulation via the duct of Cuvier [203,204]. Melong et al. inoculated androgen-sensitive LNCaP cells into zebrafish and observed the effect of testosterone on the growth. Administration of exogenous testosterone increased the proliferation of PCa cells [205]. Further, the growth-promoting effect of testosterone was reversed by the anti-androgen receptor drug, enzalutamide. The invasive potential of PC3 cells overexpressing the calcitonin receptor (CTR) has also been evaluated in the zebrafish model [206]. The zebrafish model has several advantages, including the fact that zebrafish are small and can generate a large number of offspring in a short time, and they are easy to maintain and observe owing to their transparency. Moreover, humans and zebrafish have 71% protein similarity, and, most importantly, zebrafish absorb molecules from water providing an additional route for drug administration.

4. Conclusions and Future Outlook

In the past years, understanding of PCa pathobiology paired with mechanistic studies has remarkably advanced the field of PCa research. This insight has only been possible because of the availability of several types of research models. These models have been extremely helpful in improving our knowledge of PCa etiology, development, and metastatic progression. The cell line models have offered an easy and inexpensive platform to study the functions of aberrantly-expressed genes and various types of genetic alterations including gene mutations, splice variants, gene rearrangements, etc. Furthermore, cell lines serve as a primary model for screening of newer drugs or drug combination and provide us data on the molecular mechanisms of therapy resistance that is crucial for drug development. Since cell lines do not completely capture the tumor heterogeneity and are not grown in a complex microenvironment that tumor cells encounter in vivo, other in vivo models play an important role in further evaluation of gene functions and drug efficacies. The 3D-tissue culture model mimics the in vivo system under in vitro settings and has proven very useful in drug screening. Further, as the field of precision medicine is developing, these models could be of great significance in patient-tailored treatment planning based on preliminary assessment. Patient-derived xenografts (PDXs) grown in mice are useful as they more closely mimic a human tumor in vivo microenvironment. Genetically engineered mouse models (GEMs) are useful as they capture the complete progression of PCa from initiation to metastatic spread under a non-immunocompromised environment. Further, these models also develop a variety of PCa tumor types although they do not have the complete molecular diversity of human tumors (Figure 3). Regardless of limitations, each model has its own importance and these models often complement each other and are often utilized in progressive sets of experiments. There is, however, a need to develop models representing PCa of different racial and ethnic groups considering racial health disparities in incidence and clinical outcomes. Our refined knowledge of tumor genetics and awareness of health disparities and technologically advances will help us make further progress and we would continue to add to our list of PCa tumor models.

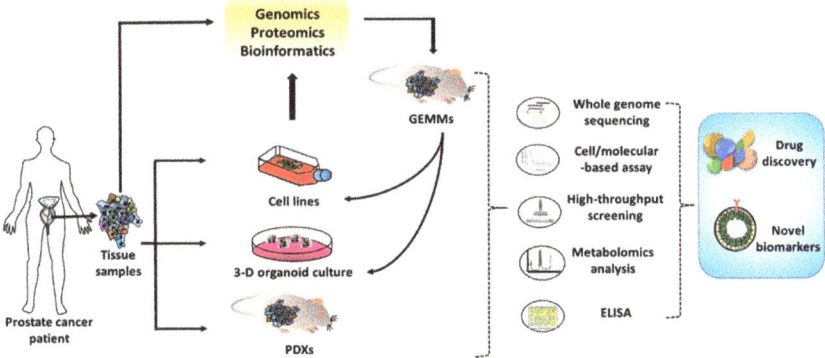

Figure 3. Application of the prostate cancer model in basic and preclinical cancer research. To develop the novel drugs or biomarkers, the prostate cancer models are required for in vitro and in vivo studies. The prostate cell lines, 3D-organiods, and patient-derived tumor xenografts (PDXs) can be generated from prostate tumor tissue from human patients. Patient tumor tissues can be also used to create genetically engineered mouse models (GEMMs). The results from research and preclinical studies are validated through several techniques such as whole genome sequencing, cell and molecular-based assays, high-throughput screening, metabolomics analysis, and ELISA. The promising drugs or biomarkers that emerge from those works will subsequently progress to preclinical and clinical studies.

Author Contributions: Conceptualization: A.P.S., S.S. (Seema Singh), S.D., S.P., S.S. (Sirin Saranyutanon), and S.K.D.; Supervision; A.P.S., S.S. (Seema Singh), and S.D.; Resources: A.P.S. and S.S. (Seema Singh); Writing, review and editing: A.P.S., S.S. (Seema Singh), S.D., S.P., S.S. (Sirin Saranyutanon), and S.K.D. All authors have read and agreed to the published version of the manuscript.

Funding: This work was supported by the National Institutes of Health/National Cancer Institute (CA185490, CA224306 (to AP Singh) and CA204801, CA231925 (to S Singh)) and the University of South Alabama Mitchell Cancer Institute.

Acknowledgments: Sirin Saranyutanon would also like to acknowledge the financial support provided by the Royal Thai Government Scholarship.

Conflicts of Interest: The authors declare no conflict of interest.

References

1. Siegel, R.L.; Miller, K.D.; Jemal, A. Cancer statistics, 2020. *CA Cancer J. Clin.* **2020**, *70*, 7–30. [CrossRef]
2. Powell, I.J. Prostate cancer and African-American men. *Oncology (Williston Park)* **1997**, *11*, 599–605.
3. Fuletra, J.G.; Kamenko, A.; Ramsey, F.; Eun, D.D.; Reese, A.C. African-American men with prostate cancer have larger tumor volume than Caucasian men despite no difference in serum prostate specific antigen. *Can. J. Urol.* **2018**, *25*, 9193–9198.
4. Humphrey, P.A. Histopathology of Prostate Cancer. *Cold Spring Harb. Perspect. Med.* **2017**, *7*, a030411. [CrossRef] [PubMed]
5. Inamura, K. Prostatic cancers: Understanding their molecular pathology and the 2016 WHO classification. *Oncotarget* **2018**, *9*, 14723–14737. [CrossRef]
6. Hoffman, R.M.; Gilliland, F.D.; Adams-Cameron, M.; Hunt, W.C.; Key, C.R. Prostate-specific antigen testing accuracy in community practice. *BMC Fam. Pract.* **2002**, *3*, 19. [CrossRef]
7. Punglia, R.S.; D'Amico, A.V.; Catalona, W.J.; Roehl, K.A.; Kuntz, K.M. Effect of verification bias on screening for prostate cancer by measurement of prostate-specific antigen. *N. Engl. J. Med.* **2003**, *349*, 335–342. [CrossRef]
8. Brawley, O.W. Prostate cancer screening: Biases and the need for consensus. *J. Natl. Cancer Inst.* **2013**, *105*, 1522–1524. [CrossRef]
9. Donnelly, B.J.; Saliken, J.C.; Brasher, P.M.; Ernst, S.D.; Rewcastle, J.C.; Lau, H.; Robinson, J.; Trpkov, K. A randomized trial of external beam radiotherapy versus cryoablation in patients with localized prostate cancer. *Cancer* **2010**, *116*, 323–330. [CrossRef]
10. Hayden, A.J.; Catton, C.; Pickles, T. Radiation therapy in prostate cancer: A risk-adapted strategy. *Curr. Oncol.* **2010**, *17* (Suppl. 2), S18–S24. [CrossRef]
11. Shipley, W.U.; Verhey, L.J.; Munzenrider, J.E.; Suit, H.D.; Urie, M.M.; McManus, P.L.; Young, R.H.; Shipley, J.W.; Zietman, A.L.; Biggs, P.J.; et al. Advanced prostate cancer: The results of a randomized comparative trial of high dose irradiation boosting with conformal protons compared with conventional dose irradiation using photons alone. *Int. J. Radiat. Oncol. Biol. Phys.* **1995**, *32*, 3–12. [CrossRef]
12. Perlmutter, M.A.; Lepor, H. Androgen deprivation therapy in the treatment of advanced prostate cancer. *Rev. Urol* **2007**, *9* (Suppl. 1), S3–S8.
13. Miller, E.T.; Chamie, K.; Kwan, L.; Lewis, M.S.; Knudsen, B.S.; Garraway, I.P. Impact of treatment on progression to castration-resistance, metastases, and death in men with localized high-grade prostate cancer. *Cancer Med.* **2017**, *6*, 163–172. [CrossRef]
14. Moreira, D.M.; Howard, L.E.; Sourbeer, K.N.; Amarasekara, H.S.; Chow, L.C.; Cockrell, D.C.; Pratson, C.L.; Hanyok, B.T.; Aronson, W.J.; Kane, C.J.; et al. Predicting Time From Metastasis to Overall Survival in Castration-Resistant Prostate Cancer: Results From SEARCH. *Clin. Genitourin. Cancer* **2017**, *15*, 60–66.e2. [CrossRef]
15. Lee, C.H.; Akin-Olugbade, O.; Kirschenbaum, A. Overview of prostate anatomy, histology, and pathology. *Endocrinol. Metab. Clin. N. Am.* **2011**, *40*, 565–575. [CrossRef]
16. McNeal, J.E. The zonal anatomy of the prostate. *Prostate* **1981**, *2*, 35–49. [CrossRef]
17. Wang, G.; Zhao, D.; Spring, D.J.; DePinho, R.A. Genetics and biology of prostate cancer. *Genes Dev.* **2018**, *32*, 1105–1140. [CrossRef]
18. Zhang, D.; Zhao, S.; Li, X.; Kirk, J.S.; Tang, D.G. Prostate Luminal Progenitor Cells in Development and Cancer. *Trends Cancer* **2018**, *4*, 769–783. [CrossRef]
19. Xin, L. Cells of origin for cancer: An updated view from prostate cancer. *Oncogene* **2013**, *32*, 3655–3663. [CrossRef]

20. Wang, Z.A.; Toivanen, R.; Bergren, S.K.; Chambon, P.; Shen, M.M. Luminal cells are favored as the cell of origin for prostate cancer. *Cell Rep.* **2014**, *8*, 1339–1346. [CrossRef]
21. Stoyanova, T.; Cooper, A.R.; Drake, J.M.; Liu, X.; Armstrong, A.J.; Pienta, K.J.; Zhang, H.; Kohn, D.B.; Huang, J.; Witte, O.N.; et al. Prostate cancer originating in basal cells progresses to adenocarcinoma propagated by luminal-like cells. *Proc. Natl. Acad. Sci. USA* **2013**, *110*, 20111–20116. [CrossRef]
22. Garber, K. A tale of two cells: Discovering the origin of prostate cancer. *J. Natl. Cancer Inst.* **2010**, *102*, 1528–1529, 1535. [CrossRef]
23. Shen, M.M.; Abate-Shen, C. Molecular genetics of prostate cancer: New prospects for old challenges. *Genes Dev.* **2010**, *24*, 1967–2000. [CrossRef] [PubMed]
24. Krajewska, M.; Krajewski, S.; Epstein, J.I.; Shabaik, A.; Sauvageot, J.; Song, K.; Kitada, S.; Reed, J.C. Immunohistochemical analysis of bcl-2, bax, bcl-X, and mcl-1 expression in prostate cancers. *Am. J. Pathol.* **1996**, *148*, 1567–1576.
25. Martignano, F.; Gurioli, G.; Salvi, S.; Calistri, D.; Costantini, M.; Gunelli, R.; De Giorgi, U.; Foca, F.; Casadio, V. GSTP1 Methylation and Protein Expression in Prostate Cancer: Diagnostic Implications. *Dis. Markers* **2016**, *2016*, 4358292. [CrossRef] [PubMed]
26. Gurel, B.; Iwata, T.; Koh, C.M.; Jenkins, R.B.; Lan, F.; Van Dang, C.; Hicks, J.L.; Morgan, J.; Cornish, T.C.; Sutcliffe, S.; et al. Nuclear MYC protein overexpression is an early alteration in human prostate carcinogenesis. *Mod. Pathol.* **2008**, *21*, 1156–1167. [CrossRef]
27. Ellwood-Yen, K.; Graeber, T.G.; Wongvipat, J.; Iruela-Arispe, M.L.; Zhang, J.; Matusik, R.; Thomas, G.V.; Sawyers, C.L. Myc-driven murine prostate cancer shares molecular features with human prostate tumors. *Cancer Cell* **2003**, *4*, 223–238. [CrossRef]
28. McMenamin, M.E.; Soung, P.; Perera, S.; Kaplan, I.; Loda, M.; Sellers, W.R. Loss of PTEN expression in paraffin-embedded primary prostate cancer correlates with high Gleason score and advanced stage. *Cancer Res.* **1999**, *59*, 4291–4296.
29. Hubbard, G.K.; Mutton, L.N.; Khalili, M.; McMullin, R.P.; Hicks, J.L.; Bianchi-Frias, D.; Horn, L.A.; Kulac, I.; Moubarek, M.S.; Nelson, P.S.; et al. Combined MYC Activation and Pten Loss Are Sufficient to Create Genomic Instability and Lethal Metastatic Prostate Cancer. *Cancer Res.* **2016**, *76*, 283–292. [CrossRef]
30. Gurel, B.; Ali, T.Z.; Montgomery, E.A.; Begum, S.; Hicks, J.; Goggins, M.; Eberhart, C.G.; Clark, D.P.; Bieberich, C.J.; Epstein, J.I.; et al. NKX3.1 as a marker of prostatic origin in metastatic tumors. *Am. J. Surg. Pathol.* **2010**, *34*, 1097–1105. [CrossRef]
31. Tomlins, S.A.; Laxman, B.; Varambally, S.; Cao, X.; Yu, J.; Helgeson, B.E.; Cao, Q.; Prensner, J.R.; Rubin, M.A.; Shah, R.B.; et al. Role of the TMPRSS2-ERG gene fusion in prostate cancer. *Neoplasia* **2008**, *10*, 177–188. [CrossRef]
32. Furusato, B.; Tan, S.H.; Young, D.; Dobi, A.; Sun, C.; Mohamed, A.A.; Thangapazham, R.; Chen, Y.; McMaster, G.; Sreenath, T.; et al. ERG oncoprotein expression in prostate cancer: Clonal progression of ERG-positive tumor cells and potential for ERG-based stratification. *Prostate Cancer Prostatic Dis.* **2010**, *13*, 228–237. [CrossRef] [PubMed]
33. Blattner, M.; Liu, D.; Robinson, B.D.; Huang, D.; Poliakov, A.; Gao, D.; Nataraj, S.; Deonarine, L.D.; Augello, M.A.; Sailer, V.; et al. SPOP Mutation Drives Prostate Tumorigenesis In Vivo through Coordinate Regulation of PI3K/mTOR and AR Signaling. *Cancer Cell* **2017**, *31*, 436–451. [CrossRef]
34. Shoag, J.; Liu, D.; Blattner, M.; Sboner, A.; Park, K.; Deonarine, L.; Robinson, B.D.; Mosquera, J.M.; Chen, Y.; Rubin, M.A.; et al. SPOP mutation drives prostate neoplasia without stabilizing oncogenic transcription factor ERG. *J. Clin. Investig.* **2018**, *128*, 381–386. [CrossRef]
35. Lara, P.N., Jr.; Heilmann, A.M.; Elvin, J.A.; Parikh, M.; de Vere White, R.; Gandour-Edwards, R.; Evans, C.P.; Pan, C.X.; Schrock, A.B.; Erlich, R.; et al. TMPRSS2-ERG fusions unexpectedly identified in men initially diagnosed with nonprostatic malignancies. *JCO Precis. Oncol.* **2017**, *2017*. [CrossRef]
36. Guo, C.C.; Dancer, J.Y.; Wang, Y.; Aparicio, A.; Navone, N.M.; Troncoso, P.; Czerniak, B.A. TMPRSS2-ERG gene fusion in small cell carcinoma of the prostate. *Hum. Pathol.* **2011**, *42*, 11–17. [CrossRef] [PubMed]
37. Gerhardt, J.; Montani, M.; Wild, P.; Beer, M.; Huber, F.; Hermanns, T.; Muntener, M.; Kristiansen, G. FOXA1 promotes tumor progression in prostate cancer and represents a novel hallmark of castration-resistant prostate cancer. *Am. J. Pathol.* **2012**, *180*, 848–861. [CrossRef] [PubMed]

38. Annala, M.; Taavitsainen, S.; Vandekerkhove, G.; Bacon, J.V.W.; Beja, K.; Chi, K.N.; Nykter, M.; Wyatt, A.W. Frequent mutation of the FOXA1 untranslated region in prostate cancer. *Commun. Biol.* **2018**, *1*, 122. [CrossRef]
39. Jamaspishvili, T.; Berman, D.M.; Ross, A.E.; Scher, H.I.; De Marzo, A.M.; Squire, J.A.; Lotan, T.L. Clinical implications of PTEN loss in prostate cancer. *Nat. Rev. Urol.* **2018**, *15*, 222–234. [CrossRef]
40. Wang, S.; Gao, J.; Lei, Q.; Rozengurt, N.; Pritchard, C.; Jiao, J.; Thomas, G.V.; Li, G.; Roy-Burman, P.; Nelson, P.S.; et al. Prostate-specific deletion of the murine Pten tumor suppressor gene leads to metastatic prostate cancer. *Cancer Cell* **2003**, *4*, 209–221. [CrossRef]
41. Chen, W.S.; Alshalalfa, M.; Zhao, S.G.; Liu, Y.; Mahal, B.A.; Quigley, D.A.; Wei, T.; Davicioni, E.; Rebbeck, T.R.; Kantoff, P.W.; et al. Novel RB1-Loss Transcriptomic Signature Is Associated with Poor Clinical Outcomes across Cancer Types. *Clin. Cancer Res.* **2019**, *25*, 4290–4299. [CrossRef] [PubMed]
42. Graham, M.K.; Meeker, A. Telomeres and telomerase in prostate cancer development and therapy. *Nat. Rev. Urol.* **2017**, *14*, 607–619. [CrossRef] [PubMed]
43. Graham, M.K.; Kim, J.; Da, J.; Brosnan-Cashman, J.A.; Rizzo, A.; Baena Del Valle, J.A.; Chia, L.; Rubenstein, M.; Davis, C.; Zheng, Q.; et al. Functional Loss of ATRX and TERC Activates Alternative Lengthening of Telomeres (ALT) in LAPC4 Prostate Cancer Cells. *Mol. Cancer Res.* **2019**, *17*, 2480–2491. [CrossRef] [PubMed]
44. Schmitz, M.; Grignard, G.; Margue, C.; Dippel, W.; Capesius, C.; Mossong, J.; Nathan, M.; Giacchi, S.; Scheiden, R.; Kieffer, N. Complete loss of PTEN expression as a possible early prognostic marker for prostate cancer metastasis. *Int. J. Cancer* **2007**, *120*, 1284–1292. [CrossRef] [PubMed]
45. Ding, Z.; Wu, C.J.; Chu, G.C.; Xiao, Y.; Ho, D.; Zhang, J.; Perry, S.R.; Labrot, E.S.; Wu, X.; Lis, R.; et al. SMAD4-dependent barrier constrains prostate cancer growth and metastatic progression. *Nature* **2011**, *470*, 269–273. [CrossRef] [PubMed]
46. Zhang, D.T.; Shi, J.G.; Liu, Y.; Jiang, H.M. The prognostic value of Smad4 mRNA in patients with prostate cancer. *Tumour Biol.* **2014**, *35*, 3333–3337. [CrossRef]
47. Lakshmikanthan, V.; Zou, L.; Kim, J.I.; Michal, A.; Nie, Z.; Messias, N.C.; Benovic, J.L.; Daaka, Y. Identification of betaArrestin2 as a corepressor of androgen receptor signaling in prostate cancer. *Proc. Natl. Acad. Sci. USA* **2009**, *106*, 9379–9384. [CrossRef]
48. Taichman, R.S.; Cooper, C.; Keller, E.T.; Pienta, K.J.; Taichman, N.S.; McCauley, L.K. Use of the stromal cell-derived factor-1/CXCR4 pathway in prostate cancer metastasis to bone. *Cancer Res.* **2002**, *62*, 1832–1837.
49. Chinni, S.R.; Sivalogan, S.; Dong, Z.; Filho, J.C.; Deng, X.; Bonfil, R.D.; Cher, M.L. CXCL12/CXCR4 signaling activates Akt-1 and MMP-9 expression in prostate cancer cells: The role of bone microenvironment-associated CXCL12. *Prostate* **2006**, *66*, 32–48. [CrossRef]
50. Wu, X.; Scott, H.; Carlsson, S.V.; Sjoberg, D.D.; Cerundolo, L.; Lilja, H.; Prevo, R.; Rieunier, G.; Macaulay, V.; Higgins, G.S.; et al. Increased EZH2 expression in prostate cancer is associated with metastatic recurrence following external beam radiotherapy. *Prostate* **2019**, *79*, 1079–1089. [CrossRef]
51. Yang, Y.A.; Yu, J. EZH2, an epigenetic driver of prostate cancer. *Protein Cell* **2013**, *4*, 331–341. [CrossRef]
52. Augello, M.A.; Den, R.B.; Knudsen, K.E. AR function in promoting metastatic prostate cancer. *Cancer Metastasis Rev.* **2014**, *33*, 399–411. [CrossRef] [PubMed]
53. Jernberg, E.; Bergh, A.; Wikstrom, P. Clinical relevance of androgen receptor alterations in prostate cancer. *Endocr. Connect.* **2017**, *6*, R146–R161. [CrossRef] [PubMed]
54. Casimiro, S.; Mohammad, K.S.; Pires, R.; Tato-Costa, J.; Alho, I.; Teixeira, R.; Carvalho, A.; Ribeiro, S.; Lipton, A.; Guise, T.A.; et al. RANKL/RANK/MMP-1 molecular triad contributes to the metastatic phenotype of breast and prostate cancer cells in vitro. *PLoS ONE* **2013**, *8*, e63153. [CrossRef] [PubMed]
55. Armstrong, A.P.; Miller, R.E.; Jones, J.C.; Zhang, J.; Keller, E.T.; Dougall, W.C. RANKL acts directly on RANK-expressing prostate tumor cells and mediates migration and expression of tumor metastasis genes. *Prostate* **2008**, *68*, 92–104. [CrossRef]
56. Srivastava, S.K.; Bhardwaj, A.; Singh, S.; Arora, S.; McClellan, S.; Grizzle, W.E.; Reed, E.; Singh, A.P. Myb overexpression overrides androgen depletion-induced cell cycle arrest and apoptosis in prostate cancer cells, and confers aggressive malignant traits: Potential role in castration resistance. *Carcinogenesis* **2012**, *33*, 1149–1157. [CrossRef] [PubMed]

57. Ganaie, A.A.; Beigh, F.H.; Astone, M.; Ferrari, M.G.; Maqbool, R.; Umbreen, S.; Parray, A.S.; Siddique, H.R.; Hussain, T.; Murugan, P.; et al. BMI1 Drives Metastasis of Prostate Cancer in Caucasian and African-American Men and Is A Potential Therapeutic Target: Hypothesis Tested in Race-specific Models. *Clin. Cancer Res.* **2018**, *24*, 6421–6432. [CrossRef]
58. Deplus, R.; Delliaux, C.; Marchand, N.; Flourens, A.; Vanpouille, N.; Leroy, X.; de Launoit, Y.; Duterque-Coquillaud, M. TMPRSS2-ERG fusion promotes prostate cancer metastases in bone. *Oncotarget* **2017**, *8*, 11827–11840. [CrossRef]
59. Tian, T.V.; Tomavo, N.; Huot, L.; Flourens, A.; Bonnelye, E.; Flajollet, S.; Hot, D.; Leroy, X.; de Launoit, Y.; Duterque-Coquillaud, M. Identification of novel TMPRSS2:ERG mechanisms in prostate cancer metastasis: Involvement of MMP9 and PLXNA2. *Oncogene* **2014**, *33*, 2204–2214. [CrossRef]
60. Stambolic, V.; Suzuki, A.; de la Pompa, J.L.; Brothers, G.M.; Mirtsos, C.; Sasaki, T.; Ruland, J.; Penninger, J.M.; Siderovski, D.P.; Mak, T.W. Negative regulation of PKB/Akt-dependent cell survival by the tumor suppressor PTEN. *Cell* **1998**, *95*, 29–39. [CrossRef]
61. Berenjeno, I.M.; Guillermet-Guibert, J.; Pearce, W.; Gray, A.; Fleming, S.; Vanhaesebroeck, B. Both p110alpha and p110beta isoforms of PI3K can modulate the impact of loss-of-function of the PTEN tumour suppressor. *Biochem. J.* **2012**, *442*, 151–159. [CrossRef] [PubMed]
62. Vocke, C.D.; Pozzatti, R.O.; Bostwick, D.G.; Florence, C.D.; Jennings, S.B.; Strup, S.E.; Duray, P.H.; Liotta, L.A.; Emmert-Buck, M.R.; Linehan, W.M. Analysis of 99 microdissected prostate carcinomas reveals a high frequency of allelic loss on chromosome 8p12-21. *Cancer Res.* **1996**, *56*, 2411–2416.
63. Emmert-Buck, M.R.; Vocke, C.D.; Pozzatti, R.O.; Duray, P.H.; Jennings, S.B.; Florence, C.D.; Zhuang, Z.; Bostwick, D.G.; Liotta, L.A.; Linehan, W.M. Allelic loss on chromosome 8p12-21 in microdissected prostatic intraepithelial neoplasia. *Cancer Res.* **1995**, *55*, 2959–2962.
64. Abdulkadir, S.A.; Magee, J.A.; Peters, T.J.; Kaleem, Z.; Naughton, C.K.; Humphrey, P.A.; Milbrandt, J. Conditional loss of Nkx3.1 in adult mice induces prostatic intraepithelial neoplasia. *Mol. Cell. Biol.* **2002**, *22*, 1495–1503. [CrossRef]
65. Qian, J.; Jenkins, R.B.; Bostwick, D.G. Genetic and chromosomal alterations in prostatic intraepithelial neoplasia and carcinoma detected by fluorescence in situ hybridization. *Eur. Urol.* **1999**, *35*, 479–483. [CrossRef]
66. Abate-Shen, C.; Shen, M.M.; Gelmann, E. Integrating differentiation and cancer: The Nkx3.1 homeobox gene in prostate organogenesis and carcinogenesis. *Differentiation* **2008**, *76*, 717–727. [CrossRef]
67. Bhatia-Gaur, R.; Donjacour, A.A.; Sciavolino, P.J.; Kim, M.; Desai, N.; Young, P.; Norton, C.R.; Gridley, T.; Cardiff, R.D.; Cunha, G.R.; et al. Roles for Nkx3.1 in prostate development and cancer. *Genes Dev.* **1999**, *13*, 966–977. [CrossRef]
68. Kim, M.J.; Bhatia-Gaur, R.; Banach-Petrosky, W.A.; Desai, N.; Wang, Y.; Hayward, S.W.; Cunha, G.R.; Cardiff, R.D.; Shen, M.M.; Abate-Shen, C. Nkx3.1 mutant mice recapitulate early stages of prostate carcinogenesis. *Cancer Res.* **2002**, *62*, 2999–3004.
69. Kim, M.J.; Cardiff, R.D.; Desai, N.; Banach-Petrosky, W.A.; Parsons, R.; Shen, M.M.; Abate-Shen, C. Cooperativity of Nkx3.1 and Pten loss of function in a mouse model of prostate carcinogenesis. *Proc. Natl. Acad. Sci. USA* **2002**, *99*, 2884–2889. [CrossRef] [PubMed]
70. Chen, H.; Liu, W.; Roberts, W.; Hooker, S.; Fedor, H.; DeMarzo, A.; Isaacs, W.; Kittles, R.A. 8q24 allelic imbalance and MYC gene copy number in primary prostate cancer. *Prostate Cancer Prostatic Dis.* **2010**, *13*, 238–243. [CrossRef] [PubMed]
71. Fromont, G.; Godet, J.; Peyret, A.; Irani, J.; Celhay, O.; Rozet, F.; Cathelineau, X.; Cussenot, O. 8q24 amplification is associated with Myc expression and prostate cancer progression and is an independent predictor of recurrence after radical prostatectomy. *Hum. Pathol.* **2013**, *44*, 1617–1623. [CrossRef]
72. Qian, J.; Jenkins, R.B.; Bostwick, D.G. Detection of chromosomal anomalies and c-myc gene amplification in the cribriform pattern of prostatic intraepithelial neoplasia and carcinoma by fluorescence in situ hybridization. *Mod. Pathol.* **1997**, *10*, 1113–1119. [PubMed]
73. Dang, C.V. MYC on the path to cancer. *Cell* **2012**, *149*, 22–35. [CrossRef] [PubMed]
74. Zanet, J.; Pibre, S.; Jacquet, C.; Ramirez, A.; de Alboran, I.M.; Gandarillas, A. Endogenous Myc controls mammalian epidermal cell size, hyperproliferation, endoreplication and stem cell amplification. *J. Cell Sci.* **2005**, *118*, 1693–1704. [CrossRef] [PubMed]

75. Dang, C.V. MYC, metabolism, cell growth, and tumorigenesis. *Cold Spring Harb. Perspect. Med.* **2013**, *3*, a014217. [CrossRef]
76. Koh, C.M.; Bieberich, C.J.; Dang, C.V.; Nelson, W.G.; Yegnasubramanian, S.; De Marzo, A.M. MYC and Prostate Cancer. *Genes Cancer* **2010**, *1*, 617–628. [CrossRef]
77. He, T.C.; Sparks, A.B.; Rago, C.; Hermeking, H.; Zawel, L.; da Costa, L.T.; Morin, P.J.; Vogelstein, B.; Kinzler, K.W. Identification of c-MYC as a target of the APC pathway. *Science* **1998**, *281*, 1509–1512. [CrossRef]
78. Wang, L.; Liu, R.; Li, W.; Chen, C.; Katoh, H.; Chen, G.Y.; McNally, B.; Lin, L.; Zhou, P.; Zuo, T.; et al. Somatic single hits inactivate the X-linked tumor suppressor FOXP3 in the prostate. *Cancer Cell* **2009**, *16*, 336–346. [CrossRef]
79. Sotelo, J.; Esposito, D.; Duhagon, M.A.; Banfield, K.; Mehalko, J.; Liao, H.; Stephens, R.M.; Harris, T.J.; Munroe, D.J.; Wu, X. Long-range enhancers on 8q24 regulate c-Myc. *Proc. Natl. Acad. Sci. USA* **2010**, *107*, 3001–3005. [CrossRef]
80. Pettersson, A.; Gerke, T.; Penney, K.L.; Lis, R.T.; Stack, E.C.; Pertega-Gomes, N.; Zadra, G.; Tyekucheva, S.; Giovannucci, E.L.; Mucci, L.A.; et al. MYC Overexpression at the Protein and mRNA Level and Cancer Outcomes among Men Treated with Radical Prostatectomy for Prostate Cancer. *Cancer Epidemiol. Biomark. Prev.* **2018**, *27*, 201–207. [CrossRef]
81. Zhou, C.K.; Young, D.; Yeboah, E.D.; Coburn, S.B.; Tettey, Y.; Biritwum, R.B.; Adjei, A.A.; Tay, E.; Niwa, S.; Truelove, A.; et al. TMPRSS2:ERG Gene Fusions in Prostate Cancer of West African Men and a Meta-Analysis of Racial Differences. *Am. J. Epidemiol.* **2017**, *186*, 1352–1361. [CrossRef]
82. Tomlins, S.A.; Rhodes, D.R.; Perner, S.; Dhanasekaran, S.M.; Mehra, R.; Sun, X.W.; Varambally, S.; Cao, X.; Tchinda, J.; Kuefer, R.; et al. Recurrent fusion of TMPRSS2 and ETS transcription factor genes in prostate cancer. *Science* **2005**, *310*, 644–648. [CrossRef] [PubMed]
83. Demichelis, F.; Fall, K.; Perner, S.; Andren, O.; Schmidt, F.; Setlur, S.R.; Hoshida, Y.; Mosquera, J.M.; Pawitan, Y.; Lee, C.; et al. TMPRSS2:ERG gene fusion associated with lethal prostate cancer in a watchful waiting cohort. *Oncogene* **2007**, *26*, 4596–4599. [CrossRef]
84. Lapointe, J.; Kim, Y.H.; Miller, M.A.; Li, C.; Kaygusuz, G.; van de Rijn, M.; Huntsman, D.G.; Brooks, J.D.; Pollack, J.R. A variant TMPRSS2 isoform and ERG fusion product in prostate cancer with implications for molecular diagnosis. *Mod. Pathol.* **2007**, *20*, 467–473. [CrossRef] [PubMed]
85. Perner, S.; Mosquera, J.M.; Demichelis, F.; Hofer, M.D.; Paris, P.L.; Simko, J.; Collins, C.; Bismar, T.A.; Chinnaiyan, A.M.; De Marzo, A.M.; et al. TMPRSS2-ERG fusion prostate cancer: An early molecular event associated with invasion. *Am. J. Surg. Pathol.* **2007**, *31*, 882–888. [CrossRef]
86. Tomlins, S.A.; Palanisamy, N.; Siddiqui, J.; Chinnaiyan, A.M.; Kunju, L.P. Antibody-based detection of ERG rearrangements in prostate core biopsies, including diagnostically challenging cases: ERG staining in prostate core biopsies. *Arch. Pathol. Lab. Med.* **2012**, *136*, 935–946. [CrossRef]
87. Edwards, J.; Krishna, N.S.; Witton, C.J.; Bartlett, J.M. Gene amplifications associated with the development of hormone-resistant prostate cancer. *Clin. Cancer Res.* **2003**, *9*, 5271–5281. [PubMed]
88. Webber, M.M.; Trakul, N.; Thraves, P.S.; Bello-DeOcampo, D.; Chu, W.W.; Storto, P.D.; Huard, T.K.; Rhim, J.S.; Williams, D.E. A human prostatic stromal myofibroblast cell line WPMY-1: A model for stromal-epithelial interactions in prostatic neoplasia. *Carcinogenesis* **1999**, *20*, 1185–1192. [CrossRef]
89. Bello, D.; Webber, M.M.; Kleinman, H.K.; Wartinger, D.D.; Rhim, J.S. Androgen responsive adult human prostatic epithelial cell lines immortalized by human papillomavirus 18. *Carcinogenesis* **1997**, *18*, 1215–1223. [CrossRef]
90. Hayward, S.W.; Dahiya, R.; Cunha, G.R.; Bartek, J.; Deshpande, N.; Narayan, P. Establishment and characterization of an immortalized but non-transformed human prostate epithelial cell line: BPH-1. *Vitr. Cell. Dev. Biol. Anim.* **1995**, *31*, 14–24. [CrossRef]
91. D'Abronzo, L.S.; Bose, S.; Crapuchettes, M.E.; Beggs, R.E.; Vinall, R.L.; Tepper, C.G.; Siddiqui, S.; Mudryj, M.; Melgoza, F.U.; Durbin-Johnson, B.P.; et al. The androgen receptor is a negative regulator of eIF4E phosphorylation at S209: Implications for the use of mTOR inhibitors in advanced prostate cancer. *Oncogene* **2017**, *36*, 6359–6373. [CrossRef] [PubMed]
92. Theodore, S.; Sharp, S.; Zhou, J.; Turner, T.; Li, H.; Miki, J.; Ji, Y.; Patel, V.; Yates, C.; Rhim, J.S. Establishment and characterization of a pair of non-malignant and malignant tumor derived cell lines from an African American prostate cancer patient. *Int. J. Oncol.* **2010**, *37*, 1477–1482. [CrossRef]

93. Sherwood, E.R.; Berg, L.A.; Mitchell, N.J.; McNeal, J.E.; Kozlowski, J.M.; Lee, C. Differential cytokeratin expression in normal, hyperplastic and malignant epithelial cells from human prostate. *J. Urol.* **1990**, *143*, 167–171. [CrossRef]
94. Horoszewicz, J.S.; Leong, S.S.; Chu, T.M.; Wajsman, Z.L.; Friedman, M.; Papsidero, L.; Kim, U.; Chai, L.S.; Kakati, S.; Arya, S.K.; et al. The LNCaP cell line–a new model for studies on human prostatic carcinoma. *Prog. Clin. Biol. Res.* **1980**, *37*, 115–132.
95. Klein, K.A.; Reiter, R.E.; Redula, J.; Moradi, H.; Zhu, X.L.; Brothman, A.R.; Lamb, D.J.; Marcelli, M.; Belldegrun, A.; Witte, O.N.; et al. Progression of metastatic human prostate cancer to androgen independence in immunodeficient SCID mice. *Nat. Med.* **1997**, *3*, 402–408. [CrossRef] [PubMed]
96. Craft, N.; Chhor, C.; Tran, C.; Belldegrun, A.; DeKernion, J.; Witte, O.N.; Said, J.; Reiter, R.E.; Sawyers, C.L. Evidence for clonal outgrowth of androgen-independent prostate cancer cells from androgen-dependent tumors through a two-step process. *Cancer Res.* **1999**, *59*, 5030–5036.
97. Korenchuk, S.; Lehr, J.E.; MClean, L.; Lee, Y.G.; Whitney, S.; Vessella, R.; Lin, D.L.; Pienta, K.J. VCaP, a cell-based model system of human prostate cancer. *Vivo* **2001**, *15*, 163–168.
98. Navone, N.M.; Olive, M.; Ozen, M.; Davis, R.; Troncoso, P.; Tu, S.M.; Johnston, D.; Pollack, A.; Pathak, S.; von Eschenbach, A.C.; et al. Establishment of two human prostate cancer cell lines derived from a single bone metastasis. *Clin. Cancer Res.* **1997**, *3*, 2493–2500.
99. Whang, Y.E.; Wu, X.; Suzuki, H.; Reiter, R.E.; Tran, C.; Vessella, R.L.; Said, J.W.; Isaacs, W.B.; Sawyers, C.L. Inactivation of the tumor suppressor PTEN/MMAC1 in advanced human prostate cancer through loss of expression. *Proc. Natl. Acad. Sci. USA* **1998**, *95*, 5246–5250. [CrossRef]
100. Kaighn, M.E.; Narayan, K.S.; Ohnuki, Y.; Lechner, J.F.; Jones, L.W. Establishment and characterization of a human prostatic carcinoma cell line (PC-3). *Investig. Urol.* **1979**, *17*, 16–23.
101. Stone, K.R.; Mickey, D.D.; Wunderli, H.; Mickey, G.H.; Paulson, D.F. Isolation of a human prostate carcinoma cell line (DU 145). *Int. J. Cancer* **1978**, *21*, 274–281. [CrossRef] [PubMed]
102. Pfitzenmaier, J.; Quinn, J.E.; Odman, A.M.; Zhang, J.; Keller, E.T.; Vessella, R.L.; Corey, E. Characterization of C4-2 prostate cancer bone metastases and their response to castration. *J. Bone Miner. Res.* **2003**, *18*, 1882–1888. [CrossRef]
103. Thalmann, G.N.; Anezinis, P.E.; Chang, S.M.; Zhau, H.E.; Kim, E.E.; Hopwood, V.L.; Pathak, S.; von Eschenbach, A.C.; Chung, L.W. Androgen-independent cancer progression and bone metastasis in the LNCaP model of human prostate cancer. *Cancer Res.* **1994**, *54*, 2577–2581. [PubMed]
104. Sramkoski, R.M.; Pretlow, T.G., 2nd; Giaconia, J.M.; Pretlow, T.P.; Schwartz, S.; Sy, M.S.; Marengo, S.R.; Rhim, J.S.; Zhang, D.; Jacobberger, J.W. A new human prostate carcinoma cell line, 22Rv1. *Vitr. Cell. Dev. Biol. Anim.* **1999**, *35*, 403–409. [CrossRef] [PubMed]
105. Zhau, H.Y.; Chang, S.M.; Chen, B.Q.; Wang, Y.; Zhang, H.; Kao, C.; Sang, Q.A.; Pathak, S.J.; Chung, L.W. Androgen-repressed phenotype in human prostate cancer. *Proc. Natl. Acad. Sci. USA* **1996**, *93*, 15152–15157. [CrossRef]
106. Sun, Y.; Schaar, A.; Sukumaran, P.; Dhasarathy, A.; Singh, B.B. TGFbeta-induced epithelial-to-mesenchymal transition in prostate cancer cells is mediated via TRPM7 expression. *Mol. Carcinog.* **2018**, *57*, 752–761. [CrossRef]
107. Millena, A.C.; Vo, B.T.; Khan, S.A. JunD Is Required for Proliferation of Prostate Cancer Cells and Plays a Role in Transforming Growth Factor-beta (TGF-beta)-induced Inhibition of Cell Proliferation. *J. Biol. Chem.* **2016**, *291*, 17964–17976. [CrossRef]
108. Hayward, S.W.; Wang, Y.; Cao, M.; Hom, Y.K.; Zhang, B.; Grossfeld, G.D.; Sudilovsky, D.; Cunha, G.R. Malignant transformation in a nontumorigenic human prostatic epithelial cell line. *Cancer Res.* **2001**, *61*, 8135–8142.
109. Lee, M.; Garkovenko, E.; Yun, J.; Weijerman, P.; Peehl, D.; Chen, L.; Rhim, J. Characterization of adult human prostatic epithelial-cells immortalized by polybrene-induced DNA transfection with a plasmid containing an origin-defective sv40-genome. *Int. J. Oncol.* **1994**, *4*, 821–830. [CrossRef]
110. Shi, X.B.; Xue, L.; Tepper, C.G.; Gandour-Edwards, R.; Ghosh, P.; Kung, H.J.; DeVere White, R.W. The oncogenic potential of a prostate cancer-derived androgen receptor mutant. *Prostate* **2007**, *67*, 591–602. [CrossRef]
111. De Launoit, Y.; Veilleux, R.; Dufour, M.; Simard, J.; Labrie, F. Characteristics of the biphasic action of androgens and of the potent antiproliferative effects of the new pure antiestrogen EM-139 on cell cycle kinetic parameters in LNCaP human prostatic cancer cells. *Cancer Res.* **1991**, *51*, 5165–5170. [PubMed]

112. Nesslinger, N.J.; Shi, X.B.; deVere White, R.W. Androgen-independent growth of LNCaP prostate cancer cells is mediated by gain-of-function mutant p53. *Cancer Res.* **2003**, *63*, 2228–2233. [PubMed]
113. van Bokhoven, A.; Varella-Garcia, M.; Korch, C.; Johannes, W.U.; Smith, E.E.; Miller, H.L.; Nordeen, S.K.; Miller, G.J.; Lucia, M.S. Molecular characterization of human prostate carcinoma cell lines. *Prostate* **2003**, *57*, 205–225. [CrossRef] [PubMed]
114. Vlietstra, R.J.; van Alewijk, D.C.; Hermans, K.G.; van Steenbrugge, G.J.; Trapman, J. Frequent inactivation of PTEN in prostate cancer cell lines and xenografts. *Cancer Res.* **1998**, *58*, 2720–2723.
115. Mitchell, S.; Abel, P.; Ware, M.; Stamp, G.; Lalani, E. Phenotypic and genotypic characterization of commonly used human prostatic cell lines. *BJU Int.* **2000**, *85*, 932–944. [CrossRef]
116. Kokontis, J.M.; Hay, N.; Liao, S. Progression of LNCaP prostate tumor cells during androgen deprivation: Hormone-independent growth, repression of proliferation by androgen, and role for p27Kip1 in androgen-induced cell cycle arrest. *Mol. Endocrinol.* **1998**, *12*, 941–953. [CrossRef]
117. Hudson, T.S.; Perkins, S.N.; Hursting, S.D.; Young, H.A.; Kim, Y.S.; Wang, T.C.; Wang, T.T. Inhibition of androgen-responsive LNCaP prostate cancer cell tumor xenograft growth by dietary phenethyl isothiocyanate correlates with decreased angiogenesis and inhibition of cell attachment. *Int. J. Oncol.* **2012**, *40*, 1113–1121. [CrossRef]
118. Arnold, J.T.; Gray, N.E.; Jacobowitz, K.; Viswanathan, L.; Cheung, P.W.; McFann, K.K.; Le, H.; Blackman, M.R. Human prostate stromal cells stimulate increased PSA production in DHEA-treated prostate cancer epithelial cells. *J. Steroid Biochem. Mol. Biol.* **2008**, *111*, 240–246. [CrossRef]
119. Craft, N.; Shostak, Y.; Carey, M.; Sawyers, C.L. A mechanism for hormone-independent prostate cancer through modulation of androgen receptor signaling by the HER-2/neu tyrosine kinase. *Nat. Med.* **1999**, *5*, 280–285. [CrossRef]
120. Garcia, R.R.; Masoodi, K.Z.; Pascal, L.E.; Nelson, J.B.; Wang, Z. Growth of LAPC4 prostate cancer xenograft tumor is insensitive to 5alpha-reductase inhibitor dutasteride. *Am. J. Clin. Exp. Urol.* **2014**, *2*, 82–91.
121. Patrawala, L.; Calhoun-Davis, T.; Schneider-Broussard, R.; Tang, D.G. Hierarchical organization of prostate cancer cells in xenograft tumors: The CD44+alpha2beta1+ cell population is enriched in tumor-initiating cells. *Cancer Res.* **2007**, *67*, 6796–6805. [CrossRef] [PubMed]
122. Tsingotjidou, A.S.; Zotalis, G.; Jackson, K.R.; Sawyers, C.; Puzas, J.E.; Hicks, D.G.; Reiter, R.; Lieberman, J.R. Development of an animal model for prostate cancer cell metastasis to adult human bone. *Anticancer Res.* **2001**, *21*, 971–978. [PubMed]
123. Nickerson, T.; Chang, F.; Lorimer, D.; Smeekens, S.P.; Sawyers, C.L.; Pollak, M. In vivo progression of LAPC-9 and LNCaP prostate cancer models to androgen independence is associated with increased expression of insulin-like growth factor I (IGF-I) and IGF-I receptor (IGF-IR). *Cancer Res.* **2001**, *61*, 6276–6280. [PubMed]
124. Lee, Y.; Schwarz, E.; Davies, M.; Jo, M.; Gates, J.; Wu, J.; Zhang, X.; Lieberman, J.R. Differences in the cytokine profiles associated with prostate cancer cell induced osteoblastic and osteolytic lesions in bone. *J. Orthop. Res.* **2003**, *21*, 62–72. [CrossRef]
125. McLean, D.T.; Strand, D.W.; Ricke, W.A. Prostate cancer xenografts and hormone induced prostate carcinogenesis. *Differentiation* **2017**, *97*, 23–32. [CrossRef] [PubMed]
126. Watson, P.A.; Chen, Y.F.; Balbas, M.D.; Wongvipat, J.; Socci, N.D.; Viale, A.; Kim, K.; Sawyers, C.L. Constitutively active androgen receptor splice variants expressed in castration-resistant prostate cancer require full-length androgen receptor. *Proc. Natl. Acad. Sci. USA* **2010**, *107*, 16759–16765. [CrossRef] [PubMed]
127. Linxweiler, J.; Korbel, C.; Muller, A.; Hammer, M.; Veith, C.; Bohle, R.M.; Stockle, M.; Junker, K.; Menger, M.D.; Saar, M. A novel mouse model of human prostate cancer to study intraprostatic tumor growth and the development of lymph node metastases. *Prostate* **2018**, *78*, 664–675. [CrossRef]
128. Wang, J.; Cai, Y.; Yu, W.; Ren, C.; Spencer, D.M.; Ittmann, M. Pleiotropic biological activities of alternatively spliced TMPRSS2/ERG fusion gene transcripts. *Cancer Res.* **2008**, *68*, 8516–8524. [CrossRef]
129. Martinez, L.A.; Yang, J.; Vazquez, E.S.; Rodriguez-Vargas Mdel, C.; Olive, M.; Hsieh, J.T.; Logothetis, C.J.; Navone, N.M. p21 modulates threshold of apoptosis induced by DNA-damage and growth factor withdrawal in prostate cancer cells. *Carcinogenesis* **2002**, *23*, 1289–1296. [CrossRef]
130. Alimonti, A.; Nardella, C.; Chen, Z.; Clohessy, J.G.; Carracedo, A.; Trotman, L.C.; Cheng, K.; Varmeh, S.; Kozma, S.C.; Thomas, G.; et al. A novel type of cellular senescence that can be enhanced in mouse models and human tumor xenografts to suppress prostate tumorigenesis. *J. Clin. Investig.* **2010**, *120*, 681–693. [CrossRef]

131. Hara, T.; Nakamura, K.; Araki, H.; Kusaka, M.; Yamaoka, M. Enhanced androgen receptor signaling correlates with the androgen-refractory growth in a newly established MDA PCa 2b-hr human prostate cancer cell subline. *Cancer Res.* **2003**, *63*, 5622–5628. [PubMed]
132. Corey, E.; Quinn, J.E.; Buhler, K.R.; Nelson, P.S.; Macoska, J.A.; True, L.D.; Vessella, R.L. LuCaP 35: A new model of prostate cancer progression to androgen independence. *Prostate* **2003**, *55*, 239–246. [CrossRef] [PubMed]
133. Gaupel, A.-C.; Wang, W.-L.W.; Mordan-McCombs, S.; Lee, E.C.Y.; Tenniswood, M. Xenograft, Transgenic, and Knockout Models of Prostate Cancer. In *Animal Models for the Study of Human Disease*; Elsevier Inc.: Amsterdam, The Netherlands, 2013.
134. Myers, J.S.; Vallega, K.A.; White, J.; Yu, K.; Yates, C.C.; Sang, Q.A. Proteomic characterization of paired non-malignant and malignant African-American prostate epithelial cell lines distinguishes them by structural proteins. *BMC Cancer* **2017**, *17*, 480. [CrossRef] [PubMed]
135. Masumori, N.; Thomas, T.Z.; Chaurand, P.; Case, T.; Paul, M.; Kasper, S.; Caprioli, R.M.; Tsukamoto, T.; Shappell, S.B.; Matusik, R.J. A probasin-large T antigen transgenic mouse line develops prostate adenocarcinoma and neuroendocrine carcinoma with metastatic potential. *Cancer Res.* **2001**, *61*, 2239–2249.
136. Attardi, B.J.; Burgenson, J.; Hild, S.A.; Reel, J.R. Steroid hormonal regulation of growth, prostate specific antigen secretion, and transcription mediated by the mutated androgen receptor in CWR22Rv1 human prostate carcinoma cells. *Mol. Cell. Endocrinol.* **2004**, *222*, 121–132. [CrossRef]
137. Knouf, E.C.; Metzger, M.J.; Mitchell, P.S.; Arroyo, J.D.; Chevillet, J.R.; Tewari, M.; Miller, A.D. Multiple integrated copies and high-level production of the human retrovirus XMRV (xenotropic murine leukemia virus-related virus) from 22Rv1 prostate carcinoma cells. *J. Virol.* **2009**, *83*, 7353–7356. [CrossRef]
138. Nagle, R.B.; Ahmann, F.R.; McDaniel, K.M.; Paquin, M.L.; Clark, V.A.; Celniker, A. Cytokeratin characterization of human prostatic carcinoma and its derived cell lines. *Cancer Res.* **1987**, *47*, 281–286. [PubMed]
139. Tai, S.; Sun, Y.; Squires, J.M.; Zhang, H.; Oh, W.K.; Liang, C.Z.; Huang, J. PC3 is a cell line characteristic of prostatic small cell carcinoma. *Prostate* **2011**, *71*, 1668–1679. [CrossRef]
140. Ravenna, L.; Principessa, L.; Verdina, A.; Salvatori, L.; Russo, M.A.; Petrangeli, E. Distinct phenotypes of human prostate cancer cells associate with different adaptation to hypoxia and pro-inflammatory gene expression. *PLoS ONE* **2014**, *9*, e96250. [CrossRef]
141. Bhardwaj, A.; Singh, S.; Srivastava, S.K.; Arora, S.; Hyde, S.J.; Andrews, J.; Grizzle, W.E.; Singh, A.P. Restoration of PPP2CA expression reverses epithelial-to-mesenchymal transition and suppresses prostate tumour growth and metastasis in an orthotopic mouse model. *Br. J. Cancer* **2014**, *110*, 2000–2010. [CrossRef]
142. Puhr, M.; Hoefer, J.; Eigentler, A.; Ploner, C.; Handle, F.; Schaefer, G.; Kroon, J.; Leo, A.; Heidegger, I.; Eder, I.; et al. The Glucocorticoid Receptor Is a Key Player for Prostate Cancer Cell Survival and a Target for Improved Antiandrogen Therapy. *Clin. Cancer Res.* **2018**, *24*, 927–938. [CrossRef] [PubMed]
143. Jarrard, D.F.; Blitz, B.F.; Smith, R.C.; Patai, B.L.; Rukstalis, D.B. Effect of epidermal growth factor on prostate cancer cell line PC3 growth and invasion. *Prostate* **1994**, *24*, 46–53. [CrossRef] [PubMed]
144. Pfeiffer, M.J.; Schalken, J.A. Stem cell characteristics in prostate cancer cell lines. *Eur. Urol.* **2010**, *57*, 246–254. [CrossRef]
145. Van Leenders, G.J.; Aalders, T.W.; Hulsbergen-van de Kaa, C.A.; Ruiter, D.J.; Schalken, J.A. Expression of basal cell keratins in human prostate cancer metastases and cell lines. *J. Pathol.* **2001**, *195*, 563–570. [CrossRef]
146. Scaccianoce, E.; Festuccia, C.; Dondi, D.; Guerini, V.; Bologna, M.; Motta, M.; Poletti, A. Characterization of prostate cancer DU145 cells expressing the recombinant androgen receptor. *Oncol. Res.* **2003**, *14*, 101–112. [CrossRef]
147. Jones, H.E.; Dutkowski, C.M.; Barrow, D.; Harper, M.E.; Wakeling, A.E.; Nicholson, R.I. New EGF-R selective tyrosine kinase inhibitor reveals variable growth responses in prostate carcinoma cell lines PC-3 and DU-145. *Int. J. Cancer* **1997**, *71*, 1010–1018. [CrossRef]
148. Sherwood, E.R.; Van Dongen, J.L.; Wood, C.G.; Liao, S.; Kozlowski, J.M.; Lee, C. Epidermal growth factor receptor activation in androgen-independent but not androgen-stimulated growth of human prostatic carcinoma cells. *Br. J. Cancer* **1998**, *77*, 855–861. [CrossRef]
149. Mickey, D.D.; Stone, K.R.; Wunderli, H.; Mickey, G.H.; Vollmer, R.T.; Paulson, D.F. Heterotransplantation of a human prostatic adenocarcinoma cell line in nude mice. *Cancer Res.* **1977**, *37*, 4049–4058. [PubMed]

150. Bastide, C.; Bagnis, C.; Mannoni, P.; Hassoun, J.; Bladou, F. A Nod Scid mouse model to study human prostate cancer. *Prostate Cancer Prostatic Dis.* **2002**, *5*, 311–315. [CrossRef]
151. Zhau, H.E.; Odero-Marah, V.; Lue, H.W.; Nomura, T.; Wang, R.; Chu, G.; Liu, Z.R.; Zhou, B.P.; Huang, W.C.; Chung, L.W. Epithelial to mesenchymal transition (EMT) in human prostate cancer: Lessons learned from ARCaP model. *Clin. Exp. Metastasis* **2008**, *25*, 601–610. [CrossRef] [PubMed]
152. Wang, R.; Chu, G.C.Y.; Mrdenovic, S.; Annamalai, A.A.; Hendifar, A.E.; Nissen, N.N.; Tomlinson, J.S.; Lewis, M.; Palanisamy, N.; Tseng, H.R.; et al. Cultured circulating tumor cells and their derived xenografts for personalized oncology. *Asian J. Urol.* **2016**, *3*, 240–253. [CrossRef] [PubMed]
153. He, H.; Yang, X.; Davidson, A.J.; Wu, D.; Marshall, F.F.; Chung, L.W.; Zhau, H.E.; Wang, R. Progressive epithelial to mesenchymal transitions in ARCaP E prostate cancer cells during xenograft tumor formation and metastasis. *Prostate* **2010**, *70*, 518–528. [CrossRef]
154. Gingrich, J.R.; Barrios, R.J.; Morton, R.A.; Boyce, B.F.; DeMayo, F.J.; Finegold, M.J.; Angelopoulou, R.; Rosen, J.M.; Greenberg, N.M. Metastatic prostate cancer in a transgenic mouse. *Cancer Res.* **1996**, *56*, 4096–4102. [PubMed]
155. Greenberg, N.M.; DeMayo, F.J.; Sheppard, P.C.; Barrios, R.; Lebovitz, R.; Finegold, M.; Angelopoulou, R.; Dodd, J.G.; Duckworth, M.L.; Rosen, J.M.; et al. The rat probasin gene promoter directs hormonally and developmentally regulated expression of a heterologous gene specifically to the prostate in transgenic mice. *Mol. Endocrinol.* **1994**, *8*, 230–239. [CrossRef] [PubMed]
156. Maroulakou, I.G.; Anver, M.; Garrett, L.; Green, J.E. Prostate and mammary adenocarcinoma in transgenic mice carrying a rat C3(1) simian virus 40 large tumor antigen fusion gene. *Proc. Natl. Acad. Sci. USA* **1994**, *91*, 11236–11240. [CrossRef] [PubMed]
157. Greenberg, N.M.; DeMayo, F.; Finegold, M.J.; Medina, D.; Tilley, W.D.; Aspinall, J.O.; Cunha, G.R.; Donjacour, A.A.; Matusik, R.J.; Rosen, J.M. Prostate cancer in a transgenic mouse. *Proc. Natl. Acad. Sci. USA* **1995**, *92*, 3439–3443. [CrossRef]
158. Wang, L.; Bonorden, M.J.; Li, G.X.; Lee, H.J.; Hu, H.; Zhang, Y.; Liao, J.D.; Cleary, M.P.; Lu, J. Methyl-selenium compounds inhibit prostate carcinogenesis in the transgenic adenocarcinoma of mouse prostate model with survival benefit. *Cancer Prev. Res. (Phila)* **2009**, *2*, 484–495. [CrossRef] [PubMed]
159. Gupta, S.; Hastak, K.; Ahmad, N.; Lewin, J.S.; Mukhtar, H. Inhibition of prostate carcinogenesis in TRAMP mice by oral infusion of green tea polyphenols. *Proc. Natl. Acad. Sci. USA* **2001**, *98*, 10350–10355. [CrossRef]
160. Gingrich, J.R.; Barrios, R.J.; Kattan, M.W.; Nahm, H.S.; Finegold, M.J.; Greenberg, N.M. Androgen-independent prostate cancer progression in the TRAMP model. *Cancer Res.* **1997**, *57*, 4687–4691.
161. Chiaverotti, T.; Couto, S.S.; Donjacour, A.; Mao, J.H.; Nagase, H.; Cardiff, R.D.; Cunha, G.R.; Balmain, A. Dissociation of epithelial and neuroendocrine carcinoma lineages in the transgenic adenocarcinoma of mouse prostate model of prostate cancer. *Am. J. Pathol.* **2008**, *172*, 236–246. [CrossRef]
162. Rickman, D.S.; Beltran, H.; Demichelis, F.; Rubin, M.A. Biology and evolution of poorly differentiated neuroendocrine tumors. *Nat. Med.* **2017**, *23*, 664–673. [CrossRef]
163. Kasper, S.; Sheppard, P.C.; Yan, Y.; Pettigrew, N.; Borowsky, A.D.; Prins, G.S.; Dodd, J.G.; Duckworth, M.L.; Matusik, R.J. Development, progression, and androgen-dependence of prostate tumors in probasin-large T antigen transgenic mice: A model for prostate cancer. *Lab. Investig.* **1998**, *78*, i–xv.
164. Klezovitch, O.; Chevillet, J.; Mirosevich, J.; Roberts, R.L.; Matusik, R.J.; Vasioukhin, V. Hepsin promotes prostate cancer progression and metastasis. *Cancer Cell* **2004**, *6*, 185–195. [CrossRef]
165. Berman-Booty, L.D.; Knudsen, K.E. Models of neuroendocrine prostate cancer. *Endocr. Relat. Cancer* **2015**, *22*, R33–R49. [CrossRef] [PubMed]
166. Di Cristofano, A.; Pesce, B.; Cordon-Cardo, C.; Pandolfi, P.P. Pten is essential for embryonic development and tumour suppression. *Nat. Genet.* **1998**, *19*, 348–355. [CrossRef] [PubMed]
167. Suzuki, A.; de la Pompa, J.L.; Stambolic, V.; Elia, A.J.; Sasaki, T.; del Barco Barrantes, I.; Ho, A.; Wakeham, A.; Itie, A.; Khoo, W.; et al. High cancer susceptibility and embryonic lethality associated with mutation of the PTEN tumor suppressor gene in mice. *Curr. Biol.* **1998**, *8*, 1169–1178. [CrossRef]
168. Podsypanina, K.; Ellenson, L.H.; Nemes, A.; Gu, J.; Tamura, M.; Yamada, K.M.; Cordon-Cardo, C.; Catoretti, G.; Fisher, P.E.; Parsons, R. Mutation of Pten/Mmac1 in mice causes neoplasia in multiple organ systems. *Proc. Natl. Acad. Sci. USA* **1999**, *96*, 1563–1568. [CrossRef]

169. Stambolic, V.; Tsao, M.S.; Macpherson, D.; Suzuki, A.; Chapman, W.B.; Mak, T.W. High incidence of breast and endometrial neoplasia resembling human Cowden syndrome in pten+/− mice. *Cancer Res.* **2000**, *60*, 3605–3611. [PubMed]
170. Li, Q.; Liu, L.; Zhang, Q.; Liu, S.; Ge, D.; You, Z. Interleukin-17 Indirectly Promotes M2 Macrophage Differentiation through Stimulation of COX-2/PGE2 Pathway in the Cancer Cells. *Cancer Res. Treat.* **2014**, *46*, 297–306. [CrossRef]
171. Zhang, Q.; Liu, S.; Zhang, Q.; Xiong, Z.; Wang, A.R.; Myers, L.; Melamed, J.; Tang, W.W.; You, Z. Interleukin-17 promotes development of castration-resistant prostate cancer potentially through creating an immunotolerant and pro-angiogenic tumor microenvironment. *Prostate* **2014**, *74*, 869–879. [CrossRef]
172. Bai, F.; Pei, X.H.; Pandolfi, P.P.; Xiong, Y. p18 Ink4c and Pten constrain a positive regulatory loop between cell growth and cell cycle control. *Mol. Cell. Biol.* **2006**, *26*, 4564–4576. [CrossRef] [PubMed]
173. Bowen, C.; Bubendorf, L.; Voeller, H.J.; Slack, R.; Willi, N.; Sauter, G.; Gasser, T.C.; Koivisto, P.; Lack, E.E.; Kononen, J.; et al. Loss of NKX3.1 expression in human prostate cancers correlates with tumor progression. *Cancer Res.* **2000**, *60*, 6111–6115. [PubMed]
174. Jayaprakash, P.; Ai, M.; Liu, A.; Budhani, P.; Bartkowiak, T.; Sheng, J.; Ager, C.; Nicholas, C.; Jaiswal, A.R.; Sun, Y.; et al. Targeted hypoxia reduction restores T cell infiltration and sensitizes prostate cancer to immunotherapy. *J. Clin. Investig.* **2018**, *128*, 5137–5149. [CrossRef] [PubMed]
175. Wang, G.; Lu, X.; Dey, P.; Deng, P.; Wu, C.C.; Jiang, S.; Fang, Z.; Zhao, K.; Konaparthi, R.; Hua, S.; et al. Targeting YAP-Dependent MDSC Infiltration Impairs Tumor Progression. *Cancer Discov.* **2016**, *6*, 80–95. [CrossRef] [PubMed]
176. Wu, X.; Wu, J.; Huang, J.; Powell, W.C.; Zhang, J.; Matusik, R.J.; Sangiorgi, F.O.; Maxson, R.E.; Sucov, H.M.; Roy-Burman, P. Generation of a prostate epithelial cell-specific Cre transgenic mouse model for tissue-specific gene ablation. *Mech. Dev.* **2001**, *101*, 61–69. [CrossRef]
177. Zhang, J.; Thomas, T.Z.; Kasper, S.; Matusik, R.J. A small composite probasin promoter confers high levels of prostate-specific gene expression through regulation by androgens and glucocorticoids in vitro and in vivo. *Endocrinology* **2000**, *141*, 4698–4710. [CrossRef]
178. McMullin, R.P.; Mutton, L.N.; Bieberich, C.J. Hoxb13 regulatory elements mediate transgene expression during prostate organogenesis and carcinogenesis. *Dev. Dyn.* **2009**, *238*, 664–672. [CrossRef]
179. Majumder, P.K.; Yeh, J.J.; George, D.J.; Febbo, P.G.; Kum, J.; Xue, Q.; Bikoff, R.; Ma, H.; Kantoff, P.W.; Golub, T.R.; et al. Prostate intraepithelial neoplasia induced by prostate restricted Akt activation: The MPAKT model. *Proc. Natl. Acad. Sci. USA* **2003**, *100*, 7841–7846. [CrossRef]
180. Ramaswamy, S.; Nakamura, N.; Vazquez, F.; Batt, D.B.; Perera, S.; Roberts, T.M.; Sellers, W.R. Regulation of G1 progression by the PTEN tumor suppressor protein is linked to inhibition of the phosphatidylinositol 3-kinase/Akt pathway. *Proc. Natl. Acad. Sci. USA* **1999**, *96*, 2110–2115. [CrossRef]
181. Gao, D.; Chen, Y. Organoid development in cancer genome discovery. *Curr. Opin. Genet. Dev.* **2015**, *30*, 42–48. [CrossRef]
182. Ben-David, U.; Beroukhim, R.; Golub, T.R. Genomic evolution of cancer models: Perils and opportunities. *Nat. Rev. Cancer* **2019**, *19*, 97–109. [CrossRef]
183. Wang, S.; Gao, D.; Chen, Y. The potential of organoids in urological cancer research. *Nat. Rev. Urol.* **2017**, *14*, 401–414. [CrossRef] [PubMed]
184. Gao, D.; Vela, I.; Sboner, A.; Iaquinta, P.J.; Karthaus, W.R.; Gopalan, A.; Dowling, C.; Wanjala, J.N.; Undvall, E.A.; Arora, V.K.; et al. Organoid cultures derived from patients with advanced prostate cancer. *Cell* **2014**, *159*, 176–187. [CrossRef] [PubMed]
185. Puca, L.; Bareja, R.; Prandi, D.; Shaw, R.; Benelli, M.; Karthaus, W.R.; Hess, J.; Sigouros, M.; Donoghue, A.; Kossai, M.; et al. Patient derived organoids to model rare prostate cancer phenotypes. *Nat. Commun.* **2018**, *9*, 2404. [CrossRef] [PubMed]
186. Choi, S.Y.; Lin, D.; Gout, P.W.; Collins, C.C.; Xu, Y.; Wang, Y. Lessons from patient-derived xenografts for better in vitro modeling of human cancer. *Adv. Drug Deliv. Rev.* **2014**, *79–80*, 222–237. [CrossRef]
187. Nguyen, H.M.; Vessella, R.L.; Morrissey, C.; Brown, L.G.; Coleman, I.M.; Higano, C.S.; Mostaghel, E.A.; Zhang, X.; True, L.D.; Lam, H.M.; et al. LuCaP Prostate Cancer Patient-Derived Xenografts Reflect the Molecular Heterogeneity of Advanced Disease and Serve as Models for Evaluating Cancer Therapeutics. *Prostate* **2017**, *77*, 654–671. [CrossRef]

188. Li, Z.G.; Mathew, P.; Yang, J.; Starbuck, M.W.; Zurita, A.J.; Liu, J.; Sikes, C.; Multani, A.S.; Efstathiou, E.; Lopez, A.; et al. Androgen receptor-negative human prostate cancer cells induce osteogenesis in mice through FGF9-mediated mechanisms. *J. Clin. Investig.* **2008**, *118*, 2697–2710. [CrossRef]
189. Lee, C.H.; Xue, H.; Sutcliffe, M.; Gout, P.W.; Huntsman, D.G.; Miller, D.M.; Gilks, C.B.; Wang, Y.Z. Establishment of subrenal capsule xenografts of primary human ovarian tumors in SCID mice: Potential models. *Gynecol. Oncol.* **2005**, *96*, 48–55. [CrossRef]
190. Okada, S.; Vaeteewoottacharn, K.; Kariya, R. Establishment of a Patient-Derived Tumor Xenograft Model and Application for Precision Cancer Medicine. *Chem. Pharm. Bull. (Tokyo)* **2018**, *66*, 225–230. [CrossRef]
191. Kopetz, S.; Lemos, R.; Powis, G. The promise of patient-derived xenografts: The best laid plans of mice and men. *Clin. Cancer Res.* **2012**, *18*, 5160–5162. [CrossRef]
192. Hoehn, W.; Schroeder, F.H.; Reimann, J.F.; Joebsis, A.C.; Hermanek, P. Human prostatic adenocarcinoma: Some characteristics of a serially transplantable line in nude mice (PC 82). *Prostate* **1980**, *1*, 95–104. [CrossRef] [PubMed]
193. Van Weerden, W.M.; de Ridder, C.M.; Verdaasdonk, C.L.; Romijn, J.C.; van der Kwast, T.H.; Schroder, F.H.; van Steenbrugge, G.J. Development of seven new human prostate tumor xenograft models and their histopathological characterization. *Am. J. Pathol.* **1996**, *149*, 1055–1062. [PubMed]
194. Kiefer, J.A.; Vessella, R.L.; Quinn, J.E.; Odman, A.M.; Zhang, J.; Keller, E.T.; Kostenuik, P.J.; Dunstan, C.R.; Corey, E. The effect of osteoprotegerin administration on the intra-tibial growth of the osteoblastic LuCaP 23.1 prostate cancer xenograft. *Clin. Exp. Metastasis* **2004**, *21*, 381–387. [CrossRef]
195. Corey, E.; Quinn, J.E.; Bladou, F.; Brown, L.G.; Roudier, M.P.; Brown, J.M.; Buhler, K.R.; Vessella, R.L. Establishment and characterization of osseous prostate cancer models: Intra-tibial injection of human prostate cancer cells. *Prostate* **2002**, *52*, 20–33. [CrossRef] [PubMed]
196. Toivanen, R.; Berman, D.M.; Wang, H.; Pedersen, J.; Frydenberg, M.; Meeker, A.K.; Ellem, S.J.; Risbridger, G.P.; Taylor, R.A. Brief report: A bioassay to identify primary human prostate cancer repopulating cells. *Stem Cells* **2011**, *29*, 1310–1314. [CrossRef]
197. Morton, C.L.; Houghton, P.J. Establishment of human tumor xenografts in immunodeficient mice. *Nat. Protoc.* **2007**, *2*, 247–250. [CrossRef]
198. Yada, E.; Wada, S.; Yoshida, S.; Sasada, T. Use of patient-derived xenograft mouse models in cancer research and treatment. *Future Sci. OA* **2018**, *4*, FSO271. [CrossRef]
199. Dunning, W.F.; Curtis, M.R.; Segaloff, A. Methylcholanthrene squamous cell carcinoma of the rat prostate with skeletal metastases, and failure of the rat liver to respond to the carcinogen. *Cancer Res.* **1946**, *6*, 256–262.
200. Tennant, T.R.; Kim, H.; Sokoloff, M.; Rinker-Schaeffer, C.W. The Dunning model. *Prostate* **2000**, *43*, 295–302. [CrossRef]
201. Pollard, M. The Lobund-Wistar rat model of prostate cancer. *J. Cell. Biochem. Suppl.* **1992**, *16H*, 84–88. [CrossRef]
202. Wertman, J.; Veinotte, C.J.; Dellaire, G.; Berman, J.N. The Zebrafish Xenograft Platform: Evolution of a Novel Cancer Model and Preclinical Screening Tool. *Adv. Exp. Med. Biol.* **2016**, *916*, 289–314. [CrossRef] [PubMed]
203. Herbomel, P.; Thisse, B.; Thisse, C. Ontogeny and behaviour of early macrophages in the zebrafish embryo. *Development* **1999**, *126*, 3735–3745.
204. Le Guyader, D.; Redd, M.J.; Colucci-Guyon, E.; Murayama, E.; Kissa, K.; Briolat, V.; Mordelet, E.; Zapata, A.; Shinomiya, H.; Herbomel, P. Origins and unconventional behavior of neutrophils in developing zebrafish. *Blood* **2008**, *111*, 132–141. [CrossRef] [PubMed]
205. Melong, N.; Steele, S.; MacDonald, M.; Holly, A.; Collins, C.C.; Zoubeidi, A.; Berman, J.N.; Dellaire, G. Enzalutamide inhibits testosterone-induced growth of human prostate cancer xenografts in zebrafish and can induce bradycardia. *Sci. Rep.* **2017**, *7*, 14698. [CrossRef] [PubMed]
206. Xu, W.; Foster, B.A.; Richards, M.; Bondioli, K.R.; Shah, G.; Green, C.C. Characterization of prostate cancer cell progression in zebrafish xenograft model. *Int. J. Oncol.* **2018**, *52*, 252–260. [CrossRef]

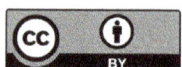

© 2020 by the authors. Licensee MDPI, Basel, Switzerland. This article is an open access article distributed under the terms and conditions of the Creative Commons Attribution (CC BY) license (http://creativecommons.org/licenses/by/4.0/).

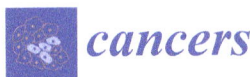

Article

The Role of Daily Adaptive Stereotactic MR-Guided Radiotherapy for Renal Cell Cancer

Shyama U. Tetar [1,†], Omar Bohoudi [1,†], Suresh Senan [1], Miguel A. Palacios [1], Swie S. Oei [1], Antoinet M. van der Wel [1], Berend J. Slotman [1], R. Jeroen A. van Moorselaar [2], Frank J. Lagerwaard [1] and Anna M. E. Bruynzeel [1,*]

1. Department of Radiation Oncology, Amsterdam University Medical Centers, 1081 HZ Amsterdam, The Netherlands; su.tetar@amsterdamumc.nl (S.U.T.); o.bohoudi@amsterdamumc.nl (O.B.); s.senan@amsterdamumc.nl (S.S.); m.palacios@amsterdamumc.nl (M.A.P.); ss.oei@amsterdamumc.nl (S.S.O.); a.vanderwel1@amsterdamumc.nl (A.M.v.d.W.); bj.slotman@amsterdamumc.nl (B.J.S.); fj.lagerwaard@amsterdamumc.nl (F.J.L.)
2. Department of Urology, Amsterdam University Medical Centers, 1081 HV Amsterdam, The Netherlands; rja.vanmoorselaar@amsterdamumc.nl
* Correspondence: ame.bruynzeel@amsterdamumc.nl; Tel.: +31-20-4440413
† These authors joined first authors.

Received: 24 July 2020; Accepted: 22 September 2020; Published: 25 September 2020

Simple Summary: Standard treatment for localized renal cell carcinoma (RCC) is surgery. Stereotactic radiotherapy given in a few high dose fractions is a promising treatment for this indication and could be an alternative option for patients unsuitable for surgery. Stereotactic MR-guided radiotherapy (MRgRT) is clinically implemented as a new technique for precise treatment delivery of abdominal tumors, like RCC. In this study, we evaluated the clinical impact of stereotactic MRgRT given in five fractions of 8 Gy and routine plan re-optimization for 36 patients with large primary RCCs. Our evaluation showed good oncological results with minimal side-effects. Even in this group with large tumors, daily plan re-optimization was only needed in a minority of patients who can be identified upfront. This is a favorable result since online MRgRT plan adaptation is a time-consuming procedure. In these patients, MRgRT delivery will be faster, and these patients could be candidates for even less fractions per treatment.

Abstract: Novel magnetic-resonance-guided radiotherapy (MRgRT) permits real-time soft-tissue visualization, respiratory-gated delivery with minimal safety margins, and time-consuming daily plan re-optimisation. We report on early clinical outcomes of MRgRT and routine plan re-optimization for large primary renal cell cancer (RCC). Thirty-six patients were treated with MRgRT in 40 Gy/5 fractions. Prior to each fraction, re-contouring of tumor and normal organs on a pretreatment MR-scan allowed daily plan re-optimization. Treatment-induced toxicity and radiological responses were scored, which was followed by an offline analysis to evaluate the need for such daily re-optimization in 180 fractions. Mean age and tumor diameter were 78.1 years and 5.6 cm, respectively. All patients completed MRgRT with an average fraction duration of 45 min. Local control (LC) and overall survival rates at one year were 95.2% and 91.2%. No grade ≥3 toxicity was reported. Plans without re-optimization met institutional radiotherapy constraints in 83.9% of 180 fractions. Thus, daily plan re-optimization was required for only a minority of patients, who can be identified upfront by a higher volume of normal organs receiving 25 Gy in baseline plans. In conclusion, stereotactic MRgRT for large primary RCC showed low toxicity and high LC, while daily plan re-optimization was required only in a minority of patients.

Keywords: MR-guided; radiotherapy; MRgRT; stereotactic ablative radiotherapy; stereotactic ablative radiation therapy (SABR); renal cell cancer; RCC; online adaptive

1. Introduction

A radical or partial nephrectomy is the preferred standard curative treatment for localized renal cell carcinoma (RCC) [1–4]. Ablative local treatment, such as radiofrequency ablation (RFA), cryoablation (CA), or microwave ablation (MWA), is an alternative in elderly patients who present with a high surgical risk due to several comorbidities [3]. Radiotherapy does not have a prominent role in current international and national guidelines in treating primary RCC [1–4]. In recent years, stereotactic ablative radiation therapy (SABR) has been evaluated in several smaller retrospective and prospective studies [5–14], usually in RCC patients unsuitable for surgery. Outcomes of a multi-institutional pool from nine institutions, utilizing either single or multi-fractionated treatment in 223 patients, have been reported by the International Radiosurgery Oncology Consortium for Kidney (IROCK) [15]. SABR for RCC was found to be well tolerated, achieved local control (LC) rates exceeding 95% at four years of follow-up and grade ≥3 toxicity rates of 1.3%, and had an average decrease in glomerular filtration rate of 5.5 mL per minute. The majority of the tumors in this pooled analysis was ≤4 cm and clinical data for larger tumors is limited. A retrospective analysis of a subgroup of 95 patients with tumors >4 cm was recently published [16], but with the exception of these data, clinical outcomes on cT1b-T2 RCC SABR are scarce. Due to the inherent limitations to a pooled analyses, the Trans-Tasman Radiation Oncology Group (TROG) and the Australian and New Zealand Urogenital and Prostate Cancer Trials Group (ANZUP) have initiated a prospective, multi-institutional phase II study in 70 patients with biopsy-confirmed medical inoperable RCC patients [17]. Full accrual has recently been completed, and the data of this trial are eagerly awaited.

Technical challenges in renal SABR include the management of intra-fractional motion, and potential solutions using an internal target volume-approach, fiducial-assisted robotic SABR or abdominal compression [18] have been described. Magnetic-resonance (MR)-guided radiotherapy (MRgRT) has been considered a promising option because of its improved visualization of kidney tumors in relation to critical adjacent organs such as a small bowel, duodenum, and stomach and the opportunity of real-time tumor tracking and automated gated delivery [18,19]. MRgRT also facilitates daily plan re-optimization as a means to reduce organs at risk (OAR) doses when abdominal organs are near the primary tumor. Furthermore, MRgRT is an outpatient treatment for which no invasive procedures or anesthesia is required. However, to the best of our knowledge, clinical data on MR-guided SABR for localized RCC have not been reported.

Stereotactic MRgRT with routine daily plan adaptation was clinically implemented at our center in 2016 for a variety of clinical indications. The aim of the current paper is to describe our technique, early clinical outcomes, and the role of daily plan adaptation in MRgRT for patients with primary large RCC.

2. Materials and Methods

Data from all patients treated with MRgRT on the MRIdian-system (ViewRay Inc., Mountain View, CA, USA) at the Amsterdam University Medical Centers are collected within a prospective institutional review board approved database. Between May 2016 and February 2020, a total of 51 patients were treated for a primary RCC ($n = 36$), local recurrences ($n = 5$), renal metastases from other primary tumors ($n = 3$), or a diagnosis of urothelial carcinoma ($n = 7$). This analysis is restricted to the remaining 36 patients who were treated for primary RCC.

All patients underwent stereotactic adaptive MRgRT delivered to a dose of 40 Gy in five fractions in a two-week period. Implanted fiducials were not required, and the adaptive workflow was similar to that which had been described previously for pancreatic tumors [20]. Briefly, for simulation, both a MR-scan (0.35T True-FISP, TR/TE: 3.37 ms/1.45 ms, FA: 60°, 17-s with 1.6 mm × 1.6 mm × 3.0 mm resolution) and computed tomography (CT)-scan (slice thickness of 2 mm) are acquired during a shallow-inspiration breath-hold. Geometric accuracy of the MRIdian system is < 0.1 cm in a sphere of 10 cm radius around the isocenter, and <0.15 cm in a sphere of 17.5 cm radius. Every patient was brought as close to the isocenter as possible for each fraction, and the maximum distance from the tumor or any other critical structure to the isocenter was always below 10 cm. Geometric accuracy was assessed with two different dedicated phantoms for spatial integrity measurements. Contouring of the primary tumor (also called gross tumor volume; GTV) and OAR is performed on breath-hold MR-images with the aid of diagnostic imaging, generally contrast-enhanced CT scans. The PTV (planning target volume) is derived from the GTV plus an isotropic 3-mm margin. A co-planar baseline plan consisting of between 30 and 42 intensity modulated radiotherapy (IMRT)-segments is generated, using the MRIdian treatment planning software. Dose calculation was executed with a VMC and EGSnrc code-based Monte-Carlo algorithm (statistical uncertainty of 1% and a grid size of 0.3 cm × 0.3 cm × 0.3 cm) using the deformed electron density map from the simulation CT scan. Institutional target coverage and OAR constraints are summarized in Table 1.

Table 1. Dose prescription for institutional target coverage and normal tissue constraints. The constraints represent the cut-off doses for radiotherapy planning with the aim of dose sparing in the surrounding organs (contralateral kidney, liver, duodenum, bowel, and stomach) while, at the same time, aiming to achieve a high dose in the tumor with the margin, which is represented as the planning target volume. Organs at risk are only re-contoured within 2 cm of the tumor and, for an adaptive setting, only the dose in these structures are optimized.

Structure	Dose to Volume			
Planning Target Volume	≥50	% at	38	Gy
	≤1	cc at	50	Gy
Kidney Contralateral	≤25	% at	12	Gy
Liver	≤50	% at	12	Gy
Duodenum, Bowel, Stomach in 2 cm	≤0.1	cc at	36	Gy
	≤1	cc at	33	Gy

We perform routine plan re-optimization using the daily pre-SABR breath-hold MR-imaging acquired in the treatment position. After rigid registration on the GTV, OAR contours are propagated to the repeat MR using deformable image registration. The ViewRay deformable image registration algorithm uses an intensity-based algorithm, which minimizes a cost function that measures the similarity between the images including a regularization term in order to obtain smoother deformation fields and prevent sharp discontinuities. The GTV and OAR contours are checked and adjusted where needed within a 2-cm distance of the PTV by the attending radiation oncologist. Next, the baseline IMRT plan is recalculated on the new anatomy ("predicted plan"), and subsequently re-optimized using the target and OAR optimization objectives of the baseline plan ("re-optimized plan"). Plan re-optimization prioritizes avoiding high doses to OARs, even when this is at the cost of decreased PTV coverage. Both the predicted and re-optimized plans are reviewed, and the re-optimized plan is selected for the actual delivery.

MRgRT delivery is performed using respiratory gating during subsequent breath-hold periods in shallow inspiration. The tracking structure for gating is either the primary tumor, or the kidney itself on a single sagittal plane (Figure 1), depending on the visibility on this sagittal plane. Gating is augmented by visual and/or auditory feedback provided to patients during treatment [21]. Visual feedback is performed with the aid of an in-room MR compatible monitor on which both the tracking structure (GTV or kidney) and the gating boundary (3 mm), generally corresponding to the PTV, is projected in real-time. The 2D MR images during treatment were acquired with a True FISP sequence with the MRIdian (0.35 T) at a frequency of four frames-per-second (TR: 2.1 ms, TE: 0.91 ms, FA: 60°).

FOV was 0.35 cm × 0.35 cm and the slice thickness was 0.7 cm. Due to the low magnetic field and low FA, "real-time" MR images of the patient were performed without interruption during the beam-on time. A previous analysis showed a treatment duty cycle efficiency between 67% and 87% for upper abdominal tumors [22].

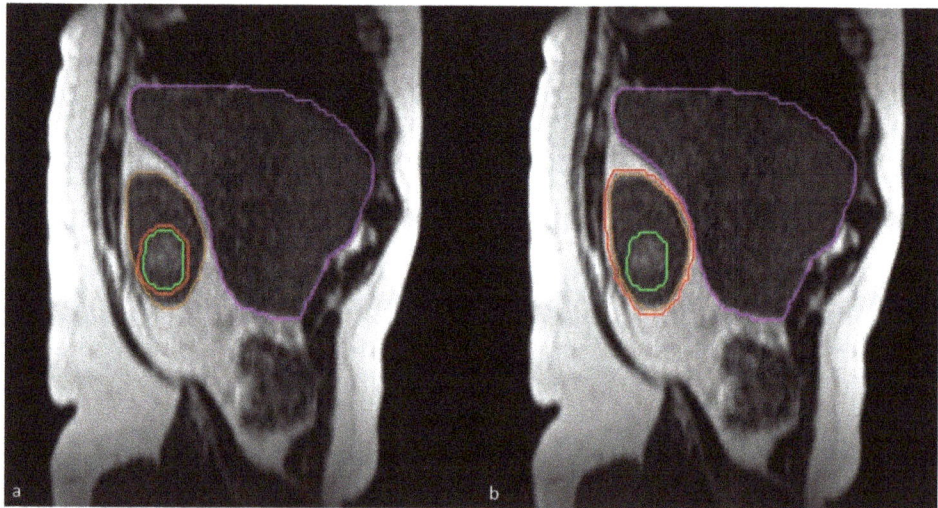

Figure 1. Sagittal plane for tumor tracking: either (**a**) tracking on gross tumor volume (green) or (**b**) tracking on the whole kidney (orange). A boundary of 3 mm (red) for gated delivery.

Baseline patient and tumor characteristics and follow-up data including LC, renal function, and toxicity were collected. Acute and late toxicity was scored using the Common Terminology Criteria for Adverse Events (CTCAE) version 4.0. Follow-up imaging was assessed by a CT-scan or ultrasound, and the tumor response was classified according to RECIST 1.1. criteria.

An offline analysis was performed to evaluate the need for daily plan re-optimization in MRgRT for RCC in a total of 180 fractions. For this purpose, predicted and re-optimized plans were analyzed for adherence with planning target objectives and OAR constraints, i.e., a V_{38Gy} of the GTV ≥ 90%, and V_{33Gy} ≤ 1 cc for stomach, duodenum, and bowel. Re-optimization was defined as "needed" when the predicted plan violated the above-mentioned GTV and/or OAR constraints, which was subsequently corrected by re-optimization. In contrast, plan re-optimization was defined as "redundant" when predicted plans already complied with the planning objectives. In addition, the value of plan re-optimization was analyzed on a patient level by studying the number of fractions per patient that were considered suboptimal.

Statistical Analysis

Descriptive statistics were used for baseline patient and tumor characteristics. The change in renal function (eGFR) from baseline versus post-treatment at the latest available time point in follow-up was evaluated using the paired sampled *t*-test. Local, regional, distant disease control and overall survival (OS) were estimated using the Kaplan-Meier method. OS was calculated as the time between the first fraction of MRgRT and the date of the last follow-up. LC was calculated as the time between the first fraction of MRgRT and the date of last imaging. Statistical analysis used for plan comparisons was performed using the Wilcoxon Signed-Rank test. A *p*-value of < 0.05 was considered to be statistically significant. Decision tree analysis (CHAID, Chi-square automatic interaction detection) was used to explore predictive pretreatment characteristics and most significant cut-off values to identify patients for whom daily re-optimization was needed. Baseline volumetric, geometric, and dosimetric parameters, i.e., GTV size (cc), laterality (left, right), location (interpolar, upper or lower pole), V_{33Gy}, V_{30Gy}, V_{25Gy}, and V_{20Gy} for each OAR structure separately or combined in one structure were used as input variables. The qualitative re-optimization benefit variable ("redundant" or "needed") was selected as the target variable for decision tree analysis. The significance level for node splitting was set at $p < 0.05$. Stopping parameters to prevent over-fitting were applied by setting the minimum number of records in a leaf to be at least 10% of the data set. The Statistical Package for the Social Sciences (SPSS) version 26 (IBM® SPSS Statistics, Armonk, NY, USA) was used to perform all statistical analyses.

3. Results

3.1. Clinical Outcomes

All 36 patients were referred for SABR after discussion in a multidisciplinary tumor board, and reasons for referral included a high surgical risk due to comorbidity ($n = 9$), which is unsuitable for other ablative therapies due to tumor size ($n = 10$) or location ($n = 5$), patient preference ($n = 5$), co-existing second malignancy ($n = 3$), use of anti-coagulants ($n = 2$), and chronic stage ≥IV kidney disease ($n = 2$). Baseline patient characteristics are summarized in Table 2. The mean age of this cohort was 78.1 years with a preponderance of men (66.7%). The mean tumor diameter was 5.6 cm (range 2.4–9.3 cm) with 86.1% of tumors measuring ≥4 cm in the largest dimension of which 23 patients have a cT1b tumor and 8 patients have a cT2a tumor. Five patients (13.9%) had metastasized renal cell carcinoma (RCC) at the time of diagnosis. Pathologic confirmation of RCC before treatment was achieved in approximately half of patients (55.6%) of which the majority was diagnosed with Fuhrman grade 2 ($n = 14$). Other patients with histology included Fuhrman grade 1 ($n = 1$), Fuhrman grade 3 ($n = 1$), a RCC with sarcomatoid features ($n = 1$), and a chromophobe tumor ($n = 1$). In two patients, no grading was available because pathologic confirmation was obtained from systemic metastases. All patients were able to complete adaptive MRgRT with an average time per fraction of 45 min. An overview of the average duration of the different components of adaptive MRgRT for RCC is shown in Figure 2. Three patients completed treatment while tracking on the kidney instead of the tumor.

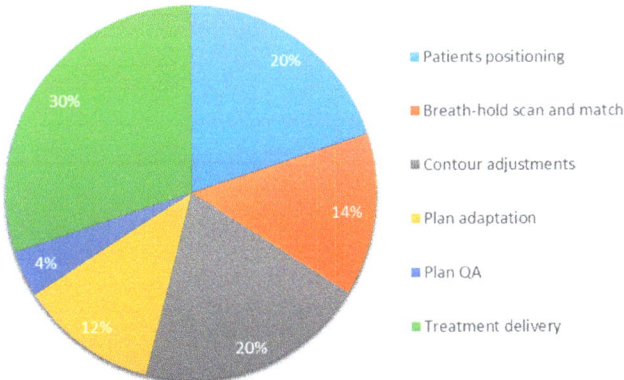

Figure 2. Pie-chart of the average duration of the different components of breath-hold gated adaptive MR-guided radiotherapy with an average time per fraction of 45 min.

Table 2. Baseline patient characteristics (n = 36). Abbreviations: RCC = renal cell carcinoma, GTV = gross tumor volume, PTV = planning target volume, CKD = chronic kidney disease.

	Mean Age (Range), Years	78.1 (58–95)
	Sex, n (%)	
	Male	24 (66.7)
	Female	12 (33.3)
	WHO performance status, n (%)	
	0	3 (7.9)
	1	21 (58.3)
	2	12 (33.3)
	Charlson comorbidity, n (%)	
	Mean (SD)	6.4 (2.5)
	2–3	3 (8.3)
	4–6	18 (50)
	7–9	10 (27.8)
	10–13	5 (13.9)
	Histology RCC, n (%)	
	Yes	20 (55.6)
	No	16 (44.4)
	Tumor Laterality, n (%)	
	Left	13 (36.1)
	Right	23 (63.9)
	Tumor location, n (%)	
	Interpolar	13 (36.1)
	Lower pole	13 (36.1)
	Upper pole	10 (27.8)
	Tumor size largest dimension, cm	
	Mean (SD)	5.6 (1.6)
	Median (range)	5.5 (2.4–9.3)
	T-stage, n (%)	
	cT1a	5 (13.9)
	cT1b	23 (63.9)
	cT2a	8 (22.2)
	GTV, cc	
	Mean (range)	79.7 (7.7–350.4)
	PTV, cc	
	Mean (range)	108.6 (14.3–445.9)
	Renal function (eGFR), ml/min/1.73 m^2	
	Mean (SD)	55.8 (20.1)
	CKD classification, n (%)	
I	Normal (eGFR ≥ 90)	0 (0)
II	Mild (eGFR ≥ 60 to < 90)	15 (41.7)
IIIa	Mild-Moderate (eGFR ≥ 45 to <60)	10 (27.8)
IIIb	Moderate-Severe (eGFR ≥ 30 to <45)	8 (22.2)
IV	Severe (eGFR < 30)	2 (5.6)
V	Kidney failure (eGFR < 15)	1 (2.8)

The median follow-up was 16.4 months. Overall survival was 91.2% at one year (Figure 3), LC was 95.2% (Figure 3), and freedom from any progression was 91% at one year. Two patients had local recurrences. One patient had progressive distant disease at recurrence for which systemic therapy was delivered, and the second patient with an isolated local recurrence underwent radiofrequency ablation as salvage. Treatment-related acute toxicity grade ≥ 2 in the form of nausea was observed in a single patient, which responded to oral ondansetron. No other acute or late grade ≥2 toxicity was reported. The mean eGFR at baseline was 55.3 (SD ±19.0) mL/min/1.73 m^2. With a mean interval of 16 months and mean eGFR post-MRgRT was 49.3 (SD ± 19.1) mL/min/1.73 m^2, which indicates a decrease of 6.0 mL/min/1.73 m^2. No patient in this cohort required dialysis during follow-up.

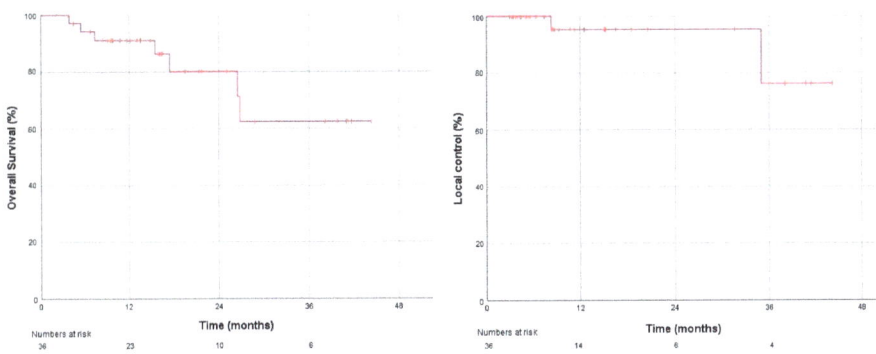

Figure 3. Kaplan-Meier plots for overall survival (left) and local control (right).

3.2. The Need for Daily Plan Re-Optimization

In 151 out of 180 fractions (83.9%), the predicted plans (without re-optimization) met all institutional target and OAR constraints. In these fractions, predicted and re-optimized plans were of similar quality with a mean GTV V_{38Gy} of 98.8% and 99.1%, respectively, and mean V_{33Gy} of 0 cc for both stomach, duodenum, and bowel. In the other 29 fractions, predicted plans were suboptimal with insufficient GTV coverage in two out of 180 fractions (1.1%) exceeding OAR constraints in 25 fractions (13.9%), and both insufficient GTV coverage and exceeded OAR constraints in another two fractions (1.1%). There was no significant difference in suboptimal predicted plans for left-sided or right-sided RCC ($p = 0.56$). For these suboptimal plans, on-couch re-optimization corrected the GTV V_{38Gy} from a mean of 88.7% (predicted) to 97.4% (re-optimized). Similarly, re-optimization corrected OAR $V_{33Gy} \leq 1$ cc violations from on average V_{33Gy} of 4.1 (predicted plans) to 0.3 cc (re-optimized plans). Analysis on a patient basis showed that the 29 insufficient predicted fractions were distributed among 11 patients (11/36, 30.6%). However, three or more suboptimal fractions were seen in only five patients (13.9%).

Decision tree analysis identified the baseline OAR V_{25Gy} (combined structure of stomach, bowel, and duodenum) as the most significant predictor variable for daily adaptive planning needs with 0.5 cc as an optimal cut-off value ($p < 0.001$). In all cases with a baseline OAR V_{25Gy} of ≤ 0.5 cc, plan adaptation was redundant as the predicted plans already complied with institutional constraints. In patients with baseline OAR V_{25Gy} of more than 0.5 cc, plan re-optimization was needed in 32.2% of fractions in order to fulfill the preset target coverage and OAR constraints (Table 3). The correct classification rate of the decision tree was 86.1% with a sensitivity of 100% and a specificity of 67.7%. The difference between re-optimized and predicted dose parameters for target (GTV $V_{95\%}$) and OAR (V_{33Gy}) stratified for split group 1 and 2 (Table 3) is shown in Figure 4.

Table 3. Results in the Chi-square automatic interaction detection (CHAID) tree table.

	Redundant n (%)	Needed n (%)	Total n (%)	Predictive Variable	Split Values	Chi-Square	df	p-Value
Parent node: all cases	151 (83.9)	29 (16.1)	180 (100)					
Split group 1	90 (100)	0 (0)	90 (100)	OAR V_{25Gy}	≤ 0.5 cc	34.6	1	<0.001
Split group 2	61 (67.8)	25 (32.2)	90 (100)	OAR V_{25Gy}	>0.5 cc	34.6	1	<0.001

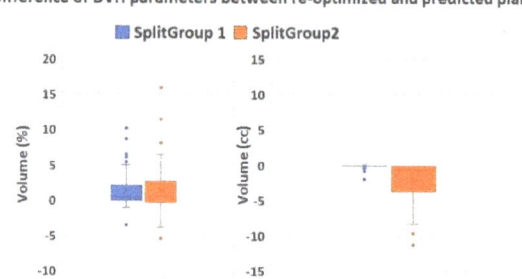

Figure 4. Difference of DVH parameters. Boxplots showing the relative volume difference in GTV $V_{95\%}$ (%) and absolute difference in OAR V_{33Gy} (cc) of the re-optimized compared to the predicted plans stratified for Split group 1 (re-optimization not needed) and 2 (re-optimization needed). Abbreviations: DVH = dose volume histogram, GTV = gross target volume, OAR = organs at risk.

4. Discussion

To the best of our knowledge, this is the first series of patients treated for primary RCC using MRgRT with routine daily plan re-optimization. We applied a commonly used fractionation scheme of 40 Gy in five fractions [18,23,24] in an overall treatment time of two weeks. Only a single patient reported nausea as acute toxicity, and no grade ≥ 2 late toxicity was observed. Despite the inclusion of large tumors, mostly T1b and T2, which had a mean tumor diameter of 5.6 cm and were generally unsuitable for other local therapies, we observed an LC rate of 95.2%. Our local response scoring has been according to the RECIST 1.1 criteria, and 83.3% had stable disease. In addition, 11.1% had partial remission, while 5.6% showed local progression. Fast tumor size regression is uncommon after SABR as previously reported by Sun and colleagues [11]. This preponderance of stable disease is in accordance with their paper. Both LC and OS are reported to be poorer for larger primary RCC than for the smaller lesions [25,26]. Despite this observation, our LC rate is within the high range of what was reported in recent systematic reviews, meta-analyses, and pooled analyses of SABR for primary RCC [15,24,27].

MRgRT with daily plan re-optimization was feasible with an average fraction duration of 45 min, even in poorer condition patients with multiple co-existing diseases. Despite this prolonged treatment duration, all patients were able to complete treatment, which indicates good tolerability. Our fractionation scheme of 40 Gy in five fractions is commonly used and seems safe without severe toxicity. With a mean interval of well over one year, the mean decline in eGFR in our study was only 6.0 (SD ± 9.8) mL/min/1.73 m². This value corresponds well with the mean decline in eGFR of 5.5 (SD ± 13.3) mL/min/1.73 m² that was described in previous SABR studies [15,28]. This limited decline in renal function in our patients with relatively large RCC may well be the result of this gated approach with small mobility boundaries, instead of using internal target volumes incorporating full tumor motion.

MRgRT also offers the advantage of using plan re-optimization for each delivered fraction at the cost of additional time. Our offline analysis showed that daily plan re-optimization was required in only 16% of fractions in which the predicted plan failed to meet the predetermined high-dose OAR constraints or target coverage objectives. Decision tree analysis showed that patients for whom daily plan re-optimization is not required can be identified upfront on the basis of a V_{25Gy} of the combined OAR of less than 0.5 cc in the baseline plan. It is, however, unlikely that an isolated single fraction violating high OAR dose or target constraints will be clinically relevant, and three out of five insufficient predicted plans were seen in only 14% of patients. Performing MRgRT without plan re-optimization indicates that the re-contouring, plan adaptation, and plan quality assurance phases can be omitted, which would enable respiratory-gated MRgRT fractions to be completed in 30 min. Furthermore, when plan adaptation is redundant, this indicates that the presence of the radiation oncologist at the MR Linac is not necessary. As a result of our analysis, we are currently introducing the found V_{25Gy} selection criterion in clinical practice.

The main limitation of our study is the relative short and unstructured patient follow-up. The limited number of RCC patients reflects the limited role of SABR in current international treatment guidelines, as only patients unsuitable for or refusing other local treatments are referred for curative radiation therapy. Another limitation includes the absence of pathology in half of our patients. Incomplete pathology confirmation is partly inherent to our patient population with generally frail elderly patients, which is unsuitable for other treatment modalities. Moreover, in a number of patients, a diagnostic biopsy was considered contra-indicated because of anticoagulant use or the anatomical location of the tumor. All patients had been discussed in a multidisciplinary tumor board with access to all available diagnostic imaging. Contrast enhanced multi-phasic CT has a high sensitivity and specificity for characterization and detection of RCC [3,29] and this specific imaging was available for all patients without pathological confirmation.

Prior to the MRgRT era, the need for radiologists to implant fiducial markers has also been an obstacle for referral for SABR. Our data show that MRgRT can be a valid alternative in patients unsuitable for the more commonly used local treatments, because of patient vitality or tumor size. The only contra-indication for MRgRT is having MR-incompatible devices. The main advantage of MRgRT is that it is an outpatient, non-invasive treatment for which not even the placement of fiducial markers is necessary. Whether MRgRT can also be considered as an alternative to partial nephrectomy or cryotherapy needs to be addressed in a prospective randomized study, which should also evaluate quality of life and cost-effectiveness. With regard to the favorable outcome in the data on SABR literature as well as the current analysis on MRgRT, a more prominent role of SABR in the treatment guidelines for RCC appears warranted.

5. Conclusions

In conclusion, hypo-fractionated MRgRT for large RCC resulted in high LC and very low toxicity rates. Gated treatment without the need for anesthesia or fiducials appeared well tolerated. Even in this group with large RCCs, daily plan re-optimization was not needed for the majority of patients, who can be identified upfront by a combined OAR V_{25Gy} of ≤ 0.5 cc in the baseline plans. This is a favorable result since online MRgRT plan adaptation is a time-consuming procedure. In this group of patients, MRgRT delivery will be faster, and these patients could be candidates for further hypofractionation [30].

Author Contributions: Conceptualization, S.U.T., O.B., F.J.L., and A.M.E.B.; Methodology, O.B. and F.J.L.; Software, O.B. and F.J.L.; Formal analysis, S.U.T., O.B., and F.J.L.; Investigation, S.U.T and O.B.; Resources, S.U.T., S.S.O., A.M.v.d.W., and A.M.E.B.; Data curation, S.U.T., O.B., and F.J.L.; Writing—original draft preparation, S.U.T., O.B., F.J.L., and A.M.E.B.; Writing—review and editing, S.S., M.A.P., S.S.O., A.M.v.d.W., R.J.A.v.M., and B.J.S.; Visualization, S.U.T. and O.B.; Supervision, F.J.L. and A.M.E.B.; Project administration, S.U.T., O.B., F.J.L., and A.M.E.B. All authors have read and agreed to the published version of the manuscript.

Funding: This research received no external funding.

Conflicts of Interest: O.B. reports personal fees from ViewRay Techonologies Inc. outside the submitted work. S.S. reports grants from ViewRay Inc, grants from Varian Medical Systems, grants and personal fees from AstraZeneca, personal fees from MSD, personal fees from Celgene, outside the submitted work. M.A.P. reports personal fees from ViewRay Technologies, Inc., outside the submitted work. B.J.S. reports grants and personal fees from ViewRay and grants from Varian Medical Systems outside the submitted work. F.J.L. reports personal fees from ViewRay outside the submitted work. A.M.E.B. reports grants from ViewRay Inc. during the conduct of the study, personal fees from ViewRay Inc., and other from ViewRay Inc. outside the submitted work.

References

1. Escudier, B.; Porta, C.; Schmidinger, M.; Rioux-Leclercq, N.; Bex, A.; Khoo, V.; Grünwald, V.; Gillessen, S.; Horwich, A.; ESMO Guidelines Committee. Renal cell carcinoma: ESMO Clinical Practice Guidelines for diagnosis, treatment and follow-up. *Ann. Oncol.* **2019**, *30*, 706–720. [CrossRef] [PubMed]

2. Campbell, S.; Uzzo, R.G.; Allaf, M.E.; Bass, E.B.; Cadeddu, J.A.; Chang, A.; Clark, P.E.; Davis, B.J.; Derweesh, I.H.; Giambarresi, L.; et al. Renal Mass and Localized Renal Cancer: AUA Guideline. *J. Urol.* **2017**, *198*, 520–529. [CrossRef] [PubMed]
3. Ljungberg, B.; Albiges, L.; Bensalah, K.; Bex, A.; Giles, R.H.; Hora, M.; Kuczyk, M.A.; Lam, T.; Marconi, L.; Merseburger, A.S.; et al. *European Association of Urology Guidelines on Renal Cell Carcinoma*; EAU Annual Congress: Amsterdam, The Netherlands, 2020; ISBN 978-94-92671-07-3.
4. Motzer, R.J.; Jonasch, E.; Agarwal, N.; Bhayani, S.; Bro, W.P.; Chang, S.S.; Choueiri, T.K.; Costello, B.A.; Derweesh, I.H.; Fishman, M.; et al. Kidney Cancer, Version 2.2017, NCCN Clinical Practice Guidelines in Oncology. *J. Natl. Compr. Canc. Netw.* **2017**, *15*, 804–834. [CrossRef] [PubMed]
5. Peddada, A.V.; Anderson, D.; Blasi, O.C.; McCollough, K.; Jennings, S.B.; Monroe, A.T. Nephron-Sparing Robotic Radiosurgical Therapy for Primary Renal Cell Carcinoma: Single-Institution Experience and Review of the Literature. *Adv. Radiat. Oncol.* **2019**, *5*, 204–211. [CrossRef] [PubMed]
6. Siva, S.; Pham, D.; Kron, T.; Bressel, M.; Lam, J.; Tan, T.H.; Chesson, B.; Shaw, M.; Chander, S.; Gill, S.; et al. Stereotactic ablative body radiotherapy for inoperable primary kidney cancer: A prospective clinical trial. *BJU Int.* **2017**, *120*, 623–630. [CrossRef]
7. Staehler, M.; Bader, M.; Schlenker, B.; Casuscelli, J.; Karl, A.; Roosen, A.; Stief, C.G.; Bex, A.; Wowra, B.; Muacevic, A. Single fraction radiosurgery for the treatment of renal tumors. *J. Urol.* **2015**, *193*, 771–775. [CrossRef]
8. Ponsky, L.; Lo, S.S.; Zhang, Y.; Schluchter, M.; Liu, Y.; Patel, R.; Abouassaly, R.; Welford, S.; Gulani, V.; Haaga, J.R.; et al. Phase I dose-escalation study of stereotactic body radiotherapy (SBRT) for poor surgical candidates with localized renal cell carcinoma. *Radiother. Oncol.* **2015**, *117*, 183–187. [CrossRef]
9. Pham, D.; Thompson, A.; Kron, T.; Foroudi, F.; Kolsky, M.S.; Devereux, T.; Lim, A.; Siva, S. Stereotactic ablative body radiation therapy for primary kidney cancer: A 3-dimensional conformal technique associated with low rates of early toxicity. *Int. J. Radiat. Oncol. Biol. Phys.* **2014**, *90*, 1061–1068. [CrossRef]
10. Kaidar-Person, O.; Price, A.; Schreiber, E.; Zagar, T.M.; Chen, R.C. Stereotactic Body Radiotherapy for Large Primary Renal Cell Carcinoma. *Clin. Genitourin. Cancer* **2017**, *15*, e851–e854. [CrossRef]
11. Sun, M.R.; Brook, A.; Powell, M.F.; Kaliannan, K.; Wagner, A.A.; Kaplan, I.D.; Pedrosa, I. Effect of Stereotactic Body Radiotherapy on the Growth Kinetics and Enhancement Pattern of Primary Renal Tumors. *AJR Am. J. Roentgenol.* **2016**, *206*, 544–553. [CrossRef]
12. Chang, J.H.; Cheung, P.; Erler, D.; Sonier, M.; Korol, R.; Chu, W. Stereotactic Ablative Body Radiotherapy for Primary Renal Cell Carcinoma in Non-surgical Candidates: Initial Clinical Experience. *Clin. Oncol.* **2016**, *28*, e109–e114. [CrossRef] [PubMed]
13. Beitler, J.J.; Makara, D.; Silverman, P.; Lederman, G. Definitive, high-dose-perfraction, conformal, stereotactic external radiation for renal cell carcinoma. *Am. J. Clin. Oncol.* **2004**, *27*, 646–648. [CrossRef] [PubMed]
14. McBride, S.M.; Wagner, A.A.; Kaplan, I.D. A phase 1 dose-escalation study of robotic radiosurgery in inoperable primary renal cell carcinoma. *Int. J. Radiat. Oncol. Biol. Phys.* **2013**, *87*, S84. [CrossRef]
15. Siva, S.; Louie, A.V.; Warner, A.; Muacevic, A.; Gandhidasan, S.; Ponsky, L.; Ellis, R.; Kaplan, I.; Mahadevan, A.; Chu, w.; et al. Pooled analysis of stereotactic ablative radiotherapy for primary renal cell carcinoma: A report from the international radiosurgery oncology consortium for kidney (IROCK). *Cancer* **2018**, *124*, 934–942. [CrossRef] [PubMed]
16. Siva, S.; Correa, R.J.; Warner, A.; Staehler, M.; Ellis, R.J.; Ponsky, L.; Kaplan, I.D.; Mahadevan, A.; Chu, W.; Gandhidasan, S.; et al. Stereotactic Ablative Radiotherapy for ≥T1b Primary Renal Cell Carcinoma: A Report from the International Radiosurgery Oncology Consortium for Kidney (IROCK). *Int. J. Radiat. Oncol. Biol. Phys.* **2020**, in press journal pre-proof. [CrossRef] [PubMed]
17. Siva, S.; Chesson, B.; Bressel, M.; Pryor, D.; Higgs, B.; Reynolds, H.M.; Hardcastle, N.; Montgomery, R.; Vanneste, B.G.; Khoo, V.; et al. TROG 15.03 Phase II Clinical Trial of Focal Ablative STereotactic Radiosurgery for Cancers of the Kidney—FASTRACK II. *BMC Cancer* **2018**, *18*, 1030. [CrossRef] [PubMed]
18. Rühle, A.; Andratschke, N.; Siva, S.; Guckenberger, M. Is there a role for stereotactic radiotherapy in the treatment of renal cell carcinoma? *Clin. Transl. Radiat. Oncol.* **2019**, *18*, 104–112. [CrossRef]
19. Corradini, S.; Alongi, F.; Andratschke, N.; Belka, C.; Boldrini, L.; Cellini, F.; Debus, J.; Guckenberger, M.; Hoerner-Rieber, J.; Lagerwaard, F.J.; et al. MR-guidance in clinical reality: Current treatment challenges and future perspectives. *Radiat. Oncol.* **2019**, *14*, 92. [CrossRef]

20. Bohoudi, O.; Bruynzeel, A.; Senan, S.; Cuijpers, J.; Slotman, B.; Lagerwaard, F.; Palacios, M. Fast and robust online adaptive planning in stereotactic MR-guided adaptive radiation therapy (SMART) for pancreatic cancer. *Radiother. Oncol.* **2017**, *125*, 439–444. [CrossRef]
21. Tetar, S.; Bruynzeel, A.; Bakker, R.; Jeulink, M.; Slotman, B.; Oei, S.; Haasbeek, C.; De Jong, K.; Senan, S.; Lagerwaard, F.J. Patient-reported Outcome Measurements on the Tolerance of Magnetic Resonance Imaging-guided Radiation Therapy. *Cureus* **2018**, *10*, e2236. [CrossRef]
22. Koste, J.R.V.S.D.; Palacios, M.A.; Bruynzeel, A.M.; Slotman, B.; Senan, S.; Lagerwaard, F.J. MR-guided Gated Stereotactic Radiation Therapy Delivery for Lung, Adrenal, and Pancreatic Tumors: A Geometric Analysis. *Int. J. Radiat. Oncol. Biol. Phys.* **2018**, *102*, 858–866. [CrossRef] [PubMed]
23. Francolini, G.; Detti, B.; Ingrosso, G.; Desideri, I.; Becherini, C.; Carta, G.A.; Pezzulla, D.; Caramia, G.; Dominici, L.; Maragna, V.; et al. Stereotactic Body Radiation Therapy (SBRT) on Renal Cell Carcinoma, an Overview of Technical Aspects, Biological Rationale and Current Literature. *Crit. Rev. Oncol. Hematol.* **2018**, *131*, 24–29. [CrossRef]
24. Siva, S.; Pham, D.; Gill, S.; Corcoran, N.M.; Foroudi, F. A systematic review of stereotactic radiotherapy ablation for primary renal cell carcinoma. *BJU Int.* **2012**, *110*, E737–E743. [CrossRef] [PubMed]
25. Siva, S.; Staehler, M.; Correa, R.; Warner, A.; Ellis, R.; Gandhidasan, S.; Ponsky, L.; Kaplan, I.; Mahadevan, A.; Chu, W.; et al. Stereotactic Body Radiotherapy for Large Primary Renal Cell Carcinoma: A Report from the International Radiosurgery Oncology Consortium for Kidney (IROCK). *Int. J. Radiat. Oncol. Biol. Phys.* **2019**, *105*, E257–E258. [CrossRef]
26. Wegner, R.E.; Abel, S.; Vemana, G.; Mao, S.; Fuhrer, R. Utilization of Stereotactic Ablative Body Radiation Therapy for Intact Renal Cell Carcinoma: Trends in Treatment and Predictors of Outcome. *Adv. Radiat. Oncol.* **2019**, *5*, 85–91. [CrossRef] [PubMed]
27. Correa, R.J.; Louie, A.V.; Zaorsky, N.G.; Lehrer, E.J.; Ellis, R.; Ponsky, L.; Kaplan, I.; Mahadevan, A.; Chu, W.; Swaminath, A.; et al. The Emerging Role of Stereotactic Ablative Radiotherapy for Primary Renal Cell Carcinoma: A Systematic Review and Meta-Analysis. *Eur. Urol. Focus* **2019**, *5*, 958–969. [CrossRef]
28. Siva, S.; Jackson, P.; Kron, T.; Bressel, M.; Lau, E.; Hofman, M.; Shaw, M.; Chander, S.; Pham, D.; Lawrentshuk, N.; et al. Impact of stereotactic radiotherapy on kidney function in primary renal cell carcinoma: Establishing a dose-response relationship. *Radiother. Oncol.* **2016**, *118*, 540–546. [CrossRef]
29. Musaddaq, B.; Musaddaq, T.; Gupta, A.; Ilyas, S.; Von Stempel, C. Renal Cell Carcinoma: The Evolving Role of Imaging in the 21st Century. *Semin. Ultrasound CT MR* **2020**, *41*, 344–350. [CrossRef]
30. Grant, S.R.; Lei, X.; Hess, K.R.; Smith, G.L.; Matin, S.F.; Wood, C.G.; Nguyen, Q.; Frank, S.J.; Anscher, M.S.; Smith, B.D.; et al. Stereotactic Body Radiation Therapy for the Definitive Treatment of Early Stage Kidney Cancer: A Survival Comparison with Surgery, Tumor Ablation, and Observation. *Adv. Radiat. Oncol.* **2020**, *5*, 495–502. [CrossRef]

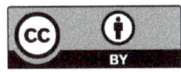

© 2020 by the authors. Licensee MDPI, Basel, Switzerland. This article is an open access article distributed under the terms and conditions of the Creative Commons Attribution (CC BY) license (http://creativecommons.org/licenses/by/4.0/).

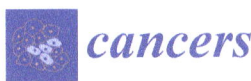

Article

Dual-Time Point [^{68}Ga]Ga-PSMA-11 PET/CT Hybrid Imaging for Staging and Restaging of Prostate Cancer

Manuela A. Hoffmann [1,2,*], Hans-Georg Buchholz [2], Helmut J Wieler [3], Florian Rosar [2,4], Matthias Miederer [2], Nicolas Fischer [5] and Mathias Schreckenberger [2]

1. Department of Occupational Health & Safety, Federal Ministry of Defense, 53123 Bonn, Germany
2. Clinic of Nuclear Medicine, Johannes Gutenberg-University, 55101 Mainz, Germany; hans-georg.buchholz@unimedizin-mainz.de (H.-G.B.); florian.rosar@uks.eu (F.R.); matthias.miederer@unimedizin-mainz.de (M.M.); mathias.schreckenberger@unimedizin-mainz.de (M.S.)
3. Clinic of Nuclear Medicine, Bundeswehr Central Hospital, 56072 Koblenz, Germany; helmut.wieler@web.de
4. Department of Nuclear Medicine, Saarland University Medical Center, 66421 Homburg, Germany
5. Department of Urology, University of Cologne, 50937 Cologne, Germany; nicolas.fischer@uk-koeln.de
* Correspondence: manuhoffmann@web.de

Received: 2 September 2020; Accepted: 25 September 2020; Published: 28 September 2020

Simple Summary: Early diagnosis and tumor characterization of prostate cancer (PCa) are important for accurate treatment. [^{68}Ga]Ga-PSMA-11 PET/CT turns out to constitute a major step toward improved diagnostic procedures to detect primary, recurrent, and metastatic PCa. The aim of our study is to evaluate the effect of a second imaging modality for the staging and restaging of PCa by possibly detecting additional PCa lesions due to the well-known increase of PSMA uptake over time. There was a significant increase in tracer uptake on delayed images in comparison to early [^{68}Ga]Ga-PSMA-11 PET/CT in our study, but the lesion positivity rate was comparable. However, in a few individual cases, additional delayed scans provided an information advantage in PCa lesion detection. The findings of our study are likely to be of major interest to clinicians as well as to researchers defining the algorithms that are necessary to implement this promising method with its specific tracer into clinical routine.

Abstract: Routine [^{68}Ga]Ga-PSMA-11 PET/CT (one hour post-injection) has been shown to accurately detect prostate cancer (PCa) lesions. The goal of this study is to evaluate the benefit of a dual-time point imaging modality for the staging and restaging of PCa patients. Biphasic [^{68}Ga]Ga-PSMA-11 PET/CT of 233 patients, who underwent early and late scans (one/three hours post-injection), were retrospectively studied. Tumor uptake and biphasic lesion detection for 215 biochemically recurrent patients previously treated for localized PCa (prostatectomized patients (P-P)/irradiated patients (P-I) and 18 patients suspected of having primary PCa (P-T) were separately evaluated. Late [^{68}Ga]Ga-PSMA-11 PET/CT imaging detected 554 PCa lesions in 114 P-P patients, 187 PCa lesions in 33 P-I patients, and 47 PCa lesions in 13 P-T patients. Most patients (106+32 P-P/P-I, 13 P-T) showed no additional PCa lesions. However, 11 PSMA-avid lesions were only detected in delayed images, and 33 lesions were confirmed as malignant by a SUVmax increase. The mean SUVmax of pelvic lymph node metastases was 25% higher ($p < 0.001$) comparing early and late PET/CT. High positivity rates from routine [^{68}Ga]Ga-PSMA-11 PET/CT for the staging and restaging of PCa patients were demonstrated. There was no decisive influence of additional late imaging with PCa lesion detection on therapeutic decisions. However, in a few individual cases, additional delayed scans provided an information advantage in PCa lesion detection due to higher tracer uptake and improved contrast.

Keywords: [^{68}Ga]Ga-PSMA PET/CT; prostate cancer; dual-time point imaging; delayed imaging; biphasic imaging; lesion positivity rate

1. Introduction

Prostate cancer (PCa) is the most commonly diagnosed cancer with an incidence of 1.276 million worldwide in 2018 [1]. Early diagnosis, accurate staging, and tumor characterization are critical for selection of optimal therapy. Molecular imaging with positron-emission tomography (PET) is regarded as a relevant diagnostic approach and has found its way into the guidelines of the European Association of Urology (EAU guidelines) on PCa [2,3]. The prostate-specific membrane antigen (PSMA) is a transmembrane glycoprotein that is significantly overexpressed in most prostate adenocarcinomas, compared with other PSMA-expressing tissues [4]. After many years of preclinical research on PSMA ligands, a breakthrough was achieved in 2011 with the clinical introduction of Glu-NH-CO-NH-Lys(Ahx)-{^{68}Ga-(N,N'-bis-[2-hydroxy-5-(carboxyethyl)benzyl]ethylen-ediamine-N,N'-diacetic-acid)}([^{68}Ga]Ga-HBED-CC-PSMA or [^{68}Ga]Ga-PSMA-11) as a ^{68}Gallium (^{68}Ga)-labeled PSMA-targeted radioligand for PET/computed tomography (CT) [5,6]. PSMA PET/CT offers an appealing combination of PCa specificity and high sensitivity at low tumor volumes [7]. Sensitive and specific imaging is a fundamental requirement for the definition of the target volume in radiotherapy planning. One of the main limitations of both CT and magnetic resonance imaging (MRI) for lymph node (LN) staging is their limited capability to detect metastatic clusters in normal sized nodes; and microscopic LNM are often not enlarged [8,9]. The accurate assessment of locoregional LN metastases (LNM) is much more sensitive with PSMA PET/CT than with MRI [9]. Whereas PSMA PET/CT can detect an LNM of diameter of 3 mm, MRI can generally only identify pathological LN when they show aberrant anatomical characteristics such as a short-axis diameter >1 cm and/or non-oval shape. However, up to 80% of metastasis-involved nodes are smaller than this threshold limit that is typically used in clinical practice [10]. Meta-analytical data for the traditional CT and MRI imaging approaches suggest sensitivity of only 39–42% and specificity of 82% [10]. Since normal lymphatic or retroperitoneal fatty tissue does not demonstrate PSMA expression, metastatic LNs can be detected with a favorable lesion-to-background ratio. [^{68}Ga]Ga-PSMA PET/CT imaging has been shown to accurately detect PCa lesions for LNM [11,12]. These characteristics have led to the evolution of PSMA PET/CT as an important diagnostic tool in nuclear medicine [7,9,13]. In 130 patients with intermediate to high-risk PCa, a sensitivity of 65.9% and a specificity of 98.9% for LN staging using [^{68}Ga]Ga-PSMA-11 PET/CT was reported by Maurer et al. [12].

It has been described that PCa metastases demonstrate an increase of PSMA ligand uptake over time [5,14]. According to the Heidelberg group [5], 70% of PCa lesions have increased uptake and contrast three hours (h) post-injectionem (p.i.) compared to one h p.i. Clarification of the special situation of pelvic LNM and the possible impact of additional delayed imaging for salvage or primary therapy would be important for improved clinical decision making.

The goal of our study is to evaluate the effect of a second (late) imaging modality for the restaging and initial staging of patients with recurrent PCa, using additional findings in the abdominopelvic area based on the well-known increase of PSMA uptake over time.

2. Results

2.1. Overall Lesion Positivity Rate

A positivity rate in 147 out of 215 restaging patients (68%) (mean prostate-specific antigen (PSA) serum level 19.2 ± 82.5 ng/mL) and in 13 out of 18 primary staging patients (72%) (mean PSA 39.1 ± 67.5 ng/mL) was shown by [^{68}Ga]Ga-PSMA-11 PET/CT. At least one lesion suspect for malignancy was detected in these patients. This retrospective study includes 147 restaging patients (prostatectomized patients (P-P) and irradiated patients (P-I)) and 13 staging patients (patients suspected of having primary PCa (P-T)), both with PSMA-positive findings (Table 1). To ensure accurate statistical analysis and a homogenous patient population, the biochemically recurrent (BC)-patients, previously treated by radical prostatectomy (patient group P-P) and those previously treated by irradiation (patient group P-I) were separately evaluated according to the definition protocol of BC patients [15].

Table 1. Patient characteristics.

Characteristics (n)	Parameters
Number of patients	233
Age (y) (233)	
Median	72
Range	47–85
Mean ± SD	70.3 ± 7.3
Primary Gleason score (228)	
≤6 (low risk + grade group 1)	16
7a, 7b (intermediate risk + grade group 2 + 3)	96
8 (high risk + grade group 4)	33
>8 (high risk + grade group 5)	83
PSA (ng/mL) (233)	
Median	2.32
Range	0.2–960
Mean ± SD	15.1 ± 71.9
Prior treatment of primary tumor (233)	
Surgery (radical prostatectomy)	178
Radiotherapy and other	37
Primary staging (pre-therapy)	18
Further treatment	
Anti-androgen therapy (x/233)	101
Lesion positivity rate (160/233)	68.7%
Restaging (PET/CT-positive/total)	147/215
Primary staging (PET/CT-positive/total)	13/18

Abbreviations: PSA, prostate-specific antigen; SD, standard deviation; n, number of patients; y, year.

2.1.1. Lesion Positivity Rate Post-Prostatectomized (P-P)

- Baseline: 551 lesions in 114 patients

In this subgroup (P-P and baseline PET/CT), the detection efficacy was 27% (33) for PSA levels of 0.2 to <0.5 ng/mL and 32% (25), 70% (27), 77% (43), and 90% (50) for PSA levels of 0.5 to <1 ng/mL, 1 to <2 ng/mL, 2 to <5 ng/mL, and ≥5 ng/mL, respectively ($p < 0.001$) (Table 2).

Patients with a PSMA-positive scan showed local recurrence in 24% (27/114) and metastases in 90%. Of the patients with metastases, 39% exhibited local metastases and 30% exhibited distant metastases, and 31% showed both. In 70% of the patients, LNM were detected, 78% of which were pelvic LNM (Table 2).

- Delayed: 554 lesions in 114 patients

Late imaging (3 h after intravenous injection (p.i.)) showed no difference in the detection efficacy when considering the patients without separate division of the number of lesions (Table 2).

Table 2. PET/CT findings: Lesion positivity rate (LPR) post-prostatectomized (P-P) related to different PSA values.

PSA (ng/mL)	0.2–<0.5	0.5–<1.0	1.0–<2.0	2.0–<5.0	≥5.0	Chi², p
Number (x/178) post-prostatectomized patients	33	25	27	43	50	
PET/CT-positive (x/114)	9	8	19	33	45	$r = 0.507; p < 0.001$
Lesion positivity rate	27.3%	32.0%	70.4%	76.6%	90.0%	
Regions:						
Local recurrence	2	0	5	6	14	$r = 0.236; p = 0.01$
Metastases	7	8	16	31	41	$r = 0.471; p < 0.001$
Site of metastases:						$r = 0.459; p < 0.001$
Local metastases	4	4	9	11	12	
Distant metastases	0	4	4	10	13	
Local + distant metastases	3	0	3	10	16	
Number of metastases:						$r = 0.536; p < 0.001$
Single metastases	3	6	7	7	2	
Multiple metastases	4	2	9	24	39	
Lymph node metastases (LNM)	7	4	12	21	28	$r = 0.296; p = 0.001$
Site of LNM:						$r = 0.297; p < 0.042$
Pelvic LNM	6	4	10	17	19	
Extra-pelvic LNM	0	0	1	1	2	
Pelvic + extra-pelvic LNM	1	0	1	3	7	
Bone metastases	2	4	5	18	24	$r = 0.355; p < 0.001$
Visceral metastases	0	0	1	1	4	$r = 0.153; p = 0.352$ *

* Fisher's exact test. Abbreviations: PSA, prostate-specific antigen; LNM, lymph node metastases; $p < 0.05$ is considered significant; r, Pearson correlation coefficient.

2.1.2. Lesion Positivity Rate Post-Irradiated (P-I)

- Baseline: 186 lesions in 33 patients

This subgroup (P-I and baseline PET/CT) showed a detection efficacy rate of 100% for PSA levels of 2 to <5 ng/mL and 94% for PSA levels of ≥5 ng/mL, respectively. Local recurrence was detected in 79% and metastases were detected in 67%. A total of 42% of the patients showed LNM, while 80% of them showed pelvic LNM. Due to the small number of patients, a statistical analysis would not have given meaningful results.

- Delayed: 187 lesions in 33 patients

The detection efficacy rates 3 h p.i. showed the same results as baseline images.

2.1.3. Lesion Positivity Rate Pre-Therapy (P-T)

All patients (13) with PSMA-positive lesions showed histopathologically (biopsy-proven) adenocarcinoma PCa.

- Baseline: 47 lesions in 13 patients

In this subgroup (P-T and baseline PET/CT), the detection efficacy was shown in 69% for PSA levels of >4 to <50 ng/mL and in 100% for PSA levels of ≥50 ng/mL. Primary tumor lesions in the prostate were detected in 100%, metastases were detected in 38%, and LNM were detected in 31%, of which pelvic LNM were shown in 75%. Statistical analysis was not done due to the small patient number.

- Delayed: 47 lesions in 13 patients

No difference in the detection efficacy was shown in late compared to baseline imaging.

2.2. Impact of Delayed Imaging on Lesion Positivity Rate

A combination of results from both scans (baseline and delayed [^{68}Ga]Ga-PSMA-11 PET/CT) revealed a total of 788 lesions (554 P-P, 187 P-I, 47 P-T) (Figures 1 and 2).

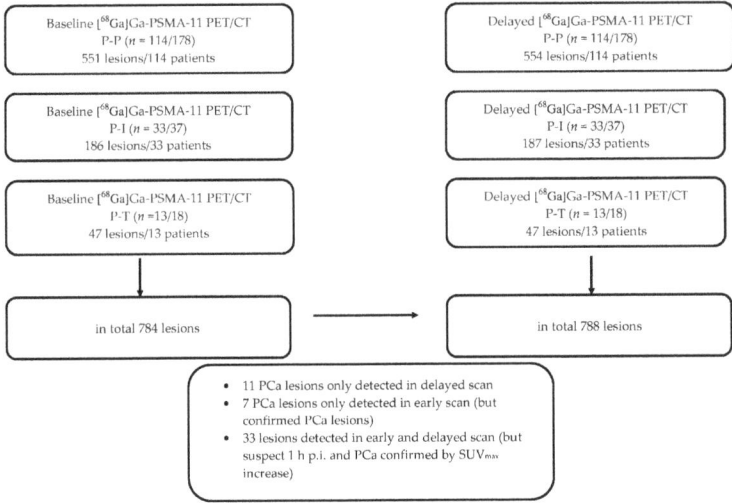

Figure 1. Flow chart showing baseline and delayed [^{68}Ga]Ga-PSMA-11 PET/CT results regarding LPR in patients.

2.2.1. Impact of Delayed Imaging on Lesion Positivity Rate P-P

A total of 551 lesions in 114 patients were detected on early scans. Twenty-nine of these lesions were local recurrent findings, and 326 were LNM (262 pelvic LNM and 64 extra-pelvic LNM). In delayed images, 328 LNM (262 pelvic LNM and 66 extra-pelvic LNM) were found. A total of 106 patients showed no additional malignant lesions in late images. Three lesions were only found in the late imaging (two extra-pelvic LNM and one bone metastasis). Comparison of tracer accumulation in pathologic lesions between baseline and delayed scans was statistically significant ($p < 0.001$ pelvic LNM, bone metastases), but this increase in maximum standardized uptake value (SUVmax) did not correspond to a significant influence of late images on the lesion positivity rates (LPR) (Table 3, Figure 1).

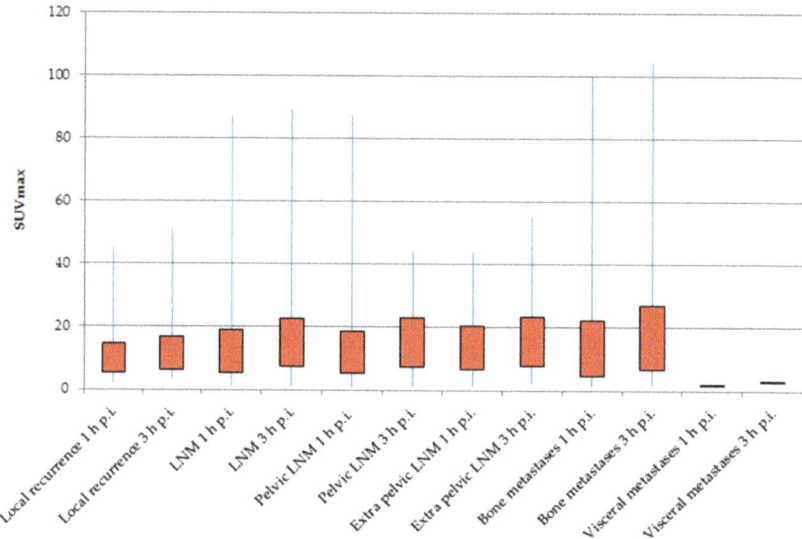

Figure 2. Comparison of baseline and delayed [^{68}Ga]Ga-PSMA-11 positron-emission tomography/computed tomography (PET/CT) regarding tracer uptake of prostate-specific membrane antigen (PSMA)-positive lesions (P-P).

Table 3. Comparison of baseline and delayed PET/CT P-P related to tracer uptake of PSMA-positive lesions.

Tumor Location	Number of Patients (x/178)	PET/CT-Positive Patients (x/114)	Number of PSMA-Positive Lesions	SUV$_{max}$ Mean ± SD Range	Wilcoxon p
Local recurrence 1 h p.i.	27	27	29	10.1 ± 9.5/2.1–45.2	
Local recurrence 3 h p.i.	27	27	29	11.7 ± 10.7/3.6–50.9	$p < 0.001$
LNM 1 h p.i.	72	72	326	12.2 ± 13.6/1.1–87.2	
LNM 3 h p.i.	72	72	328	15.0 ± 15.1/1.2–89.2	$p < 0.001$
Pelvic LNM 1 h p.i.	68	68	262	12.0 ± 13.7/0.9–87.2	
Pelvic LNM 3 h p.i.	68	68	262	15.2 ± 15.5/1.2–89.2	$p < 0.001$
Extra-pelvic LNM 1 h p.i.	16	16	64	13.8 ± 13.8/1.2–44.2	
Extra-pelvic LNM 3 h p.i.	16	16	66	15.6 ± 15.6/2.0–55.5	$p < 0.005$
Bone metastases 1 h p.i.	53	53	195	13.5 ± 18.0/1.3–100.1	
Bone metastases 3 h p.i.	53	53	196	17.0 ± 20.2/1.8–104.5	$p < 0.001$
Visceral metastases 1 h p.i.	1	1	1	2.1	
Visceral metastases 3 h p.i.	1	1	1	3.2	

Abbreviations: LNM, lymph node metastases; SUVmax, maximum standardized uptake value; $p < 0.05$ is considered significant.

2.2.2. Impact of Delayed Imaging on Lesion Positivity Rate P-I

In 33 patients, 186 lesions were found in baseline PET/CT (Figure 1). By comparison, the 33 patients showed 187 findings in late imaging. No additional PCa lesions were shown in 32 patients. In total, a single lesion in one patient was noted 3 h p.i. (one local recurrent PCa lesion in the prostate bed). The comparison of SUVmax in pathologic lesions between early and late images was statistically significant ($p = 0.008$ pelvic LNM). However, there was no significant impact of delayed imaging on LPR.

2.2.3. Impact of Delayed Imaging on Lesion Positivity Rate P-T

All 13 [^{68}Ga]Ga-PSMA-11 PET/CT-positive patients showed 47 lesions (Figure 1). No additional PCa lesions were identified by late imaging.

2.2.4. Total Comparison of Biphasic Lesion Detection

Eleven patients with discordant results showed 51 discordant lesions. All unclear lesions (33 lesions moderately suspicious of malignancy) detected by [^{68}Ga]Ga-PSMA-11 PET/CT on standard imaging (1 h p.i.) could be clarified by additional late images (3 h p.i.). The decision to classify the lesions as malignant was made on the basis of various criteria such as a higher tracer uptake with increased SUVmax in the late images compared to the early images (Table 3), and an improved contrast as well as presentation of the lesions with a more focal character. The assessment was carried out by nuclear medicine and radiological specialists with several years of diagnostic experience with regard to the analysis of oncologic PET/CT imaging of PCa foci.

- LPR on PET, but not on CT:

By comparison of PET and CT imaging separately, nine LNM with high PSMA avidity were detected on PET, but these were not suspect of malignancy on CT alone.

- Lesions only detected on early imaging:

Seven PSMA-avid lesions (five LNM and two bone metastases) were only shown on early imaging (two P-P and zero P-I). These findings could not be confirmed as PCa lesions on delayed images.

- Lesions only detected on delayed imaging:

In this study, 11 lesions suspicious of malignancy were detected exclusively by delayed imaging (eight P-P and one P-I).

- Additional impact of delayed imaging:

A total of 33 PSMA-avid lesions (of which 15 were LNM, eight were bone metastases, and five were lesions in the prostate bed) suspected of being malignant were confirmed as malignant by increased tracer uptake in the delayed scans.

- No additional impact of delayed imaging/concordant lesions:

In 222 of 233 evaluable patients (95%), the baseline PET/CT and the delayed PET/CT were concordant.

- Time dependency of LPR:

PSMA avidity in pelvic LNM was related more often to scan time than in other metastases (e.g., extra-pelvic LNM, bone metastases, visceral metastases) ($p < 0.001$). Comparing early and late PET/CT imaging, the mean SUVmax of pelvic LNM was 25% higher ($p < 0.001$) and the mean SUVmax of extra-pelvic LNM was 14% higher ($p = 0.003$), respectively.

2.3. SUVmax

An increase of tracer accumulation over time was observed in patient groups P-P, P-I, and P-T. The SUV_{max} values of the detected sites of PCa lesions of the late scans were higher than those of the baseline scans. Overall, the SUV_{max} values of tumor lesions in the late PET/CT scans was higher in 22.1% (P-P), 22.5% (P-I), and 17.8% (P-T) than the SUV_{max} values in the baseline scans (each $p < 0.001$) (Table 3).

2.3.1. SUV$_{max}$ of Malignant Lesions (P-P)

The Wilcoxon test showed a statistically significant difference in SUVmax between baseline and delayed scans. SUVmax was the highest in bone metastases (mean + standard deviation/SD: 17.0 ± 20.2 3 h p.i.; $p < 0.001$) and lowest in local recurrence in the prostate bed (10.1 ± 9.5 1 h p.i./11.7 ± 10.7 3 h p.i.; $p < 0.001$). The SUVmax of LNM showed high values of 15.2 ± 15.5 3 h p.i. for pelvic LNM ($p < 0.001$) and 15.6 ± 15.6 3 h p.i. for extra-pelvic LNM ($p < 0.005$) (Table 3, Figure 2).

2.3.2. SUV$_{max}$ of Malignant Lesions (P-I)

The greatest increase of tracer uptake over time was seen in bone metastases: at 1 h p.i. SUVmax 24.3 ± 44.6 vs. at 3 h p.i. SUVmax 29.3 ± 48.6 ($p = 0.002$).

2.3.3. SUV$_{max}$ of Malignant Lesions (P-T)

In P-T patients, an increase of tracer accumulation was also observed in bone metastases, but these data were not statistically significant ($p = 0.068$).

2.4. Gleason Score

The LPR showed a clear differentiation depending on the primary histological starting situation, which is expressed by the evaluation system for determining the aggressiveness of PCa. According to previous studies, PCa with a Gleason score (GS) of 7b (4 + 3) has a significantly worse prognosis than PCa with a GS of 7a (3 + 4). For this reason, 7a is classified as grade group 2 and 7b is classified as grade group 3, although they belong to the same group of intermediate-risk PCa. In our study, 11% of the PSMA-positive subgroup P-P was previously categorized as low-risk PCa (GS < 7) with grade 1 according to the International Society of Urological Pathology (ISUP) and intermediate-risk with grade 2 (GS 7a), whereas a categorization of PCa grade 3 to grade 5 (GS 7b, 8 and >8; intermediate up to high-risk) was found in 89% (Table 4) [3,16,17]. By comparison of the LNM-LPR of grade group 1 to 2 PCa-patients (GS ≤ 7a) with that of grade group 3 to 5 (GS ≥7b), a statistically significant difference ($p = 0.029$) was noted (12% vs. 88% respectively) (Table 4).

Table 4. Gleason score in relation to [^{68}Ga]Ga-PSMA-11 PET/CT LPR P-P.

n = 178	GS < 7 (11)	GS 7a (33)	GS 7b (51)	GS 8 (26)	GS > 8 (57)	Chi² r, p Value
PSMA-positive (xx/114)	1	11	38	25	39	0.326; $p < 0.001$
Local recurrence (xx/27)	1	4	5	6	11	0.112; $p = 0.446$
Metastases (xx/103)	0	9	34	23	37	0.346; $p < 0.001$
LNM (xx/68)	0	8	22	17	21	0.186; $p = 0.029$

Abbreviations: GS, Gleason score; n, number of patients; $p < 0.05$ is considered significant; r, Pearson correlation coefficient.

When comparing grade 1 to 2 PCa patients (GS ≤ 7a) with grade 3 to 5 PCa patients (GS ≥ 7b) in the subgroup P-I, we evaluated an LNM-LPR in 10% for grade 1 to 2 and in 80% for grade 3 to 5. In the subgroup P-T, all PSMA-avid LNM belong to grade group 3 to 5 (GS ≥ 7b). However, these results were not statistically significant.

2.5. Subpopulation

Based on EAU guidelines, which suggest the examination of PSMA PET/CT in patients with PSA serum values of ≥1 ng/mL and based on the definition of BC (PSA is >0.2 ng/mL in prostatectomized patients), we highlighted and examined the patient collective of restaging patients (P-P) in the range from 0.2 to <1 ng/mL as particularly assessable [3,15]. In baseline PET/CT, 33% (58/178) of patients (P-P) showed PSA values in the range of 0.2 to <1 ng/mL, of which 29% were PSMA-positive and 14%

showed local metastases ($p < 0.001$) (Table 5). There was no difference in the results determined by delayed PET/CT images.

In one of our previous studies, we determined an optimal PSA cutoff level of 1.24 ng/mL for distinguishing between positive and negative PSMA PET/CT results for BC patients after primary prostatectomy (P-P) [13]. In this study, P-P patients in baseline shots, with PSA < 1.24 ng/mL, showed an overall positivity in 34% (24/71), PSMA-avid local metastases in 13% (9/71), and distant metastases in 10% (7/71), compared to 84% (90/107), 29% (31/107), and 22% (24/107) in patients with PSA ≥ 1.24 ng/mL ($p < 0.001$) (Table 5). The results were comparable in delayed images.

Table 5. Baseline PET/CT: LPR P-P of different subgroups related to PSA subgroups.

PSA Range (ng/mL)	Overall Positivity	Chi² p/r Value	Single Metastases	Multiple Metastases	Chi² p/r Value
0.2 to <1 (58)	17 (29.3%)		9 (15.5%)	6 (10.3%)	
<1.24 (71)	24 (33.8%)		12 (16.9%)	9 (12.7%)	
≥1.24 (107)	90 (84.1%)		13 (12.1%)	69 (64.5%)	
Total (178)	114 (64%)	$p < 0.001$ r 0.513	25	78	$p < 0.001$ r 0.522

PSA Range (ng/mL)	Local Recurrence	p/r Value	Local Metastases	Distant Metastases	Local + Distant Metastases	p/r Value
0.2 to <1 (58)	2 (3.4%)		8 (13.8%)	4 (6.9%)	3 (5.2%)	
<1.24 (71)	3 (4.2%)		9 (12.7%)	7 (9.9%)	5 (7.0%)	
≥1.24 (107)	24 (22.4%)		31 (29.0%)	24 (22.4%)	27 (25.2%)	
Total (178)	27	$p = 0.001$ r 0.249	40	31	32	$p < 0.001$ r 0.412

Abbreviations: PSA, prostate-specific-antigen; $p < 0.05$ is considered significant; r, Pearson correlation coefficient.

3. Discussion

In this study, the biphasic [^{68}Ga]Ga-PSMA-11 PET/CT of 233 patients was retrospectively studied. A total of 178 prostatectomized patients and 37 irradiated patients as well as 18 pre-therapy patients were assessed, and their data (e.g. tumor uptake, biphasic LPR) were separately evaluated. As reported in other studies, we also found high LPR from baseline [^{68}Ga]Ga-PSMA-11 PET/CT for the staging (72%) and restaging (68%) of PCa patients [11,13,18].

A recently published prospective, randomized, multi-center study from Australia [9] including 300 men with biopsy-proven PCa found that [^{68}Ga]Ga-PSMA PET/CT yielded 92% accuracy in identifying those with distant metastatic or pelvic nodal disease compared with 65% accuracy from traditional imaging (CT, bone scan). Furthermore, conventional imaging had more equivocal findings, fewer management changes, and higher radiation doses (19.2 mSv vs. 8.4 mSv; $p < 0.001$) [9]. In addition to improving detection, PSMA PET/CT will have a significant impact on a patient's treatment plan and disease management in future guidelines [9,11].

Several acquisition protocols with different acquisition times, including early dynamic to 3 h p.i. imaging, have been proposed for [^{68}Ga]Ga-PSMA PET/CT studies [18–22]. Time activity curves acquired from PCa lesions showed a continuously increasing tracer accumulation during early dynamic PET acquisition, which also supports the essential role of additional late imaging [22]. The addition of delayed scans has been considered to offer substantial advantages for the discrimination of PCa versus non-PCa lesions, as the malignant foci usually show a further increase in tracer accumulation on the late scans. Benign lesions, on the other hand, usually show a decrease in SUV [18–22]. The optimal time point for the various currently available tracers for PSMA PET/CT imaging and the potential of additional late images have been and are currently being investigated. In the present study, we evaluated the incremental value of [^{68}Ga]Ga-PSMA-11 PET delayed imaging, especially abdominopelvic imaging.

As described by previous studies, there is a significant increase in SUVmax of PCa lesions on delayed images when evaluating dual time point [^{68}Ga]Ga-PSMA-11 PET/CT imaging [18,21,23,24]. Beheshti et al. reported that this increase relates to suspicious lesions ($p < 0.001$) in the prostate bed (11.6 ± 8.2 to 14.8 ± 1.0) as well as to LNs (9.7 ± 5.9 to 12.3 ± 8.8) [23]. Nevertheless, lesions' tracer accumulation on early imaging has been sufficient for diagnosis [23], which is consistent with our results.

Afshar-Oromieh et al. reported a mixed pattern of tracer behavior (increase/decrease of SUVmax in metastases) in the same patient in 11.6% (8/69 patients), whereas six of 69 patients (8.7%) showed a consistent decrease in metastatic uptake [20]. We did not find similar results in our patient group. Another study showed a SUVmax decrease in 26 out of 157 lesions [23]. Beheshti et al. reported [23] an increase of SUVmax over time in most lesions, which was also in agreement with our findings. Delayed images could confirm malignancy of 33 moderately PSMA-avid lesions, which were suspicious of being malignant on early scans, due to the increase of tracer uptake. However, some of the findings were ambiguous (11 lesions only detected in delayed scan, seven lesions only detected in early scan), but all of them were characteristic for PCa in follow-up (such as PSMA PET/CT, PSMA PET/MRI, CT, MRI), which support the results of a previous study that demonstrated [^{68}Ga]Ga-PSMA PET/CT to be a helpful tool to determine malignancy in ambiguous lesions [24]. These different results might be explained by various tumor cell biologies. Afshar et al. suspect that individual lesions may have a decreased rate of internalization of the PSMA ligand [20]. We speculate that miscellaneous and mixed patient populations may also account for at least some of the different findings that have been reported in the literature. In the large patient group with recurrent PCa, the role of primary treatment (e.g., prostatectomy, radiation therapy) could be an important factor as well.

In our study, the clinically most important group (P-P) of recurrent PCa-patients ($n = 114/178$) showed no significant difference in LPR (551 lesions early vs. 554 late). However, a statistically significant increase of tumor uptake in PCa lesions detected by baseline PET/CT compared with delayed PET/CT was shown. As described by previous PSMA PET studies, the standardized uptake values (SUVs) of LNs are significantly higher 3 h p.i. than 1 h p.i., and nearly all LNM of PCa show high PSMA expression [18,25]. The increase of SUVmax values between baseline and delayed scan in our study also did not significantly raise the number of pathological findings in the P-I and in the P-T-groups, especially for LN lesions, which are of important clinical interest for therapy planning. Due to the fact that microscopic LNs uploaded with metastatic tumor cells are frequently non-enlarged, LN staging and restaging by CT and MRI alone is limited [8], and PSMA PET/CT or PET/MRI is preferred [9,11,12,26]. In a series of PCa patients, the authors found 72% [25] of [^{68}Ga]Ga-PSMA-avid LNs to be metastatic in normal-sized LNs (<1 cm) [25,26]. Our data demonstrated nine LNM with high PSMA avidity on PET, which showed no signs of malignancy on CT alone. Aside from the overexpressed PSMA avidity in prostate tumor cells, the LPR of microscopic LNs could improve in the near future as the next generation of scanners (including time-of-flight technique) results in increased spatial resolution, which—compared to the older scanner systems—leads to a higher contrast as well as a higher intrinsic sensitivity [24,27].

A just published comprehensive literature search [28], including nine retrospective and two prospective studies, reported detection rates of [^{68}Ga]Ga-PSMA-PET in recurrent patients for PSA <0.2 ng/mL, for 0.2–0.49 ng/mL, and for PSA 0.5 to <1.0 ng/mL ranged from 11% to 50%, 20% to 73%, and 25% to 88%. Our results match those of Luiting et al. We had LPR values of 27% for 0.2 to <0.5 ng/mL and 32% for 0.5 to <1.0 ng/mL. The subgroup of patients with PSA < 0.2 ng/mL was excluded in our study, because they do not belong to BC patients per definition [15]. The authors [28] observed high specificity rates of [^{68}Ga]Ga-PSMA-PET imaging for pelvic LNM detection in primary staging as well as in restaging, while sensitivity was modest, and they concluded that [^{68}Ga]Ga-PSMA PET has a high impact in patient management concerning the salvage setting [11,28,29]. In our study, we found LNM in 70% of the PSMA-avid metastases, 78% of which were pelvic LNM in restaging patients (P-P). In primary tumor staging, LNM were detected in 31%, of which pelvic LNM were shown in 75%. Previous studies report the dynamic uptake of PSMA in ganglia (e.g., celiac ganglia) [18,30]. However, none of the patients in the present study showed PSMA-positive celiac ganglia, neither 1 h p.i. nor 3 h p.i.

The impact of delayed imaging in our patient groups (P-P, P-I, P-T) was limited due to the lack of significantly increased rates of pathological findings 3 h p.i. Our findings were consistent with the results of a study by Derlin et al. [31] using [^{68}Ga]Ga-THP-PSMA, who also found that delayed imaging did not increase the number of detected metastases significantly (two out of 99 patients). In contrast, Afshar-Oromieh et al. [32], using [^{68}Ga]Ga-PSMA-11, found a 3-h delay as an optimal time point for imaging, as the majority of cancer lesions could be detected then. However, their patient cohort was very small ($n = 4$). It is known from early pharmacokinetic studies that the background activity decreases significantly between 1 and 3 h p.i., resulting in an improved tumor/background (T/B) ratio [5]. However, in the present study, these higher T/B ratios or contrasts to lesions' tracer accumulation did not result in significantly higher LPR on delayed images, compared to other authors [21]. It must be taken into account here that due to the ^{68}Ga's relatively short half-life of 68 minutes, the count statistics in the 3-hour measurement are significantly lower. Most PC lesions (97%) in our study were already detected early in the imaging process, which sheds some doubt on the need for a second late examination in clinical routine. However, sometimes, it can also be useful to perform late images, e.g., if the effect of urinary activity in assessing pelvic PCa lesions remains unclear in baseline scans [26,33]. In this setting, imaging with ^{18}F-labeled compounds (PSMA-based radiopharmaceuticals such as [^{18}F]PSMA-1007) should be considered [34], since it offers advantages in late imaging due to the longer half-life of 110 minutes and the significantly lower positron range with improved resolution and the detection of small LNs. However, with regard to a theranostic approach, therapies with [^{177}Lu]Lu-PSMA make a pre-therapeutic PET/CT with [^{68}Ga]Ga-PSMA appear more meaningful [6,35]. From our theranostic point of view, dual-time point imaging definitely has an important teaching value. The results of our study do not really support a routine performance of supplementary late images for every PSMA PET/CT examination. However, delayed imaging is useful to confirm or rule out a suspicious abnormality seen in early images in individual cases. An important point to emphasize is that additional late images are useful for clearing up unclear lesions whose signs of malignancy would lead to a change in the therapeutic approach.

4. Materials and Methods

4.1. Patient Characteristics

The clinical characteristics of the 233 included patients are summarized in Table 1. From 2015 to 2018, 233 patients for staging and restaging were retrospectively evaluated. [^{68}Ga]Ga-PSMA-11 PET/CT of 215 BC patients who had previously undergone either radical prostatectomy (178, patient group P-P, PSA elevation to >0.2 ng/mL by definition) or radiation therapy (37, patient group P-I, PSA elevation to >2 ng/mL above nadir by definition) and 18 patients with elevated PSA serum level of >4.0 ng/mL, highly suspicious of having primary PCa (group P-T) were separately assessed [15]. All PSMA-positive lesions of P-T were histopathologically confirmed as PCa by biopsy. In case of BC (P-P, P-I), when the biopsy or surgery of PSMA-avid lesions was not possible or considered too invasive for the patients (e.g., bone metastases), we rated the increase of PSA before therapy and decrease after therapy as a tumor confirmation and marker. Additionally, we have included the findings of follow-up examinations (such as PSMA PET/CT, PSMA PET/MRI, CT, MRI).

This retrospective study was done in accordance with the Declaration of Helsinki. All reported investigations were conducted according to the national regulations (German Medical Products Act, AMG § 13.2b). The protocol was approved by the Ethics Committee of Laek Rlp (2018-13390).

All patients signed an informed consent (including participation in the study and for evaluation and publication of their anonymized data).

4.2. Imaging Protocol and Analysis

^{68}Ga-labeled PSMA ligand, Glu-urea-Lys(Ahx)-HBED-CC ([^{68}Ga]Ga-PSMA-11), was synthesized using sterile methods as previously described by Eder et al. [36]. The included patients underwent imaging on a Biograph 64 TruePoint (True V HD) PET/CT scanner (Siemens/Erlangen/Germany) 60 ± 10 min (whole body; baseline scan) p.i. of 195.5 ± 48.3 MBq (median activity: 193 MBq, range: 97–299 MBq) and 180 ± 10 min. p.i. (pelvic, abdominal, and suspicious regions; delayed scan). The following parameters were used: three-dimensional acquisition mode (168 × 168); acquisition time of three min. per bed position; axial field of view (FOV): 21.8 cm; random, scatter, and decay correction; ordered-subsets expectation maximization method (OSEM) for PET image reconstruction (two iterations, 14 subsets, Gaussian filtering, 4.2 mm transaxial resolution, full-width at half-maximum). Attenuation corrections were performed using the low-dose non-enhanced CT data (120 kV, 20–60 mAs, CT transverse scan-field 50 cm, 70 cm extended FOV, resolution 1.0 s, 0.6 mm) or the contrast-enhanced CT data (140 kV, 100–400 mAs, dose modulation). The images were assessed by nuclear medicine clinicians and radiologists (each with more than 5 years experience in PET/CT imaging) and reviewed visually in consensus by two board-certified nuclear medicine clinicians and one board-certified radiologist. The term "lesion positivity rate" is used based on the imaging result and its interpretation by the nuclear medicine and radiological expert team in relation to the PSMA-positive tumor lesions. Any lesion with an increased radiotracer uptake (measured with SUV_{max}) above physiological uptake was considered suspicious of malignancy, and biphasic lesion detection (baseline and delayed images) was taken into account. If no consensus could be found between the board-certified nuclear medicine clinicians and the board-certified radiologist, these lesions were classified as moderately suspicious of malignancy. However, in this case, all the experts classified the lesions as abnormal and probably malignant. SUV_{max} of PSMA-avid lesions detected by baseline and by delayed scan were compared. There have been extensive efforts to develop quantitative criteria for the analysis of oncologic PET images. The measures proposed are based on the SUV in a certain volume of interest (VOI) enclosing the lesion. The principle of the SUV was introduced by Strauss and Conti [37]. For a defined VOI, the mean SUV value (SUV_{mean}) of all included pixels is usually calculated as a representative measure of tracer uptake. As a result of the VOI definition dependence, the SUV_{mean} suffers from a limited reproducibility. To overcome this problem, the SUV_{max} has been introduced, which is the maximal SUV value in the lesion. Thus, we have only used the SUV_{max} in the present study. LNM were divided into two groups based on their location (pelvic LNM: iliac and/or pararectal) and extra-pelvic distant LNM (retroperitoneal and/or above the iliac bifurcation).

4.3. Statistical Analysis

Data were analyzed using IPM SPSS Statistics version 23.0 (IBM Corporation, Ehningen, Germany). First, variables were tested for normal distribution using the Shapiro–Wilk test. To compare normally distributed values of two patient groups, Student's-*t*-test was used. The Mann–Whitney U-test was used for non-normally distributed continuous variables. For further analysis, we evaluated PSA-stratified LPR and evaluated categorical differences by Chi-square test and Pearson correlation. For comparing values of baseline and delayed imaging, i.e., SUV_{max} of PET-positive lesions, the Wilcoxon-signed-rank-test was used. Mean and SD are given if normality was observed. Additionally, for non-normal distributed variables, median and range were evaluated. p values < 0.05 were considered statistically significant.

5. Conclusions

Although there was a significant increase in SUVmax on delayed images in pelvic and extra-pelvic LNM in comparison to early [^{68}Ga]Ga-PSMA PET/CT in our study, the LPR was comparable, especially in the assessment of small subcentimeter pelvic PCa lesions in patients with multiple metastases.

The few additional findings, respectively, the confirmed lesions in the late images, had no effect on staging or restaging of PCa, as they did not lead to any modification of the final interpretation or TNM classification and did not change patient management. However, in a few individual cases, additional late scans provided an information advantage in PCa lesion detection due to a higher tracer uptake and an improved contrast.

Author Contributions: Conceptualization, M.A.H., H.-G.B., H.J.W., M.M. and M.S.; methodology, M.A.H., H.-G.B., H.J.W., M.M., F.R. and M.S.; software, M.A.H., H.-G.B. and N.F.; validation, M.A.H., H.-G.B., H.J.W., M.M., F.R., N.F. and M.S.; formal analysis, M.A.H., H.-G.B., H.J.W., M.M., F.R. and N.F.; investigation, M.A.H., H.J.W. and M.M.; resources, M.A.H., H.-G.B., H.J.W. and M.M.; data curation, H.J.W., M.M. and M.S.; writing—original draft preparation, M.A.H., H.-G.B., H.J.W., M.M. and M.S.; writing—review and editing, H.J.W., M.M., F.R., N.F. and M.S.; visualization, M.A.H., H.-G.B. and M.S.; supervision, M.M. and M.S.; project administration, H.J.W., M.M. and M.S. All authors have read and agreed to the published version of the manuscript.

Funding: This research received no external funding.

Acknowledgments: The authors wish to express their gratitude to Ed Michaelson, MD, Fort Lauderdale, Florida, USA for language revision and to Rainer Arenz, Wolken, Germany, for technical support.

Conflicts of Interest: The authors declare no conflict of interest.

References

1. Ferlay, J.; Colombet, M.; Soerjomataram, I.; Mathers, C.; Parkin, D.M.; Piñeros, M.; Znaor, A.; Bray, F. Estimating the global cancer incidence and mortality in 2018: GLOBOCAN sources and methods. *Int. J. Cancer* **2019**, *144*, 1941–1953. [CrossRef] [PubMed]
2. Wibmer, A.G.; Burger, I.A.; Sala, E.; Hricak, H.; Weber, W.A.; Vargas, H.A. Molecular Imaging of Prostate Cancer. *Radiographics* **2016**, *36*, 142–159. [CrossRef] [PubMed]
3. Mottet, N.; Bellmunt, J.; Bolla, M.; Briers, E.; Cumberbatch, M.G.; De Santis, M.; Fossati, N.; Gross, T.; Henry, A.M.; Joniau, S.; et al. EAU-ESTRO-SIOG Guidelines on Prostate Cancer. Part 1: Screening, Diagnosis, and Local Treatment with Curative Intent. *Eur Urol.* **2017**, *71*, 618–629. [CrossRef] [PubMed]
4. Ghosh, A.; Heston, W.D. Tumor target prostate specific membrane antigen (PSMA) and its regulation in prostate cancer. *J. Cell. Biochem.* **2004**, *91*, 528–539. [CrossRef]
5. Afshar-Oromieh, A.; Malcher, A.; Eder, M.; Eisenhut, M.; Linhart, H.G.; Hadaschik, B.A.; Holland-Letz, T.; Giesel, F.L.; Kratochwil, C.; Haufe, S.; et al. PET imaging with a [^{68}Ga]gallium-labelled PSMA ligand for the diagnosis of prostate cancer: Biodistribution in humans and first evaluation of tumour lesions. *Eur. J. Nucl. Med. Mol. Imaging* **2013**, *40*, 486–495. [CrossRef]
6. Coenen, H.H.; Gee, A.D.; Adam, M.; Antoni, G.; Cutler, C.S.; Fujibayashi, Y.; Jeong, J.M.; Mach, R.H.; Mindt, T.L.; Pike, V.W.; et al. Open letter to journal editors on: International Consensus Radiochemistry Nomenclature Guidelines. *EJNMMI Radiopharm. Chem.* **2019**, *4*, 7. [CrossRef]
7. Sanli, Y.; Sanli, O.; Has Simsek, D.; Subramaniam, R.M. ^{68}Ga-PSMA PET/CT and PET/MRI in high-risk prostate cancer patients. *Nucl. Med. Commun.* **2018**, *39*, 871–880. [CrossRef]
8. Grubnic, S.; Vinnicombe, S.J.; Norman, A.R.; Husband, J.E. MR evaluation of normal retroperitoneal and pelvic lymph nodes. *Clin. Radiol.* **2002**, *57*, 193–200. [CrossRef]
9. Hofman, M.S.; Lawrentschuk, N.; Francis, R.J.; Tang, C.; Vela, I.; Thomas, P.; Rutherford, N.; Martin, J.M.; Frydenberg, M.; Shakher, R.; et al. Prostate-specific membrane antigen PET-CT in patients with high-risk prostate cancer before curative-intent surgery or radiotherapy (proPSMA): A prospective, randomised, multicentre study. *Lancet* **2020**, *395*, 1208–1216. [CrossRef]
10. Hövels, A.M.; Heesakkers, R.A.; Adang, E.M.; Jager, G.J.; Strum, S.; Hoogeveen, Y.L.; Severens, J.L.; Barentsz, J.O. The diagnostic accuracy of CT and MRI in the staging of pelvic lymph nodes in patients with prostate cancer: A meta-analysis. *Clin. Radiol.* **2008**, *63*, 387–395. [CrossRef]

11. Hoffmann, M.A.; Wieler, H.J.; Baues, C.; Kuntz, N.J.; Richardsen, I.; Schreckenberger, M. The Impact of ^{68}Ga-PSMA PET/CT and PET/MRI on the Management of Prostate Cancer. *Urology* **2019**, *130*, 1–12. [CrossRef] [PubMed]
12. Maurer, T.; Gschwend, J.E.; Rauscher, I.; Souvatzoglou, M.; Haller, B.; Weirich, G.; Wester, H.J.; Heck, M.; Kübler, H.; Beer, A.J.; et al. Diagnostic Efficacy of (^{68})Gallium-PSMA Positron Emission Tomography Compared to Conventional Imaging for Lymph Node Staging of 130 Consecutive Patients with Intermediate to High Risk Prostate Cancer. *J. Urol.* **2016**, *195*, 1436–1443. [CrossRef]
13. Hoffmann, M.A.; Buchholz, H.G.; Wieler, H.J.; Miederer, M.; Rosar, F.; Fischer, N.; Müller-Hübenthal, J.; Trampert, L.; Pektor, S.; Schreckenberger, M. PSA and PSA Kinetics Thresholds for the Presence of ^{68}Ga-PSMA-11 PET/CT-Detectable Lesions in Patients with Biochemical Recurrent Prostate Cancer. *Cancers* **2020**, *12*, 398. [CrossRef] [PubMed]
14. Herrmann, K.; Bluemel, C.; Weineisen, M.; Schottelius, M.; Wester, H.J.; Czernin, J.; Eberlein, U.; Beykan, S.; Lapa, C.; Riedmiller, H.; et al. Biodistribution and radiation dosimetry for a probe targeting prostate-specific membrane antigen for imaging and therapy. *J. Nucl. Med.* **2015**, *56*, 855–861. [CrossRef] [PubMed]
15. Cornford, P.; Bellmunt, J.; Bolla, M.; Briers, E.; De Santis, M.; Gross, T.; Henry, A.M.; Joniau, S.; Lam, T.B.; Mason, M.D.; et al. EAU-ESTRO-SIOG Guidelines on Prostate Cancer. Part II: Treatment of Relapsing, Metastatic, and Castration-Resistant Prostate Cancer. *Eur. Urol.* **2017**, *71*, 630–642. [CrossRef]
16. Hoffmann, M.A.; Miederer, M.; Wieler, H.J.; Ruf, C.; Jakobs, F.M.; Schreckenberger, M. Diagnostic performance of ^{68}Gallium-PSMA-11 PET/CT to detect significant prostate cancer and comparison with ^{18}FEC PET/CT. *Oncotarget* **2017**, *14*, 111073–111083. [CrossRef]
17. Epstein, J.I.; Egevad, L.; Amin, M.B.; Delahunt, B.; Srigley, J.R.; Humphrey, P.A.; Grading Committee. The 2014 International Society of Urological Pathology (ISUP) Consensus Conference on Gleason Grading of Prostatic Carcinoma: Definition of Grading Patterns and Proposal for a New Grading System. *Am. J. Surg. Pathol.* **2016**, *40*, 244–252. [CrossRef]
18. Alberts, I.; Sachpekidis, C.; Dijkstra, L.; Prenosil, G.; Gourni, E.; Boxler, S.; Gross, T.; Thalmann, G.; Rahbar, K.; Rominger, A.; et al. The role of additional late PSMA-ligand PET/CT in the differentiation between lymph node metastases and ganglia. *Eur. J. Nucl. Med. Mol. Imaging* **2020**, *47*, 642–651. [CrossRef]
19. Fendler, W.P.; Eiber, M.; Beheshti, M.; Bomanji, J.; Ceci, F.; Cho, S.; Giesel, F.; Haberkorn, U.; Hope, T.A.; Kopka, K.; et al. ^{68}Ga-PSMA PET/CT: Joint EANM and SNMMI procedure guideline for prostate cancer imaging: Version 1.0. *Eur. J. Nucl. Med. Mol. Imaging* **2017**, *44*, 1014–1024. [CrossRef]
20. Afshar-Oromieh, A.; Sattler, L.P.; Mier, W.; Hadaschik, B.A.; Debus, J.; Holland-Letz, T.; Kopka, K.; Haberkorn, U. The Clinical Impact of Additional Late PET/CT Imaging with ^{68}Ga-PSMA-11 (HBED-CC) in the Diagnosis of Prostate Cancer. *J. Nucl. Med.* **2017**, *58*, 750–755. [CrossRef]
21. Schmuck, S.; Nordlohne, S.; von Klot, C.A.; Henkenberens, C.; Sohns, J.M.; Christiansen, H.; Wester, H.J.; Ross, T.L.; Bengel, F.M.; Derlin, T. Comparison of standard and delayed imaging to improve the detection rate of [^{68}Ga]PSMA I&T PET/CT in patients with biochemical recurrence or prostate-specific antigen persistence after primary therapy for prostate cancer. *Eur. J. Nucl. Med. Mol. Imaging* **2017**, *44*, 960–968. [CrossRef] [PubMed]
22. Schmuck, S.; Mamach, M.; Wilke, F.; von Klot, C.A.; Henkenberens, C.; Thackeray, J.T.; Sohns, J.M.; Geworski, L.; Ross, T.L.; Wester, H.J.; et al. Multiple Time-Point ^{68}Ga-PSMA I&T PET/CT for Characterization of Primary Prostate Cancer: Value of Early Dynamic and Delayed Imaging. *Clin. Nucl. Med.* **2017**, *42*, 286–293. [CrossRef]
23. Beheshti, M.; Paymani, Z.; Brilhante, J.; Geinitz, H.; Gehring, D.; Leopoldseder, T.; Wouters, L.; Pirich, C.; Loidl, W.; Langsteger, W. Optimal time-point for ^{68}Ga-PSMA-11 PET/CT imaging in assessment of prostate cancer: Feasibility of sterile cold-kit tracer preparation? *Eur. J. Nucl. Med. Mol. Imaging* **2018**, *45*, 1188–1196. [CrossRef] [PubMed]
24. Sahlmann, C.O.; Meller, B.; Bouter, C.; Ritter, C.O.; Ströbel, P.; Lotz, J.; Trojan, L.; Meller, J.; Hijazi, S. Biphasic ^{68}Ga-PSMA-HBED-CC-PET/CT in patients with recurrent and high-risk prostate carcinoma. *Eur. J. Nucl. Med. Mol. Imaging* **2016**, *43*, 898–905. [CrossRef]
25. Freitag, M.T.; Radtke, J.P.; Hadaschik, B.A.; Kopp-Schneider, A.; Eder, M.; Kopka, K.; Haberkorn, U.; Roethke, M.; Schlemmer, H.P.; Afshar-Oromieh, A. Comparison of hybrid (^{68})Ga-PSMA PET/MRI and (^{68})Ga-PSMA PET/CT in the evaluation of lymph node and bone metastases of prostate cancer. *Eur. J. Nucl. Med. Mol. Imaging* **2016**, *43*, 70–83. [CrossRef]

26. Kunikowska, J.; Kujda, S.; Królicki, L. ^{68}Ga-PSMA PET/CT in Recurrence Prostate Cancer. Should We Perform Delayed Image in Cases of Negative 60 Minutes Postinjection Examination? *Clin. Nucl. Med.* **2020**, *45*, e213–e214. [CrossRef]
27. Rosar, F.; Buchholz, H.G.; Michels, S.; Hoffmann, M.A.; Piel, M.; Waldmann, C.M.; Rösch, F.; Reuss, S.; Schreckenberger, M. Image quality analysis of 44Sc on two preclinical PET scanners: A comparison to ^{68}Ga. *EJNMMI Phys.* **2020**, *7*, 16. [CrossRef]
28. Luiting, H.B.; van Leeuwen, P.J.; Busstra, M.B.; Brabander, T.; van der Poel, H.G.; Donswijk, M.L.; Vis, A.N.; Emmett, L.; Stricker, P.D.; Roobol, M.J. Use of gallium-68 prostate-specific membrane antigen positron-emission tomography for detecting lymph node metastases in primary and recurrent prostate cancer and location of recurrence after radical prostatectomy: An overview of the current literature. *BJU Int.* **2020**, *125*, 206–214. [CrossRef]
29. Han, S.; Woo, S.; Kim, Y.J.; Suh, C.H. Impact of ^{68}Ga-PSMA PET on the Management of Patients with Prostate Cancer: A Systematic Review and Meta-analysis. *Eur. Urol.* **2018**, *74*, 179–190. [CrossRef]
30. Krohn, T.; Verburg, F.A.; Pufe, T.; Neuhuber, W.; Vogg, A.; Heinzel, A.; Mottaghy, F.M.; Behrendt, F.F. [(^{68}Ga)]PSMA-HBED uptake mimicking lymph node metastasis in coeliac ganglia: An important pitfall in clinical practice. *Eur. J. Nucl. Med. Mol. Imaging* **2015**, *42*, 210–214. [CrossRef]
31. Derlin, T.; Schmuck, S.; Juhl, C.; Zörgiebel, J.; Schneefeld, S.M.; Walte, A.C.A.; Hueper, K.; von Klot, C.A.; Henkenberens, C.; Christiansen, H.; et al. PSA-stratified detection rates for [^{68}Ga]THP-PSMA, a novel probe for rapid kit-based ^{68}Ga-labeling and PET imaging, in patients with biochemical recurrence after primary therapy for prostate cancer. *Eur. J. Nucl. Med. Mol. Imaging* **2018**, *45*, 913–922. [CrossRef] [PubMed]
32. Afshar-Oromieh, A.; Hetzheim, H.; Kübler, W.; Kratochwil, C.; Giesel, F.L.; Hope, T.A.; Eder, M.; Eisenhut, M.; Kopka, K.; Haberkorn, U. Radiation dosimetry of (^{68})Ga-PSMA-11 (HBED-CC) and preliminary evaluation of optimal imaging timing. *Eur. J. Nucl. Med. Mol. Imaging* **2016**, *43*, 1611–1620. [CrossRef] [PubMed]
33. Haupt, F.; Dijkstra, L.; Alberts, I.; Sachpekidis, C.; Fech, V.; Boxler, S.; Gross, T.; Holland-Letz, T.; Zacho, H.D.; Haberkorn, U.; et al. ^{68}Ga-PSMA-11 PET/CT in patients with recurrent prostate cancer-a modified protocol compared with the common protocol. *Eur. J. Nucl. Med. Mol. Imaging* **2020**, *47*, 624–631. [CrossRef]
34. Annunziata, S.; Pizzuto, D.A.; Treglia, G. Diagnostic Performance of PET Imaging Using Different Radiopharmaceuticals in Prostate Cancer According to Published Meta-Analyses. *Cancers* **2020**, *12*, 2153. [CrossRef]
35. Werner, R.A.; Derlin, T.; Lapa, C.; Sheikbahaei, S.; Higuchi, T.; Giesel, F.L.; Behr, S.; Drzezga, A.; Kimura, H.; Buck, A.K.; et al. 18F-Labeled, PSMA-Targeted Radiotracers: Leveraging the Advantages of Radiofluorination for Prostate Cancer Molecular Imaging. *Theranostics* **2020**, *10*, 1–16. [CrossRef]
36. Eder, M.; Neels, O.; Müller, M.; Bauder-Wüst, U.; Remde, Y.; Schäfer, M.; Hennrich, U.; Eisenhut, M.; Afshar-Oromieh, A.; Haberkorn, U.; et al. Novel Preclinical and Radiopharmaceutical Aspects of [^{68}Ga]Ga-PSMA-HBED-CC: A New PET Tracer for Imaging of Prostate Cancer. *Pharmaceuticals* **2014**, *7*, 779–796. [CrossRef]
37. Strauss, L.G.; Conti, P.S. The applications of PET in clinical oncology. *J. Nucl. Med.* **1991**, *32*, 623–648.

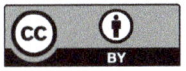

© 2020 by the authors. Licensee MDPI, Basel, Switzerland. This article is an open access article distributed under the terms and conditions of the Creative Commons Attribution (CC BY) license (http://creativecommons.org/licenses/by/4.0/).

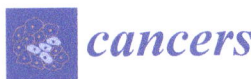

Article

Analysis of CXCL9, PD1 and PD-L1 mRNA in Stage T1 Non-Muscle Invasive Bladder Cancer and Their Association with Prognosis

Jennifer Kubon [1,†], Danijel Sikic [1,†,‡], Markus Eckstein [2,‡], Veronika Weyerer [2,‡], Robert Stöhr [2,‡], Angela Neumann [1], Bastian Keck [1,‡], Bernd Wullich [1,‡], Arndt Hartmann [2,‡], Ralph M. Wirtz [3,‡], Helge Taubert [1,*,‡,§] and Sven Wach [1,‡,§]

1. Department of Urology and Pediatric Urology, University Hospital Erlangen, Friedrich-Alexander Universität Erlangen-Nürnberg, 91054 Erlangen, Germany; jennifer.kubon@fau.de (J.K.); danijel.sikic@uk-erlangen.de (D.S.); Angela.Neumann@uk-erlangen.de (A.N.); bastian.keck@web.de (B.K.); Bernd.Wullich@uk-erlangen.de (B.W.); sven.wach@uk-erlangen.de (S.W.)
2. Institute of Pathology, University Hospital Erlangen, Friedrich-Alexander Universität Erlangen-Nürnberg, 91054 Erlangen, Germany; Markus.Eckstein@uk-erlangen.de (M.E.); veronika.weyerer@uk-erlangen.de (V.W.); robert.stoehr@uk-erlangen.de (R.S.); arndt.hartmann@uk-erlangen.de (A.H.)
3. STRATIFYER Molecular Pathology GmbH, 50935 Cologne, Germany; ralph.wirtz@stratifyer.de
* Correspondence: helge.taubert@uk-erlangen.de; Tel.: +49-9131-8523-373; Fax: +49-9131-852-3374
† These authors share equal contribution.
‡ Authors belong to Bridge Consortium, 12049 Berlin, Germany.
§ These authors share equal senior authorship.

Received: 3 September 2020; Accepted: 24 September 2020; Published: 29 September 2020

Simple Summary: Non-muscle invasive bladder cancer (NMIBC) patients possess a high rate of recurrences and very long treatment times, which remains a major unresolved problem for them and the health care system. We analyzed the mRNA of three immune markers, *CXCL9*, *PD1* and *PD-L1*, in 80 NMIBC by qRT-PCR. Lower *CXCL9* mRNA appeared to be an independent prognostic parameter for reduced OS and RFS. Furthermore, low *PD-L1* mRNA was an independent prognostic factor for DSS and RFS. In univariate Cox's regression analysis, the stratification of patients revealed that low *CXCL9* or *PD1* mRNA was associated with reduced RFS in the patient group younger than 72 years. Low *CXCL9* or *PD-L1* was associated with shorter RFS in patients with higher tumor cell proliferation or without instillation therapy. In conclusion, the characterization of mRNA levels of the immune markers *CXCL9*, *PD1* and *PD-L1* differentiates NIMBC patients with respect to prognosis.

Abstract: Non-muscle invasive bladder cancer (NMIBC), which is characterized by a recurrence rate of approximately 30% and very long treatment times, remains a major unresolved problem for patients and the health care system. The immunological interplay between tumor cells and the immune environment is important for tumor development. Therefore, we analyzed the mRNA of three immune markers, *CXCL9*, *PD1* and *PD-L1*, in NMIBC by qRT-PCR. The results were subsequently correlated with clinicopathological parameters and prognostic data. Altogether, as expected, higher age was an independent prognostic factor for overall survival (OS) and disease-specific survival (DSS), but not for recurrence-free survival (RFS). Lower *CXCL9* mRNA was observed in multivariate Cox's regression analysis to be an independent prognostic parameter for reduced OS (relative risk; RR = 2.08; $p = 0.049$), DSS (RR = 4.49; $p = 0.006$) and RFS (RR = 2.69; $p = 0.005$). In addition, *PD-L1* mRNA was an independent prognostic factor for DSS (RR = 5.02; $p = 0.042$) and RFS (RR = 2.07; $p = 0.044$). Moreover, in univariate Cox's regression analysis, the stratification of patients revealed that low *CXCL9* or low *PD1* mRNA was associated with reduced RFS in the younger patient group (≤71 years), but not in the older patient group (>71 years). In addition, low *CXCL9* or low *PD-L1* was associated with shorter RFS in patients with higher tumor cell proliferation and in patients without instillation therapy. In conclusion, the characterization of mRNA levels of immune markers differentiates NIMBC patients with respect to prognosis.

Keywords: *CXCL9*; *PD1*; *PD-L1*; stage T1 NMIBC; prognosis

1. Introduction

Urothelial bladder cancer (BCa) accounts for approximately 3% of global cancer diagnoses. It was recently reported to be the 10th most commonly diagnosed cancer and the 13th leading cause of cancer-related death worldwide [1]. Approximately 25% of BCas are categorized as muscle-invasive BCa (MIBC) and 75% as non-muscle invasive BCa (NMIBC) [2]. NMIBC treatment comprises transurethral resection of the bladder (TURB) and, depending on the risk of progression, instillation with bacillus Calmette-Guerin (BCG) or mitomycin [3–5]. However, high-risk NMIBC remains a challenge because 30% to 60% of patients with stage pT1 NMIBC develop local recurrence, and up to 20% experience disease progression to MIBC [6–8]. There is heterogeneity in stage pT1 NMIBC, and its risk stratification is based only on clinicopathological parameters that necessitate lifelong follow-up [9]. Altogether, bladder cancers, including NMIBC, impose the highest costs on society among cancers per patient from diagnosis to death [10]. However, bladder tumor markers cannot yet definitively replace cystoscopy in surveillance regimens [10]. Therefore, the continued search for biomarkers in bladder cancer is necessary.

The tumor biology of BCa, including NMIBC, is related to cell lineage and cell proliferation [11–13]. Therefore, we included an analysis of the mRNA of keratin 5 (*KRT5*; basal-like lineage), keratin 20 (*KRT20*; luminal-like lineage) and marker of proliferation KI67 (*MKI67, KI67*) in this study. Furthermore, studies conducted by other groups, as well as our own previous studies, showed that gene expression can differentiate NMIBCs into subsets that possess different risk profiles, and may impact treatment decisions in the future [14,15].

In the current study, we investigated the expression of genes associated with tumor immune status and their association with prognosis in stage pT1 NMIBC. Recently, we reported that a cytotoxic T-cell-related gene expression signature containing three genes (*CXCL9*, *CD3 Z*, *CD8*) correlates with immune cell infiltration, and predicts improved survival in MIBC patients after radical cystectomy and adjuvant chemotherapy [16]. All three immune signature genes were strongly associated with each other, which is why we chose only *CXCL9* for the current analysis. Additionally, we chose programmed cell death 1 gene (*PD1/PDCD1*) and programmed cell death ligand 1 (*PD-L1/CD274/B7-H1*) since they are also very prominent in the immune response of MIBC, and represent therapeutic targets for MIBC [16–18]. *CXCL9* (*SCYB9/MIG*) and *CXCL10* (*SCYB10*) genes are located in chromosome band 4 q21 [19], and belong to the CXC family of chemokines [20]. *CXCL9* encodes a T-cell chemoattractant that is significantly induced by interferon gamma, which mediates a T-cell-driven antitumoral immune response [21]. *CXCL9* has not been previously studied in NMIBC. The *PD1* gene has been mapped to the chromosome region 2 q37.3 by the Honyo group [22]. It encodes a cell surface receptor on T-cells and tumor-associated macrophages (TAMs), and is a member of the B7 superfamily involved in immunomodulation. PD1 acts as an inhibitory molecule on T-cells/TAMs after interacting with its ligand PD-L1 [23,24]. The *PD-L1* gene is located on chromosome 9 p24.1 and codes for a costimulatory molecule that negatively regulates cell-mediated immune responses [23,25]. PD-L1 is expressed by both tumor cells and tumor-associated antigen-presenting cells [26]. Le Goux et al. [27] did not find an association between *PD1* or *PD-L1* gene expression and prognosis (RFS and progression-free survival) in NMIBC. We recently demonstrated in an NMIBC cohort that increased *PD-L1* mRNA was an independent prognostic indicator for both RFS and DSS [28]. However, in that study, *PD1* mRNA was not associated with prognosis [28].

In this study, we analyzed a new independent cohort of NMIBC patients with extended follow-up periods to reassess the long-term association of PD-L1 mRNA with disease prognosis, and to determine whether the two immune markers CXCL9 and PD1 are associated with survival.

2. Results

2.1. Correlations of CXCL9, PD1, PD-L1, KRT5 and KRT20 mRNA with Each Other and with Clinicopathological Parameters

CXCL9 mRNA negatively correlated with the incidence of recurrence (correlation coefficient; $r_s = -0.374$; $p = 0.001$) and with mRNA of KRT20 ($r_s = -0.305$; $p = 0.006$) and KRT5 ($r_s = -0.230$; $p = 0.040$), and is positively correlated with mRNA of PD1 ($r_s = 0.639$; $p < 0.001$) and PD-L1 ($r_s = 0.601$; $p < 0.001$) (Table 1). PD1 mRNA was negatively correlated with mRNA of KRT20 ($r_s = -0.253$; $p = 0.024$) and KI67 ($r_s = -0.222$; $p = 0.047$), and positively correlated with time of RFS ($r_s = 0.298$; $p = 0.007$) and PD-L1 mRNA ($r_s = 0.459$; $p < 0.001$). PD-L1 mRNA negatively correlated with KRT20 ($r_s = -0.233$; $p = 0.038$) (Table 1).

Table 1. Bivariate correlations for mRNA of CXCL9, KRT20, KRT5, PD1, PD-L1 and KI67 with clinicopathological parameters.

Bivariate Correlations		KRT20	KRT5	PD1	PD-L1	KI67	Fu_Recurr	Recurr
CXCL9	Correlation coefficient	−0.305	−0.230	0.639	0.601	−0.136	0.208	−0.374
	Sig. (2-sided)	**0.006**	0.040	**<0.001**	**<0.001**	0.228	0.065	**0.001**
KRT20	Correlation coefficient		−0.042	−0.253	−0.233	0.356	−0.152	0.116
	Sig. (2-sided)		0.714	0.024	0.038	**0.001**	0.178	0.304
KRT5	Correlation coefficient			−0.212	0.036	−0.070	0.039	0.067
	Sig. (2-sided)			0.059	0.753	0.537	0.733	0.557
PD1	Correlation coefficient				0.459	−0.222	0.298	−0.204
	Sig. (2-sided)				**<0.001**	0.047	**0.007**	0.070
PD-L1	Correlation coefficient					0.001	0.096	−0.215
	Sig. (2-sided)					0.994	0.397	0.055
KI67	Correlation coefficient						−0.152	0.138
	Sig. (2-sided)						0.177	0.222
fu_recurr	Correlation coefficient							−0.562
	Sig. (2-sided)							**<0.001**

Abbreviation: fu recur—follow-up recurrence (time until occurrence of recurrence); recur.—recurrence. Bonferroni correction results in $\alpha = 0.00714$. Significance at the α level is marked in bold.

2.2. Association of CXCL9, PD1, PD-L1, KRT5 and KRT20 mRNA with NMIBC Prognosis

The association of mRNA in the 80 tumor samples with patient survival was examined by Kaplan–Meier analysis. As expected, age was associated with both OS and DSS ($p = 0.019$ and $p = 0.025$). However, CXCL9, PD1 and PD-L1 mRNA was not associated with OS or DSS (Table 2).

Interestingly, higher CXCL9 ($p < 0.001$), PD1 ($p = 0.023$) or PD-L1 ($p = 0.007$) mRNA were associated with increased RFS (all Kaplan–Meier analyses, Table 2; Figure 1).

Table 2. Kaplan–Meier analysis of the association of age, *CXCL9*, *PD1* and *PD-L1* mRNA with prognosis.

Parameter	Kaplan–Meier Analysis								
	n	OS Months	*p*	*n*	DSS Months	*p*	*n*	RFS Months	*p*
Age									
≤71 vs. >71 year	40 vs. 40	124.8 vs. 84.5	**0.019**	40 vs. 40	170.2 vs. 108.3	**0.025**	40 vs. 40	n.s.	n.s.
CXCL9									
low vs. high	32 vs. 48	n.s.	n.s.	25 vs. 55	n.s.	n.s.	32 vs. 48	38.7 vs. 87.4	**<0.001**
PD1									
low vs. high	40 vs. 40	n.s.	n.s.	40 vs. 40	n.s.	n.s.	53 vs. 27	62.0 vs. 99.5	**0.023**
PD-L1									
low vs. high	24 vs. 56	n.s.	n.s.	46 vs. 34	n.s.	n.s.	46 vs. 34	58.6 vs. 102.7	**0.007**

Significant values are in bold face. Abbreviation: n.s., not significant.

(A) (B) (C)

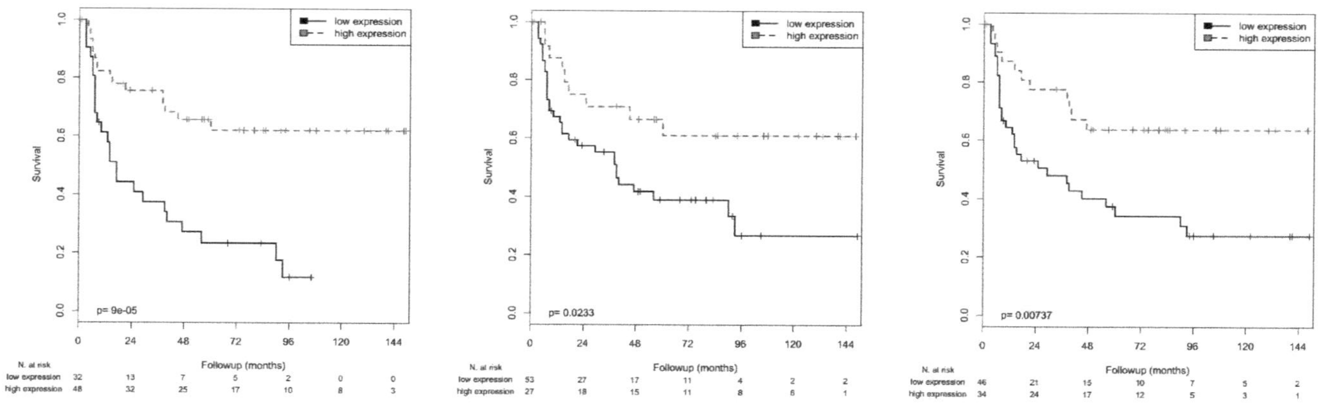

Figure 1. Kaplan–Meier analysis of the association of *CXCL9*, *PD1* or *PD-L1* mRNA with RFS. Gene expression was significantly associated with RFS for the genes. (**A**): *CXCL9* ($p < 0.001$). (**B**): *PD1* ($p = 0.023$). (**C**): *PD-L1* ($p = 0.007$).

In univariate Cox's regression analysis, the clinicopathological parameters of histological grade, tumor stage (pT1 with/without presence of cis), intravesical therapy and gender, and the molecular parameters KI67, KRT5 and KRT20, were not associated with prognosis (OS, DSS, RFS), and therefore were not included in further multivariate Cox's regression analysis (data not shown).

As expected, in univariate Cox's regression analysis, higher age (RR = 2.29; p = 0.022) was associated with an increased risk of shorter OS. Furthermore, higher age (RR = 3.44; p = 0.034) was associated with increased risk of shorter DSS (Table 3).

Table 3. Univariate Cox's regression analysis for the association of age and CXCL9, PD1 and PD-L1 mRNA with prognosis.

Parameter	n	Univariate Cox's Regression Analysis							
		OS RR	p	n	DSS RR	p	n	RFS RR	p
Age ≤71 vs. >71 year	40 vs. 40	2.29	0.022	40 vs. 40	3.44	0.034	40 vs. 40	n.s.	n.s.
CXCL9 low vs. high	32 vs. 48	n.s.	n.s.	25 vs. 55	n.s.	n.s.	21 vs. 59	3.30	<0.001
PD1 low vs. high	40 vs. 40	n.s.	n.s.	40 vs. 40	n.s.	n.s.	53 vs. 27	2.31	0.027
PD-L1 low vs. high	24 vs. 56	n.s.	**n.s.**	46 vs. 34	n.s.	n.s.	46 vs. 34	2.51	0.009

Significant values are in bold face. Abbreviation: n.s., not significant.

In univariate Cox's regression analysis, lower CXCL9 (RR = 3.30; p < 0.001), lower PD1 (RR = 2.31; p = 0.027) and lower PD-L1 (RR = 2.51; p = 0.009) mRNA showed an increased risk for shorter RFS. However, age was not associated with an increased risk of shorter RFS (Table 3).

In multivariate Cox's regression analysis (adjusted for age and the molecular parameters PD1, PD-L1 and CXCL9), an association with OS was found for higher age (RR = 2.31; p = 0.021) and lower CXCL9 (RR = 2.08; p = 0.049) mRNA (Table 4). Multivariate analysis (adjusted for age and the molecular parameters PD1, PD-L1 and CXCL9) revealed associations with DSS for higher age (RR = 4.47; p = 0.014), lower CXCL9 (RR = 4.49; p = 0.006) and lower PD-L1 (RR = 5.02; p = 0.042) mRNA (Table 4).

Table 4. Multivariate Cox's regression analysis for the association of age and CXCL9, PD1 and PD-L1 mRNA with prognosis.

Parameter	n	Multivariate Cox's Regression Analysis							
		OS RR	p	n	DSS RR	p	n	RFS RR	p
Age ≤71 vs. >71 year	40 vs. 40	2.31	0.021	40 vs. 40	4.47	0.014	40 vs. 40	n.s.	n.s.
CXCL9 low vs. high	32 vs. 48	2.08	0.049	25 vs. 55	4.49	0.006	21 vs. 59	2.69	0.005
PD1 low vs. high	40 vs. 40	n.s	n.s	40 vs. 40	n.s.	n.s.	53 vs. 27	n.s.	n.s.
PD-L1 low vs. high	24 vs. 56	n.s.	n.s.	46 vs. 34	5.02	0.042	46 vs. 34	2.07	0.044

Significant values are in bold face. Abbreviation: n.s., not significant.

Furthermore, in the multivariate Cox's regression analysis, associations with shorter RFS were found for lower CXCL9 (RR = 2.69; p = 0.005) and lower PD-L1 (RR = 2.07; p = 0.044) mRNA (Table 4).

Altogether, as expected, higher age was an independent prognostic factor for OS and DSS, but not for RFS. CXCL9 mRNA was as independent prognostic parameter for OS, DSS and RFS. In addition, PD-L1 mRNA was an independent prognostic factor for DSS and RFS.

2.3. Association of CXCL9, PD1, PD-L1, KRT5 and KRT20 mRNA with RFS Stratified by Clinicopathological Parameters or mRNA

2.3.1. Stratification by Age

Using the median age of 71 years as a cut-off to define the two age groups (≤71 vs. >71 years), age itself was not associated with RFS (Table 4). In the univariate Cox's regression analysis in the younger age group, low CXCL9 (RR = 6.21; $p = < 0.001$) was associated with an increased risk of recurrence (Table 5). This finding is in accordance with the above mentioned results for all patients, but it indicates the greater relevance of CXCL9 mRNA in younger patients. Low PD1 mRNA was only associated with a risk of shorter RFS in the younger patient group (RR = 4.93; $p = 0.035$). Altogether, the higher risks of recurrence for CXCL9 and low PD1 levels were only relevant to the younger age group (Table 5).

Table 5. Univariate Cox's regression analysis for stratification by clinicopathological or molecular parameters: the association of CXCL9, PD1 and PD-L1 mRNA with RFS.

		Univariate Cox's Regression Analysis	
Parameter by Stratification	n	RFS RR	p
Strata age: young patients	40		
CXCL9 low vs. high	15 vs. 25	6.21	**<0.001**
PD1 low vs. high	27 vs.13	4.93	**0.035**
Strata KRT5 low	40		
CXCL9 low vs. high	13 vs. 27	3.76	**0.004**
Strata KRT5 high	40		
CXCL9 low vs. high	19 vs. 21	3.33	**0.013**
PD-L1 low vs. high	22 vs. 18	3.68	**0.012**
Strata KRT20 low	40		
CXCL9 low vs. high	13 vs. 27	3.04	**0.019**
Strata KRT20 high	40		
CXCL9 low vs. high	19 vs. 21	3.28	**0.007**
PD-L1 low vs. high	25 vs. 15	4.23	**0.009**
Strata KI67 high	40		
CXCL9 low vs. high	19 vs. 21	4.54	**<0.001**
PD-L1 low vs. high	25 vs. 15	7.49	**0.001**
Strata: no intravesical	39		
CXCL9 low vs. high	15 vs. 24	10.33	**<0.001**
PD1 low vs. high	23 vs. 16	5.31	**0.010**
PD-L1 low vs. high	22 vs. 17	4.36	**0.022**

Significant values are in bold face.

2.3.2. Stratification by KRT5 or KRT20 Expression

KRT5 or KRT20 mRNA is considered a characteristic feature for a basal or luminal lineage, respectively, in bladder cancer [11]. We utilized the expressions of both mRNA markers as proxies to define a more basal or more luminal-like gene expression pattern, respectively. The expression of both markers was separated by median expression into two groups with low/high KRT5 (≤36.78 vs. >36.78) or low/high KRT20 (≤37.47 vs. >37.47) mRNA level. In low and high KRT20 groups, CXCL9 mRNA was associated with a shorter RFS (RR = 3.04; $p = 0.019$ and RR = 3.28, respectively; $p = 0.007$) (Table 5). Similarly, low CXCL9 mRNA was associated with a shorter RFS in the low and high KRT5 groups (RR = 3.76; $p = 0.004$ and RR = 3.33; $p = 0.013$, respectively; Table 5). These results were expected since they reflected findings for all patients. In the high KRT5 and high KRT20 groups, low PD-L1 mRNA was associated with shorter RFS (RR = 3.68; $p = 0.012$ and RR = 4.23, respectively; $p = 0.009$; Table 5), but this was not so in the low KRT5 or low KRT20 group.

2.3.3. Stratification by KI67

KI67 characterizes the proliferation activity of tumor cells [29]. *KI67* expression was separated into two groups (low vs. high expression) by median mRNA (≤33.10 vs. >33.10). In the high *KI67* expression group, low *CXCL9* (RR = 4.54; $p < 0.001$) mRNA and low *PD-L1* (RR = 7.49; $p = 0.001$; Table 5) mRNA were associated with a higher risk of shorter RFS, but these associations were not observed in the low *KI67* group.

2.3.4. Stratification by Intravesical Therapy

Intravesical therapy was not associated with RFS in this study group. In the group with no intravesical therapy, low *CXCL9* (RR = 10.33; $p < 0.001$), low *PD1* (RR = 5.31; $p = 0.010$) and low *PD-L1* (RR = 4.36; $p = 0.022$; Table 5) mRNA was associated with the increased risk of shorter RFS, but no associations were observed with RFS in the intravesical group.

Altogether, *CXCL9* mRNA was associated with RFS in all stratification approaches. Interestingly, the increased risk of shorter RFS in low *CXCL9* mRNA patients was substantiated in the young patient group, the high *KI67* group and in patients without instillation, but it showed no association with RFS in the older patient group, the low *KI67* group or the instillation group.

In addition, the increased risk observed with low *PD1* levels was assigned to the younger patient group and the no instillation group, with no association with RFS being observed in the older patient group or the instillation patient group.

For the third marker, *PD-L1*, an increased risk of shorter RFS with low *PD-L1* mRNA was detected only in the high *KRT5* and high *KRT20* groups, but not in the low *KRT5* or low *KRT20* groups. In addition, this risk was found in the high *KI67* and the no instillation group, but not in the low *KI67* group or the instillation group.

3. Discussion

In this study, we investigated the mRNA of the immune markers CXCL9, PD1 and PD-L1. First, we correlated mRNA data with clinicopathological data and with each other. We observed that *CXCL9* mRNA was positively correlated with transcript levels of *PD1* and *PD-L1*, but negatively correlated with incidence of recurrence, as well as *KRT5* and *KRT20* mRNA. In addition, PD1 was positively correlated with *PD-L1* mRNA and time to RFS, while being negatively correlated with *KRT20* mRNA. *PD-L1* mRNA was additionally negatively correlated with *KRT20* mRNA.

Similar to Huang et al. we showed a correlation between the mRNA of *PD-L1* and *C-C chemokines* (*CCL2, CCL3, CCL8* and *CCL18*) [30,31]. A correlation between *PD1* and *PD-L1* mRNA was previously shown by both Huang et al. [31] and by us [28]. These correlations can all be explained by the common expression of these factors by immune cells, i.e., leukocytes such as T-cells and macrophages.

In this study, multivariate Cox's regression analyses revealed that high *CXCL9* mRNA was associated with longer OS and DSS, and high *PD-L1* mRNA was correlated with longer DSS. In addition, the high mRNA of *CXCL9* or *PD-L1* was significantly associated with longer RFS. Huang and colleagues found that elevated *PD-L1* mRNA was associated with reduced patient survival (OS, DSS), but they studied a mixed cohort of NMIBC and MIBC where the association could have been influenced by MIBC patients, and further, they did not examine RFS [31]. We previously found that increased *PD-L1* mRNA expression was associated with longer DSS and RFS in pT1 NMIBC [28]. In this study, we confirmed the association of high *PD-L1* mRNA with DSS and RFS. However, the impact of *PD-L1* on OS, DSS and RFS need to be evaluated further in prospective studies.

PD1 was previously not described to be associated with RFS [28], but in this study, we observed an association between increased *PD1* mRNA and longer RFS. Although both studies were performed in consecutive patients, in this study, observation time was longer (62 vs. 42 months), and the numbers of recurrences (51.3% vs. 33.4%) were higher than in the previous study, which may explain the differential results.

CXCL9 mRNA level has not been previously described in NMIBC to be associated with OS, DSS or RFS. The effect of an immune intravesical therapy with bacillus Calmette-Guérin (BCG) on *CXCL9* mRNA was controversially discussed. BCG therapy upregulates the mRNA of different chemokines, including *CXCL9*, in an in vivo mouse model [32]. Interestingly, using an in vitro approach in established human BCa cell lines, Özcan et al. demonstrated that BCG treatment reduced *CXCL9* mRNA [33]. This supports the assumption that the tumor microenvironment is responsible for the chemokine reaction following BCG therapy. A recent review reports that the CXCL9/CXCL10/CXCL11/CXCR3 axis is responsible for angiogenesis inhibition, and the activation and migration of immune cells such as cytotoxic lymphocytes and natural killer cells into the tumor microenvironment, to prevent tumor progression in BCa [34].

Next, we were interested in whether the association of *CXCL9*, *PD1* and *PD-L1* mRNA with RFS could be further stratified by clinicopathological parameter (age) or other parameters applied for lineage differentiation, such as *KRT5* or *KRT20* mRNA, proliferation activity (*KI67*), or therapeutic application (instillation therapy). Interestingly, after separating patients by their median age (≤71 vs. >71 years), only in the younger age group (≤71 years) was higher *CXCL9* or higher *PD1* mRNA associated with longer RFS. This finding could be simply related to the fact that the immune system is more active in younger than in older persons, in whom immunosenescence has been reported [35]. Increasing multi morbidity affecting health status in elderly patients may also play a role in shorter RFS, although time to recurrence was not significantly different between the age groups (data not shown).

KRT5 and *KRT20* are considered intrinsic markers for basal and luminal subtypes of muscle-invasive bladder cancer, respectively [11,36,37]. Interestingly, high *PD-L1* mRNA was associated with longer RFS in both high *KRT5* and high *KRT20* groups, but not in the low *KRT5* or low *KRT20* groups. This finding suggests that high *PD-L1* mRNA is favorable for longer RFS in both basal and luminal subtypes of NMIBC. We previously showed that high *KRT20* mRNA was associated with shorter RFS [38]. In this context, *PD-L1* mRNA further distinguishes the unfavorable RFS group (high *KRT20*) in patients with longer RFS (*PD-L1* high) or shorter RFS (*PD-L1* low).

High KI67 expression has been described as a prognostic factor for poor OS, DSS, RFS and PFS in a meta-analysis of NMIBC patients [12]. In the high *KI67* group, high *CXCL9* and high *PD-L1* mRNA were associated with longer RFS, but this association was not observed in the low *KI67* group. In this way, within the unfavorable high *KI67* group, patients with longer RFS (high *CXCL9* or high *PD-L1*) and with shorter RFS (low *CXCL9* or low *PD-L1*) could be distinguished.

Intravesical therapy with either BCG or cytostatic drugs, like mitomycin, is mostly standard therapy for intermediate or high risk NMIBC, but its application differs between several guidelines [3,5]. Interestingly, only in the no instillation group was high *CXCL9*, high *PD1* or high *PD-L1* associated with longer RFS compared to the instillation group. One explanation for this finding could be that BCG therapy affects the immune response of patients, and *CXCL9*, *PD1* and *PD-L1* reflect intrinsic immune status. In this way, both the expression of the immune markers and the intravesical therapy may influence each other. As mentioned above, the BCG exposure of established BCa cell lines devoid of any tumor microenvironment reduced *CXCL9* mRNA in vitro [33]. Furthermore, increases in PD-L1 protein levels, which are considered a negative prognostic marker, have been reported after BCG therapy compared to before BCG treatment [39].

4. Material and Methods

4.1. Patients and Tumor Material

In this study, we retrospectively analyzed clinical and histopathological data from 80 patients treated with TURB at the Department of Urology and Pediatric Urology of the University Hospital Erlangen between 2000 and 2015 who were initially diagnosed with stage pT1 NMIBC (Table 6). All patients received a Re-TURB within six to eight weeks after the initial TURB. All patients were treated with a bladder-preserving approach. Tissue from formalin-fixed paraffin embedded (FFPE) tumor samples from all patients was evaluated for pathological stage according to the 2010 TNM classification [40], and was graded according to the common grading systems [41,42] by two experienced uropathologists (M.E., A.H.). All specimens contained at least 20% tumor cells. All procedures were performed in accordance with the ethical standards established in the 1964 Declaration of Helsinki and its later amendments. All patients treated after 2008 provided informed consent. For samples collected prior to 2008, the Ethics Committee in Erlangen waived the need for informed individual consent. This study was approved by the Ethics Committee of the University Hospital Erlangen (No. 3755; 2008).

Table 6. Clinicopathological and survival data.

Clinicopathological and Survival Parameters	Patients (Percentage)
Total	80
Gender	
female	19 (23.7)
male	61 (76.3)
Age (years)	
range	46.0–97.0
mean	70.5
median	71.5
Tumor Stage	
pT1	52 (65.0)
pT1 with cis	28 (35.0)
Tumor Grade 1973	
G1	3 (3.7)
G2	28 (35.0)
G3	48 (60.0)
unknown	1 (1.3)
Tumor Grade 2004	
low grade	3 (3.7)
high grade	76 (95.0)
unknown	1 (1.3)
Intravesical Therapy	
yes	41 (51.3)
no	39 (48.7)
Survival/observation Time (months)	
range	0–189.0
mean	71.6
median	62.0
Overall Survival (OS)	
alive	44 (55.0)
dead	36 (45.0)
Disease-Specific Survival (DSS)	
alive	64 (80.0)
dead	16 (20.0)
Recurrence-Free Survival Time (months)	
range	0–149
mean	46.7
median	38.5
Recurrence-Free Survival (RFS)	
without recurrence	39 (48.7)
with recurrence	41 (51.3)

4.2. Assessment of mRNA by qRT-PCR

Tumor specimens were assessed by qRT-PCR as previously described [43]. In short, RNA was extracted from a single 10 µm curl of FFPE tissue and processed according to a commercially available bead-based extraction method (Xtract kit; Stratifyer Molecular Pathology GmbH, Cologne, Germany). RNA was eluted with 100 µL of elution buffer. DNA was digested, and RNA eluates were then stored at −80 °C until use.

The mRNA levels of CXCL9, PD1, PD-L1, KRT5, KRT20, KI67 and the reference genes *Calmodulin2* (*CALM2*) and *Beta-2 microglobulin* (*B2 M*) were determined by a one-step qRT-PCR using the SuperScript III RT-qPCR system (Invitrogen, Waltham, MA, USA) and gene specific primer-probe combinations (Stratifyer). Each patient sample or control was analyzed in duplicate in an ABI Step One PCR System (ThermoFisher, Darmstadt, Germany) according to the manufacturers' instructions. Gene expression was quantified with a modification of the method by Schmittgen and Livak by calculating 40-ΔCt, whereas ΔCt was calculated as the difference in Ct between the test gene and the mean of the reference genes [38,44].

4.3. Statistical Methods

Correlations between the mRNA of CXCL9, PD1, PD-L1, KRT5, KRT20 and KI67 and clinicopathological data were calculated using Spearman's bivariate correlation. Optimized cut-off values for dichotomizing each marker with respect to survival were defined using Youden's index on the receiver operating characteristic (ROC). Detailed information about the calculated optimal cut-off values, the associated area under the ROC curve and internal validation using bootstrapping are provided in Tables S1 and S2. Following standard practice in retrospective survival analysis, the common time point zero for all patients was the date of the first TURB. The associations of mRNA with recurrence-free survival (RFS), overall survival (OS) and cancer-specific survival (CSS) were determined by univariate (Kaplan–Meier analysis and Cox's regression hazard models) and multivariate (Cox's regression hazard models, adjusted for age and the molecular parameters PD1, PD-L1 and CXCL9) analyses. A p-value < 0.05 was considered statistically significant. Statistical analyses were performed with the SPSS 21.0 software package (SPSS Inc., Chicago, IL, USA) and R V3.2.1 (The R foundation for statistical computing, Vienna, Austria).

5. Conclusions

Altogether, we confirmed that high PD-L1 mRNA is associated with increased DSS and RFS. Furthermore, we demonstrated for the first time that CXCL9 mRNA is associated with a longer OS, DSS and RFS. Associations with RFS were also identified or further pinpointed to special groups, including the younger age group (CXCL9, PD1), the high KRT5 or high KRT20 group (CXCL9, PD-L1), the high KI67 group (CXCL9, PD-L1) or the no instillation group (CXCL9, PD-L1).

An increased mRNA for PD1, PD-L1 and CXCL9 being associated with a better prognosis may mirror the host–tumor interaction. In this way, we suggest that the increased mRNA levels of all three genes may reflect the immune response of the host.

Our finding of associations between these immune markers and prognosis may aid in future therapeutic options and decisions.

Supplementary Materials: The following are available online at http://www.mdpi.com/2072-6694/12/10/2794/s1. Table S1: Optimized Ct cutoff values and internal validation and Table S2: Area under the ROC curve and internal validation.

Author Contributions: D.S., H.T., S.W., R.M.W. and B.K. designed the study. D.S., J.K., S.W., V.W., R.S., A.H. and B.W. acquired the clinical samples and patient information. A.H. and M.E. performed the pathological review of all cases. J.K. and A.N. performed qRT-PCR experiments. H.T., S.W., D.S. and J.K. performed statistical analyses, and H.T., S.W., J.K., D.S., M.E. prepared the tables and figures. H.T., S.W., D.S., B.W., M.E. and A.H. wrote the main manuscript. All authors reviewed the manuscript and approved the final version of the manuscript.

Funding: This study was funded by the ELAN Fund (ELAN 18"C08-18"C1-Sikic) and was supported by the Interdisciplinary Center for Clinical Research (IZKF) at the University Hospital of the Friedrich-Alexander University Erlangen-Nuremberg. We thank the Rudolf und Irmgard Kleinknecht-Stiftung for supporting H.T., and the Johannes und Frieda Marohn-Stiftung and the Wilhelm Sander-Stiftung for supporting S.W. and H.T.

Acknowledgments: The present work was performed in (partial) fulfillment of the requirements for obtaining the degree "Dr. med." (M.D.) of the Friedrich-Alexander-Universität Erlangen-Nürnberg, Medizinische Fakultät for Jennifer Kubon. The authors thank Johannes Breyer (University of Regensburg) and Philipp Erben (Heidelberg University) for helpful discussion. We thank American Journal Experts for editing the manuscript. The authors also acknowledge support from Deutsche Forschungsgemeinschaft and Friedrich-Alexander-Universität Erlangen-Nürnberg within the funding program Open Access Publishing.

Conflicts of Interest: The authors declare that there are no financial and/or nonfinancial conflicts of interest.

Abbreviations

BCa	bladder cancer
CXCL9	Chemokine, CXC motif, ligand 9
DSS	disease-free survival
Fu recur	follow up recurrence
KI67	Proliferation marker KI67
KRT5	Cytokeratin 5
KRT20	Cytokeratin 20
MIBC	muscle invasive bladder cancer
NMIBC	non-muscle invasive bladder cancer
OS	overall survival
n.s.	not significant
n.d.	not determined
PD1	programmed cell death 1
PD-L1	programmed cell death ligand 1
PFS	progression-free survival
pT	pathological tumor stage
pN	pathological lymph node stage
qRT-PCR	quantitative real-time PCR
RFS	recurrence-free survival

References

1. Bray, F.; Ferlay, J.; Soerjomataram, I.; Siegel, R.L.; Torre, L.A.; Jemal, A. Global cancer statistics 2018: GLOBOCAN estimates of incidence and mortality worldwide for 36 cancers in 185 countries. *CA Cancer J. Clin.* **2018**, *68*, 394–424. [CrossRef] [PubMed]
2. Burger, M.; Catto, J.W.; Dalbagni, G.; Grossman, H.B.; Herr, H.; Karakiewicz, P.; Kassouf, W.; Kiemeney, L.A.; La Vecchia, C.; Shariat, S.; et al. Epidemiology and risk factors of urothelial bladder cancer. *Eur. Urol.* **2013**, *63*, 234–241. [CrossRef] [PubMed]
3. Babjuk, M.; Bohle, A.; Burger, M.; Capoun, O.; Cohen, D.; Comperat, E.M.; Hernandez, V.; Kaasinen, E.; Palou, J.; Roupret, M.; et al. EAU Guidelines on Non-Muscle-invasive Urothelial Carcinoma of the Bladder: Update 2016. *Eur. Urol.* **2017**, *71*, 447–461. [CrossRef] [PubMed]
4. Novotny, V.; Froehner, M.; Ollig, J.; Koch, R.; Zastrow, S.; Wirth, M.P. Impact of Adjuvant Intravesical Bacillus Calmette-Guerin Treatment on Patients with High-Grade T1 Bladder Cancer. *Urol. Int.* **2016**, *96*, 136–141. [CrossRef] [PubMed]
5. Zhang, J.; Wang, Y.; Weng, H.; Wang, D.; Han, F.; Huang, Q.; Deng, T.; Wang, X.; Jin, Y. Management of non-muscle-invasive bladder cancer: Quality of clinical practice guidelines and variations in recommendations. *BMC Cancer* **2019**, *19*, 1054. [CrossRef] [PubMed]
6. D'Andrea, D.; Hassler, M.R.; Abufaraj, M.; Soria, F.; Ertl, I.E.; Ilijazi, D.; Mari, A.; Foerster, B.; Egger, G.; Shariat, S.F. Progressive tissue biomarker profiling in non-muscle-invasive bladder cancer. *Expert Rev. Anticancer Ther.* **2018**, *18*, 695–703. [CrossRef]
7. Stein, J.P.; Penson, D.F. Invasive T1 bladder cancer: Indications and rationale for radical cystectomy. *BJU Int.* **2008**, *102*, 270–275. [CrossRef]

8. Thalmann, G.N.; Markwalder, R.; Shahin, O.; Burkhard, F.C.; Hochreiter, W.W.; Studer, U.E. Primary T1G3 bladder cancer: Organ preserving approach or immediate cystectomy? *J. Urol.* **2004**, *172*, 70–75. [CrossRef]
9. van Rhijn, B.W.; Burger, M.; Lotan, Y.; Solsona, E.; Stief, C.G.; Sylvester, R.J.; Witjes, J.A.; Zlotta, A.R. Recurrence and progression of disease in non-muscle-invasive bladder cancer: From epidemiology to treatment strategy. *Eur. Urol.* **2009**, *56*, 430–442. [CrossRef]
10. Hong, Y.M.; Loughlin, K.R. Economic impact of tumor markers in bladder cancer surveillance. *Urology* **2008**, *71*, 131–135. [CrossRef]
11. Choi, W.; Porten, S.; Kim, S.; Willis, D.; Plimack, E.R.; Hoffman-Censits, J.; Roth, B.; Cheng, T.; Tran, M.; Lee, I.L.; et al. Identification of distinct basal and luminal subtypes of muscle-invasive bladder cancer with different sensitivities to frontline chemotherapy. *Cancer Cell* **2014**, *25*, 152–165. [CrossRef] [PubMed]
12. Ko, K.; Jeong, C.W.; Kwak, C.; Kim, H.H.; Ku, J.H. Significance of Ki-67 in non-muscle invasive bladder cancer patients: A systematic review and meta-analysis. *Oncotarget* **2017**, *8*, 100614–100630. [CrossRef] [PubMed]
13. Robertson, A.G.; Kim, J.; Al-Ahmadie, H.; Bellmunt, J.; Guo, G.; Cherniack, A.D.; Hinoue, T.; Laird, P.W.; Hoadley, K.A.; Akbani, R.; et al. Comprehensive Molecular Characterization of Muscle-Invasive Bladder Cancer. *Cell* **2017**, *171*, 540–556. [CrossRef] [PubMed]
14. Dyrskjot, L.; Ingersoll, M.A. Biology of nonmuscle-invasive bladder cancer: Pathology, genomic implications, and immunology. *Curr. Opin. Urol.* **2018**, *28*, 598–603. [CrossRef] [PubMed]
15. Hedegaard, J.; Lamy, P.; Nordentoft, I.; Algaba, F.; Hoyer, S.; Ulhoi, B.P.; Vang, S.; Reinert, T.; Hermann, G.G.; Mogensen, K.; et al. Comprehensive Transcriptional Analysis of Early-Stage Urothelial Carcinoma. *Cancer Cell* **2016**, *30*, 27–42. [CrossRef] [PubMed]
16. Eckstein, M.; Strissel, P.; Strick, R.; Weyerer, V.; Wirtz, R.; Pfannstiel, C.; Wullweber, A.; Lange, F.; Erben, P.; Stoehr, R.; et al. Cytotoxic T-cell-related gene expression signature predicts improved survival in muscle-invasive urothelial bladder cancer patients after radical cystectomy and adjuvant chemotherapy. *J. Immunother. Cancer* **2020**, *8*. [CrossRef]
17. Jiang, Z.; Hsu, J.L.; Li, Y.; Hortobagyi, G.N.; Hung, M.C. Cancer Cell Metabolism Bolsters Immunotherapy Resistance by Promoting an Immunosuppressive Tumor Microenvironment. *Front. Oncol.* **2020**, *10*, 1197. [CrossRef]
18. Pfannstiel, C.; Strissel, P.L.; Chiappinelli, K.B.; Sikic, D.; Wach, S.; Wirtz, R.M.; Wullweber, A.; Taubert, H.; Breyer, J.; Otto, W.; et al. The Tumor Immune Microenvironment Drives a Prognostic Relevance That Correlates with Bladder Cancer Subtypes. *Cancer Immunol. Res.* **2019**, *7*, 923–938. [CrossRef]
19. Lee, H.H.; Farber, J.M. Localization of the gene for the human MIG cytokine on chromosome 4q21 adjacent to INP10 reveals a chemokine "mini-cluster". *Cytogenet. Cell Genet.* **1996**, *74*, 255–258. [CrossRef]
20. Do, H.T.T.; Lee, C.H.; Cho, J. Chemokines and their Receptors: Multifaceted Roles in Cancer Progression and Potential Value as Cancer Prognostic Markers. *Cancers* **2020**, *12*, 287. [CrossRef]
21. Farber, J.M. HuMig: A new human member of the chemokine family of cytokines. *Biochem. Biophys. Res. Commun.* **1993**, *192*, 223–230. [CrossRef] [PubMed]
22. Shinohara, T.; Taniwaki, M.; Ishida, Y.; Kawaichi, M.; Honjo, T. Structure and chromosomal localization of the human PD-1 gene (PDCD1). *Genomics* **1994**, *23*, 704–706. [CrossRef] [PubMed]
23. Freeman, G.J.; Long, A.J.; Iwai, Y.; Bourque, K.; Chernova, T.; Nishimura, H.; Fitz, L.J.; Malenkovich, N.; Okazaki, T.; Byrne, M.C.; et al. Engagement of the PD-1 immunoinhibitory receptor by a novel B7 family member leads to negative regulation of lymphocyte activation. *J. Exp. Med.* **2000**, *192*, 1027–1034. [CrossRef] [PubMed]
24. Gordon, S.R.; Maute, R.L.; Dulken, B.W.; Hutter, G.; George, B.M.; McCracken, M.N.; Gupta, R.; Tsai, J.M.; Sinha, R.; Corey, D.; et al. PD-1 expression by tumour-associated macrophages inhibits phagocytosis and tumour immunity. *Nature* **2017**, *545*, 495–499. [CrossRef] [PubMed]
25. Dong, H.; Zhu, G.; Tamada, K.; Chen, L. B7-H1, a third member of the B7 family, co-stimulates T-cell proliferation and interleukin-10 secretion. *Nat. Med.* **1999**, *5*, 1365–1369. [CrossRef]
26. Bardhan, K.; Anagnostou, T.; Boussiotis, V.A. The PD1:PD-L1/2 Pathway from Discovery to Clinical Implementation. *Front. Immunol.* **2016**, *7*, 550. [CrossRef]
27. Le Goux, C.; Damotte, D.; Vacher, S.; Sibony, M.; Delongchamps, N.B.; Schnitzler, A.; Terris, B.; Zerbib, M.; Bieche, I.; Pignot, G. Correlation between messenger RNA expression and protein expression of immune checkpoint-associated molecules in bladder urothelial carcinoma: A retrospective study. *Urol. Oncol.* **2017**, *35*, 257–263. [CrossRef]

28. Breyer, J.; Wirtz, R.M.; Otto, W.; Erben, P.; Worst, T.S.; Stoehr, R.; Eckstein, M.; Denzinger, S.; Burger, M.; Hartmann, A. High PDL1 mRNA expression predicts better survival of stage pT1 non-muscle-invasive bladder cancer (NMIBC) patients. *Cancer Immunol. Immunother.* **2018**, *67*, 403–412. [CrossRef]
29. Gerdes, J.; Schwab, U.; Lemke, H.; Stein, H. Production of a mouse monoclonal antibody reactive with a human nuclear antigen associated with cell proliferation. *Int. J. Cancer* **1983**, *31*, 13–20. [CrossRef]
30. Eckstein, M.; Epple, E.; Jung, R.; Weigelt, K.; Lieb, V.; Sikic, D.; Stohr, R.; Geppert, C.; Weyerer, V.; Bertz, S.; et al. CCL2 Expression in Tumor Cells and Tumor-Infiltrating Immune Cells Shows Divergent Prognostic Potential for Bladder Cancer Patients Depending on Lymph Node Stage. *Cancers* **2020**, *12*, 1253. [CrossRef]
31. Huang, Y.; Zhang, S.D.; McCrudden, C.; Chan, K.W.; Lin, Y.; Kwok, H.F. The prognostic significance of PD-L1 in bladder cancer. *Oncol. Rep.* **2015**, *33*, 3075–3084. [CrossRef] [PubMed]
32. Seow, S.W.; Rahmat, J.N.; Bay, B.H.; Lee, Y.K.; Mahendran, R. Expression of chemokine/cytokine genes and immune cell recruitment following the instillation of Mycobacterium bovis, bacillus Calmette-Guerin or Lactobacillus rhamnosus strain GG in the healthy murine bladder. *Immunology* **2008**, *124*, 419–427. [CrossRef] [PubMed]
33. Ozcan, Y.; Caglar, F.; Celik, S.; Demir, A.B.; Ercetin, A.P.; Altun, Z.; Aktas, S. The role of cancer stem cells in immunotherapy for bladder cancer: An in vitro study. *Urol. Oncol.* **2020**, *38*, 476–487. [CrossRef] [PubMed]
34. Nazari, A.; Ahmadi, Z.; Hassanshahi, G.; Abbasifard, M.; Taghipour, Z.; Falahati-Pour, S.K.; Khorramdelazad, H. Effective Treatments for Bladder Cancer Affecting CXCL9/CXCL10/CXCL11/CXCR3 Axis: A Review. *Oman Med. J.* **2020**, *35*, e103. [CrossRef] [PubMed]
35. Morgia, G.; Russo, G.I.; Berretta, M.; Privitera, S.; Kirkali, Z. Genito-urological cancers in elderly patients. *Anticancer Agents Med. Chem.* **2013**, *13*, 1391–1405. [CrossRef]
36. Damrauer, J.S.; Hoadley, K.A.; Chism, D.D.; Fan, C.; Tiganelli, C.J.; Wobker, S.E.; Yeh, J.J.; Milowsky, M.I.; Iyer, G.; Parker, J.S.; et al. Intrinsic subtypes of high-grade bladder cancer reflect the hallmarks of breast cancer biology. *Proc. Natl. Acad. Sci. USA* **2014**, *111*, 3110–3115. [CrossRef]
37. Lerner, S.P.; McConkey, D.J.; Hoadley, K.A.; Chan, K.S.; Kim, W.Y.; Radvanyi, F.; Hoglund, M.; Real, F.X. Bladder Cancer Molecular Taxonomy: Summary from a Consensus Meeting. *Bladder Cancer* **2016**, *2*, 37–47. [CrossRef]
38. Breyer, J.; Wirtz, R.M.; Otto, W.; Erben, P.; Kriegmair, M.C.; Stoehr, R.; Eckstein, M.; Eidt, S.; Denzinger, S.; Burger, M.; et al. In stage pT1 non-muscle-invasive bladder cancer (NMIBC), high KRT20 and low KRT5 mRNA expression identify the luminal subtype and predict recurrence and survival. *Virchows Arch.* **2017**, *470*, 267–274. [CrossRef]
39. Hashizume, A.; Umemoto, S.; Yokose, T.; Nakamura, Y.; Yoshihara, M.; Shoji, K.; Wada, S.; Miyagi, Y.; Kishida, T.; Sasada, T. Enhanced expression of PD-L1 in non-muscle-invasive bladder cancer after treatment with Bacillus Calmette-Guerin. *Oncotarget* **2018**, *9*, 34066–34078. [CrossRef]
40. Sobin, L.H.; Gospodarowicz, M.K.; Wittekind, C. *TNM Classification of Malignant Tumours*, 7th ed.; Wiley-Blackwell: Oxford, UK, 2010.
41. Mostofi, F.K.; Sobin, L.H.; Torloni, H. *Histological Typing of Urinary Bladder Tumours*; World Health Organization: Geneva, Switzerland, 1973.
42. Eble, J.N.; Sauter, G.; Epstein, J.I.; Sesterhenn, I.A. *Pathology and Genetics of Tumours of the Urinary System*; IARCPress: Lyon, France, 2004.
43. Sikic, D.; Breyer, J.; Hartmann, A.; Burger, M.; Erben, P.; Denzinger, S.; Eckstein, M.; Stohr, R.; Wach, S.; Wullich, B.; et al. High Androgen Receptor mRNA Expression Is Independently Associated with Prolonged Cancer-Specific and Recurrence-Free Survival in Stage T1 Bladder Cancer. *Transl. Oncol.* **2017**, *10*, 340–345. [CrossRef]
44. Schmittgen, T.D.; Livak, K.J. Analyzing real-time PCR data by the comparative C(T) method. *Nat. Protoc.* **2008**, *3*, 1101–1108. [CrossRef] [PubMed]

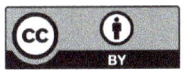

© 2020 by the authors. Licensee MDPI, Basel, Switzerland. This article is an open access article distributed under the terms and conditions of the Creative Commons Attribution (CC BY) license (http://creativecommons.org/licenses/by/4.0/).

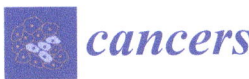

Article

Epidemiological Characteristics and Survival in Patients with De Novo Metastatic Prostate Cancer

Carlo Cattrini [1,2,*], Davide Soldato [1,3], Alessandra Rubagotti [3,4], Linda Zinoli [3], Elisa Zanardi [1,3], Paola Barboro [3], Carlo Messina [5], Elena Castro [6], David Olmos [2] and Francesco Boccardo [1,3]

1. Department of Internal Medicine and Medical Specialties (DIMI), School of Medicine, University of Genoa, 16132 Genoa, Italy; davide.soldato@gmail.com (D.S.); elisa.zanardi@unige.it (E.Z.); fboccardo@unige.it (F.B.)
2. Prostate Cancer Clinical Research Unit, Spanish National Cancer Research Centre (CNIO), 28029 Madrid, Spain; dolmos@cnio.es
3. Academic Unit of Medical Oncology, IRCCS Ospedale Policlinico San Martino, 16132 Genoa, Italy; alessandra.rubagotti@unige.it (A.R.); datamanager.omb@unige.it (L.Z.); paola.barboro@hsanmartino.it (P.B.)
4. Department of Health Sciences (DISSAL), School of Medicine, University of Genoa, 16132 Genoa, Italy
5. Department of Medical Oncology, Santa Chiara Hospital, 38122 Trento, Italy; carlo.messina@apss.tn.it
6. CNIO-IBIMA Genitourinary Cancer Unit, Hospitales Universitarios Virgen de la Victoria y Regional de Málaga, Instituto de Investigación Biomédica de Málaga, 29010 Malaga, Spain; ecastro@ext.cnio.es
* Correspondence: ccattrini@cnio.es

Received: 22 September 2020; Accepted: 1 October 2020; Published: 3 October 2020

Simple Summary: In randomized trials, both chemotherapy and androgen-receptor signaling inhibitors provided significant survival benefits in patients with metastatic prostate cancer (mPCa). However, it is largely unknown to what extent these therapeutic advances have impacted the general, real-world survival of patients with de novo mPCa. Here, we analyzed more than 26,000 patients included in the U.S. Surveillance, Epidemiology, and End Results (SEER) database to describe potential recent improvements in overall and cancer-specific survival. We found that patients diagnosed in the latest years showed a modest reduction in the risk of death and cancer-specific death, compared with those diagnosed in 2000–2003 and 2004–2010. Although our analysis was not adjusted for many confounders, the overall population of patients diagnosed in 2011–2014 only showed a survival gain of 4 months. Patients' ineligibility or refusal of anticancer treatments, insurance issues, intrinsic disease aggressiveness, or prior unavailability of drugs in a hormone-sensitive setting might contribute to these disappointing results.

Abstract: The real-world outcomes of patients with metastatic prostate cancer (mPCa) are largely unexplored. We investigated the trends in overall survival (OS) and cancer-specific survival (CSS) in patients with de novo mPCa according to distinct time periods. The U.S. Surveillance, Epidemiology, and End Results (SEER) Research Data (2000–2017) were analyzed using the SEER*Stat software. The Kaplan– Meier method and Cox regression were used. Patients with de novo mPCa were allocated to three cohorts based on the year of diagnosis: A (2000–2003), B (2004–2010), and C (2011–2014). The maximum follow-up was fixed to 5 years. Overall, 26,434 patients were included. Age, race, and metastatic stage (M1) significantly affected OS and CSS. After adjustment for age and race, patients in Cohort C showed a 9% reduced risk of death (hazard ratio (HR): 0.91 (95% confidence interval [CI] 0.87–0.95), $p < 0.001$) and an 8% reduced risk of cancer-specific death (HR: 0.92 (95% CI 0.88–0.96), $p < 0.001$) compared with those in Cohort A. After adjustment for age, race, and metastatic stage, patients in Cohort C showed an improvement in OS and CSS compared with Cohort B (HR: 0.94 (95% CI 0.91–0.97), $p = 0.001$; HR: 0.89 (95% CI 0.85–0.92), $p < 0.001$). Patients with M1c disease had a more pronounced improvement in OS and CSS compared with the other stages. No differences were found between Cohorts B and C. In conclusion, the real-world survival of de novo mPCa remains poor, with a median OS and CSS improvement of only 4 months in the latest years.

Keywords: prostatic neoplasms/mortality; prostatic neoplasms/epidemiology; SEER Program

1. Introduction

The treatment landscape of metastatic prostate cancer (mPCa) has completely changed over the last decades. In 2004, docetaxel was the first drug to demonstrate an overall survival (OS) benefit of 2.4 months in mPCa, compared with mitoxantrone, and was approved for the treatment of men with metastatic castration-resistant prostate cancer (mCRPC) [1]. Cabazitaxel showed a similar OS increase compared with mitoxantrone and became a second-line treatment option for mCRPC in 2010 [2]. Subsequently, abiraterone acetate and enzalutamide were approved in both post-docetaxel [3,4] (2011–2012) and pre-docetaxel mCRPC [5,6] (2013–2014), reporting OS advantages between 4.0 and 4.8 months compared with placebo (Figure 1). Docetaxel was also introduced for the hormone-sensitive phase of mPCa (mHSPC) in 2015 [7]. Several androgen-receptor signaling inhibitors (ARSi)—abiraterone, enzalutamide, and apalutamide—were then approved for the treatment of mHSPC [8].

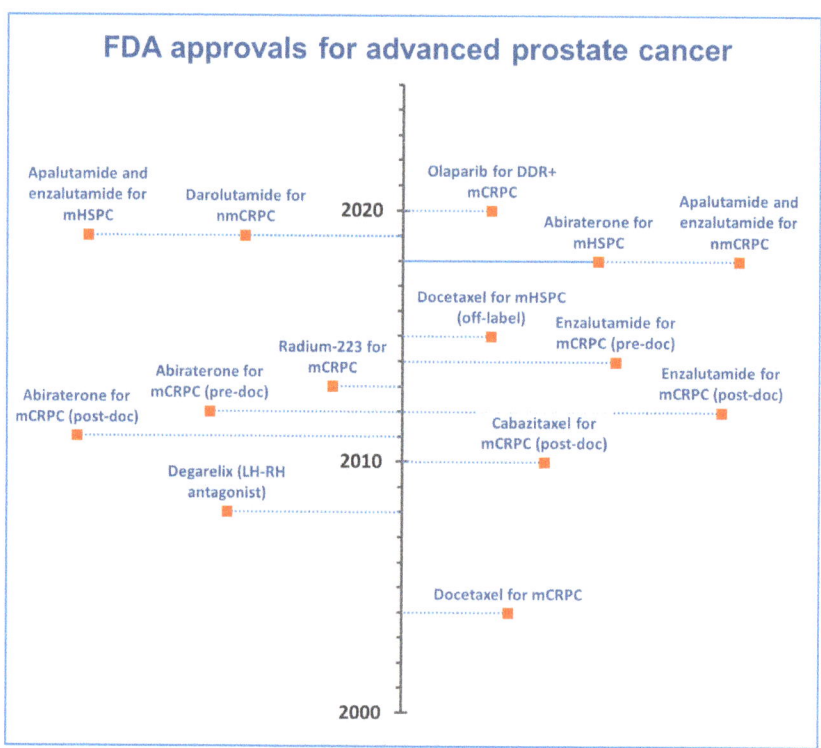

Figure 1. Regulatory timeline of approvals in advanced prostate cancer therapies. DDR+: DNA damage response genes mutated; mHSPC: metastatic hormone-sensitive prostate cancer; mCRPC: metastatic castration-resistant prostate cancer; nmCRPC: nonmetastatic castration-resistant prostate cancer; post-doc: post-docetaxel; pre-doc: pre-docetaxel.

Although the aforementioned randomized trials showed significant survival improvements in the first- and second-line of mCRPC, the real-world survival benefit in the population of patients outside of clinical trials is largely unexplored. The ideal population of patients enrolled in clinical trials might overestimate the true benefit induced by approved drugs in the general population of patients with newly diagnosed mPCa. For example, not all patients can receive chemotherapy. Although no specific advice is included in the U.S. National Comprehensive Cancer Network guidelines, the European Association of Urology guidelines recommend that docetaxel should be only offered to mHSPC patients who are fit enough for chemotherapy [9]. Of note, the STAMPEDE trial of docetaxel in mHSPC only included patients fit for chemotherapy and without significant cardiovascular history. Many patients with mPCa in the real-world are elderly with many comorbidities, and they cannot receive chemotherapy [10]. In addition, patients with poor general conditions or poor performance status are often not suitable for aggressive anticancer therapies. Moreover, although some retrospective data have been reported [11], no randomized trial has ever assessed the long-term, cumulative benefit on survival that can derive from the temporal sequence of different treatment strategies. Finally, the U.S. insurance policies or limited access to healthcare services could contribute to producing a discrepancy between the expected survival gain and the real-world data [12].

Here, we investigated the survival trends and prognostic variables in patients with de novo mPCa included in the U.S. Surveillance, Epidemiology, and End Results (SEER) database. Given the introduction of chemotherapy in 2004 and of ARSi in 2011, we hypothesized that a significant difference in OS and cancer-specific survival (CSS) was detectable in patients diagnosed in three time periods: 2000–2003 (Cohort A), 2004–2010 (Cohort B), and 2011–2014 (Cohort C). Of note, our study should not be intended to provide data on the efficacy of the newer treatments, but to provide epidemiological results about the survival trends in patients with de novo mPCa diagnosed in the United States in the last two decades.

2. Results

2.1. Study Cohort

Our selection criteria identified 26,434 patients with de novo mPCa diagnosed between 2000 and 2014. Of these, 6047 were diagnosed between 2000 and 2003 (Cohort A), 11,815 between 2004 and 2010 (Cohort B), and 8572 between 2011 and 2014 (Cohort C). The main characteristics of the study population are summarized in Table 1. Overall, 68.3% of patients were ≥65 years. The percentage of patients younger than 75 years was higher in Cohort C compared to Cohorts B and A (64.8% vs. 61.1% vs. 58.3%, respectively). The majority of patients were white (62.7%), followed by black (19.4%) and Hispanic (11.6%). Metastatic classification (American Joint Committee on Cancer (AJCC), 6th edition) was available for Cohorts B and C. The majority of patients were M1b (72.7%), with a significant difference between Cohorts B (70.1%) and C (76.4%). The full contingency table with the comparison of baseline characteristics among the cohorts is available in Table S1. The median follow-up was 25, 26, and 29 months in Cohorts A, B, and C, respectively, with a median follow-up of censored patients of 60, 60, and 51 months.

2.2. Clinical Outcome and Prognostic Variables

In the 26,434 patients analyzed for OS, the median values for OS in Cohorts A, B, and C were 26 (95% confidence interval (CI) 25.0–27.0), 26 (95% CI 25.3–26.7), and 30 (95% CI 29.1–30.9) months (Figure 2A). In the 26,032 patients analyzed for CSS, the median values of CSS were 31 (95% CI 29.7–32.3), 31 (95% CI 30.1–31.9), and 35 months (95% CI 32.4–33.6) in Cohorts A, B, and C, respectively (Figure 2B). The detailed age-standardized 1- to 5-year OS and CSS are shown in Figure 3.

Table 1. Basal characteristics of patients.

Variables		Number of Patients (%)			
		Total	2000–2003	2004–2010	2011–2014
Age (years)	15–54	2087 (7.9)	474 (7.8)	970 (8.2)	643 (7.5)
	55–64	6323 (23.9)	1250 (20.7)	2857 (24.2)	2216 (25.9)
	65–74	7892 (29.9)	1804 (29.8)	3391 (28.7)	2697 (31.5)
	75–84	7099 (26.9)	1862 (30.8)	3268 (27.7)	1969 (23.0)
	≥85	3033 (11.5)	657 (10.9)	1329 (11.2)	1047 (12.2)
	Total	26,434 (100)	6047 (100)	11,815 (100)	8572 (100)
Race	White	16,513 (62.7)	3830 (63.5)	7361 (62.5)	5322 (62.3)
	Black	5111 (19.4)	1227 (20.3)	2279 (19.3)	1605 (18.8)
	Am. Indian/Alaska Native	170 (0.6)	31 (0.5)	76 (0.6)	63 (0.7)
	Asian or Pacific Islander	1484 (5.6)	329 (5.4)	680 (5.8)	475 (5.6)
	Hispanic	3066 (11.6)	614 (10.2)	1377 (11.7)	1075 (12.6)
	Total	26,344 (100)	6031 (100)	11,773 (100)	8540 (100)
Metastatic stage	M1a	1097 (5.6)	-	610 (5.3)	487 (5.9)
	M1b	14,301 (72.7)	-	8011 (70.1)	6290 (76.4)
	M1c	4265 (21.7)	-	2811 (24.6)	1454 (17.7)
	Total	19,663 (100)	-	11,432 (100)	8231 (100)

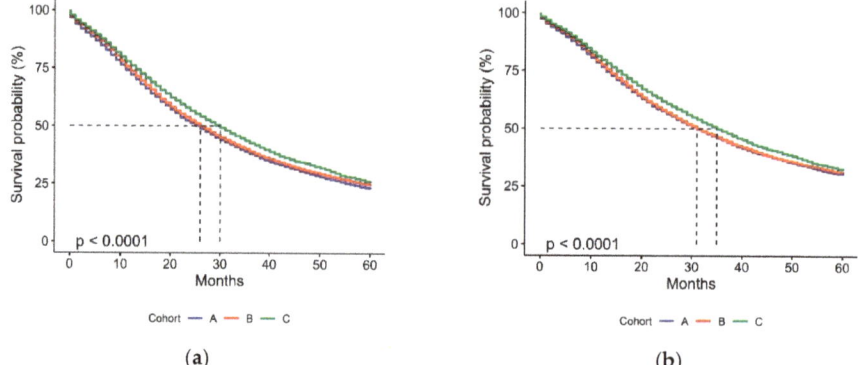

Figure 2. Kaplan–Meier estimations of overall survival (OS) (a) and cancer-specific survival (CSS) (b) according to cohort allocation. p-value from log-rank test.

Age, race, and metastatic stage (the latter was only analyzed in Cohorts B and C) were identified as significant prognostic factors at univariate analysis (data not shown) and were included in the multivariable models.

2.3. Multivariable Models

The multivariable models for OS and CSS showed a substantially increased risk of death according to age, with the highest risk in patients ≥85 (Tables 2 and 3). Black patients showed a slightly higher risk of death compared to white, whereas Asians/Pacific Islanders showed better outcomes compared to white. A 9% decreased risk of death and an 8% decreased risk of cancer-specific death were found in Cohort C compared with Cohort A (hazard ratio (HR): 0.91 (95% CI 0.87–0.95), $p < 0.001$ for OS; HR: 0.92 (95% CI 0.88–0.96), $p < 0.001$ for CSS), whereas no statistically significant differences in OS and CSS were found between Cohorts A and B. Exploratory multivariable models were also performed in Cohorts B and C to include the metastatic stage classification (AJCC, 6th edition), which was found to be associated with distinct OS and CSS outcomes (Tables S2 and S3). In these multivariable models, significant OS and CSS advantages were reported in Cohort C compared with Cohort B (HR: 0.94 (95% CI 0.91–0.97), $p = 0.001$ for OS; HR: 0.89 (95% CI 0.85–0.92), $p < 0.001$ for CSS). In the exploratory subgroup analysis comparing the OS and CSS of Cohort C with Cohort B, a significant interaction was found among the subgroups of the AJCC metastatic classification. More pronounced OS and CSS advantages in Cohort C were shown in M1c patients compared with patients with metastases that were limited to nodes or bone (M1c HR: 0.87 (95% CI 0.81–0.94), interaction $p = 0.014$ for OS; M1c HR: 0.81 (0.75–0.88), interaction $p = 0.015$ for CSS) (Table 4).

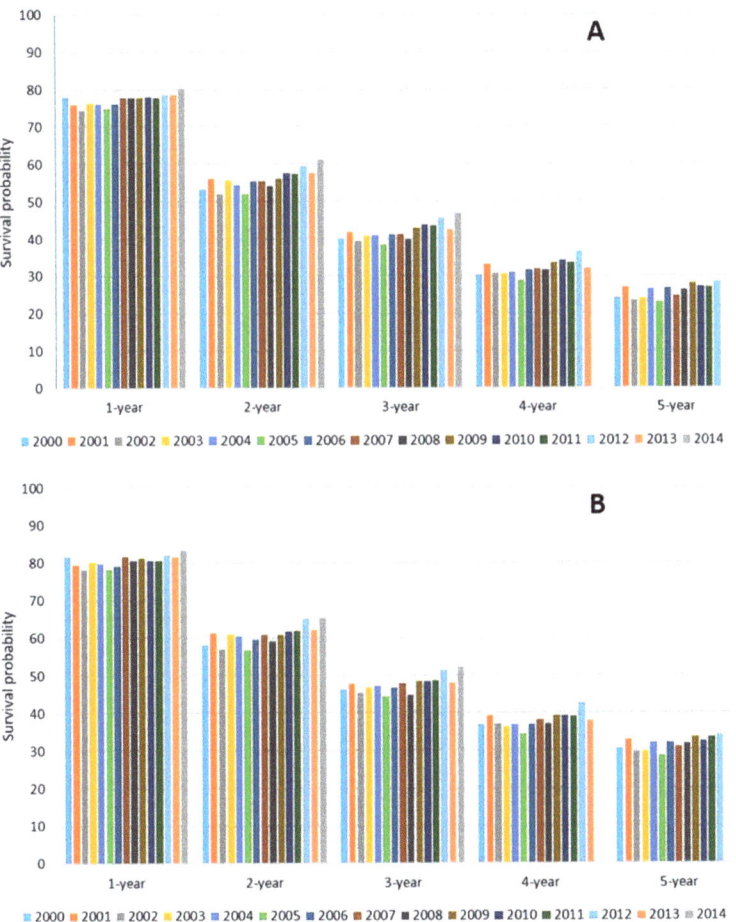

Figure 3. Age-standardized 1- to 5-year OS (**A**) and CSS (**B**) of patients according to year of diagnosis.

Table 2. Multivariable analysis for OS.

Variables		Number of Patients	HR	95% CI Lower	95% CI Upper	p
Age (years)	15–54	2081				<0.001
	55–64	6300	0.98	0.92	1.04	0.515
	65–74	7857	1.03	0.97	1.09	0.286
	75–84	7078	1.42	1.34	1.50	<0.001
	≥85	3028	2.18	2.04	2.32	<0.001
Race	White	16,513				<0.001
	Black	5111	1.10	1.06	1.14	<0.001
	Am. Indian/Alaska Native	170	1.08	0.91	1.28	0.393
	Asian or Pacific Islander	1484	0.74	0.69	0.79	<0.001
	Hispanic	3066	0.94	0.90	0.98	0.010
Year of diagnosis	2000–2003 (Cohort A)	6031				<0.001
	2004–2010 (Cohort B)	11,773	0.97	0.94	1.01	0.145
	2011–2014 (Cohort C)	8540	0.91	0.87	0.95	<0.001

Table 3. Multivariable analysis for CSS.

Variables		Number of Patients	HR	95% CI Lower	95% CI Upper	p
Age (years)	15–54	2049				<0.001
	55–64	6216	0.94	0.88	0.99	0.048
	65–74	7720	0.93	0.88	0.99	0.033
	75–84	6979	1.20	1.12	1.27	<0.001
	≥85	2987	1.74	1.62	1.87	<0.001
Race	White	16,376				<0.001
	Black	5053	1.09	1.04	1.13	<0.001
	Am. Indian/Alaska Native	167	1.01	0.83	1.23	0.922
	Asian or Pacific Islander	1423	0.73	0.67	0.78	<0.001
	Hispanic	2932	0.95	0.91	1.00	0.076
Year of diagnosis	2000–2003 (Cohort A)	5928				<0.001
	2004–2010 (Cohort B)	11,599	0.99	0.95	1.03	0.596
	2011–2014 (Cohort C)	8424	0.92	0.88	0.96	<0.001

Table 4. Subgroup analysis of OS and CSS between Cohorts C and B.

2011–2014 (Cohort C) vs. 2004–2010 (Cohort B)		Number of Patients	HR	95% CI		p
				Lower	Upper	
OS Metastatic Stage	M1a	1088	1.09	0.93	1.28	0.014 *
	M1b	14,250	0.96	0.92	0.99	
	M1c	4254	0.87	0.81	0.94	
	All [1]	19,592	0.94	0.91	0.97	0.001
CSS Metastatic Stage	M1a	1069	1.01	0.85	1.20	0.015 *
	M1b	14,050	0.91	0.87	0.95	
	M1c	4189	0.81	0.75	0.88	
	All [1]	19,308	0.89	0.85	0.92	<0.001

Multivariable models including age and race were used to compute the hazard ratios (HR) and their 95% confidence intervals (CI) for OS and CSS in the metastatic subgroups of patients diagnosed in 2011–2014 vs. 2004–2010. * p-value for interaction; [1] Multivariable model including age, race and metastatic stage for OS and CSS (Cohort C vs. Cohort B).

3. Discussion

Several randomized trials demonstrated that both chemotherapy and ARSi provided a significant survival benefit in mPCa [1–8]. However, the real-world survival outcomes of patients with de novo mPCa remain largely unexplored.

A recent analysis compared 590 patients with mCRPC, who were diagnosed and treated in two treatment eras (2004–2007 vs. 2010–2013) at the Dana–Farber Cancer Institute [11]. The authors demonstrated a 41% decreased risk of death in the newer treatment era, with a median OS gain of 6 months. In addition, the cumulative benefit from the newer therapies was more pronounced in longer-term survivors and de novo patients. Although this study provided useful information, all patients had castration-resistant disease, only 216 had de novo mPCa, and they were all managed in a top-level institution.

In another study, Helgstrand and colleagues analyzed the incidence and mortality data of patients with de novo mPCa included in the SEER database and in the Danish Prostate Cancer Registry [13]. In patients diagnosed between 2000 and 2009, the median OS was 22 months in SEER and 30 months in the Danish Registry. The five-year overall mortality was 80.0% in both registries in the period of 2000–2004, remained stable (80.5%) according to SEER in 2005–2008, and decreased to 73.2% according to the Danish Registry in 2005–2009.

Although the monocentric experience of the Dana–Farber Cancer Institute and the Danish data confirmed the potential survival gain offered by newer treatments, the SEER analysis by Helgstrand and colleagues did not show substantial survival changes after 2004.

In the present SEER-based analysis, we investigated whether the introduction of both chemotherapy and ARSi in mCRPC had substantially changed the real-world OS and CSS in the population of patients with de novo mPCa diagnosed in the United States of America in three different time periods (2000–2003—Cohort A, 2004–2010—Cohort B, 2011–2014—Cohort C). Although the patients were allocated to these cohorts regardless of having received a specific treatment, we highlight that docetaxel was approved by the FDA for the treatment of mCRPC in 2004, whereas ARSi was approved from 2011 onwards (Figure 1).

More than 26,000 patients diagnosed between 2000 and 2014 were included in our analysis; of these, 6047 were allocated to Cohort A, 11,815 to Cohort B, and 8572 to Cohort C (Table 1). We found that age had a significant impact on patients' OS and CSS (Tables 2 and 3). In the multivariable model, patients older than 85 showed a double risk of dying compared with patients between 15 and 54 years old, and the hazard ratio for death was also significantly unfavorable in patients aged 75–84. Although this figure might be at least in part attributable to the reduced expected survival, older patients may also be less likely to receive the same treatments as their younger counterparts, especially chemotherapy.

We did not find a significant difference in the OS and CSS between Cohort A and Cohort B (Figure 2). Conversely, we observed a statistically significant improvement in the OS and CSS of patients included in Cohort C, who showed a decreased risk of death of 9%, a decreased risk of cancer-specific death of 8%, and a median OS gain of 4 months compared with Cohort A. The comparison of Cohort C with Cohort B, adjusted for the metastatic stage, also demonstrated an OS improvement of 6% and a CSS improvement of 11%. When compared with the other metastatic stages, we found that patients with M1c disease showed the worst survival, but had a more pronounced OS and CSS improvement in the newer ARSi era compared with M1a or M1b patients (Table 4). Although the reason for this observation remains unknown, the presence of visceral metastases might lead to more aggressive pharmaceutical approaches and more adherence to treatment that could result in increased benefit compared with the other stages.

The median OS gain of chemotherapy and ARSi in randomized trials for mCRPC was 2–4 months in first-line [1,5,6] and 4–5 months in second-line [3,4]. Although our study was not designed to demonstrate the potential benefit of chemotherapy or ARSi, a more robust OS and CSS improvement would have been expected in patients diagnosed in 2011–2014, after the introduction of several agents in clinical practice (Figure 1). A median OS improvement of 4 months in Cohort C compared with Cohort A appears to be quite discouraging. Regardless of cohort analysis, the probability of survival after 3 years from diagnosis was 40.0% in 2000 and 46.8% in 2014 (Figure 3). Similarly, the five-year probability of survival was 24.0% in 2000 and 28.2% in 2012. Several reasons might explain these disappointing results.

First, the degree of benefit seen in clinical trials does not necessarily translate into the real-world setting. Screen failure rates on trials are relatively high and can easily affect the ultimate generalizability of trial results to the real-world population.

Second, our study was based on patients diagnosed with de novo mHSPC who were supposed to receive androgen-deprivation therapy (ADT) as a first-line treatment for metastatic disease, and subsequently docetaxel or ARSi as a first-line treatment for mCRPC. The number of patients who died without receiving a first-line treatment for mCRPC or refused therapies for mCRPC was unknown. The information on the number of lines of treatment, type of treatment, disease burden, number and site of metastases, body mass index, performance status, and comorbidities was not available in the SEER database, and these potential confounders were not included in our analysis. In addition, we acknowledge that some patients could have received chemotherapy or ARSi outside of the defined cohort allocation in the context of clinical trials or some years after mPCa diagnosis.

Third, the medical costs and the health insurance policies might have significantly reduced the extensive use of ARSi and chemotherapy in the general population of patients with de novo mPCa diagnosed and treated in the United States, affecting their survival outcomes. Ramsey and colleagues reported that the cumulative incidence of bankruptcy in the first 5 years after prostate cancer diagnosis is 38% (nearly 50% in metastatic stage), and the risk of mortality is almost twice as high among patients with prostate cancer who file for bankruptcy compared with those who do not [12]. Further studies should investigate whether insurance policies or limited access to healthcare services could contribute to such disappointing survival gains observed in the SEER registry after the introduction of chemotherapy and ARSi.

Fourth, patients with de novo mPCa showed worse time to castration and survival compared with those who relapsed after local therapy, irrespective of treatment received [14,15]. Therefore, the intrinsic aggressiveness of de novo mPCa could have also led to decreased survival gains in this patient population. Although discouraged by international guidelines in recent years, possible premature discontinuation of ARSi and chemotherapy based on PSA progression without clinical or radiographic progression could have also affected the outcome data of patients diagnosed between 2004 and 2014 [16].

Finally, we acknowledge that our study excludes the possible benefit induced by docetaxel or ARSi in mHSPC, given their approval for this setting in the latest years (Figure 1). The earlier use of these agents provided OS gains that exceeded 12 months in randomized trials for mHSPC [8]. Future analyses could also detect additional survival benefits that might be provided by an increased knowledge in the sequencing of agents for mCRPC and by the biomarker-driven selection of patients suitable for specific drugs (i.e., poly (ADP-ribose) polymerase (PARP) inhibitors) [17–19].

4. Patients and Methods

The SEER*Stat software was used to select all patients with de novo mPCa from the SEER Research Data 2000–2017 [20]. Patients were assigned to three cohorts based on the year of diagnosis (2000–2003: Cohort A; 2004–2010: Cohort B; 2011–2014: Cohort C). Patients with prostate cancer were identified using the codes for malignant adenocarcinoma (8140/3) and prostate gland (C61.9). Only patients with a single tumor in medical history were selected. Metastatic patients were identified using a combination of the American Joint Committee on Cancer (AJCC) classification from the 3rd and 6th editions. According to the November 2019 submission of SEER data, the study cut-off for survival data was 31 December 2017. In order to minimize potential bias related to different follow-up among the cohorts, the maximum follow-up was fixed to 5 years, and patients diagnosed from 2015 onwards were excluded. OS was defined as the time from mPCa diagnosis to death from any cause. CSS was defined as the time from mPCa diagnosis to death from prostate cancer. Patient age (SEER standard for survival in prostate cancer: 15–54, 55–64, 65–74, 75–84, 85+), race, year of mPCa diagnosis, metastatic stage, and outcome data were included in the case listing session of SEER*Stat. The variables described were analyzed in univariate analysis using Kaplan–Meier curves and a log-rank test. A p-value ≤ 0.05 was considered statistically significant. Cox proportional hazards models were used to test the effects of covariates on OS and CSS. Only patients who had known values for the variables of interest were included. The chi-square statistic was applied to compare groups. The IBM software Statistical Package for Social Sciences (SPSS) Version 23 and RStudio Version 1.2.5001 were used for data analysis.

5. Conclusions

Our large-scale, retrospective study suggested that the real-world OS and CSS have not drastically changed during the last two decades in patients with de novo mPCa diagnosed in the United States. The median OS of these patients remained poor and did not exceed 2.5 years. Although we acknowledge that several potential confounding factors have not been adjusted in our analysis, our study highlighted that a significant discrepancy might exist between the benefit observed in randomized trials and the real-world data. Several reasons might explain this discrepancy, such as a lack of access to cancer cares, patients' ineligibility or refusal of treatments, insurance issues, or intrinsic aggressiveness of de novo disease. However, given that patients were not allocated according to the receipt of specific treatments, our results should not be used to draw conclusions about the potential efficacy of systemic therapies.

Supplementary Materials: The following are available online at http://www.mdpi.com/2072-6694/12/10/2855/s1, Table S1: Baseline characteristics—contingency table; Table S2: multivariable model for OS in Cohorts B and C; Table S3: multivariable model for CSS in Cohorts B and C.

Author Contributions: Conceptualization, C.C.; methodology, D.O., A.R.; formal analysis, C.C., A.R., L.Z.; data curation, L.Z., C.M.; writing—original draft preparation, C.C., D.S.; writing—review and editing, P.B., C.M., E.C., E.Z., D.S.; supervision, F.B., D.O., E.C.; project administration, L.Z. All authors have read and agreed to the published version of the manuscript.

Funding: This research received no external funding.

Acknowledgments: C.C. is supported by an ESMO Clinical Research Fellowship (2019–2020). This work has been awarded with a Conquer Cancer Foundation of ASCO Merit Award at 2020 ASCO–GU.

Conflicts of Interest: E.Z.: advisory board from Janssen. E.C.: honoraria from Astellas Pharma, AstraZeneca, Bayer, Janssen-Cilag, Pfizer; consulting or advisory role from Astellas Pharma, Astra Zeneca, Bayer, Janssen, Merk; Research Funding from AstraZeneca (Inst), Bayer (Inst), Janssen (Inst); travel, accommodations, expenses from Astellas Pharma, Astra Zeneca, Bayer, Janssen, Roche. D.O.: honoraria from Astellas Pharma (Inst), Bayer, Janssen; consulting or advisory role from AstraZeneca (Inst), Bayer, Bayer (Inst), Clovis Oncology, Janssen, Janssen (Inst); research funding from Astellas Medivation (Inst), AstraZeneca (Inst), Bayer (Inst), Genentech/Roche (Inst), Janssen

(Inst), Pfizer (Inst), Tokai Pharmaceuticals (Inst); travel, accommodations, expenses from Astellas Pharma, Bayer, Ipsen, Janssen. The other authors have no conflicts of interest to declare.

References

1. Tannock, I.F.; de Wit, R.; Berry, W.R.; Horti, J.; Pluzanska, A.; Chi, K.N.; Oudard, S.; Theodore, C.; James, N.D.; Turesson, I.; et al. Docetaxel plus prednisone or mitoxantrone plus prednisone for advanced prostate cancer. *N. Engl. J. Med.* **2004**, *351*, 1502–1512. [CrossRef]
2. De Bono, J.S.; Oudard, S.; Ozguroglu, M.; Hansen, S.; Machiels, J.P.; Kocak, I.; Gravis, G.; Bodrogi, I.; Mackenzie, M.J.; Shen, L.; et al. Prednisone plus cabazitaxel or mitoxantrone for metastatic castration-resistant prostate cancer progressing after docetaxel treatment: A randomised open-label trial. *Lancet* **2010**, *376*, 1147–1154. [CrossRef]
3. De Bono, J.S.; Logothetis, C.J.; Molina, A.; Fizazi, K.; North, S.; Chu, L.; Chi, K.N.; Jones, R.J.; Goodman, O.B., Jr.; Saad, F.; et al. Abiraterone and increased survival in metastatic prostate cancer. *N. Engl. J. Med.* **2011**, *364*, 1995–2005. [CrossRef] [PubMed]
4. Scher, H.I.; Fizazi, K.; Saad, F.; Taplin, M.E.; Sternberg, C.N.; Miller, K.; de Wit, R.; Mulders, P.; Chi, K.N.; Shore, N.D.; et al. Increased survival with enzalutamide in prostate cancer after chemotherapy. *N. Engl. J. Med.* **2012**, *367*, 1187–1197. [CrossRef] [PubMed]
5. Ryan, C.J.; Smith, M.R.; de Bono, J.S.; Molina, A.; Logothetis, C.J.; de Souza, P.; Fizazi, K.; Mainwaring, P.; Piulats, J.M.; Ng, S.; et al. Abiraterone in metastatic prostate cancer without previous chemotherapy. *N. Engl. J. Med.* **2013**, *368*, 138–148. [CrossRef] [PubMed]
6. Beer, T.M.; Armstrong, A.J.; Rathkopf, D.E.; Loriot, Y.; Sternberg, C.N.; Higano, C.S.; Iversen, P.; Bhattacharya, S.; Carles, J.; Chowdhury, S.; et al. Enzalutamide in metastatic prostate cancer before chemotherapy. *N. Engl. J. Med.* **2014**, *371*, 424–433. [CrossRef] [PubMed]
7. Sweeney, C.J.; Chen, Y.H.; Carducci, M.; Liu, G.; Jarrard, D.F.; Eisenberger, M.; Wong, Y.N.; Hahn, N.; Kohli, M.; Cooney, M.M.; et al. Chemohormonal Therapy in Metastatic Hormone-Sensitive Prostate Cancer. *N. Engl. J. Med.* **2015**, *373*, 737–746. [CrossRef] [PubMed]
8. Cattrini, C.; Castro, E.; Lozano, R.; Zanardi, E.; Rubagotti, A.; Boccardo, F.; Olmos, D. Current Treatment Options for Metastatic Hormone-Sensitive Prostate Cancer. *Cancers* **2019**, *11*, 1355. [CrossRef] [PubMed]
9. Mottet, N.; Bellmunt, J.; Briers, E.; Bolla, M.; Bourke, L.; Cornford, P.; De Santis, M.; Henry, A.; Joniau, S.; Lam, T. *Members of the EAU–ESTRO–ESUR–SIOG Prostate Cancer Guidelines Panel. EAU–ESTRO–ESUR–SIOG Guidelines on Prostate Cancer*; Presented at the EAU Annual Congress Amsterdam 2020. 978-94-92671-07-3; EAU Guidelines Office: Arnhem, The Netherlands, 2020.
10. Thompson, A.L.; Sarmah, P.; Beresford, M.J.; Jefferies, E.R. Management of metastatic prostate cancer in the elderly: Identifying fitness for chemotherapy in the post-STAMPEDE world. *Bju Int.* **2017**, *120*, 751–754. [CrossRef] [PubMed]
11. Francini, E.; Gray, K.P.; Shaw, G.K.; Evan, C.P.; Hamid, A.A.; Perry, C.E.; Kantoff, P.W.; Taplin, M.E.; Sweeney, C.J. Impact of new systemic therapies on overall survival of patients with metastatic castration-resistant prostate cancer in a hospital-based registry. *Prostate Cancer Prostatic Dis.* **2019**, *22*, 420–427. [CrossRef] [PubMed]
12. Ramsey, S.D.; Bansal, A.; Fedorenko, C.R.; Blough, D.K.; Overstreet, K.A.; Shankaran, V.; Newcomb, P. Financial Insolvency as a Risk Factor for Early Mortality among Patients with Cancer. *J. Clin. Oncol.* **2016**, *34*, 980–986. [CrossRef] [PubMed]
13. Helgstrand, J.T.; Roder, M.A.; Klemann, N.; Toft, B.G.; Lichtensztajn, D.Y.; Brooks, J.D.; Brasso, K.; Vainer, B.; Iversen, P. Trends in incidence and 5-year mortality in men with newly diagnosed, metastatic prostate cancer-A population-based analysis of 2 national cohorts. *Cancer* **2018**, *124*, 2931–2938. [CrossRef] [PubMed]
14. Francini, E.; Gray, K.P.; Xie, W.; Shaw, G.K.; Valenca, L.; Bernard, B.; Albiges, L.; Harshman, L.C.; Kantoff, P.W.; Taplin, M.E.; et al. Time of metastatic disease presentation and volume of disease are prognostic for metastatic hormone sensitive prostate cancer (mHSPC). *Prostate* **2018**, *78*, 889–895. [CrossRef] [PubMed]
15. Finianos, A.; Gupta, K.; Clark, B.; Simmens, S.J.; Aragon-Ching, J.B. Characterization of Differences Between Prostate Cancer Patients Presenting with De Novo Versus Primary Progressive Metastatic Disease. *Clin. Genitourin. Cancer* **2017**, *16*, 85–89. [CrossRef] [PubMed]

16. Becker, D.J.; Iyengar, A.D.; Punekar, S.R.; Ng, J.; Zaman, A.; Loeb, S.; Becker, K.D.; Makarov, D. Treatment of Metastatic Castration-resistant Prostate Cancer with Abiraterone and Enzalutamide Despite PSA Progression. *Anticancer Res.* **2019**, *39*, 2467–2473. [CrossRef] [PubMed]
17. De Wit, R.; de Bono, J.; Sternberg, C.N.; Fizazi, K.; Tombal, B.; Wulfing, C.; Kramer, G.; Eymard, J.C.; Bamias, A.; Carles, J.; et al. Cabazitaxel versus Abiraterone or Enzalutamide in Metastatic Prostate Cancer. *N. Engl. J. Med.* **2019**, *381*, 2506–2518. [CrossRef] [PubMed]
18. De Bono, J.; Mateo, J.; Fizazi, K.; Saad, F.; Shore, N.; Sandhu, S.; Chi, K.N.; Sartor, O.; Agarwal, N.; Olmos, D.; et al. Olaparib for Metastatic Castration-Resistant Prostate Cancer. *N. Engl. J. Med.* **2020**, *382*, 2091–2102. [CrossRef] [PubMed]
19. Messina, C.; Cattrini, C.; Soldato, D.; Vallome, G.; Caffo, O.; Castro, E.; Olmos, D.; Boccardo, F.; Zanardi, E. BRCA Mutations in Prostate Cancer: Prognostic and Predictive Implications. *J. Oncol.* **2020**, *2020*, 4986365. [CrossRef] [PubMed]
20. Surveillance, Epidemiology, and End Results (SEER) Program (www.seer.cancer.gov) SEER*Stat Database: Incidence-SEER Research Data, 18 Registries, Nov 2019 Sub (2000–2017)-Linked to County Attributes-Time Dependent (1990–2017) Income/Rurality, 1969–2017 Counties; National Cancer Institute, DCCPS, Surveillance Research Program, Released April 2020, Based on the November 2019 Submission. Available online: https://seer.cancer.gov/data/citation.html (accessed on 3 October 2020).

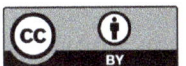

© 2020 by the authors. Licensee MDPI, Basel, Switzerland. This article is an open access article distributed under the terms and conditions of the Creative Commons Attribution (CC BY) license (http://creativecommons.org/licenses/by/4.0/).

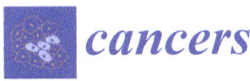

Review

Consensus Definition and Prediction of Complexity in Transurethral Resection or Bladder Endoscopic Dissection of Bladder Tumours

Mathieu Roumiguié [1], Evanguelos Xylinas [2], Antonin Brisuda [3], Maximillian Burger [4], Hugh Mostafid [5], Marc Colombel [6], Marek Babjuk [3], Joan Palou Redorta [7], Fred Witjes [8] and Bernard Malavaud [1,*]

[1] Department of Urology, Institut Universitaire du Cancer, 31059 Toulouse CEDEX 9, France; Roumiguie.Mathieu@iuct-oncopole.fr
[2] Department of Urology, Hôpital Cochin, APHP, 75014 Paris, France; evanguelos.xylinas@aphp.fr
[3] Department of Urology, 2nd Faculty of Medicine, Charles University, Teaching Hospital Motol, 15006 Prague, Czech Republic; antonin.brisuda@fnmotol.cz (A.B.); Marek.Babjuk@fnmotol.cz (M.B.)
[4] St. Josef, Klinik für Urologie, Caritas-Krankenhaus, 93053 Regensburg, Germany; mburger@caritasstjosef.de
[5] Department of Urology, Royal Surrey County Hospital, Surrey, Guildford GU2 7RF, UK; hugh.mostafid@nhs.net
[6] Department of Urology, Hôpital Edouard Herriot, 69437 Lyon, France; marc.colombel@chu-lyon.fr
[7] Department of Urology, Fundacio Puigvert, 08025 Barcelona, Spain; jpalou@fundacio-puigvert.es
[8] Department of Urology, Radboud UMC, 6525 GA Nijmegen, The Netherlands; Fred.Witjes@radboudumc.nl
* Correspondence: malavaud.bernard@iuct-oncopole.fr

Received: 5 September 2020; Accepted: 6 October 2020; Published: 20 October 2020

Simple Summary: Transurethral resection of bladder tumours may be technically challenging. Complexity was defined by consensus from the literature by a panel of ten senior urologists as "any TURBT/En-bloc dissection that results in incomplete resection and/or prolonged surgery (>1 h) and/or significant (Clavien-Dindo ≥ 3) perioperative complications". Patient and tumour's characteristics that suggested to by the panel to relate to complex surgery were collected and then ranked by Delphi consensus. They were tested in the prediction of complexity in 150 clinical scenarios. After univariate and logistic regression analyses, significant characteristics were organized into a checklist that predicts complexity. Receiver operating characteristics (ROC) curves of the regression model and the corresponding calibration curve showed adequate discrimination (AUC = 0.916) and good calibration. The resulting Bladder Complexity Checklist can be used to deliver optimal preoperative information and personalise the organisation of surgery.

Abstract: Ten senior urologists were interrogated to develop a predictive model based on factors from which they could anticipate complex transurethral resection of bladder tumours (TURBT). Complexity was defined by consensus. Panel members then used a five-point Likert scale to grade those factors that, in their opinion, drove complexity. Consensual factors were highlighted through two Delphi rounds. Respective contributions to complexity were quantitated by the median values of their scores. Multivariate analysis with complexity as a dependent variable tested their independence in clinical scenarios obtained by random allocation of the factors. The consensus definition of complexity was "any TURBT/En-bloc dissection that results in incomplete resection and/or prolonged surgery (>1 h) and/or significant (Clavien-Dindo ≥ 3) perioperative complications". Logistic regression highlighted five domains as independent predictors: patient's history, tumour number, location, and size and access to the bladder. Receiver operating characteristic (ROC) analysis confirmed good discrimination (AUC = 0.92). The sum of the scores of the five domains adjusted to their regression coefficients or Bladder Complexity Score yielded comparable performance (AUC = 0.91, C-statistics, $p = 0.94$) and good calibration. As a whole, preoperative factors identified by expert judgement were organized to quantitate the risk of a complex TURBT, a crucial requisite to personalise patient information, adapt human and technical resources to individual situations and address TURBT variability in clinical trials.

Keywords: bladder cancer; transurethral resection; en-bloc resection

1. Introduction

Bladder cancer is the seventh most prevalent cancer worldwide [1] and the sixth leading cause of cancer in the EU, where it entails a significant burden in healthcare organization and cost [2]. Most patients present with non-muscle invasive bladder cancer (NMIBC), for which endoscopic resection or en-bloc dissection of bladder tumours, collectively referred to as transurethral resection of bladder tumour (TURBT), initiate the treatment and inform the risks of recurrence and progression. Pathology also provides information on the adequacy of surgery that is visually complete resection and presence of muscle at the resection base [3]. Although this is the most common procedure in oncologic urology, with over 120,000 new cases across Europe annually [2], few reports have addressed how individual characteristics may challenge the successful completion of surgery [4,5]. In addition, the reported variability of residual disease [6] and higher performances of experienced surgeons [7] emphasize the demands of "good-quality" TURBT [7]. Moreover, quality represents latent information for the non-expert, contrary to clinical complications that are self-evident, closely monitored by the public and insurers and used as proxy for quality metrics [8].

Any system capable to document how individual presentations influence surgical outcomes would be of high clinical relevance. Therefore, the objective of the present consensus was to detail and organize the factors based on which experienced urologists anticipate a complex TURBT.

2. Results

2.1. Step 1: Definition of Complexity

A PubMed search of "transurethral resection" (of) "bladder" and "morbidity" or "complication", or "mortality" or "death" yielded 585, 664, 9 and 95 articles, respectively. Of these, 89 articles relevant to the process of defining complexity were analysed, obtaining 36 articles (Table S(1) which were instrumental in highlighting adequacy, operative time and morbidity as the three drivers that characterize a complex surgery, as opposed to an uneventful procedure [4,8–42].

After a single round of circulation, all panellists validated the following definition of a complex TURBT: "any TURBT/En-bloc dissection that results in incomplete resection and/or prolonged surgery (>1 h) and/or significant (Clavien-Dindo ≥ 3) perioperative complications".

2.2. Step 2: Items That Drive Complexity

Eighty-five characteristics that were suggested by the panellists to influence surgery were organized into six chapters consistent with standard medical practice: patient's characteristics and history, tumour characteristics, access to the bladder, bladder anatomy and surgical environment.

Their relevance was researched in two Delphi rounds, which showed consensus for 42 characteristics in the first round (Figures S1–S4) and 83 in the second (Figures 1–4). For any characteristic or item, the median opinion of the panel (Figures 1–4) was then used as the metrics to weight its individual contribution to complexity.

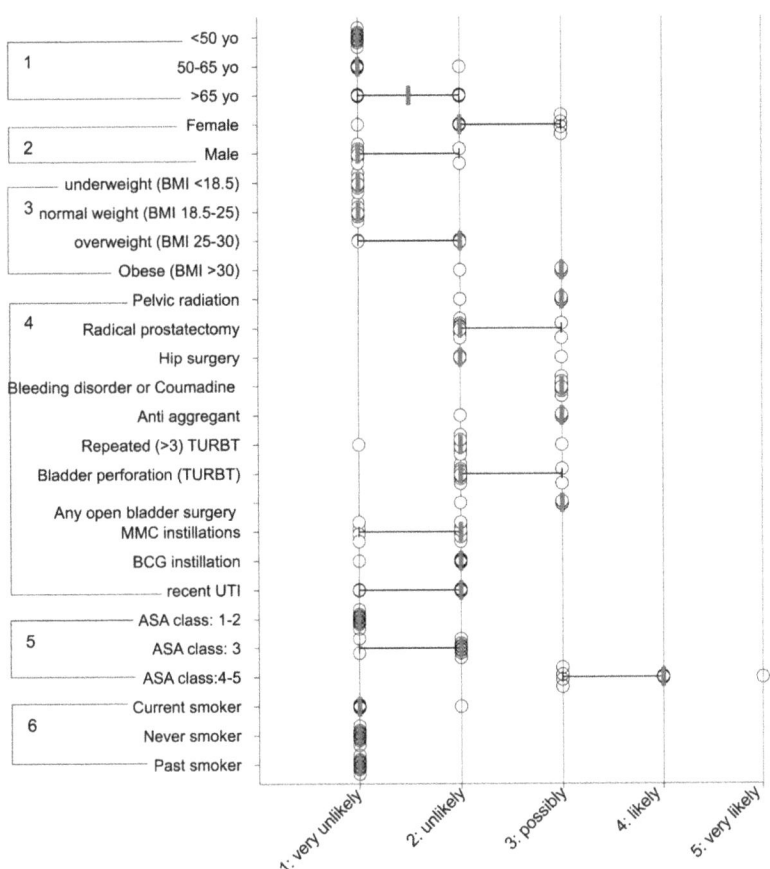

Figure 1. Distribution of the scores regarding the likelihood of incomplete resection and/or prolonged surgery (>1 h) and/or significant (Clavien-Dindo ≥ 3) perioperative complications according to patient's characteristics. ((1) age, (2) sex, (3) weight and body mass index (BMI), (4) patient's history, (5) American Society of Anaesthesiologists' (ASA) physical status classification, (6) tobacco smoking. MMC: Mitomycin C, Bacille Calmette Guérin (BCG), TURBT: transurethral resection of bladder tumour.

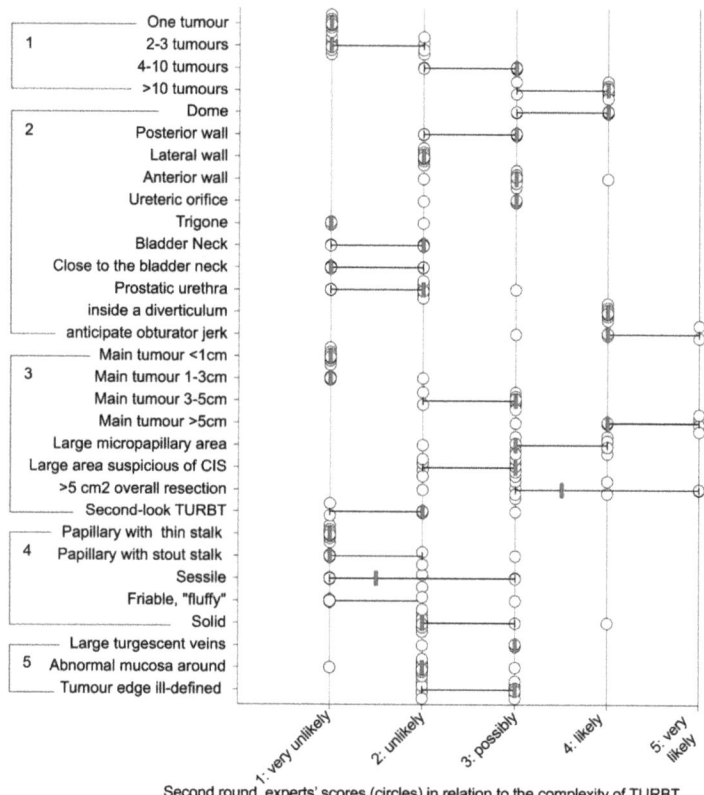

Figure 2. Distribution of the scores regarding the likelihood of incomplete resection and/or prolonged surgery (>1 h) and/or significant (Clavien-Dindo ≥ 3) perioperative complications according to tumour's characteristics: ((1) number, (2) location, (3) size, (4) structure, (5) surroundings. CIS: carcinoma in situ.

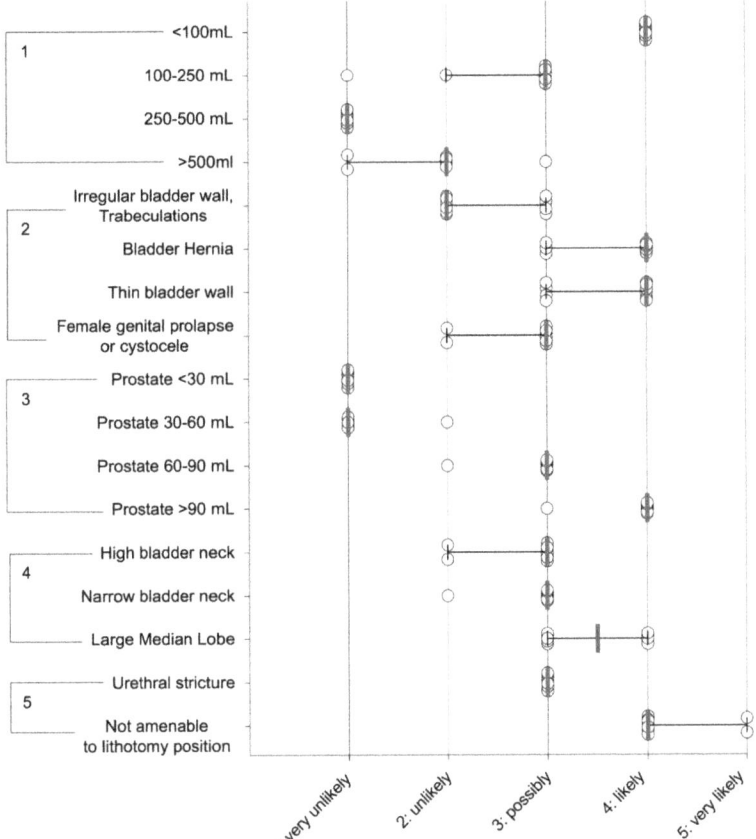

Figure 3. Distribution of the scores regarding the likelihood of incomplete resection and/or prolonged surgery (>1 h) and/or significant (Clavien-Dindo ≥ 3) perioperative complications according to bladder characteristics and access to the bladder cavity: ((1) bladder capacity, (2) bladder structure, (3) prostate volume, (4) bladder neck, (5) others.

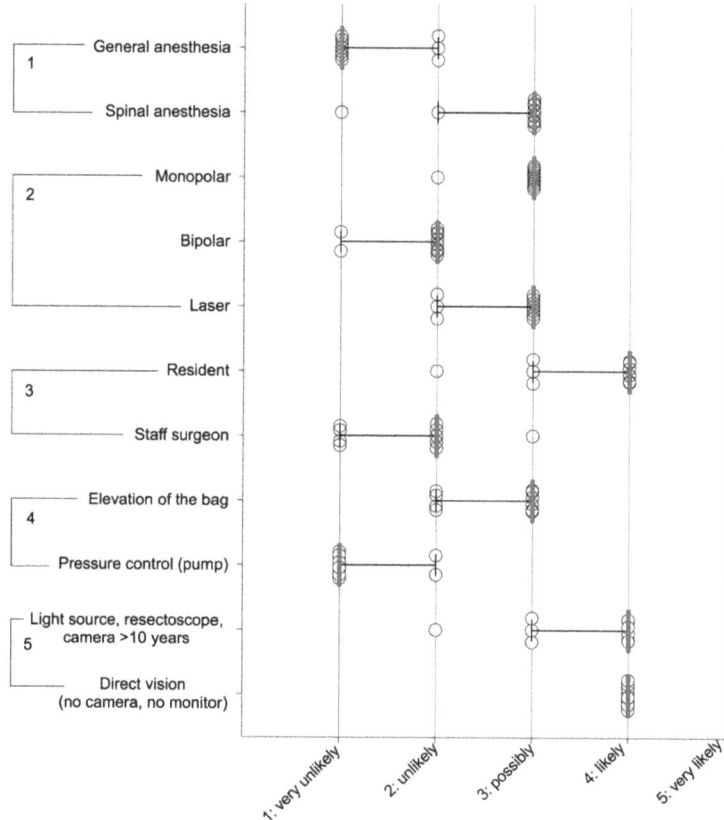

Second round, experts' scores (circles) in relation to the complexity of TURBT
Median (red) & 95% CI (black line)

Figure 4. Distribution of the scores regarding the likelihood of incomplete resection and/or prolonged surgery (>1 h) and/or significant (Clavien-Dindo ≥ 3) perioperative complications according to the surgical environment: ((1) anaesthesia, (2) energy, (3) operator, (4) bladder irrigation, (5) instruments.

2.3. Step 3: Construction, Discrimination and Accuracy of the Bladder Complexity Checklist Sum

2.3.1. Clinical Scenarios

Smoking, underweight, normal weight and American Society of Anaesthesiologists (ASA) class 1–2 or 3 that in the panel's opinions did not relate to the complexity of TURBT were not included in the scenarios, although age and sex that were also considered of little influence were retained, as they are standards in medical reporting. Although the surgical environment was consistently considered to have bearing on the odds of a complex surgery, the corresponding items were not included in the scenarios, as they were considered circumstantial rather than constitutive of the case. As a whole, 150 scenarios that included 9 items organized 5 five domains (Table 1) were presented to the panel. The members were strongly consistent in their anticipation of complexity, as consensus was observed for 131/150 (87.3%) scenarios that were by design confirmed for univariate and multivariate analysis.

Table 1. Univariate analysis of the scores of preoperative characteristics in a cohort of 131 random scenarios for which the panel was consistent in its anticipation of complexity.

Domain of Interest	Feature	Number of Items	Median Score, (95%CI)		Mann–Whitney U-Test
			TURBT Unlikely to Be Complex (n = 73)	TURBT Likely to Be Complex (n = 58)	
Patient's characteristics	Age	3	1 (1–(1)	1 (1–(1)	n.s. ($p = 0.85$)
	Sex	2	1 (1–(1)	1 (1–2)	n.s. ($p = 0.72$)
Patient's history		12	1 (1–2)	2 (1–2)	n.s. ($p = 0.07$)
Tumour's characteristics	Number	3	1 (1–(1)	3 (3–4)	$p = 0.002$
	Location	10	3 (2–3)	4 (3–4)	$p < 0.0001$
	Size	5	2 (1–3)	3 (3–3)	$p < 0.0001$
	Structure	5	2 (2–3)	2 (2–3)	n.s. ($p = 0.97$)
Bladder Anatomy		8	3 (2–3)	3 (2–3)	n.s. ($p = 0.82$)
Access to the Bladder cavity		13	1 (1–3)	3 (3–4)	$p < 0.0001$

n.s. not significant.

2.3.2. Discrimination and Accuracy

In univariate analysis, the items that informed the tumour characteristics (number, location, size) and access to the bladder were significantly associated with complexity (Table 1). Patient's history that did not reach statistical relevance still qualified for multivariate analysis ($p = 0.07$).

Five domains (Table 2) that in logistic regression were independent predictors of complexity, i.e., history, tumour number, location, and size and access to the bladder cavity, were used to develop the probability function that modelled the probability of a complex surgery.

Table 2. Logistic regression analysis showing independent relationships between the complexity of TURBT and patient history, tumour number, main tumour location and size and factors restraining the access to the bladder cavity.

Independent Variables	Regression Coefficient	Std. Error	z	$p > |z|$	95% CI of the Regression Coefficient	
Patient History	0.99	0.32	3.11	0.002	0.37	1.61
Tumour Number	0.96	0.23	4.18	0.000	0.51	1.41
Main Tumour Location	1.44	0.33	4.42	0.000	0.80	2.09
Main Tumour Size	1.04	0.26	3.98	0.000	0.53	1.55
Access	1.10	0.26	4.31	0.000	0.60	1.60
Intercept value	−13.34	2.31	−5.77	0.000	−17.87	−8.81

$$p(complex) = \frac{1}{1+\exp(13.34-0.99xHistory-0.96xTuNumber-1.44xMainTuLocation-1.04xMainTuSize-1.1xAccess)} \quad (1)$$

This function showed good discrimination (AUC: 0.92 (95%CI: 0.87–0.96)) in receiver operating characteristic (ROC) analysis (Figure 5).

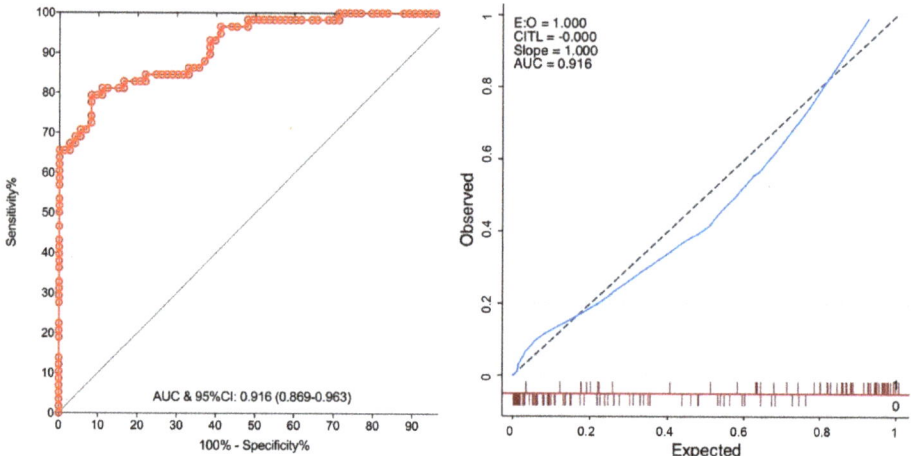

Figure 5. Receiver operating characteristics (ROC) curves of the regression model with the corresponding calibration curve showing adequate discrimination (AUC = 0.916) and good calibration, with calibration slope of 1 and calibration in the large (CITL) of 0, indicating that the predicted prevalence of complexity was in keeping with the observed prevalence (CITL) and that the model was not over fitted (slope).

The simplification offered by the Bladder Complexity Checklist Sum (BCCS, Table 3) yielded comparable performance (C-Statistics $p = 0.94$, Figure 6).

Table 3. Checklist detailing the five domains related to the prediction of a complex transurethral resection of bladder tumours by the panel. The Bladder Complexity Score (BCS) was calculated as the sum of the weight-adjusted scores. Increments in BCS relate to the positive and negative predictive values of experiencing a complex surgery, that is, "any TURBT/En-bloc dissection that results in incomplete resection and/or prolonged surgery (>1 h) and/or significant (Clavien-Dindo ≥ 3) perioperative complications".

Weight-Adjusted Scores	Patient's Characteristics			Tumour's Characteristics		
	Medical History	Bladder Access	Number	Size	Location
1	No Relevant History	No relevant features	1–3	<3 cm	
1.5					Trigon
2	Hip Surgery Radical Prostatectomy Repeated TURBT (>3) Prior Bladder perforation MMC or BCG instillations UTI	Large bladder (>500 mL) Irregular bladder wall, Trabeculations		Recent TURBT (second-look)	
3	Obese BMI > 30 Pelvic Radiation Any open bladder surgery Bleeding disorder or Coumadin or Anti-aggregant	Urethral stricture High or narrow bladder neck Large Median lobe Large prostate (60–90 mL) Small bladder (100–250 mL) Female prolapse or cystocele	4–10	3–5 cm Large micropapillary area or suspicious for CIS (>5 cm²)	Prostatic urethra Bladder neck Lateral wall
4	ASA class 4–5	Not amenable to lithotomy position Very small bladder (<100 mL) Very large prostate (>90 mL) Bladder hernia Thin bladder wall	>10	>5 cm	
4.5					Posterior or Anterior wall Ureteric orifice
6					Dome Anticipate obturator jerk Diverticulum

Abbreviations: UTI: urinary tract infection.

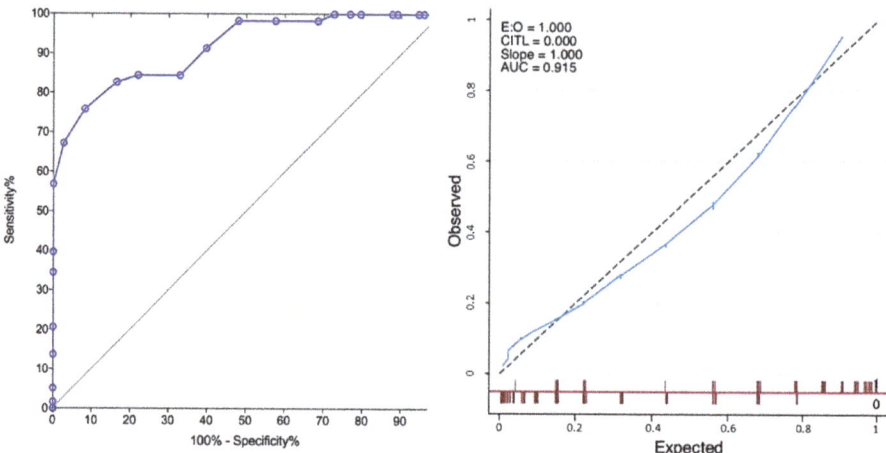

Figure 6. ROC curves of the Bladder Complexity Checklist Sum (BCCS) and the corresponding calibration curve showing similar discrimination and calibration performances compared to the regression model.

Both instruments showed good calibration (Figure 3, Figure 4).

Figure 7 illustrates the balance between positive and negative predictive values according to increments in BCCS.

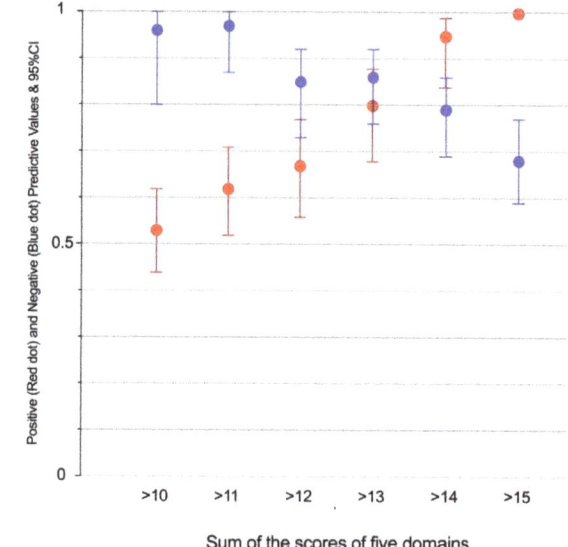

Figure 7. Negative (**blue**) and positive (**red**) predictive values (NPV and PPV) of increments in the BCCS.

3. Discussion

Anticipation is essential to adapt staff and technical resources to individual challenges of clinical situations. The adoption of standardized instruments of evaluation for major urological procedures [43] spurred us to develop similar instruments for TURBT, the most common procedure in oncologic urology [2].

The first step contextualized complexity, a concept adapted to the rationalization of healthcare [44]. A PubMed search highlighted three dimensions that characterize a complex surgery, as opposed to a satisfactory and uneventful procedure. Adequacy was recently introduced in the European Association of Urology (EAU) guidelines to insist on the importance of complete resection of all visible tumours with the detrusor muscle in the specimen, a surrogate marker of resection quality that controls the risk of early recurrence [9] and may impact adjuvant treatment [11]. Surgery longer than one hour was included following a large population-based report from the American College of Surgeons National Surgical Quality Improvement Program (NSQIP), where it related to postoperative complications independently from age, comorbidities, tumour size and ASA classification [31]. Lastly, postoperative complications requiring surgical, endoscopic or radiological intervention—that is, Grade III and higher in the recently TURBT-adapted Clavien–Dindo classification [29]—were also considered, as they were recently shown [33] to affect a significant minority of patients (8.1%, of which 15% were Grade III and higher). Reminiscent of other major oncologic procedures (e.g., trifecta in kidney and prostate surgery), the consensus therefore encompassed the three reported qualifiers of complexity, oncological, procedural and postoperative into a multidimensional definition.

The second step researched robust clinical predictors. To that end, we relayed on expert judgement, a valuable instrument when other methods are intractable for scientific or practicable reasons [45]. TURBT appears to fall in that category, as although many factors are known to impact surgery and its outcomes [4,5,46], some important ones were not detailed in population-based series (e.g., position of the tumour) or were so infrequent as to elude detection (e.g., diverticulum). Conversely, experienced urologists are bound to encounter them along their career and to drive some operational conclusions as to the influence they may have on their management. This was confirmed by the extensive list of items drawn from experience and by the broad consensus of the panel on their relative contributions to complexity.

Most of the items that carried a "possibly", "likely" or "very likely" risk of complication were consistent with the current literature. Conversely, some that had eluded cohorts [33] and population-based registries [4,31] made sense to the practising physician, notably, the access to the bladder cavity or the position of the tumours, with TURBT at the dome considered as "likely" to result in visually incomplete, lengthy or morbid surgery, compared to "very unlikely" for the trigon. The increments in scores with tumour sizes presented according to the current US procedural terminology (Figure 2) were in keeping with the increasing risks of complication and 30-day reoperation rates reported in two large NSQIP population-based studies [4,31]. A similar correlation was observed for the number of tumours, that is also a central parameter in the EAU/European Organisation for Research and Treatment of Cancer (EORTC) risk stratification of progression and recurrence [3].

Overall, high consistency between the literature or the practical constraints of surgery and the Delphi scores vindicated the present approach to anticipate complex TURBT.

However relevant, no single factor could possibly drive the entirety of the surgical challenge, which spurred us to the third step to analyse their respective contributions in random scenarios. Although the panel acknowledged the influence of technology in TURBT (Figure 4), elements pertaining to the surgical environment that were considered as adaptive rather than constitutive were not considered in the scenarios. Consistent with the format of clinical presentations, scenarios included age and sex, although they are considered of little bearing in TURBT (Figure 1). To account for the risk of cognitive overload [47], only four aspects were considered: patient's history, tumour and bladder anatomy and access. Although this resulted in a high prevalence of complex cases (58/131 (44.2%) scenarios were classified as "possibly", "likely" or "very likely" to result in incomplete resection or prolonged surgery (>1 h) or significant complications), random scenarios were preferred to collecting real-life clinical cases in the construction of the score, as this ensured that even rare situations were not overlooked.

On univariate analysis, tumour number, size, and location and access to the bladder cavity significantly related to complexity (Table 1). Although not significant in univariate analysis ($p = 0.07$), patient's history still qualified for multivariate analysis, where all five aspects independently related to complexity.

As measured by their regression coefficients (Table 2), although patients' history and bladder contributed to a lesser extent, tumour characteristics carried most of the information, thereby emphasizing the classical emphasis on thorough preoperative evaluation. The regression model showed excellent discrimination on ROC analysis (AUC: 0.92), while the calibration curve confirmed its accuracy (Figure 5).

The Bladder Complexity Checklist was then developed to facilitate the recording of significant characteristics in the clinic (Table 3). For illustration purposes, the case of a 75-year-old female patient with a thin bladder wall, showing a single 3 cm tumour of the dome would yield a sum of 15, consistent with a predictive value for complexity (PPV) of 100% (Figure 7). Summing the weight-adjusted scores of the Bladder Complexity Checklist carried similar discrimination and accuracy as the logistic model (Figure 4). This is to our knowledge the first effort to quantitatively inform with a simple clinical instrument the multidimensional complexity of TURBT. It could readily complement the other checklists proposed to control the quality of the procedure [37] or the step-by-step management of NMIBC [14].

Overall, the present methodology highlighted the factors that drove the anticipation by experienced surgeons of a complex TURBT. It would be amenable to other procedures where the surgical outcome relates to a large number of factors accessible to preoperative evaluation (e.g., radical prostatectomy, kidney transplantation). It also emphasized the variability in complexity of a procedure that is still widely regarded as menial.

The ability to anticipate and document complexity has important practical consequences. First, the Bladder Complexity Checklist could be instrumental in personalising the human and technical resources required for the most common procedure in oncologic urology [2]. This has become an absolute requisite in the current era of value-based care [48], where most procedural terminologies and reimbursement policies for TURBT consider the size and number of tumours compounded by comorbidity indexes, but overlook essential predictors such as the position of the tumour, a key descriptor of complexity in the present consensus. The Bladder Complexity Checklist Sum that organises and quantitates all relevant clinical information could also be used to drive the adaptation of health resources according to increments of complexity and support complexity-adapted coverage from health insurances.

Second, quantitating the difficulties entailed by a "good-quality" TURBT [7] would offer a solid ground to confront the morbidity and oncological outcome of a potentially complex procedure. Documenting variability is also important when analysing the benefits of different systems of resection or evaluating adjuvant treatments in research protocols [11]. Although all controlled trials to date overlooked the bias of complexity, we believe that crucial information such as the complexity score or, at the very least, a minimal dataset including size, number and position of the tumours should be documented and balanced in clinical research.

Third, measuring complexity that amounts to weighting the risks of the procedure would constitute an important instrument to inform the patient and therefore control part of his anxiety [49]. The constraints of information also include the training and experience of the surgical staff [50]. A large study from the NSQIP concluded that residents' involvement in urology procedures was not associated with increased complications, although it significantly increased the operative time [27].

Regarding TURBT, the relation between time and complications [31] and surgeon experience and the presence of the detrusor muscle in the specimen [9] vindicated the panel's prudent assessment of residents' participation (Figure 4). This observation also has direct bearing on the organisation of care in academic hospitals, in terms not only of informed consent [50] but also of organizing the list so that cases showing high complexity receive proper attention in terms of consultant supervision and position on the surgical list [50].

Several limitations should be considered. First, it is recommended for health indicators to include panellists of different origins, from public health experts to patients' representatives [51]. Here, the sole urologists' perspective was adopted, which certainly contributed to the high degree of consensus and the strong consistency with clinicians' experience. With 10 experts, the panel positioned at the first quartile of the distribution of panellists in a systematic review [51] of the Delphi methodology and was in line with the number of experts invited to develop other multidimensional instruments in urology [43].

Second, the model was not validated in the clinics, where a lower prevalence of complex cases may be anticipated. However, the review of 416 diagnostic studies showed that a lower prevalence improved specificity and had no systemic effect on sensitivity [52], suggesting that the current model would retain its relevance in the real-life setting. Third, important predictors such as the position or the multiplicity of tumours are best defined by preoperative flexible cystoscopy [53], which is optional when the diagnosis can be ascertained by medical imaging [3]. Last, the process yielded a large number of items (Table 3) that may require streamlining after the first returns of clinical experience.

4. Materials and Methods

The present Delphi method followed the recommendations of a systematic review for the development of healthcare quality indicators [51]. Six urologists designed the study into three separate work packages: definition of complexity, outline of the factors that drive complexity and evaluation of their respective contributions in clinical scenarios. Four panellists were then invited to broaden the scope of ages and experiences (Table 4). As a whole, the panel comprised 10 board-certified urologists with over 202 years of combined experience.

Table 4. Panel participants' characteristics and experience in urology.

Expert	Country	Age	Urology * (Years)	Oncology * (Years)	FEBU	PhD	Head of Urology **	National Association of Urology	European Association of Urology
1	F	36	4	2	-	-	0	Member NMIBC guidelines panel	Member
2	F	38	5	3	Yes	Yes	-	Board member NMIBC guidelines panel	Chairman YAU Board member YOU & ESOU
3	CZ	39	14	-	Yes	Yes	-	Member	Member
4	D	45	19	14	Yes	Yes	6	Board Member in charge of Research	Vice-Chairman NMIBC guidelines panel
5	UK	53	20	20	Yes	-	0	Member	Member NMIBC guidelines panel
6	F	58	26	26	-	Yes	-	Member	Board Member ESOU
7	CZ	58	27	22	-	Yes	10	President of National Urological Society	Chairman NMIBC guidelines panel Member Education office of the ESU

Table 4. Cont.

Expert	Country	Age	Urology * (Years)	Oncology * (Years)	FEBU	PhD	Head of Urology **	National Association of Urology	European Association of Urology
8	F	59	26	25	Yes	Yes	5	Member	EAU Board Member ESU Member
9	E	61	33	20	Yes	Yes	2	Member	EAU Board member Director of ESU NMIBC Guidelines panel
10	NL	62	28	28	-	Yes	22	Chairman bladder cancer guidelines office	Chairman MIBC guidelines panel, ESU Member

* Years since board certification, that is, 202 years of combined experience in urology and 160 years in oncology.
** Years since head of department or unit. FEBU: Fellow of the European Board of Urology, ESU European School of Urology, YAU: Young Academic Urologists, ESOU: European Society of Oncologic Urology, NMIBC: non-muscle invasive bladder cancer, MIBC: muscle-invasive bladder cancer.

4.1. Step 1: Consensus Definition of Complexity

Reports on morbidity or mortality of TURBT were researched in the PubMed database (English language, 4/2009–4/2019, key words: "transurethral resection (of) bladder", "morbidity", "complication" "mortality" or "death"). A senior author (BM) reviewed all abstracts and analysed the articles of potential relevance before proposing to the panel a working definition of complexity in TURBT (Table S1).

4.2. Step 2: Listing the Items That Drive Complexity

4.2.1. Collection of the Factors Related to Complexity

Experts collected the factors that in their opinion could impact TURBT. All suggested items were considered and organized into domains, consistent with the medical usage and segmented according to the literature into a comprehensive list of items.

4.2.2. Delphi Validation

The panellists scored the items using a five-point Likert scale, classifying from "very unlikely" to "very likely" the risk of complexity entailed by the individual items (Table 5). After the first Delphi round, they were informed of the panel's distribution of the scores and requested in the second round to confirm or adjust their personal evaluation.

Consensus on an item was reached when the opinions across the panel were so consistent that the 95% confidence interval of their distribution was bounded within two consecutive scores. In subsequent analyses, the median value of the opinions or Median Opinion (MO) was used to weight the contribution of an item to complexity.

Table 5. Questions and Likert scores for complexity and patient and tumour's characteristics and surgical environment.

Domains	Question	Likert Scores
Patient and tumour and bladder characteristics	How likely is this characteristic to negatively impact TURBT, that is, to result in incomplete resection or prolonged surgery (>1 h) or significant intra- or postoperative complications (Clavien-Dindo Grade III and higher)?	(1) It is VERY UNLIKELY to impact TURBT (2) It is UNLIKELY to impact TURBT (3) It may OCCASIONALLY impact TURBT (4) It is LIKELY to impact TURBT (5) It is VERY LIKELY to impact TURBT
Surgical Environment	How likely is the following element of the surgical environment to influence the risk of TURBT resulting in either three situations, i.e., incomplete resection according to the operator, or prolonged surgery (>1 h) or significant intra- (bleeding that requires transfusion, laparotomy) or postoperative complications (Clavien-Dindo Grade III and higher)?	(1) It is VERY LIKELY TO REDUCE the risk (2) It is LIKELY TO REDUCE the risk (3) It is NOT EXPECTED TO INFLUENCE the risk in either way (4) It is LIKELY TO INCREASE the risk (5) It is VERY LIKELY TO INCREASE the risk
Clinical scenarios	In the following scenario, will TURBT result in incomplete resection or prolonged surgery (>1 h) or significant intra- or postoperative complications (Clavien-Dindo Grade III and higher)?	(1) This is VERY UNLIKELY to happen (2) This is UNLIKELY to happen (3) This may OCCASIONALLY happen (4) This is LIKELY to happen (5) This is VERY LIKELY to happen

4.3. Step 3: Construction of the Bladder Complexity Checklist

4.3.1. Construction of Clinical Scenarios

To acknowledge the multifactorial nature of complexity in medicine, items that reached consensus were then organized along clinical scenarios constructed by their random allocation within their respective domains of interest: patient's history, tumour number, main tumour size, location, and structure, access to the bladder cavity. One hundred and fifty scenarios were constructed (Table S2) and validated for clinical consistency (e.g., refuting the association of 30 mL prostate and female genital prolapse) by a senior author (B.M.). In keeping with the epidemiology of bladder cancer, twice as many scenarios were developed for male than female patients [54].

The panellists were requested to follow an adapted five-point Likert scale (Table 5) to answer the question: in the following scenario will TURBT result in incomplete resection or prolonged surgery (>1 h) or significant intra or postoperative complications (Clavien-Dindo Grade III and higher)?

Consensus was reached when the 95% confidence interval of the answers strictly showed "unlikely" as the upper bound (concluded as a scenario unlikely to be complex) or "possibly" as the lower bound (concluded as a possibly complex scenario). Otherwise, the answers were considered inconclusive, and the scenario was not considered for further analyses.

4.3.2. Discrimination of Individual Items in the Prediction of Complexity

On univariate analysis, the two-tailed Mann–Whitney U-test tested in the 150 scenarios the relationship between the domains of interest and complexity, dichotomized as "very unlikely or unlikely" or "possibly, likely or very likely".

Logistic regression was conducted, with the domains showing $p < 0.1$ on univariate analyses as predictors and complexity as a dependent variable. The probability of a complex surgery was estimated from the probability function. In keeping with the logistic regression model [55], it acknowledges the contributions of all independent domains (Table 2) by their respective regression coefficients adjusted to the specifics of the case by the median opinions of the panel (e.g., the respective contributions to complexity of a single tumour compared to 4 to 10 tumours were 0.96 and 0.96 × 3, respectively, as shown in Figure 2).

Following the structure of the probability function:

$$probability = \frac{1}{1 + \exp(-x)} \qquad (2)$$

where x is the sum of the intercept value of the logistic regression and of the scores of the independent domains multiplied by their regression coefficients, for any domain, the product of its regression coefficient by the score of its descriptor correlates with the probability of a complex surgery. This was used to simplify the function into a checklist (Table 3) where the respective inputs of the items were similarly quantitated by the product of the regression coefficient of their domains by the scores summarizing the median opinions of the panel (e.g., location on the anterior wall of the bladder; median opinion: 3 (Figure 2), regression coefficient of tumour location: 1.44 (Table 2), product: 3 × 1.44, approximated for ease of use to 4.5).

In any clinical situation, recording the most significant item in patient's history and access to the bladder, in complement to the tumour number, main tumour location and size, calculated the Bladder Complexity Checklist Sum.

ROC curves of the model and of the Bladder Complexity Checklist Sum were compared by the C-statistics. Ultimately, calibration curves illustrated their accuracies in the estimation of the probability of complexity in individual scenarios [56].

STATA/MP was used for statistics (StataCorp, College Station, TX-USA), significance was set at $p < 0.05$.

5. Conclusions

Preoperative factors that relate to complex TURBT were identified by expert judgement and organized into the Bladder Complexity Checklist to facilitate the evaluation of the risk of a complex TURBT, a crucial requisite to personalise patient's information, adapt human and technical resources to individual situations and address TURBT variability in clinical trials.

Supplementary Materials: The following are available online at http://www.mdpi.com/2072-6694/12/10/3063/s1, Figure S1: First-round distribution of the experts' scores regarding the influence of the characteristics of the patient on the likelihood of complex TURBT; Figure S2: First-round distribution of the experts' scores regarding the influence of the characteristics of the tumour on the likelihood of complex TURBT; Figure S3: First-round distribution of the experts' scores regarding the influence on the likelihood of complex TURBT of bladder characteristics and access; Figure S4: First-round distribution of the experts' scores regarding the influence of the surgical environment on the risk of TURBT or En-Bloc resection resulting in either three situations: incomplete resection according to the operator, prolonged surgery (>1 h) or significant intra- (bleeding that requires transfusion, laparotomy) or postoperative complications (Clavien-Dindo Grade III and higher); Table S1: Articles (English language, 4/2009-4/2019) found relevant to the definition of complexity in transurethral resection of bladder tumours; Table S2: 150 scenarios constructed for univariate and multivariate analyses of clinical features in relation to complexity.

Author Contributions: Conceptualization: E.X., M.C., M.B. (Marek Babjuk), J.P.R., F.W., B.M.; methodology M.R., B.M.; investigations: M.R., E.X., A.B., M.B. (Maximillian Burger), H.M., M.C., M.B. (Marek Babjuk), J.P.R., F.W., B.M.; writing—original draft preparation: M.R., B.M.; writing—review and editing: B.M.; supervision: B.M. All authors have read and agreed to the published version of the manuscript.

Funding: This research received no external funding.

Acknowledgments: The authors express their gratitude to Doctor Thomas Filleron for critical discussion on the methodology and to Professor Laurent Boccon-Gibod for his comments and review of the manuscript.

Conflicts of Interest: The Authors declare no conflict of interest.

References

1. Bray, F.; Ferlay, J.; Soerjomataram, I.; Siegel, R.L.; Torre, L.A.; Jemal, A. Global cancer statistics 2018: GLOBOCAN estimates of incidence and mortality worldwide for 36 cancers in 185 countries. *CA Cancer J. Clin.* **2018**, *68*, 394–424. [CrossRef] [PubMed]
2. Leal, J.; Luengo-Fernandez, R.; Sullivan, R.; Witjes, J.A. Economic Burden of Bladder Cancer Across the European Union. *Eur. Urol.* **2016**, *69*, 438–447. [CrossRef] [PubMed]
3. Babjuk, M.; Burger, M.; Comperat, E.M.; Gontero, P.; Mostafid, A.H.; Palou, J.; van Rhijn, B.W.G.; Rouprêt, M.; Shariat, S.F.; Sylvester, R.; et al. European Association of Urology Guidelines on Non-muscle-invasive Bladder Cancer (TaT1 and Carcinoma In Situ) - 2019 Update. *Eur. Urol.* **2019**, *76*, 639–657. [CrossRef] [PubMed]
4. Pereira, J.F.; Pareek, G.; Mueller-Leonhard, C.; Zhang, Z.; Amin, A.; Mega, A.; Tucci, C.; Golijanin, D.; Gershman, B. The Perioperative Morbidity of Transurethral Resection of Bladder Tumor: Implications for Quality Improvement. *Urology* **2019**, *125*, 131–137. [CrossRef] [PubMed]
5. Hollenbeck, B.K.; Miller, D.C.; Taub, D.; Dunn, R.L.; Khuri, S.F.; Henderson, W.G.; Montie, J.E.; Underwood, W.; Wei, J.T., 3rd; Wei, J.T. Risk factors for adverse outcomes after transurethral resection of bladder tumors. *Cancer* **2006**, *106*, 1527–1535. [CrossRef]
6. Cumberbatch, M.G.K.; Foerster, B.; Catto, J.W.F.; Kamat, A.M.; Kassouf, W.; Jubber, I.; Shariat, S.F.; Sylvester, R.J.; Gontero, P. Repeat Transurethral Resection in Non-muscle-invasive Bladder Cancer: A Systematic Review. *Eur. Urol.* **2018**, *73*, 925–933. [CrossRef]
7. Mariappan, P.; Finney, S.M.; Head, E.; Somani, B.K.; Zachou, A.; Smith, G.; Mishriki, S.F.; N'Dow, J.; Grigor, K.M.; Edinburgh Urological Cancer G. Good quality white-light transurethral resection of bladder tumours (GQ-WLTURBT) with experienced surgeons performing complete resections and obtaining detrusor muscle reduces early recurrence in new non-muscle-invasive bladder cancer: Validation across time and place and recommendation for benchmarking. *BJU Int.* **2012**, *109*, 1666–1673.
8. Ghali, F.; Moses, R.A.; Raffin, E.; Hyams, E.S. What factors are associated with unplanned return following transurethral resection of bladder tumor? An analysis of a large single institution's experience. *Scand. J. Urol.* **2016**, *50*, 370–373. [CrossRef]

9. Mariappan, P.; Zachou, A.; Grigor, K.M.; Edinburgh Uro-Oncology Group. Detrusor muscle in the first, apparently complete transurethral resection of bladder tumour specimen is a surrogate marker of resection quality, predicts risk of early recurrence, and is dependent on operator experience. *Eur. Urol.* **2010**, *57*, 843–849. [CrossRef]
10. Gan, C.; Patel, A.; Fowler, S.; Catto, J.; Rosario, D.; O'Brien, T. Snapshot of transurethral resection of bladder tumours in the United Kingdom Audit (STUKA). *BJU Int.* **2013**, *112*, 930–935. [CrossRef]
11. Prasad, N.N.; Muddukrishna, S.N. Quality of transurethral resection of bladder tumor procedure influenced a phase III trial comparing the effect of KLH and mitomycin C. *Trials* **2017**, *18*, 123. [CrossRef] [PubMed]
12. Skrzypczyk, M.A.; Nyk, L.; Szostek, P.; Szemplinski, S.; Borowka, A.; Dobruch, J. The role of endoscopic bladder tumour assessment in the management of patients subjected to transurethral bladder tumour resection. *Eur. J. Cancer Care (Engl.)* **2017**, *26*. [CrossRef] [PubMed]
13. Del Rosso, A.; Pace, G.; Masciovecchio, S.; Saldutto, P.; Galatioto, G.P.; Vicentini, C. Plasmakinetic bipolar versus monopolar transurethral resection of non-muscle invasive bladder cancer: A single center randomized controlled trial. *Int. J. Urol.* **2013**, *20*, 399–403. [CrossRef] [PubMed]
14. Pan, D.; Soloway, M.S. The importance of transurethral resection in managing patients with urothelial cancer in the bladder: Proposal for a transurethral resection of bladder tumor checklist. *Eur. Urol.* **2012**, *61*, 1199–1203. [CrossRef]
15. Venkatramani, V.; Panda, A.; Manojkumar, R.; Kekre, N.S. Monopolar versus bipolar transurethral resection of bladder tumors: A single center, parallel arm, randomized, controlled trial. *J. Urol.* **2014**, *191*, 1703–1707. [CrossRef]
16. Wu, Y.P.; Lin, T.T.; Chen, S.H.; Xu, N.; Wei, Y.; Huang, J.B.; Sun, X.L.; Zheng, Q.S.; Xue, X.Y.; Li, X.D. Comparison of the efficacy and feasibility of en bloc transurethral resection of bladder tumor versus conventional transurethral resection of bladder tumor: A meta-analysis. *Medicine (Baltimore)* **2016**, *95*, e5372. [CrossRef]
17. Zhang, K.Y.; Xing, J.C.; Li, W.; Wu, Z.; Chen, B.; Bai, D.Y. A novel transurethral resection technique for superficial bladder tumor: Retrograde en bloc resection. *World J. Surg. Oncol.* **2017**, *15*, 125. [CrossRef]
18. Herkommer, K.; Hofer, C.; Gschwend, J.E.; Kron, M.; Treiber, U. Gender and body mass index as risk factors for bladder perforation during primary transurethral resection of bladder tumors. *J. Urol.* **2012**, *187*, 1566–1570. [CrossRef]
19. Golan, S.; Baniel, J.; Lask, D.; Livne, P.M.; Yossepowitch, O. Transurethral resection of bladder tumour complicated by perforation requiring open surgical repair—Clinical characteristics and oncological outcomes. *BJU Int.* **2011**, *107*, 1065–1068. [CrossRef]
20. Carmignani, L.; Picozzi, S.; Stubinski, R.; Casellato, S.; Bozzini, G.; Lunelli, L.; Arena, D. Endoscopic resection of bladder cancer in patients receiving double platelet antiaggregant therapy. *Surg. Endosc.* **2011**, *25*, 2281–2287. [CrossRef]
21. Zhao, C.; Tang, K.; Yang, H.; Xia, D.; Chen, Z. Bipolar Versus Monopolar Transurethral Resection of Nonmuscle-Invasive Bladder Cancer: A Meta-Analysis. *J. Endourol.* **2016**, *30*, 5–12. [CrossRef] [PubMed]
22. Sugihara, T.; Yasunaga, H.; Horiguchi, H.; Matsui, H.; Nishimatsu, H.; Nakagawa, T.; Fushimi, K.; Kattan, M.W.; Homma, Y. Comparison of perioperative outcomes including severe bladder injury between monopolar and bipolar transurethral resection of bladder tumors: A population based comparison. *J. Urol.* **2014**, *192*, 1355–1359. [CrossRef] [PubMed]
23. Allard, C.B.; Meyer, C.P.; Gandaglia, G.; Chang, S.L.; Chun, F.K.; Gelpi-Hammerschmidt, F.; Hanske, J.; Kibel, A.S.; Preston, M.A.; Trinh, Q.D. The Effect of Resident Involvement on Perioperative Outcomes in Transurethral Urologic Surgeries. *J. Surg. Educ.* **2015**, *72*, 1018–1025. [CrossRef] [PubMed]
24. Patel, H.D.; Ball, M.W.; Cohen, J.E.; Kates, M.; Pierorazio, P.M.; Allaf, M.E. Morbidity of urologic surgical procedures: An analysis of rates, risk factors, and outcomes. *Urology* **2015**, *85*, 552–559. [CrossRef]
25. Avallone, M.A.; Sack, B.S.; El-Arabi, A.; Charles, D.K.; Herre, W.R.; Radtke, A.C.; Davis, C.M.; See, W.A. Ten-Year Review of Perioperative Complications After Transurethral Resection of Bladder Tumors: Analysis of Monopolar and Plasmakinetic Bipolar Cases. *J. Endourol.* **2017**, *31*, 767–773. [CrossRef]
26. Rambachan, A.; Matulewicz, R.S.; Pilecki, M.; Kim, J.Y.; Kundu, S.D. Predictors of readmission following outpatient urological surgery. *J. Urol.* **2014**, *192*, 183–188. [CrossRef]

27. Matulewicz, R.S.; Pilecki, M.; Rambachan, A.; Kim, J.Y.; Kundu, S.D. Impact of resident involvement on urological surgery outcomes: An analysis of 40,000 patients from the ACS NSQIP database. *J. Urol.* **2014**, *192*, 885–890. [CrossRef]
28. Picozzi, S.; Marenghi, C.; Ricci, C.; Bozzini, G.; Casellato, S.; Carmignani, L. Risks and complications of transurethral resection of bladder tumor among patients taking antiplatelet agents for cardiovascular disease. *Surg. Endosc.* **2014**, *28*, 116–121. [CrossRef]
29. De Nunzio, C.; Franco, G.; Cindolo, L.; Autorino, R.; Cicione, A.; Perdona, S.; Falsaperla, M.; Gacci, M.; Leonardo, C.; Damiano, R.; et al. Transuretral resection of the bladder (TURB): Analysis of complications using a modified Clavien system in an Italian real life cohort. *Eur. J. Surg. Oncol.* **2014**, *40*, 90–95. [CrossRef]
30. Valerio, M.; Cerantola, Y.; Fritschi, U.; Hubner, M.; Iglesias, K.; Legris, A.S.; Lucca, I.; Vlamopoulos, Y.; Vaucher, L.; Jichlinski, P. Comorbidity and nutritional indices as predictors of morbidity after transurethral procedures: A prospective cohort study. *Can. Urol. Assoc. J.* **2014**, *8*, E600–E604. [CrossRef]
31. Matulewicz, R.S.; Sharma, V.; McGuire, B.B.; Oberlin, D.T.; Perry, K.T.; Nadler, R.B. The effect of surgical duration of transurethral resection of bladder tumors on postoperative complications: An analysis of ACS NSQIP data. *Urol. Oncol.* **2015**, *33*, e19–e24. [CrossRef] [PubMed]
32. Di Paolo, P.L.; Vargas, H.A.; Karlo, C.A.; Lakhman, Y.; Zheng, J.; Moskowitz, C.S.; Al-Ahmadie, H.A.; Sala, E.; Bochner, B.H.; Hricak, H. Intradiverticular bladder cancer: CT imaging features and their association with clinical outcomes. *Clin. Imaging* **2015**, *39*, 94–98. [CrossRef] [PubMed]
33. Gregg, J.R.; McCormick, B.; Wang, L.; Cohen, P.; Sun, D.; Penson, D.F.; Smith, J.A.; Clark, P.E.; Cookson, M.S.; Barocas, D.A.; et al. Short term complications from transurethral resection of bladder tumor. *Can. J. Urol.* **2016**, *23*, 8198–8203.
34. Cornu, J.N.; Herrmann, T.; Traxer, O.; Matlaga, B. Prevention and Management Following Complications from Endourology Procedures. *Eur. Urol. Focus* **2016**, *2*, 49–59. [CrossRef]
35. Bolat, D.; Gunlusoy, B.; Degirmenci, T.; Ceylan, Y.; Polat, S.; Aydin, E.; Aydogdu, O.; Kozacioglu, Z. Comparing the short-term outcomes and complications of monopolar and bipolar transurethral resection of non-muscle invasive bladder cancers: A prospective, randomized, controlled study. *Arch. Esp. Urol.* **2016**, *69*, 225–233. [CrossRef]
36. Bansal, A.; Sankhwar, S.; Goel, A.; Kumar, M.; Purkait, B.; Aeron, R. Grading of complications of transurethral resection of bladder tumor using Clavien-Dindo classification system. *Indian. J. Urol.* **2016**, *32*, 232–237. [CrossRef] [PubMed]
37. Anderson, C.; Weber, R.; Patel, D.; Lowrance, W.; Mellis, A.; Cookson, M.; Lang, M.; Barocas, D.; Chang, S.; Newberger, E.; et al. A 10-Item Checklist Improves Reporting of Critical Procedural Elements during Transurethral Resection of Bladder Tumor. *J. Urol.* **2016**, *196*, 1014–1020. [CrossRef]
38. Konishi, T.; Washino, S.; Nakamura, Y.; Ohshima, M.; Saito, K.; Arai, Y.; Miyagawa, T. Risks and complications of transurethral resection of bladder tumors in patients receiving antiplatelet and/or anticoagulant therapy: A retrospective cohort study. *BMC Urol.* **2017**, *17*, 118. [CrossRef]
39. Prader, R.; De Broca, B.; Chevallier, D.; Amiel, J.; Durand, M. Outcome of Transurethral Resection of Bladder Tumor: Does Antiplatelet Therapy Really Matter? Analysis of a Retrospective Series. *J. Endourol.* **2017**, *31*, 1284–1288. [CrossRef]
40. Caras, R.J.; Lustik, M.B.; Kern, S.Q.; McMann, L.P.; Sterbis, J.R. Preoperative Albumin Is Predictive of Early Postoperative Morbidity and Mortality in Common Urologic Oncologic Surgeries. *Clin. Genitourin. Cancer* **2017**, *15*, e255–e262. [CrossRef]
41. Naspro, R.; Lerner, L.B.; Rossini, R.; Manica, M.; Woo, H.H.; Calopedos, R.J.; Cracco, C.M.; Scoffone, C.M.; Herrmann, T.R.; de la Rosette, J.J.; et al. Perioperative antithrombotic therapy in patients undergoing endoscopic urologic surgery: Where do we stand with current literature? *Minerva. Urol. Nefrol.* **2018**, *70*, 126–136.
42. Suskind, A.M.; Zhao, S.; Walter, L.C.; Boscardin, W.J.; Finlayson, E. Mortality and Functional Outcomes After Minor Urological Surgery in Nursing Home Residents: A National Study. *J. Am. Geriatr. Soc.* **2018**, *66*, 909–915. [CrossRef]
43. Ficarra, V.; Novara, G.; Secco, S.; Macchi, V.; Porzionato, A.; De Caro, R.; Artibani, W. Preoperative aspects and dimensions used for an anatomical (PADUA) classification of renal tumours in patients who are candidates for nephron-sparing surgery. *Eur. Urol.* **2009**, *56*, 786–793. [CrossRef] [PubMed]

44. Broer, T.; Bal, R.; Pickersgill, M. Problematisations of Complexity: On the Notion and Production of Diverse Complexities in Healthcare Interventions and Evaluations. *Sci. Cult. (Lond.)* **2017**, *26*, 135–160. [CrossRef] [PubMed]
45. Werner, C.; Bedford, T.; Cooke, R.M.; Hanea, A.M.; Morales-Napoles, O. Expert judgement for dependence in probabilistic modelling: A systematic literature review and future research directions. *Eur. J. Operat. Res.* **2017**, *258*, 801–819. [CrossRef]
46. Fernandez, M.I.; Brausi, M.; Clark, P.E.; Cookson, M.S.; Grossman, H.B.; Khochikar, M.; Kiemeney, L.A.; Malavaud, B.; Sanchez-Salas, R.; Soloway, M.S.; et al. Epidemiology, prevention, screening, diagnosis, and evaluation: Update of the ICUD-SIU joint consultation on bladder cancer. *World J. Urol.* **2019**, *37*, 3–13. [CrossRef] [PubMed]
47. Croskerry, P. From mindless to mindful practice—Cognitive bias and clinical decision making. *N. Engl. J. Med.* **2013**, *368*, 2445–2448. [CrossRef]
48. Peard, L.; Goodwin, J.; Hensley, P.; Dugan, A.; Bylund, J.; Harris, A.M. Examining and Understanding Value: The Impact of Preoperative Characteristics, Intraoperative Variables, and Postoperative Complications on Cost of Robot-Assisted Laparoscopic Radical Prostatectomy. *J. Endourol.* **2019**, *33*, 541–548. [CrossRef]
49. Bromwich, D. Plenty to worry about: Consent, control, and anxiety. *Am. J. Bioeth.* **2012**, *12*, 35–36. [CrossRef]
50. Wiseman, O.J.; Wijewardena, M.; Calleary, J.; Masood, J.; Hill, J.T. 'Will you be doing my operation doctor?' Patient attitudes to informed consent. *Ann. R. Coll. Surg. Engl.* **2004**, *86*, 462–464. [CrossRef]
51. Boulkedid, R.; Abdoul, H.; Loustau, M.; Sibony, O.; Alberti, C. Using and reporting the Delphi method for selecting healthcare quality indicators: A systematic review. *PLoS ONE* **2011**, *6*, e20476. [CrossRef] [PubMed]
52. Leeflang, M.M.; Rutjes, A.W.; Reitsma, J.B.; Hooft, L.; Bossuyt, P.M. Variation of a test's sensitivity and specificity with disease prevalence. *CMAJ* **2013**, *185*, E537–E544. [CrossRef] [PubMed]
53. Dalgaard, L.P.; Zare, R.; Gaya, J.M.; Redorta, J.P.; Roumiguie, M.; Filleron, T.; Malavaud, B. Prospective evaluation of the performances of narrow-band imaging flexible videoscopy relative to white-light imaging flexible videoscopy, in patients scheduled for transurethral resection of a primary NMIBC. *World J. Urol.* **2019**, *37*, 1615–1621. [CrossRef] [PubMed]
54. Cumberbatch, M.G.K.; Jubber, I.; Black, P.C.; Esperto, F.; Figueroa, J.D.; Kamat, A.M.; Kiemeney, L.; Lotan, Y.; Pang, K.; Silverman, D.T.; et al. Epidemiology of Bladder Cancer: A Systematic Review and Contemporary Update of Risk Factors in 2018. *Eur. Urol.* **2018**, *74*, 784–795. [CrossRef] [PubMed]
55. Vollmer, R.T. Multivariate statistical analysis for pathologist. Part I, The logistic model. *Am. J. Clin. Pathol.* **1996**, *105*, 115–126. [CrossRef]
56. Steyerberg, E.W.; Vickers, A.J.; Cook, N.R.; Gerds, T.; Gonen, M.; Obuchowski, N.; Pencina, M.J.; Kattan, M.W. Assessing the performance of prediction models: A framework for traditional and novel measures. *Epidemiology* **2010**, *21*, 128–138. [CrossRef]

Publisher's Note: MDPI stays neutral with regard to jurisdictional claims in published maps and institutional affiliations.

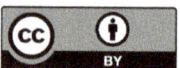

© 2020 by the authors. Licensee MDPI, Basel, Switzerland. This article is an open access article distributed under the terms and conditions of the Creative Commons Attribution (CC BY) license (http://creativecommons.org/licenses/by/4.0/).

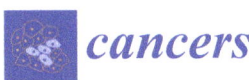

Article

CPT1A Over-Expression Increases Reactive Oxygen Species in the Mitochondria and Promotes Antioxidant Defenses in Prostate Cancer

Molishree Joshi [1], Jihye Kim [2], Angelo D'Alessandro [3,4], Emily Monk [2], Kimberley Bruce [5], Hanan Elajaili [6], Eva Nozik-Grayck [6], Andrew Goodspeed [1,4], James C. Costello [1,4] and Isabel R. Schlaepfer [2,*]

[1] Department of Pharmacology, University of Colorado Anschutz Medical Campus, Aurora, CO 80045, USA; Molishree.Joshi@cuanschutz.edu (M.J.); Andrew.Goodspeed@cuanschutz.edu (A.G.); James.Costello@cuanschutz.edu (J.C.C.)
[2] Division of Medical Oncology, University of Colorado Anschutz Medical Campus, Aurora, CO 80045, USA; Jihye.Kim@cuanschutz.edu (J.K.); Emily.Monk@cuanschutz.edu (E.M.)
[3] Department of Biochemistry, University of Colorado Anschutz Medical Campus, Aurora, CO 80045, USA; Angelo.Dalessandro@cuanschutz.edu
[4] University of Colorado Comprehensive Cancer Center, Anschutz Medical Campus, Aurora, CO 80045, USA
[5] Division of Endocrinology, Metabolism and Diabetes, University of Colorado Anschutz Medical Campus, Aurora, CO 80045, USA; Kimberley.Bruce@cuanschutz.edu
[6] Department of Pediatrics Critical Care, University of Colorado Anschutz Medical Campus, Aurora, CO 80045, USA; Hanan.Elajaili@cuanschutz.edu (H.E.); Eva.Nozik@cuanschutz.edu (E.N.-G.)
* Correspondence: Isabel.Schlaepfer@cuanschutz.edu

Received: 6 October 2020; Accepted: 9 November 2020; Published: 18 November 2020

Simple Summary: Prostate cancer (PCa) is the most common cancer in men and the second highest contributor to cancer deaths. Targeting lipid catabolism enzymes in PCa may offer new avenues for therapeutic approaches. During the last decade, carnitine palmitoyl transferase I (CPT1A) has been identified as a potential therapeutic target for a growing list of cancers. In this study, we have tested the hypothesis that excess CPT1A plays a key role in supporting adaptation to stress and antioxidant defense production in PCa cells. Specifically, we have studied molecular differences between CPT1A gain and loss of function models, revealing genetic and metabolic vulnerabilities that could be targeted to avoid progression to neuroendocrine differentiation, a lethal form of the disease. Examining public datasets, we have also found that excess CPT1A expression leads to worse progression-free survival in PCa patients.

Abstract: Cancers reprogram their metabolism to adapt to environmental changes. In this study, we examined the consequences of altered expression of the mitochondrial enzyme carnitine palmitoyl transferase I (CPT1A) in prostate cancer (PCa) cell models. Using transcriptomic and metabolomic analyses, we compared LNCaP-C4-2 cell lines with depleted (knockdown (KD)) or increased (overexpression (OE)) CPT1A expression. Mitochondrial reactive oxygen species (ROS) were also measured. Transcriptomic analysis identified ER stress, serine biosynthesis and lipid catabolism as significantly upregulated pathways in the OE versus KD cells. On the other hand, androgen response was significantly downregulated in OE cells. These changes associated with increased acyl-carnitines, serine synthesis and glutathione precursors in OE cells. Unexpectedly, OE cells showed increased mitochondrial ROS but when challenged with fatty acids and no androgens, the Superoxide dismutase 2 (SOD2) enzyme increased in the OE cells, suggesting better antioxidant defenses with excess CPT1A expression. Public databases also showed decreased androgen response correlation with increased serine-related metabolism in advanced PCa. Lastly, worse progression free survival was observed with increased lipid catabolism and decreased androgen response. Excess CPT1A is associated with a ROS-mediated stress phenotype that can support PCa disease progression. This study provides a rationale for targeting lipid catabolic pathways for therapy in hormonal cancers.

Keywords: CPT1A; prostate cancer; fatty acids; serine; androgen response; ROS; oxidative stress

---

1. Introduction

Prostate cancer (PCa) is the most common cancer in men and the second highest contributor to cancer deaths [1]. Although initially highly effective as a treatment for metastatic PCa, androgen deprivation therapy is characterized by a predictable emergence of resistance, a disease state termed castration-resistant prostate cancer (CRPC) [2]. An important feature of CRPC is the reactivation of androgen receptor (AR) signaling, an event reflected by progressive rises in serum prostate-specific antigen (PSA), a gene product regulated by the androgen receptor (AR) [3]. Substantial evidence has documented that the majority of AR-regulated genes (androgen-response hallmark genes) are re-expressed in most CRPCs, and several mechanisms capable of maintaining AR activity have been established [4,5]. Alternatively, disease progression can arise in the absence of a functional AR as an extremely aggressive and metastatic variant called small cell or neuroendocrine PCa [6,7]. Although genetic alterations are known to promote this aggressive state of the disease [8], we currently lack mechanistic insight as to which metabolic pathways play important roles in PCa plasticity, resistance and progression to lethal disease.

Mitochondrial fatty acid β-oxidation is the major pathway for the catabolism of fatty acids, and it plays an essential role in maintaining whole body energy homeostasis. The transfer of fatty acids into the mitochondria for oxidation happens in an organized, controlled way. The enzyme carnitine palmitoyl transferase I (CPT1A) resides in the outer mitochondrial membrane and catalyzes the reversible transfer of acyl groups between coenzyme A (CoA) and L-carnitine, converting acyl-CoA esters into acyl-carnitine esters. These acyl-carnitines can then enter the matrix where β-oxidation takes place [9]. The activity of CPT1A produces a greater number of acetyl groups, which can be used for energy, de novo lipid synthesis and acetylation reactions, including histone acetylation in the nucleus [10].

Support for a strong association between specific dietary lipids and PCa is still unclear. For example, a recent paper showed that a high fat diet promotes metastatic prostate cancer [11]. Although this is a great step forward in understanding the clinical role of dietary lipids promoting metastatic PCa, it does not address how tumor cells use the lipids to their benefit. Particularly, it is not clear how CPT1A activity could promote a metabolic environment conducive to cell transformation, cancer progression and drug resistance [12].

Targeting lipid catabolism enzymes in PCa may offer new avenues for therapeutic approaches [13]. During the last decade, CPT1A has been identified as a potential therapeutic target for a growing list of cancers [14]. In these cancers, CPT1A expression is increased, and/or its inhibition has been reported to have antitumor effects. Our group has shown that fatty acid oxidation is an important pathway in cancer metabolism in PCa cells when using the CPT1 inhibitor etomoxir [15–17]. The blockade of CPT1A with etomoxir produced unresolved endoplasmic reticulum (ER) stress leading to cell apoptosis and decreased tumor growth in vivo. Indeed, lipid oxidation in the mitochondria of aggressive cancer cells can provide adaptation to stress by promoting the generation of antioxidant molecules, like Nicotinamide adenine dinucleotide phosphate (NADPH) [18].

Loss of balance between the antioxidant defense and oxidant production in the cells, which commonly occurs as a secondary feature in many diseases, is loosely termed "oxidative stress". This balance is important because the intracellular redox environment must be more reducing than oxidizing to maintain optimal cell function. Oxidative stress and ER stress are linked to multiple pathologies, including metabolic, neurodegenerative, immune, and neoplastic diseases. Studies on these two cellular stresses have not only contributed to our understanding of disease, but also opened new avenues to next-generation therapies for these illnesses [19,20]. Their exact role in supporting cancer survival and drug resistance remains unknown.

Since oxidative stress is usually coupled with ER stress [21], the unfolded protein response (UPR) has evolved to handle both proteins folding defects and oxidative challenge. In fact, excess nutrients are proposed to induce ER stress and oxidative stress in pancreatic beta-cells, including glucotoxicity and lipotoxicity. For example, chronic excess glucose induces the pro-apoptotic UPR and oxidative stress in beta-cells cells in vitro and in mice models [22]. In addition, free fatty acids, such as palmitate, induce ER stress and oxidative stress and cause apoptosis in β cells [23]. Cancer cells, especially hormone-dependent cancers, like PCa, exploit these stress responses to deal with the oncogenic and metabolic reprograming, making them more adaptable to affront the insults from drug cancer therapies. Indeed, conditional knockout of the ER chaperone GRP78 (HSPA5) in the prostate of mice with PTEN inactivation suppressed prostate cancer growth [24]. The role of CPT1A in supporting adaptive ER stress responses and redox regulation has not been studied.

In this study, we have tested the hypothesis that excess CPT1A plays a key role in supporting adaptation to stress and antioxidant defense production in CRPC cells. We have used the LNCap-C4-2 model as it represents advanced CRPC that can grow in androgen depleted conditions and form metastasis [25]. We have also explored publicly available clinical databases to support our findings. Specifically, we have studied molecular differences between CPT1A gain and loss of function C4-2 models, revealing metabolic vulnerabilities that could be targeted to avoid progression to neuroendocrine differentiation.

2. Results

2.1. Cells with Overexpression of CPT1A Show a Lipid Catabolic Phenotype and Increased Growth When Supplemented with Fatty Acids

CPT1A fuels lipid beta-oxidation in PCa cells by producing acyl-carnitines in the mitochondria [9]. To characterize the biochemical changes in the newly described knockdown (KD) and overexpression (OE) C4-2 models [10], we used lipid-based assays and metabolomics. Figure 1A shows that CPT1A is significantly increased in the OE cells and this is associated with a significant increase in intracellular lipase activity, a step which liberates fatty acids from triglyceride stores which can then be used for beta oxidation [26] (Figure 1B). Metabolomic analysis of the OE versus KD C4-2 cells showed significant increases in most of the acyl-carnitine identified, from the short and medium-chain (Figure 1C) to the long-chain species (Figure 1D). Furthermore, the KD cells (blue bars) showed decreased production of the abundant long-chain C16:0 (palmitic) and C18:1 (Oleic) species as expected from the decreased activity of CPT1A in these cells. The use of the CPT1 inhibitor etomoxir, also resulted in decreased production of acyl carnitines in C4-2 parental cells treated with the inhibitor for 48 h (Figure 1E). We next studied the effects of fatty acid availability on the colony growth of OE and KD cells (Figure 1F–I). Fatty acids were conjugated to bovine serum albumin (BSA) and growth was normalized to BSA-only treatment for each cell line. Dodecanoate (C12) treatment showed increased growth in OE compared to empty virus (EV) control cells (Figure 1G), and this effect was not observed in the KD cells (Figure 1F). Similar results were obtained with C16:0 supplementation, where OE cells increased in growth (Figure 1I) but not in KD cells (Figure 1H). The addition of other medium- and long-chain fatty acids also produced significant increases in growth in OE cells compared to controls (Figure S1), except for C18:1, which promoted growth in both KD and EV cells. These results may reflect the lipid droplet-inducing effects of oleic acid supplementation in cancer cells, promoting growth and survival [27,28].

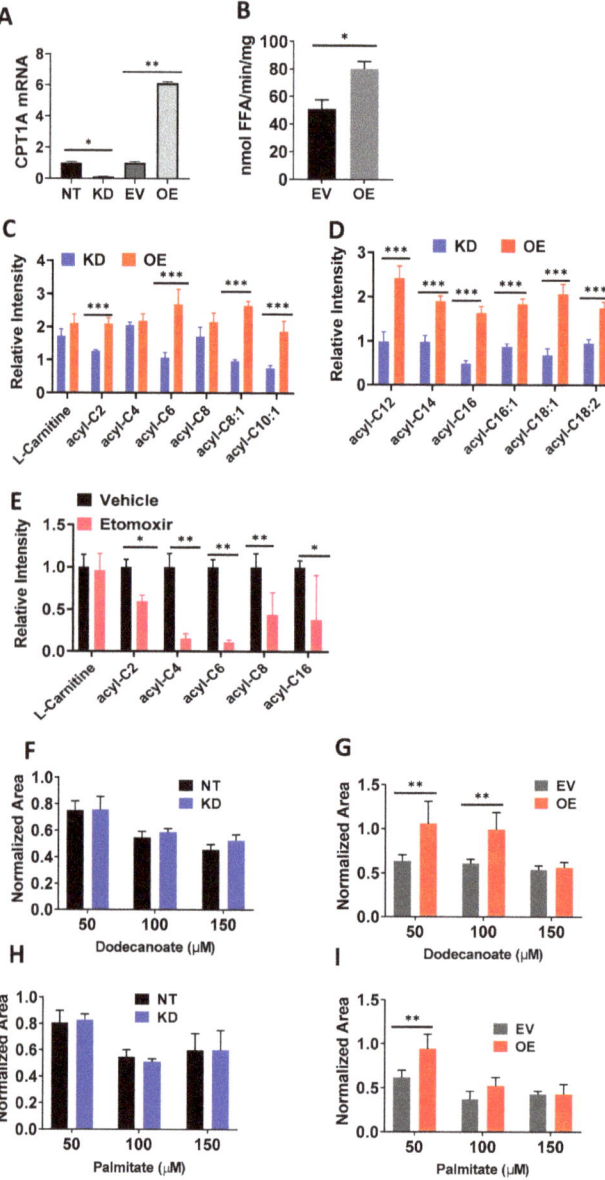

Figure 1. Cells with overexpression of carnitine palmitoyl transferase I (CPT1A) show a lipid catabolic phenotype and increased growth when supplemented with fatty acids. (**A**) mRNA expression of C4-2 cells with decreased (knockdown (KD)) and overexpression (OE) of CPT1A cells and their respective controls (non-targeting (NT) and empty virus (EV)). (**B**) Intracellular triglyceride lipase assay in OE cells. (**C,D**) Short and medium (**C**) and long chain (**D**) acyl carnitine content in OE (red) versus KD (blue), normalized to their own controls. (**E**) Acyl carnitine changes in C4-2 parental cells treated with etomoxir (100 µM) for 48 h. (**F,G**) Colony growth after treatment with C12:0 fatty acid conjugated to BSA for 14 days and normalized to BSA-only treatment. (**H,I**) Colony growth after treatment with C16:0 fatty acid conjugated to BSA for 14 days and normalized to BSA-only treatment. * $p < 0.05$, ** $p < 0.01$, *** $p < 0.001$.

2.2. RNAseq Analysis of CPT1A OE Cells Shows Increased ER Stress Response, Serine Metabolism and Less AR Signaling

To identify the molecular signatures associated with CPT1A expression, we performed RNAseq in the C4-2 KD and OE cells. Figure 2 and Table S1 show the results of our analysis comparing the OE cells to the KD cells. Briefly, we normalized each cell line to its respective control (Figure 2A), and then we used limma to compare the gene expression differences between OE and KD [29]. Overall, we found 1157 genes upregulated and 1385 genes downregulated when comparing the OE cells to the KD cells. Genes were filtered by an adjusted p-value of 0.0001. Using gene set enrichment analysis (GSEA), we found that ER stress and UPR response were some of the most significant pathways increased in the OE cells, pointing to possible lipid-mediated oxidative stress (Figure 2B). Cell division, mitosis and E2F targets pathways were significantly decreased in OE cells, which is in agreement with their decreased growth rate compared to their control line [10]. The androgen response hallmark gene set was significantly decreased in the OE cells and it reflects less dependency of OE cells on AR signaling, which is something we have observed and reported previously [10]. As expected from our metabolic observations, the lipid catabolic process pathway, including the CPT1A gene, was significantly increased in OE cells compared to KD cells. Figure 2C shows a heatmap of genes from the leading-edge analysis in Figure 2B associated with lipid catabolism, response to cellular stress and androgen response pathways. Enrichment plots for these pathways are shown in Figure S2. Examination of the significant genes in these pathways (Figure 2D–F), showed opposite directions of change between OE and KD cells. For most of the genes, the KD cells showed decreases in gene expression when compared to OE cells.

2.3. Excess CPT1A Is Associated with Serine and Glycine Metabolism and Glutathione Homeostasis Metabolites

To understand the type of stress imposed in the CPT1A OE cells, we performed global, non-targeted metabolomics in the four cells lines: non-targeting (NT), KD, EV, and OE cells. In parallel to the RNAseq analysis, we focused on the metabolic pathway differences between OE and KD cells after controlling for their respective control lines (EV and NT respectively). Analysis of the top 25 significant pathways revealed that lipid metabolism, glycine and serine metabolism, and glutathione homeostasis were the most significantly changed pathways (Figure 3A and Figure S3). Glycolysis was also significantly different across groups, with the OE cells showing less glycolysis compared to KD cells (Figure S3).

Considering the RNAseq data, we next analyzed the metabolites corresponding to the serine/glycine metabolism. The serine, glycine and one carbon metabolism pathway are a metabolic network upregulated in tumors and of high clinical relevance [30,31]. Except glucose, individual metabolites of the serine/glycine pathway were not changed significantly in OE versus KD (Figure 3B). However, the OE cells showed more intracellular glucose being shunted towards de novo serine biosynthesis compared to control EV cells (Figure S3A). In fact, less glucose seemed to be used for glycolysis in the OE cells. These results correlated with significantly increased expression of key serine/glycine pathway genes: D-3-phosphoglycerate dehydrogenase (PHGDH), phosphohydroxythreonine aminotransferase (PSAT1), and Serine hydroxymethyltransferase (SHMT2) (Figures 2E and 3B). SHMT2 is a mitochondrial enzyme that converts serine (3 carbons) into glycine (2 carbons), transferring one carbon to tetrahydrofolate (mitochondrial folate cycle). The increased dimethylglycine and cystathionine levels in OE cells compared to KD cells supports a higher folate cycle activity in these cells (Figure 3B,C).

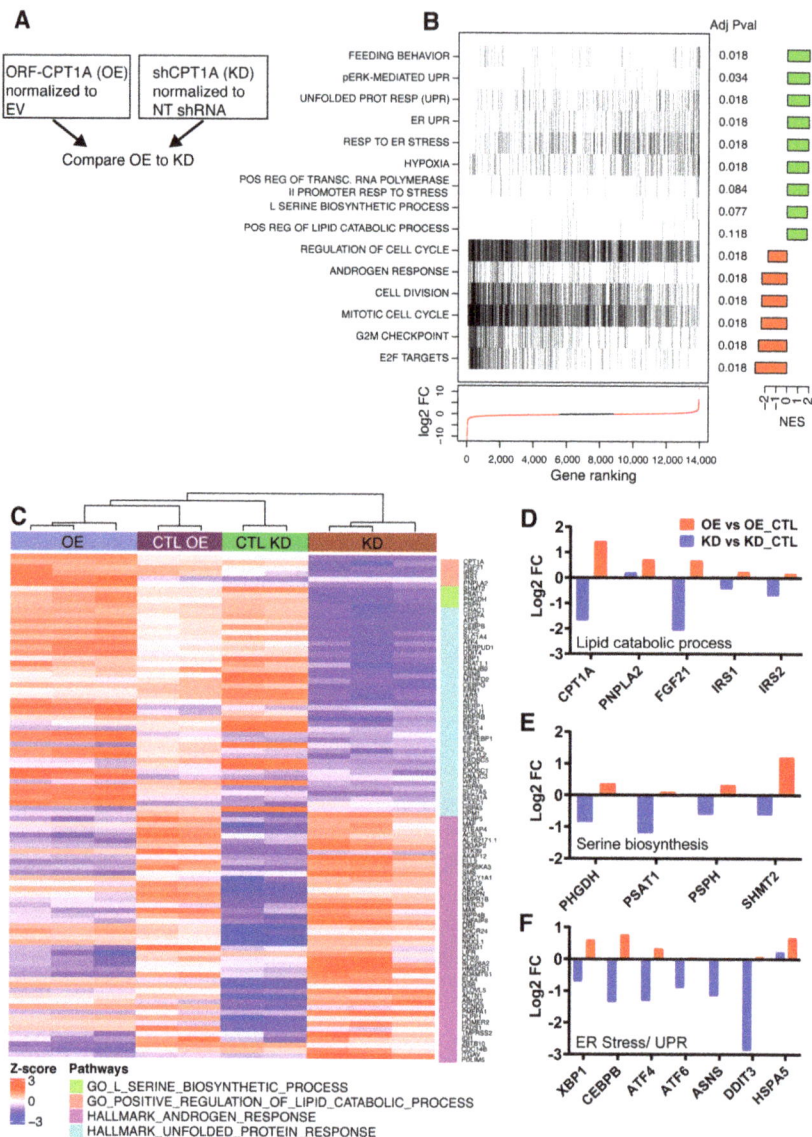

Figure 2. RNAseq analysis of CPT1A OE cells shows increased endoplasmic reticulum (ER) stress response, serine metabolism, and less androgen receptor (AR) signaling. (**A**) Schematic of the RNAseq analysis paradigm with the CPT1A-KD and OE cells. (**B**) Gene set enrichment analysis was performed on the fold change of the comparison. Normalized Enrichment Scores (NES) and False discovery rate (FDR) adjusted p-values are shown for select pathways, as well as the rank of those genes in fold change ranking, are plotted. (**C**) Heatmap of the leading-edge genes for select pathways. (**D**–**F**) Gene expression graphs of significant genes associated with lipid catabolism (**D**), serine biosynthesis (**E**) and ER stress (**F**) in OE versus KD comparison after adjustment to their respective control cell lines. Adj p value < 0.001.

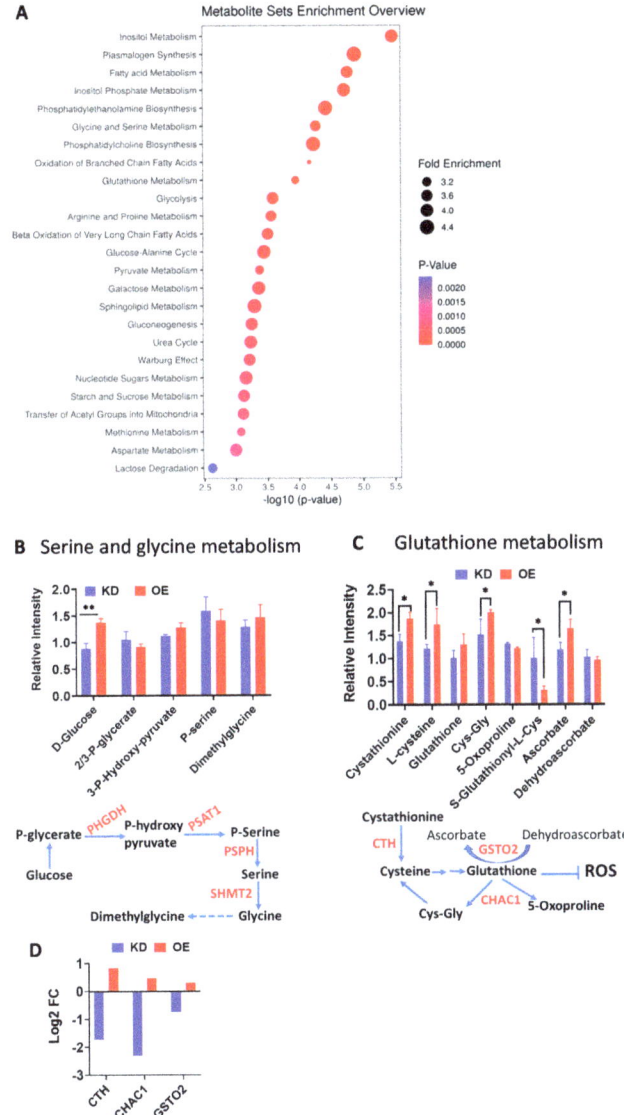

Figure 3. Excess CPT1A is associated with serine and glycine metabolism pathway and glutathione homeostasis metabolites. (**A**) Metabolite set enrichment analysis of OE metabolites versus KD cell metabolites after normalization to their own controls. The *p*-value is defined by the color scale, and the enrichment by the size of the circle. (**B**) Relative abundance of metabolites associated with the serine and glycine biosynthesis via the SHMT2 gene in the mitochondria. A scheme of the pathway is shown under the graphs, highlighting the sequence of events from glucose to synthesis of serine, glycine and the one carbon metabolism compound dimethylglycine. The genes significantly altered in OE cells from the RNAseq analysis involved in the pathway are shown in red. (**C**) Relative abundance of metabolites associated glutathione (GSH) homeostasis. The S-glutathionyl-L-Cys metabolite is associated with ineffective handling of oxidative stress. A scheme to the pathway is shown below. * $p < 0.05$, ** $p < 0.01$. (**D**) Gene expression analysis of OE versus KD cells for CTH ($p = 6.29 \times 10^{-13}$), CHAC1 ($p = 3.6 \times 10^{-12}$) and GSTO2 ($p = 0.003$) genes (adj *p*-value).

Metabolites involved in Glutathione (GSH) homeostasis were also significantly changed in the OE cells compared to the KD cells (Figure 3C), suggesting better antioxidant defense. Particularly, cystathionine and cysteine were significantly increased in OE versus KD cells, and between OE cells and controls, suggesting increased cysteine synthesis and availability to generate glutathione. These increases are associated with increased expression of CTH, a cystathionine gamma lyase that breaks down cystathionine to generate cysteine [32], Figure 3D. Unexpectedly, we also observed increased generation of two breakdown products of glutathione via the ChaC Glutathione Specific Gamma-Glutamylcyclotransferase 1 (CHAC1) enzyme. These enzymes are gamma-glutamyl cyclotransferases, which are induced by ER stress and have specific activity towards glutathione [33]. CHAC1 has been shown to break glutathione into 5-oxoproline and cysteinyl-glycine (Cys-Gly), promoting the depletion of glutathione and stress-induced apoptosis in cysteine deprived cancer cells [34]. However, we did not observe a depletion of glutathione in OE cells with higher CHAC1 expression (Figure 3C), suggesting that metabolite recycling mechanisms or compensatory increased production of glutathione may exist in OE cells [35]. Another indication that OE may have more antioxidant defense than KD cells comes from the increased ratio of ascorbate to dehydroascorbate, which is likely maintained by the dehydroascorbate activity of Glutathione S-Transferase Omega 2 (GSTO2) [36], which is significantly upregulated in the OE cells and can recycle the glutathione to a reduced state, Figure 3C,D.

2.4. Mitochondrial Reactive Oxygen Species (ROS) Are Increased in CPT1A-OE Cells

Since GSH homeostasis was significantly changed in OE cells, we reasoned that mitochondrial ROS production could be altered in response to increased CPT1A expression. Thus, we next studied the amount of ROS produced in the mitochondria of the cell models. Figure 4A shows the stacked traces of the Electron Paramagnetic Resonance (EPR) assay, highlighting the increased amplitude of the signal in the OE cells compared to all the other samples. Quantification of the signals is shown in Figure 4B, with the OE cells having a 4-fold increase in mitochondrial ROS production compared to KD cells. Examination of the RNAseq data indicated that SOD2, the mitochondrial superoxide dismutase, was significantly decreased in OE cells compared to KD cells (1.4-fold less $p < 0.0007$, Figure 4C). The cytosolic counterpart SOD1 was not significantly changed between OE and KD cells, while the extracellular SOD3 mRNA was significantly increased in the KD compared to the OE cells ($p = 0.01$). Thus, less SOD2 expression in the OE cells likely accounted for the increase in mitochondrial ROS in these cells. Since the OE cells did not show signs of apoptosis induced by excess ROS we next challenged the cells with long chain lipids (oleic and palmitate mixture at 25 µM each) in the presence or absence of androgens, using regular fetal bovine serum (FBS) or charcoal stripped serum (CSS) devoid of steroid hormones. This fatty acid mixture was used because it represents the most common fatty acids circulating in blood and they are substrates for CPT1A activity (Figure 1D). Figure 4D,E and Figure S4, show that SOD2 did not change in response to the lipid stimulation (Figure 4D), but it decreased in the KD cells compared to the OE cells with androgen withdraw conditions (Figure 4E). Thus, in the presence of lipids and androgen deprivation conditions, CPT1A OE cells are likely to cope with the excess mitochondrial ROS from fat oxidation (Figure 4F).

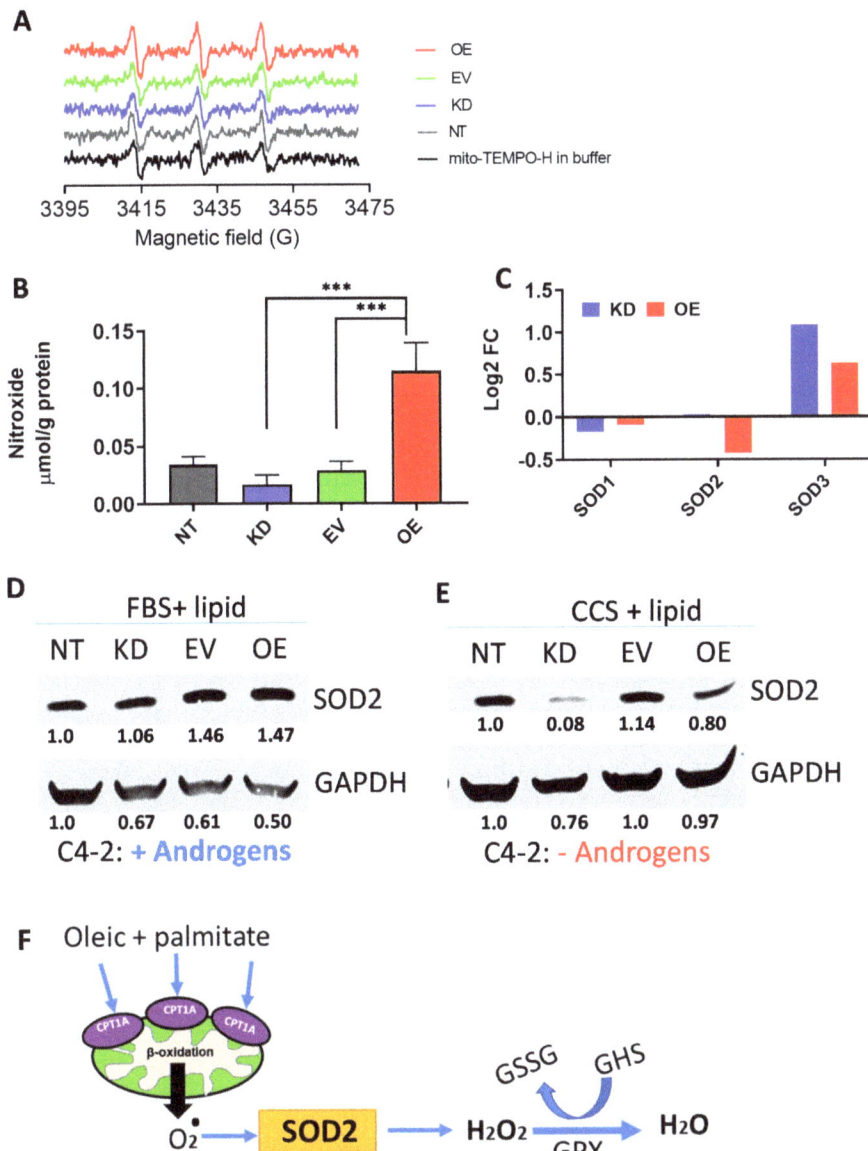

Figure 4. Mitochondrial reactive oxygen species (ROS) are increased in CPT1A-OE cells. (**A**) Electron paramagnetic resonance spectroscopy (EPR) traces of the four cell lines tested, including the mitochondrial probe by itself. Amplitude and linewidth provide information of the amount of ROS. The concentration was acquired by Spin Fit followed by SpinCount module (Bruker). (**B**) Quantification of the EPR traces normalized to protein content. *** $p < 0.001$. (**C**) Gene expression analysis of OE versus KD cells for SOD1 ns), SOD2 ($p = 6.9 \times 10^{-4}$), and SOD3 ($p = 0.015$). Only SOD2 is a mitochondrial enzyme. (**D,E**) Western blots of SOD2 expression after incubation with fatty acids (Oleic and palmitate mixture; 25 µM each) in FBS (**D**) or charcoal stripped serum (CSS) (**E**) for 48 h. (**F**) Schematic of the role of SOD2 in metabolizing superoxide and the role of glutathione in eliminating H_2O_2. GPX = Glutathione peroxide. GSSG = oxidized glutathione.

2.5. Lipid and Serine Metabolism Genes Are Associated with Less Androgen Signaling and a More Neuroendocrine Phenotype

Gene set enrichment analysis of our RNAseq showed decreased expression of androgen response genes CPT1A OE cells (Figure 5A). Since decreased AR signaling is associated with changes to a neuroendoendocrine phenotype [7], we next looked for markers of neuronal-like differentiation and identified Enolase 2 (ENO2), Synaptophysin (SYP), Neural Cell Adhesion Molecule 2 (NCAM2), and Neurexophilin 4 (NXPH4) genes significantly upregulated in OE versus KD cells. The ENO2 and SYP genes are markers associated with neuroendocrine PCa (NEPC). To investigate the possibility that CPT1A overexpression (OE) is associated with more aggressive disease, we searched previous transcriptome analysis in the public databases. Particularly, we searched for studies that compared adenocarcinoma with aggressive disease like small cell NEPC and focused on serine and one carbon metabolism, CPT1A and AR expression in clinical data.

Using the dataset from GSE32967 [37], we compared gene expression between small cell carcinoma (a subset of NEPC) and adenocarcinoma patient derived PCa xenografts. GSE Analysis showed that the androgen response hallmark was significantly decreased in the NEPC samples, while significant increases were observed in the serine metabolism and one carbon (tetrahydrofolate) metabolism pathways (Figure 5C). Several of serine and tetrahydrofolate leading-edge genes increased in our RNAseq analysis were also increased in the GSE32967 dataset (Figure 5D). Addition of CPT1A and AR gene expression to the heatmap showed that one NEPC sample had low AR as expected, but modest increased CPT1A associated with increased SHMT2, MTHFD2 and PSPH expression. Conversely, one sample with adenocarcinoma features showed less CPT1A associated with less SHMT2, MTHFD2, and PSAT1 expression (Figure 5D). We further investigated the direction of the relationship between CPT1A and AR expression in metastatic disease (Figure S5), using the Taylor et al. dataset [38]. A positive correlation was observed in the primary tumors, as expected from the role of androgens in regulating lipid metabolism [39]. However, this positive correlation was lost in the metastatic samples ($R = -0.28$, $p = 0.25$), where AR expression was significantly increased compared to primary tumors (Wilcoxon $p = 1.1 \times 10^{-7}$). The possibility that a strong anti-androgen blockade in these metastatic samples could reverse the correlation to less AR and more CPT1A expression, as it happens in NEPC, warrants further investigation.

2.6. Increased Lipid Catabolism and Decreased Androgen Response Is Associated with Poorer Progression-Free Survival

To further validate the role of CPT1A and lipid catabolism in advanced PCa, we turned to publicly accessible TCGA (The Cancer Genome Atlas) Firehose Legacy dataset (492 samples). Pathways were scored in each patient using GSEA and grouped according by median split of each pathway. Examination of the same GSEA pathways identified in our RNAseq data (Figure 2C) showed that the lipid catabolic process (Figure 6A), and the androgen response hallmark (Figure 6B), were significantly associated with progression free survival (PFS) but in opposite directions. The increase in lipid catabolism genes and the decrease in androgen response genes shortened the PFS. We did not observe significant PFS changes with the GO serine metabolism and the unfolded protein response hallmark pathways (Figure S6).

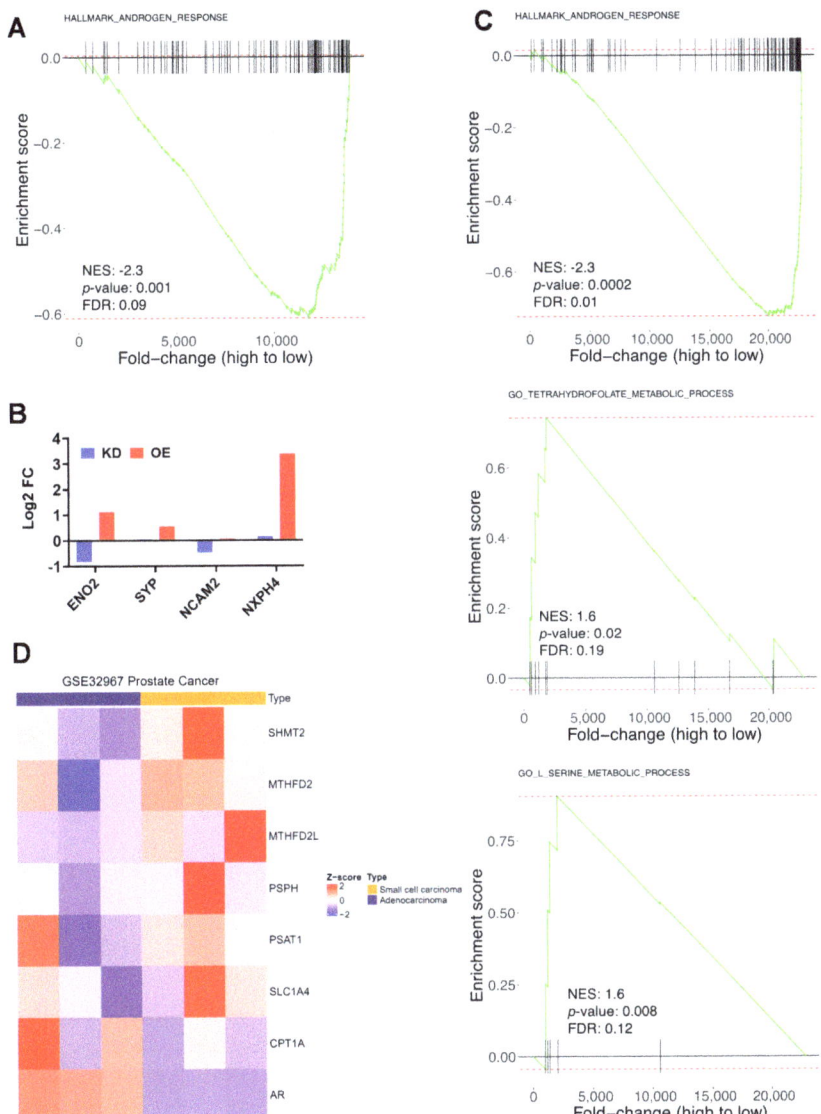

Figure 5. Lipid and serine metabolism genes are associated with less androgen signaling and a neuroendocrine phenotype. (**A**) Gene set enrichment analysis (GSEA) plot of the OE versus KD analysis showing the decrease in the androgen response hallmark in OE cells. (**B**) Gene expression analysis of OE versus KD cells for neuronal-like markers like ENO2 ($p = 6.1 \times 10^{-10}$), SYP (p = ns), NCAM2 ($p = 4.14 \times 10^{-5}$), NXPH4 ($p = 1.6 \times 10^{-17}$). (**C**) GSEA plots of the public GSE32967 dataset showing the comparison between small cell carcinoma ($n = 3$) versus adenocarcinoma ($n = 3$) patient xenografts for the Hallmark Androgen Response; GO_Serine and GO_Tetrahydrofolate pathways. Normalized enrichment scores (NES) and statistical significance are indicated in the plots. (**D**) Heatmap of the leading-edge genes from the serine and tetrahydrofolate functional GSEA plots shown in panel C, which are also genes increased in the OE cells compared to KD cells. CPT1A and AR are also included and show an inverse correlation in one of the samples of each subtype of PCa studied.

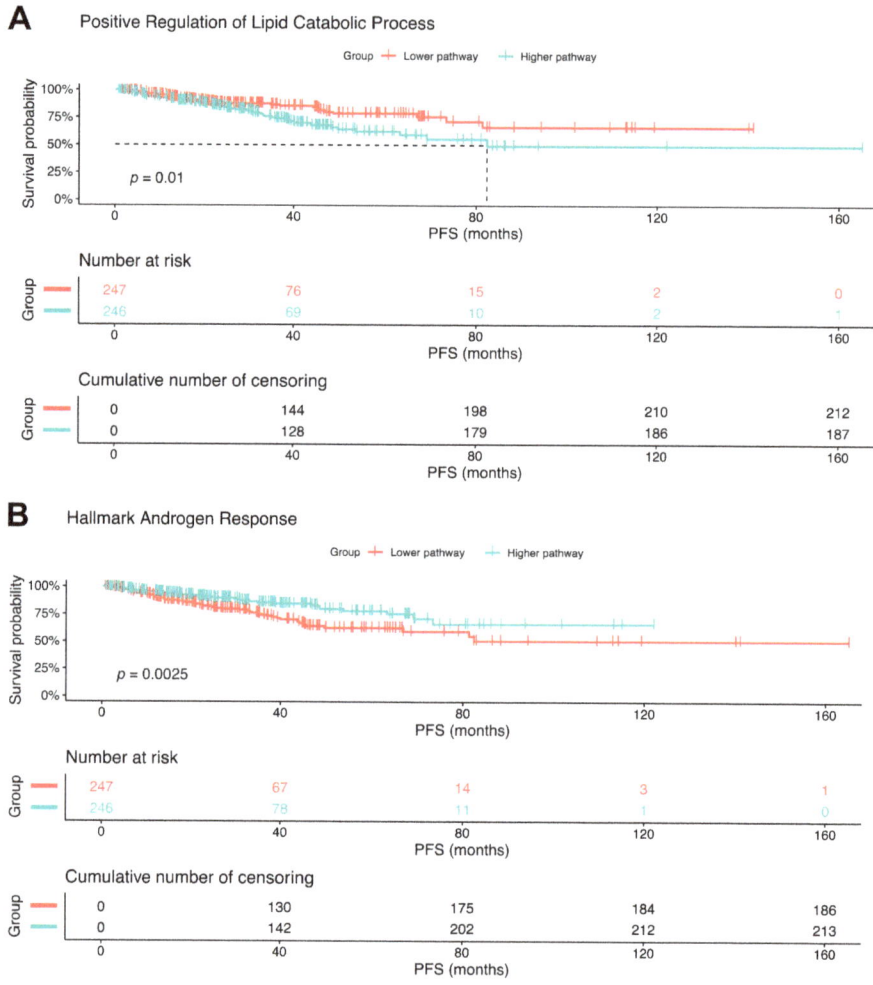

Figure 6. Increased lipid catabolism and decreased androgen response is associated with less progression-free survival. The TCGA prostate adenocarcinoma (PRAD) Firehose legacy dataset ($n = 492$) was divided by median split into high and low pathway scores. Pathways from our OE versus KD RNAseq analyses (Figure 2C) were then studied for progression free survival (PFS) in the TCGA PRAD dataset. Kaplan–Meier (KM) plots for Lipid Catabolism Process (**A**) and Androgen Response Hallmark (**B**), with the number at risk and p-value (logrank test) are shown.

3. Discussion

This study reports on the connection between CPT1A overexpression (OE) and the metabolic and genetic consequences of its increased activity. Particularly, we found that CPT1A OE cells produced a significant number of acyl-carnitines that promote growth and resistance to stress insults, like excess lipids and androgen withdrawal. These later conditions are characteristic of advanced PCa, where androgen deprivation and excess circulating lipids frequently exists [40].

At the molecular level, this work provides insights into the metabolic changes precipitated by the excess use of lipid oxidation in the mitochondria, particularly the upregulation of the overall lipid catabolic process. As expected, not only CPT1A was increased, but also the ability to hydrolyze lipid stores via PNPLA2 (triglyceride lipase or ATGL) to increase the supply of fatty acids for the mitochondria (Figures 1B and 2D). It is possible that new inhibitors for ATGL could be of therapeutic value for cancers with increased CPT1A activity [41]. Another molecular aspect of the increased CPT1A activity was the re-wiring of metabolism towards the serine biosynthesis pathway, which has been recently shown to be important in supporting mitochondrial function [30], and a driver in NEPC [42]. These unexpected amino acid metabolism changes are likely promoted by the strong activation of the adaptive ER Stress response, as indicated by the transcriptional upregulation of genes linked to the ER stress response, Figure 2. In fact, ATF4 is a key transcription factor translationally induced upon activation of the unfolded protein response or UPR [43]. This induction triggers an anti-stress response that promotes adaptation, or in the case of a chronic unresolved stress, it can promote cell death. Increased ATF4 regulates serine and glycine metabolism genes to drive de novo serine and glycine production, which can be used for antioxidant defense and glutathione production [44]. In the CPT1A-OE cells, the mitochondrial SHMT2 gene was significantly increased in OE versus KD cells, suggesting a strong induction of serine/glycine synthesis in the mitochondria. This is likely to provide antioxidant defense via the mitochondrial folate cycle that can generate NADPH [45], and carbon units to produce cystathionine, an intermediate in the synthesis of cysteine and ultimately glutathione (Figure 3).

The ER stress observed in the OE cells compared to the KD cells is likely a response to the high ROS production in the mitochondria and low SOD2 expression. This is a known mechanism to promote cancer growth [46]. This was an unexpected result considering the OE cells did not show signs of distressed or fragmented mitochondria. A possible explanation is the upregulation of the glutathione homeostasis pathway. We found that the glutathione-degrading and ER response gene CHAC1 (cation transport regulator homolog1) was increased in OE cells. This gene was discovered in a co-regulated group of genes enriched for components of the ATF4 pathway, including CCAAT/enhancer-binding protein beta (CEBPB), which also binds to the CHAC1 promoter [47,48]. All this evidence would suggest that increased expression of a glutathione-degrading enzyme and activation of the ER stress pathway will lead to cancer cell death. However, we did not observe such changes in the OE cells as the levels of glutathione did not change and cells were able to grow in the presence of exogenously added lipids (Figures 1 and 4). Other studies in breast and ovarian cancer have shown that CHAC1 expression correlates with tumor differentiation and survival [49], suggesting that the observed ER stress in our models is likely stress-resolving and can promote disease progression. In fact, when we challenged the cells with commonly circulating fatty acids in the absence of androgens (a stressful environment), more SOD2 expression was observed in the OE cells and less on the KD cells. This underscores the increased antioxidant response capabilities of the OE cells and potential for survival and growth. This environment may promote adaptation of the OE cells to androgen deprivation, supporting progression to lethal disease. Recent studies have also shown that increased SOD2 activity can protect prostate cells when exposed to radiation [50].

How oxidative changes in the mitochondria connect with ER stress remains unknown. ER and oxidative stress have overlapping and intertwined functions in cancer [21]. Both promote epithelial mesenchymal transition, a key step of metastasis and tissue invasion of many tumor cells. In addition, detachment from the extracellular matrix activates the ATF4-HSPA5 branch of the UPR, which protects from anoikis by stimulating both autophagy and antioxidative stress responses [51]. As the CPT1A-OE cells prefer to grow in suspension [10], they might be using the ER stress response and the mitochondrial oxidative environment to transform to more aggressive tumors [52].

This study and the public databases provide evidence that lipid catabolism driven by CPT1A is associated with more aggressive disease. CPT1A-OE cells showed more SYP and ENO2 neuroendocrine marker expression compared to the KD cells. This suggests that in CRPC tumors, CPT1A activity can rewire metabolism to promote growth and transformation via activation of serine biosynthesis, folate cycle, and glutathione homeostasis, all geared to maintain an adequate redox balance in the cancer cells. The role of mitochondrial ROS in activating these pro-tumor antioxidant pathways warrants further investigation.

4. Materials and Methods

4.1. Cell Lines Fatty Acids and Drugs

LNCaP-C4-2 cells were purchased from the University of Texas MD Anderson Cancer Center (Houston, TX, USA). Cells were used at low passage number and grown in RPMI containing 10% FBS supplemented with amino acids and Insulin (Gibco, ThermoFisher, Walthman, MA, USA). Charcoal stripped serum (CSS) was used for androgen-deprived conditions. Lentiviral particles for shRNA and complete cDNA specific to CPT1A were prepared at the Functional Genomics facility at the University of Colorado. For transfection, the following shRNAs from the Sigma (St. Louis, MO, USA) library were used: For knockdown (KD), TRCN0000036279 (CPT1A-sh1, [17]) and control shRNA (NTshRNA) SHC202 were used. This specific shRNA has been used by us successfully in several models of cancer [10,15–17,52,53]. For CPT1A overexpression (OE), we used the ccsbBroad304-00359 clone from the CCSB-Broad lentiviral library as described [10]. Lentiviral transduction and selection were performed according to Sigma's MISSION protocol. Puromycin (1 µg/mL) and blasticidin (5 µg/mL) from Sigma were used for KD and OE cell line drug selection, respectively. Fatty acids were purchased from Sigma, resuspended in ethanol for a stock solution of 10 mM and stored at −80 °C. Fatty acids were conjugated to albumin, (A7030, Sigma), before use at a 2 mM: 5% (Fatty acid:BSA) ratio in RPMI media. Etomoxir-HCL (CPT1 inhibitor) was purchased from Sigma and resuspended in PBS to 33.4 mM and stored at −20 °C.

4.2. Reverse-Transcriptase-PCR

For RT-PCR analysis, cDNA was synthesized (Applied Biosystems, Foster City, CA, USA) and quantified by real-time PCR using SYBR green (BioRad, Hercules, CA, USA) detection. Results were normalized to the housekeeping gene RPL13A mRNA and expressed as arbitrary units of $2^{-\Delta\Delta CT}$ relative to the control group. Primer sequences:
RPL13A-F: 5-CCTGGAGGAGAAGAGGAAAGAGA.
RPL13A-R 5-TTGAGGACCTCTGTGTATTTGTCAA.
CPT1A-F: 5-TGGATCTGCTGTATATCCTTC.
CPT1A-R: 5-AATTGGTTTGATTTCCTCCC.

4.3. Western Blot Analysis

Protein extracts of 20 µg were separated on a 4–20% SDS-PAGE gel and transferred to nitrocellulose membranes as described [10]. Band signals were obtained and visualized with the LI-COR Biosciences system (Lincoln, NE, USA). Antibodies: CPT1A: 15184-1-AP, (Proteintech, Rosemont, IL, USA); GAPDH: CST 5174, (Cell Signaling Technology, Beverly, MA, USA); SOD2: CST 13141, Cell Signaling Technology.

4.4. Metabolomics and Acyl Carnitine Analysis

Cells were grown to 80% confluency before trypsinization and collection in 2×10^6 aliquots. Samples were processed at Biological Mass Spectrometry Facility at the University of Colorado AMC (Aurora, CO, USA) using standard protocols. For the measurement of acyl-carnitines, samples were extracted in a solution of methanol, acetonitrile, and water (5:3:2) at a concentration of 1 million cells/mL in presence of acyl-carnitines, deuterated standards (NSK-B, Cambridge Isotope Laboratories, Tewksbury, MA, USA). Samples were analyzed via UHPLC-MS (Vanquish-Q Exactive, ThermoFisher, Walthman, MA, USA) as previously described [54]. Analysis of the most significant pathways was performed with the MetaboAnalyst web-based analytical program [55].

4.5. Intracellular Lipase Analysis

The enzymatic activity of intracellular lipase was measured using a substrate containing 3H Triolein (Perkin Elmer, Waltham, MA, USA) and human serum as a source of ApoC2 as described previously [56]. In brief, LNCaP-C4-2 cells overexpressing CPT1A (OE) and controls (EV) were grown to 80% confluence. Intracellular lipase was made accessible by lysing the cells in heparin containing M-PER cell lysis buffer (Pierce, Rockford, IL, USA). Intracellular lipase activity was determined by incubation with 3H Triolein substrate for 45 min at 37 °C. The protein concentration of the lysate was determined to calculate the Lipase-dependent hydrolysis (FFA release) of 3H Triolein per mg, per min.

4.6. Electron Paramagnetic Resonance Spectroscopy

Mitochondrial ROS production was measured by EPR using the mitochondrial-targeted spin probe 1-hydroxy-4-[2-triphenylphosphonio)-acetamido]-2,2,6,6-tetramethyl-piperidine,1-hydroxy-2,2,6,6-tetramethyl-4-[2-(triphenylphosphonio)acetamido] piperidinium dichloride (mito-TEMPO-H) as previously reported [57]. Cells were grown to 80% confluency prior to the EPR measurements. The mito-TEMPO-H probe was prepared in deoxygenated 50 mM phosphate buffer. Cells were washed and treated with mito-TEMPO-H 0.25 mM in Krebs-HEPES buffer (KHB) containing 100 µM of a metal chelator DTPA to avoid direct oxidation with metal ion or hydroxyl radical generation by Fenton reaction. Cells were incubated for 50 min at 37 °C, placed on ice, then gently scraped. 50 µL of cell suspension was loaded in an EPR capillary tube and EPR measurements were performed at room temperature using Bruker EMXnano X-band spectrometer [57]. EPR acquisition parameters were: microwave frequency = 9.6 GHz; center field = 3432 G; modulation amplitude = 2.0 G; sweep width = 80 G; microwave power = 19.9 mW; total number of scans = 10; sweep time = 12.11 s; and time constant = 20.48 ms. mito-TEMPO. Nitroxide radicals concentration was obtained by simulating the spectra using the SpinFit module incorporated in the Xenon software of the bench-top EMXnano EPR spectrometer followed by the SpinCount module (Bruker, Billerica, MA, USA). Total protein was extracted from analyzed samples and quantified with a Bio-Rad DC protein assay kit (Bio-Rad, Hercules, CA, USA), and nitroxide concentrations were normalized to total protein.

4.7. Statistics

Student t-tests or ANOVA tests were used to compare between groups, followed by post hoc tests when appropriate, alpha = 0.05. Analysis was carried out with GraphPad Prism software v8 (GraphPad Software, San Diego, CA, USA). All data represent mean ± SD, unless otherwise indicated.

4.8. RNAseq and Pathway Analysis

All cells (KD, OE, and their respective controls) were grown to 80% confluency before RNA isolation. RNA was extracted using a RNeasy Plus Mini Kit (Qiagen, Valencia, CA, USA). RNA quality was verified using a High Sensitivity ScreenTape Assay on the Tape Station 4200 (Agilent Technologies, Santa Clara, CA, USA) and measured with a Tecan Plate Reader (Thermo Fisher Scientific, Waltham, MA, USA). Library construction was performed using the Universal Plus mRNA Library Kit (NuGen Technologies, Redwood City, CA, USA), and sequencing was performed on the NovaSeq 6000 instrument (Illumina, San Diego, CA, USA) using paired-end sequencing (150 bp) by the University of Colorado Cancer Center Genomics and Microarray Core. Illumina adapters were removed using BBDuk (sourceforge.net/projects/bbmap) and reads <50 bp after trimming were discarded. Reads were aligned and quantified using STAR (2.6.0a) [58]) to the Ensembl human transcriptome (hg38.p12, release 96). Normalization and differential expression were calculated using the limma R package [29]. An interaction model within limma used to directly compare the OE and the KD. Gene set enrichment analysis was performed using the fGSEA R package (v1.10.0) with 10,000 permutations and the Hallmarks and GO Biological Processes gene set collections from the Molecular Signatures Database [59]. Heatmaps were generated with the ComplexHeatmap R package [60] following z-score transformation. RNA-sequencing data have been deposited into the NCBI Gene Expression Omnibus database (accession number GSE161243).

4.9. Public Database Analysis

RMA normalized prostate cancer microarray data was downloaded from GEO (GSE32967, [37]). Only the first replicate for each sample was used for the analysis to deal with uneven sample replicates. The most variable probe was selected to represent each gene. The limma R package was used to compare small cell carcinoma ($n = 4$) to adenocarcinoma ($n = 3$) prostate cancer. TPM normalized gene expression and clinical data from The Cancer Genome Atlas PRAD dataset (Firehose Legacy) [61], was downloaded from cBioPortal [62]. Gene Set Variation Analysis (GSVA) was performed using the GSVA R package [63], to score several gene sets with a Poisson distribution. Patients were classified into high and low pathway groups by median score splitting. The survival (https://cran.r-project.org/web/packages/survival/citation.html) and survminer R packages (https://rpkgs.datanovia.com/survminer/index.html) were used to generate Kaplan-Meier curves and perform log rank tests. For the CPT1A and AR gene expression correlations, Log2 normalized whole transcript mRNA expression values from Taylor et al. [38] prostate cancer samples were downloaded from cBioPortal [62]. Expression of AR and CPT1A between primary and metastatic samples were compared using a Wilcoxon rank sum test. Pearson correlation was calculated for the correlation between AR and CPT1A expression in either primary or metastatic tumors.

5. Conclusions

The overall goal of this study is to understand the lipid metabolic underpinnings of advanced prostate cancer so that metabolic therapies can be designed effectively. Overall, we provide evidence that CPT1A activity may have a relevant role in advanced PCa, including transformation to NEPC. Etomoxir is a potent inhibitor of CPT1 that has been used in clinical trials in Europe [64], but it is not currently being used in the USA. Considering all the toxic chemotherapeutic agents used in cancer treatments, the potential for drugs like etomoxir to impact cancer growth and drug response warrants investigation.

Supplementary Materials: The following are available online at http://www.mdpi.com/2072-6694/12/11/3431/s1, Figure S1: Colony growth after treatment with different chain fatty acids, Figure S2: Enrichment score plots of the pathways and Gene ontology (GO) pathways shown in Figure 2, Figure S3: Metabolomic enrichment analysis, Figure S4: Uncropped western blots of SOD2 expression and densitometry graphs, Figure S5: cBioportal database correlations of CPT1A and AR expression, Figure S6: Additional progression-free survival plots, Table S1: RNA seq analysis results from comparing the OE cells to the KD cells.

Author Contributions: Conceptualization, I.R.S.; Formal analysis, J.K., K.B., E.N.-G., A.G., J.C.C. and I.R.S.; Funding acquisition, I.R.S. and J.C.C.; Investigation, H.E. and A.G.; Methodology, A.D., E.M., K.B., and H.E.; Software, A.G. and J.C.C.; Supervision, I.R.S.; Writing–original draft, I.R.S.; Writing–review & editing, M.J., A.D., A.G., E.N.-G., J.C.C., and I.R.S. All authors have read and agreed to the published version of the manuscript.

Funding: This study was supported by the American Cancer Society (129846-RSG-16-256), NIH Bioinformatics and Biostatistics Shared Resource Core, Genomics Shared Resource, Functional Genomics Shared Resource and Cancer Center Support Grant (P30CA046934), NIH U01, (CA231978), Cancer league of Colorado (AWD-193286), Nutrition and Obesity Research Center (NORC).

Acknowledgments: We are grateful from the technical support from Maren Salzmann-Sullivan, Gergana Stoykova, and Juliana Oviedo. We are also thankful to Kristofer Fritz for the advice on SOD2 antibodies.

Conflicts of Interest: The authors declare no conflict of interest. The funders had no role in the design of the study; in the collection, analyses, or interpretation of data; in the writing of the manuscript, or in the decision to publish the results.

References

1. Auchus, R.J.; Sharifi, N. Sex hormones and prostate cancer. *Annu. Rev. Med.* **2020**, *71*, 33–45. [CrossRef] [PubMed]
2. Sharp, A.; Coleman, I.; Yuan, W.; Sprenger, C.; Dolling, D.; Rodrigues, D.N.; Russo, J.W.; Figueiredo, I.; Bertan, C.; Seed, G.; et al. Androgen receptor splice variant-7 expression emerges with castration resistance in prostate cancer. *J. Clin. Investig.* **2019**, *129*, 192–208. [CrossRef] [PubMed]

3. Nevedomskaya, E.; Baumgart, S.J.; Haendler, B. Recent advances in prostate cancer treatment and drug discovery. *Int. J. Mol. Sci.* **2018**, *19*, 1359. [CrossRef] [PubMed]
4. Carver, B.S.; Chapinski, C.; Wongvipat, J.; Hieronymus, H.; Chen, Y.; Chandarlapaty, S.; Arora, V.K.; Le, C.; Koutcher, J.; Scher, H.; et al. Reciprocal feedback regulation of PI3K and androgen receptor signaling in PTEN-deficient prostate cancer. *Cancer Cell* **2011**, *19*, 575–586. [CrossRef]
5. Dehm, S.M.; Tindall, D.J. Alternatively spliced androgen receptor variants. *Endocr. Relat. Cancer* **2011**, *18*, R183–R196. [CrossRef]
6. Beltran, H.; Prandi, D.; Mosquera, J.M.; Benelli, M.; Puca, L.; Cyrta, J.; Marotz, C.; Giannopoulou, E.; Chakravarthi, B.V.; Varambally, S.; et al. Divergent clonal evolution of castration-resistant neuroendocrine prostate cancer. *Nat. Med.* **2016**, *22*, 298–305. [CrossRef]
7. Conteduca, V.; Oromendia, C.; Eng, K.W.; Bareja, R.; Sigouros, M.; Molina, A.; Faltas, B.M.; Sboner, A.; Mosquera, J.M.; Elemento, O.; et al. Clinical features of neuroendocrine prostate cancer. *Eur. J. Cancer* **2019**, *121*, 7–18. [CrossRef]
8. Ku, S.Y.; Rosario, S.; Wang, Y.; Mu, P.; Seshadri, M.; Goodrich, Z.W.; Goodrich, M.M.; Labbé, D.P.; Gomez, E.C.; Wang, J.; et al. Rb1 and Trp53 cooperate to suppress prostate cancer lineage plasticity, metastasis, and antiandrogen resistance. *Science* **2017**, *355*, 78–83. [CrossRef]
9. Schlaepfer, I.R.; Joshi, M. CPT1A-mediated fat oxidation, mechanisms, and therapeutic potential. *Endocrinology* **2020**, *161*, 161. [CrossRef]
10. Joshi, M.; Stoykova, G.E.; Salzmann-Sullivan, M.; Dzieciatkowska, M.; Liebman, L.N.; Deep, G.; Schlaepfer, I.R. CPT1A supports castration-resistant prostate cancer in androgen-deprived conditions. *Cells* **2019**, *8*, 1115. [CrossRef]
11. Chen, M.; Zhang, J.; Sampieri, K.; Clohessy, J.G.; Mendez, L.; Gonzalez-Billalabeitia, E.; Liu, X.S.; Lee, Y.R.; Fung, J.; Katon, J.M.; et al. An aberrant SREBP-dependent lipogenic program promotes metastatic prostate cancer. *Nat. Genet.* **2018**, *50*, 206–218. [CrossRef]
12. Yao, C.H.; Liu, G.Y.; Wang, R.; Moon, S.H.; Gross, R.W.; Patti, G.J. Identifying off-target effects of etomoxir reveals that carnitine palmitoyltransferase I is essential for cancer cell proliferation independent of beta-oxidation. *PLoS Biol.* **2018**, *16*, e2003782. [CrossRef] [PubMed]
13. Carracedo, A.; Cantley, L.C.; Pandolfi, P.P. Cancer metabolism: Fatty acid oxidation in the limelight. *Nat. Rev. Cancer* **2013**, *13*, 227–232. [CrossRef] [PubMed]
14. Qu, Q.; Zeng, F.; Liu, X.; Wang, Q.J.; Deng, F. Fatty acid oxidation and carnitine palmitoyltransferase I: Emerging therapeutic targets in cancer. *Cell Death Dis.* **2016**, *7*, e2226. [CrossRef] [PubMed]
15. Schlaepfer, I.R.; Glode, L.M.; Hitz, C.A.; Pac, C.T.; Boyle, K.E.; Maroni, P.; Deep, G.; Agarwal, R.; Lucia, S.M.; Cramer, S.D.; et al. Inhibition of lipid oxidation increases glucose metabolism and enhances 2-deoxy-2-[f]fluoro-d-glucose uptake in prostate cancer mouse xenografts. *Mol. Imaging Biol.* **2015**, *17*, 529–538. [CrossRef]
16. Schlaepfer, I.R.; Nambiar, D.K.; Ramteke, A.; Kumar, R.; Dhar, D.; Agarwal, C.; Bergman, B.; Graner, M.; Maroni, P.; Singh, R.P.; et al. Hypoxia induces triglycerides accumulation in prostate cancer cells and extracellular vesicles supporting growth and invasiveness following reoxygenation. *Oncotarget* **2015**, *6*, 22836–22856. [CrossRef] [PubMed]
17. Schlaepfer, I.R.; Rider, L.; Rodrigues, L.U.; Gijon, M.A.; Pac, C.T.; Romero, L.; Cimic, A.; Sirintrapun, S.J.; Glode, L.M.; Eckel, R.H.; et al. Lipid catabolism via CPT1 as a therapeutic target for prostate cancer. *Mol. Cancer Ther.* **2014**, *13*, 2361–2371. [CrossRef]
18. Pike, L.S.; Smift, A.L.; Croteau, N.J.; Ferrick, D.A.; Wu, M. Inhibition of fatty acid oxidation by etomoxir impairs NADPH production and increases reactive oxygen species resulting in ATP depletion and cell death in human glioblastoma cells. *Biochim. Biophys. Acta* **2011**, *1807*, 726–734. [CrossRef]
19. Yun, J.; Mullarky, E.; Lu, C.; Bosch, K.N.; Kavalier, A.; Rivera, K.; Roper, J.; Chio, I.I.C.; Giannopoulou, E.G.; Rago, C.; et al. Vitamin C selectively kills KRAS and BRAF mutant colorectal cancer cells by targeting GAPDH. *Science* **2015**, *350*, 1391–1396. [CrossRef]
20. Schafer, Z.T.; Grassian, A.R.; Song, L.; Jiang, Z.; Gerhart-Hines, Z.; Irie, H.Y.; Gao, S.; Puigserver, P.; Brugge, J.S. Antioxidant and oncogene rescue of metabolic defects caused by loss of matrix attachment. *Nature* **2009**, *461*, 109–113. [CrossRef]
21. Cao, S.S.; Kaufman, R.J. Endoplasmic reticulum stress and oxidative stress in cell fate decision and human disease. *Antioxid. Redox Signal.* **2014**, *21*, 396–413. [CrossRef] [PubMed]

22. Scheuner, D.; Vander Mierde, D.; Song, B.; Flamez, D.; Creemers, J.W.; Tsukamoto, K.; Ribick, M.; Schuit, F.C.; Kaufman, R.J. Control of mRNA translation preserves endoplasmic reticulum function in beta cells and maintains glucose homeostasis. *Nat. Med.* **2005**, *11*, 757–764. [CrossRef] [PubMed]
23. Lin, N.; Chen, H.; Zhang, H.; Wan, X.; Su, Q. Mitochondrial reactive oxygen species (ROS) inhibition ameliorates palmitate-induced INS-1 beta cell death. *Endocrine* **2012**, *42*, 107–117. [CrossRef] [PubMed]
24. Fu, Y.; Wey, S.; Wang, M.; Ye, R.; Liao, C.P.; Roy-Burman, P.; Lee, A.S. Pten null prostate tumorigenesis and AKT activation are blocked by targeted knockout of ER chaperone GRP78/BiP in prostate epithelium. *Proc. Natl. Acad. Sci. USA* **2008**, *105*, 19444–19449. [CrossRef] [PubMed]
25. Thalmann, G.N.; Anezinis, P.E.; Chang, S.M.; Zhau, H.E.; Kim, E.E.; Hopwood, V.L.; Pathak, S.; von Eschenbach, A.C.; Chung, L.W. Androgen-independent cancer progression and bone metastasis in the LNCaP model of human prostate cancer. *Cancer Res.* **1994**, *54*, 2577–2581.
26. Das, S.K.; Eder, S.; Schauer, S.; Diwoky, C.; Temmel, H.; Guertl, B.; Gorkiewicz, G.; Tamilarasan, K.P.; Kumari, P.; Trauner, M.; et al. Adipose triglyceride lipase contributes to cancer-associated cachexia. *Science* **2011**, *333*, 233–238. [CrossRef]
27. Englinger, B.; Laemmerer, A.; Moser, P.; Kallus, S.; Röhrl, C.; Pirker, C.; Baier, D.; Mohr, T.; Niederstaetter, L.; Meier-Menches, S.M.; et al. Lipid droplet-mediated scavenging as novel intrinsic and adaptive resistance factor against the multikinase inhibitor ponatinib. *Int. J. Cancer* **2020**, *147*, 1680–1693. [CrossRef]
28. Schlaepfer, I.R.; Hitz, C.A.; Gijon, M.A.; Bergman, B.C.; Eckel, R.H.; Jacobsen, B.M. Progestin modulates the lipid profile and sensitivity of breast cancer cells to docetaxel. *Mol. Cell. Endocrinol.* **2012**, *363*, 111–121. [CrossRef]
29. Ritchie, M.E.; Phipson, B.; Wu, D.; Hu, Y.; Law, C.W.; Shi, W.; Smyth, G.K. Limma powers differential expression analyses for RNA-sequencing and microarray studies. *Nucleic Acids Res.* **2015**, *43*, e47. [CrossRef]
30. Gao, X.; Lee, K.; Reid, M.A.; Sanderson, S.M.; Qiu, C.; Li, S.; Liu, J.; Locasale, J.W. Serine availability influences mitochondrial dynamics and function through lipid metabolism. *Cell Rep.* **2018**, *22*, 3507–3520. [CrossRef]
31. Gao, X.; Locasale, J.W.; Reid, M.A. Serine and methionine metabolism: Vulnerabilities in lethal prostate cancer. *Cancer Cell* **2019**, *35*, 339–341. [CrossRef] [PubMed]
32. Wang, Y.H.; Huang, J.T.; Chen, W.L.; Wang, R.H.; Kao, M.C.; Pan, Y.R.; Chan, S.H.; Tsai, K.W.; Kung, H.J.; Lin, K.T.; et al. Dysregulation of cystathionine γ-lyase promotes prostate cancer progression and metastasis. *EMBO Rep.* **2019**, *20*, e45986. [CrossRef] [PubMed]
33. Kumar, A.; Tikoo, S.; Maity, S.; Sengupta, S.; Sengupta, S.; Kaur, A.; Bachhawat, A.K. Mammalian proapoptotic factor ChaC$_1$ and its homologues function as γ-glutamyl cyclotransferases acting specifically on glutathione. *EMBO Rep.* **2012**, *13*, 1095–1101. [CrossRef] [PubMed]
34. Chen, M.S.; Wang, S.F.; Hsu, C.Y.; Yin, P.H.; Yeh, T.S.; Lee, H.C.; Tseng, L.M. CHAC1 degradation of glutathione enhances cystine-starvation-induced necroptosis and ferroptosis in human triple negative breast cancer cells via the GCN2-eIF2α-ATF4 pathway. *Oncotarget* **2017**, *8*, 114588–114602. [CrossRef] [PubMed]
35. Bachhawat, A.K.; Yadav, S. The glutathione cycle: Glutathione metabolism beyond the γ-glutamyl cycle. *IUBMB Life* **2018**, *70*, 585–592. [CrossRef]
36. Schmuck, E.M.; Board, P.G.; Whitbread, A.K.; Tetlow, N.; Cavanaugh, J.A.; Blackburn, A.C.; Masoumi, A. Characterization of the monomethylarsonate reductase and dehydroascorbate reductase activities of Omega class glutathione transferase variants: Implications for arsenic metabolism and the age-at-onset of Alzheimer's and Parkinson's diseases. *Pharm. Genom.* **2005**, *15*, 493–501. [CrossRef]
37. Tzelepi, V.; Zhang, J.; Lu, J.F.; Kleb, B.; Wu, G.; Wan, X.; Hoang, A.; Efstathiou, E.; Sircar, K.; Navone, N.M.; et al. Modeling a lethal prostate cancer variant with small-cell carcinoma features. *Clin. Cancer Res.* **2012**, *18*, 666–677. [CrossRef]
38. Taylor, B.S.; Schultz, N.; Hieronymus, H.; Gopalan, A.; Xiao, Y.; Carver, B.S.; Arora, V.K.; Kaushik, P.; Cerami, E.; Reva, B.; et al. Integrative genomic profiling of human prostate cancer. *Cancer Cell* **2010**, *18*, 11–22. [CrossRef]
39. Mah, C.Y.; Nassar, Z.D.; Swinnen, J.V.; Butler, L.M. Lipogenic effects of androgen signaling in normal and malignant prostate. *Asian J. Urol.* **2020**, *7*, 258–270. [CrossRef]
40. Collier, A.; Ghosh, S.; McGlynn, B.; Hollins, G. Prostate cancer, androgen deprivation therapy, obesity, the metabolic syndrome, type 2 diabetes, and cardiovascular disease: A review. *Am. J. Clin. Oncol.* **2012**, *35*, 504–509. [CrossRef]

41. Schweiger, M.; Romauch, M.; Schreiber, R.; Grabner, G.F.; Hütter, S.; Kotzbeck, P.; Benedikt, P.; Eichmann, T.O.; Yamada, S.; Knittelfelder, O.; et al. Pharmacological inhibition of adipose triglyceride lipase corrects high-fat diet-induced insulin resistance and hepatosteatosis in mice. *Nat. Commun.* **2017**, *8*, 14859. [CrossRef] [PubMed]
42. Reina-Campos, M.; Linares, J.F.; Duran, A.; Cordes, T.; L'Hermitte, A.; Badur, M.G.; Bhangoo, M.S.; Thorson, P.K.; Richards, A.; Rooslid, T.; et al. Increased serine and one-carbon pathway metabolism by PKCλ/ι deficiency promotes neuroendocrine prostate cancer. *Cancer Cell* **2019**, *35*, 385–400. [CrossRef] [PubMed]
43. Balsa, E.; Soustek, M.S.; Thomas, A.; Cogliati, S.; García-Poyatos, C.; Martín-García, E.; Jedrychowski, M.; Gygi, S.P.; Enriquez, J.A.; Puigserver, P. ER and nutrient stress promote assembly of respiratory chain supercomplexes through the PERK-eIF2α axis. *Mol. Cell* **2019**, *74*, 877–890. [CrossRef] [PubMed]
44. DeNicola, G.M.; Chen, P.H.; Mullarky, E.; Sudderth, J.A.; Hu, Z.; Wu, D.; Tang, H.; Xie, Y.; Asara, J.M.; Huffman, K.E.; et al. NRF2 regulates serine biosynthesis in non-small cell lung cancer. *Nat. Genet.* **2015**, *47*, 1475–1481. [CrossRef]
45. Fan, J.; Ye, J.; Kamphorst, J.J.; Shlomi, T.; Thompson, C.B.; Rabinowitz, J.D. Quantitative flux analysis reveals folate-dependent NADPH production. *Nature* **2014**, *510*, 298–302. [CrossRef]
46. Zhu, C.H.; Huang, Y.; Oberley, L.W.; Domann, F.E. A family of AP-2 proteins down-regulate manganese superoxide dismutase expression. *J. Biol. Chem.* **2001**, *276*, 14407–14413. [CrossRef]
47. Crawford, R.R.; Prescott, E.T.; Sylvester, C.F.; Higdon, A.N.; Shan, J.; Kilberg, M.S.; Mungrue, I.N. Human CHAC$_1$ protein degrades glutathione, and mRNA induction is regulated by the transcription factors ATF$_4$ and ATF$_3$ and a bipartite ATF/CRE regulatory element. *J. Biol. Chem.* **2015**, *290*, 15878–15891. [CrossRef]
48. Gargalovic, P.S.; Imura, M.; Zhang, B.; Gharavi, N.M.; Clark, M.J.; Pagnon, J.; Yang, W.P.; He, A.; Truong, A.; Patel, S.; et al. Identification of inflammatory gene modules based on variations of human endothelial cell responses to oxidized lipids. *Proc. Natl. Acad. Sci. USA* **2006**, *103*, 12741–12746. [CrossRef]
49. Goebel, G.; Berger, R.; Strasak, A.M.; Egle, D.; Müller-Holzner, E.; Schmidt, S.; Rainer, J.; Presul, E.; Parson, W.; Lang, S.; et al. Elevated mRNA expression of CHAC$_1$ splicing variants is associated with poor outcome for breast and ovarian cancer patients. *Br. J. Cancer* **2012**, *106*, 189–198. [CrossRef]
50. Shrishrimal, S.; Chatterjee, A.; Kosmacek, E.A.; Davis, P.J.; McDonald, J.T.; Oberley-Deegan, R.E. Manganese porphyrin, MnTE-2-PyP, treatment protects the prostate from radiation-induced fibrosis (RIF) by activating the NRF2 signaling pathway and enhancing SOD2 and sirtuin activity. *Free Radic. Biol. Med.* **2020**, *152*, 255–270. [CrossRef]
51. Avivar-Valderas, A.; Salas, E.; Bobrovnikova-Marjon, E.; Diehl, J.A.; Nagi, C.; Debnath, J.; Aguirre-Ghiso, J.A. PERK integrates autophagy and oxidative stress responses to promote survival during extracellular matrix detachment. *Mol. Cell. Biol.* **2011**, *31*, 3616–3629. [CrossRef] [PubMed]
52. Sawyer, B.T.; Qamar, L.; Yamamoto, T.M.; McMellen, A.; Watson, Z.L.; Richer, J.K.; Behbakht, K.; Schlaepfer, I.R.; Bitler, B.G. Targeting fatty acid oxidation to promote anoikis and inhibit ovarian cancer progression. *Mol. Cancer Res.* **2020**, *18*, 1088–1098. [CrossRef] [PubMed]
53. Flaig, T.W.; Salzmann-Sullivan, M.; Su, L.J.; Zhang, Z.; Joshi, M.; Gijon, M.A.; Kim, J.; Arcaroli, J.J.; Van Bokhoven, A.; Lucia, M.S.; et al. Lipid catabolism inhibition sensitizes prostate cancer cells to antiandrogen blockade. *Oncotarget* **2017**, *8*, 56051–56065. [CrossRef] [PubMed]
54. Reisz, J.A.; Zheng, C.; D'Alessandro, A.; Nemkov, T. Untargeted and semi-targeted lipid analysis of biological samples using mass spectrometry-based metabolomics. In *Methods in Molecular Biology*; Humana Press: Totowa, NJ, USA, 2019; Volume 1978, pp. 121–135. [CrossRef]
55. Xia, J.; Wishart, D.S. Web-based inference of biological patterns, functions and pathways from metabolomic data using MetaboAnalyst. *Nat. Protoc.* **2011**, *6*, 743–760. [CrossRef]
56. Bruce, K.D.; Gorkhali, S.; Given, K.; Coates, A.M.; Boyle, K.E.; Macklin, W.B.; Eckel, R.H. Lipoprotein lipase is a feature of alternatively-activated microglia and may facilitate lipid uptake in the CNS during demyelination. *Front. Mol. Neurosci.* **2018**, *11*, 57. [CrossRef]
57. Elajaili, H.B.; Hernandez-Lagunas, L.; Ranguelova, K.; Dikalov, S.; Nozik-Grayck, E. Use of electron paramagnetic resonance in biological samples at ambient temperature and 77 K. *J. Vis. Exp. JoVE* **2019**, e58461. [CrossRef]
58. Dobin, A.; Davis, C.A.; Schlesinger, F.; Drenkow, J.; Zaleski, C.; Jha, S.; Batut, P.; Chaisson, M.; Gingeras, T.R. STAR: Ultrafast universal RNA-seq aligner. *Bioinformatics* **2013**, *29*, 15–21. [CrossRef]

59. Liberzon, A.; Subramanian, A.; Pinchback, R.; Thorvaldsdóttir, H.; Tamayo, P.; Mesirov, J.P. Molecular signatures database (MSigDB) 3.0. *Bioinformatics* **2011**, *27*, 1739–1740. [CrossRef]
60. Gu, Z.; Eils, R.; Schlesner, M. Complex heatmaps reveal patterns and correlations in multidimensional genomic data. *Bioinformatics* **2016**, *32*, 2847–2849. [CrossRef]
61. The Cancer Genome Atlas Research Network. The molecular taxonomy of primary prostate cancer. *Cell* **2015**, *163*, 1011–1025. [CrossRef]
62. Cerami, E.; Gao, J.; Dogrusoz, U.; Gross, B.E.; Sumer, S.O.; Aksoy, B.A.; Jacobsen, A.; Byrne, C.J.; Heuer, M.L.; Larsson, E.; et al. The cBio cancer genomics portal: An open platform for exploring multidimensional cancer genomics data. *Cancer Discov.* **2012**, *2*, 401–404. [CrossRef] [PubMed]
63. Hänzelmann, S.; Castelo, R.; Guinney, J. GSVA: Gene set variation analysis for microarray and RNA-Seq data. *BMC Bioinform.* **2013**, *14*, 7. [CrossRef] [PubMed]
64. Holubarsch, C.J.; Rohrbach, M.; Karrasch, M.; Boehm, E.; Polonski, L.; Ponikowski, P.; Rhein, S. A double-blind randomized multicentre clinical trial to evaluate the efficacy and safety of two doses of etomoxir in comparison with placebo in patients with moderate congestive heart failure: The ERGO (etomoxir for the recovery of glucose oxidation) study. *Clin. Sci.* **2007**, *113*, 205–212. [CrossRef] [PubMed]

Publisher's Note: MDPI stays neutral with regard to jurisdictional claims in published maps and institutional affiliations.

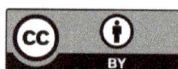

© 2020 by the authors. Licensee MDPI, Basel, Switzerland. This article is an open access article distributed under the terms and conditions of the Creative Commons Attribution (CC BY) license (http://creativecommons.org/licenses/by/4.0/).

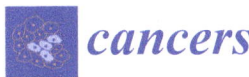

Article

Downstream Neighbor of SON (DONSON) Expression Is Enhanced in Phenotypically Aggressive Prostate Cancers

Niklas Klümper [1,2,3], Marthe von Danwitz [1,2], Johannes Stein [1,2], Doris Schmidt [1,2], Anja Schmidt [1,2], Glen Kristiansen [2,4], Michael Muders [2,4], Michael Hölzel [2,3], Manuel Ritter [1,2], Abdullah Alajati [1,2,*,†] and Jörg Ellinger [1,2,*,†]

1. Department of Urology, University Hospital Bonn, 53127 Bonn, Germany; niklas.kluemper@ukbonn.de (N.K.); s4mavond@uni-bonn.de (M.v.D.); johannes.stein@ukbonn.de (J.S.); doris.schmidt@ukbonn.de (D.S.); Anja.Schmidt@ukbonn.de (A.S.); mritter@ukbonn.de (M.R.)
2. Center for Integrated Oncology, University Hospital Bonn, 53127 Bonn, Germany; glen.kristiansen@ukbonn.de (G.K.); michael.muders@ukbonn.de (M.M.); michael.hoelzel@ukbonn.de (M.H.)
3. Institute of Experimental Oncology, University Hospital Bonn, 53127 Bonn, Germany
4. Institute of Pathology, University Hospital Bonn, 53127 Bonn, Germany
* Correspondence: abdullah.alajati@ukbonn.de (A.A.); joerg.ellinger@ukbonn.de (J.E.); Tel.: +49-22828712630 (J.E.)
† Joint senior authors.

Received: 3 November 2020; Accepted: 16 November 2020; Published: 19 November 2020

Simple Summary: Downstream neighbor of SON (DONSON) plays a crucial role in cell cycle progression and in maintaining genomic stability. We identified DONSON to be associated with an aggressive histopathological phenotype and unfavorable survival in prostate cancer (PCa) in different transcriptomic cohorts and on the protein level in our tissue microarray cohort. DONSON expression in the primary tumor was particularly strong in locally advanced, metastasized, and dedifferentiated carcinomas (TNM Stage, Gleason). Highly proliferating tumors exhibited a significant correlation to DONSON expression, and DONSON expression was notably upregulated in distant metastases and androgen-deprivation resistant metastases. In vitro, specific DONSON-knockdown significantly reduced the migration capacity in PC-3 and LNCaP, which further suggests a tumor-promoting role of DONSON in PCa. The results of our comprehensive expression analyses, as well as the functional data obtained after DONSON-depletion, lead us to the conclusion that DONSON is a promising prognostic biomarker with oncogenic properties in PCa.

Abstract: Downstream neighbor of Son (DONSON) plays a crucial role in cell cycle progression and in maintaining genomic stability, but its role in prostate cancer (PCa) development and progression is still underinvestigated. Methods: DONSON mRNA expression was analyzed with regard to clinical-pathological parameters and progression using The Cancer Genome Atlas (TCGA) and two publicly available Gene Expression Omnibus (GEO) datasets of PCa. Afterwards, DONSON protein expression was assessed via immunohistochemistry on a comprehensive tissue microarray (TMA). Subsequently, the influence of a DONSON-knockdown induced by the transfection of antisense-oligonucleotides on proliferative capacity and metastatic potential was investigated. DONSON was associated with an aggressive phenotype in the PCa TCGA cohort, two GEO PCa cohorts, and our PCa TMA cohort as DONSON expression was particularly strong in locally advanced, metastasized, and dedifferentiated carcinomas. Thus, DONSON expression was notably upregulated in distant and androgen-deprivation resistant metastases. In vitro, specific DONSON-knockdown significantly reduced the migration capacity in the PCa cell lines PC-3 and LNCaP, which further suggests a tumor-promoting role of DONSON in PCa. In conclusion, the results of our comprehensive expression analyses, as well as the functional data obtained after DONSON-depletion, lead us to the conclusion that DONSON is a promising prognostic biomarker with oncogenic properties in PCa.

Keywords: prostate carcinoma; DONSON; Downstream Neighbor of SON; biomarker; metastatic spread

1. Introduction

Prostate cancer (PCa) is the most common malignancy in men and contributes significantly to the overall mortality of malignant diseases [1]. Critical steps in PCa progression are the development of castration resistance and metastatic spread. The therapy of these advanced and castration-resistant PCa (CRPC) has improved considerably in recent years, but mortality remains high with limited therapy options in end-stage carcinomas [2,3]. A better understanding of the biology of this multi-facetted carcinoma can help to further improve the therapy of our PCa patients.

The Cancer Genome Atlas (TCGA) platform is a reliable source and an invaluable tool for cancer research [4]. A large cohort of primary PCa (pPCa) has already been comprehensively investigated by the TCGA Research Network, which has certainly contributed to a deeper understanding of this disease [5]. We hypothesized that genes that show a correlation to an unfavorable clinical course, and therefore to particularly aggressive tumors, represent interesting research targets. In an investigative approach, the PCa TCGA dataset was used to determine prognostically relevant genes [4,6], and in the present study, Downstream Neighbor of SON (DONSON) was identified as an interesting target gene for further analyses in PCa. Of note, in a comprehensive pan-cancer analysis of 30 distinct tumor entities using TCGA datasets, we recently found DONSON overexpression to be associated with unfavorable overall survival in diverse entities, suggesting tumor-independent oncogenic properties of this largely unknown gene [7]. Thus, DONSON was found to be a robust biomarker for risk stratification in clear cell renal cell carcinoma (ccRCC), and in vitro, DONSON was linked to a malignant phenotype in ccRCC cell culture models [7,8]. Mechanistically, it is known that DONSON represents a critical replication fork protein required for physiological DNA replication [9]. DONSON is pivotal for genome stability and integrity as severe replication-associated DNA damage was observed after depletion of DONSON [10]. Further, DONSON plays an important role in cell-cycle regulation and the DNA damage response pathway (DDR) signaling cascade [11]. Regulated cell division and the preservation of genomic integrity are essential to maintain cellular homeostasis, and disorders can lead to tumor formation [12].

Considering the apparently decisive role of DONSON on genome integrity and as DONSON seems to be associated with an aggressive PCa phenotype in the transcriptomic TCGA dataset, the question arises whether DONSON also plays an important role in the progression of PCa. However, a differentiated analysis of the role of this gene in PCa is still pending. Therefore, the aim of this study was to thoroughly analyze the expression pattern of DONSON in PCa cohorts and, subsequently, its functional role in vitro in established PCa cell culture models.

2. Results

2.1. Downstream Neighbor of SON (DONSON) mRNA Expression is Associated with Aggressive PCa

In order to analyze the relevance of the DONSON in PCa, we comprehensively associated clinical-pathological parameters and the patients' clinical course with the DONSON mRNA expression using the PCa TCGA dataset ($n = 532$). DONSON expression was significantly enhanced in the carcinoma samples compared to normal adjacent prostatic tissue (NAT) (Figure 1A). DONSON was associated with enhanced local tumor expansion (pT-stage, Figure 1B) and lymphonodal metastatic dissemination (pN-stage, Figure 1C). Furthermore, a strong association of the DONSON expression with the ISUP grading, derived from the PCa-specific grading parameter Gleason score [13], was evident (Figure 1D). After dichotomizing the PCa cohort using the median DONSON expression, there was a strongly reduced progression-free survival (PFS) for the DONSON overexpressing subgroup (Figure 1E). DONSON remained an independent predictor of unfavorable PFS in the PCA TCGA cohort after adjustment for co-variables (TNM; age) using a Cox regression model ($p = 0.001$; HR = 1.87, 95% CI (1.31; 2.68); Table 1). Since PCa with a Gleason score of 7 is particularly difficult to stratify in terms of aggressiveness, we next investigated whether DONSON would have additive prognostic value in this subgroup. In this clinically highly relevant patient cohort, DONSON expression was again significantly associated with shortened PFS and remained an independent predictor of unfavorable clinical course in a multivariate Cox analysis ($p = 0.01$; HR = 3.82, 95% CI [1.44; 10.2]; Table 1) (Figure 1F). Of note, the proliferation marker Ki67 expression had no prognostic value in the Gleason 7 subgroup in univariate and multivariate Cox regression analyses, and DONSON remained an independent predictor of unfavorable PFS after co-adjusting for Ki67 additionally to TNM and age ($p = 0.01$; HR = 4.03, 95% CI [1.49; 10.9]). DONSON overexpression was also associated with worse overall survival (OS). However, the low number of events in the PCa TCGA cohort ($n = 10$) only permits a limited consideration of this important endpoint (Supplementary Figure S1A and Table S1).

Table 1. Multivariate Cox Regression Analyses in the evaluated prostate cancer (PCa) cohorts regarding progression-free survival (PFS).

Clinical-Pathological Parameters	p Value	Hazard Ratio (95% CI Low/High)
Multivariate Cox Regression Analyses (TNM, Age)		
PCa TCGA cohort		
DONSON	0.001	1.87 (1.31; 2.68)
T-Stage	0.002	2.11 (1.31; 3.37)
N-Stage	0.60	1.15 (0.69; 1.91)
Age	0.68	1.01 (0.98; 1.04)
PCa TCGA cohort (Gleason = 7)		
DONSON	0.01	3.82 (1.44; 10.2)
T-Stage	0.73	1.16 (0.50; 2.72)
N-Stage	0.52	1.53 (0.42; 5.54)
Age	0.47	1.03 (0.96; 1.10)
PCa TMA cohort		
DONSON	0.13	1.48 (0.89; 2.47)
T-Stage	0.16	1.71 (0.80; 3.65)
N-Stage	0.62	0.76 (0.26; 2.25)
Age	0.98	1.00 (0.94; 1.07)

PC—Prostate cancer, TCGA—The Cancer Genome Atlas, TMA—Tissue microarray, DONSON—Downstream Neighbor of SON.

Since the PCa TCGA dataset set only contains the expression profiles of primary carcinomas, we wanted to investigate further data sets to more precisely examine the role of DONSON during tumor progression. Of note, in a publicly available PCa progression cohort (GSE21032) [14], DONSON expression was strongly upregulated in the metastatic samples compared to pPCA, which might hint towards a role DONSON plays during the metastatic process (Figure 2A). Interestingly, comparing the sites of the metastatic samples, DONSON expression was significantly enhanced in locally extensive and distant metastatic samples (bone, brain, lung) compared to lymphonodal metastases (LNPC) (Figure 2B). In accordance with this, DONSON expression was strongly enhanced in $n = 25$ androgen-deprivation resistant metastatic samples (Met(CRPC)) compared to pPCa in a second PCa progression cohort (GSE6919, Figure 2C) [15–17]. It is known that fast-growing carcinomas indicate a particularly aggressive phenotype. The proliferation marker Ki-67 is therefore evaluated for assessing tumor aggressiveness, e.g., in breast carcinoma [18], and was also described as a risk stratifier in PCa patients [19]. Of note, we observed a significant positive correlation between DONSON and the proliferative activity of the carcinomas measured by Ki-67 in all of the three independent cohorts (Figure 2D–F).

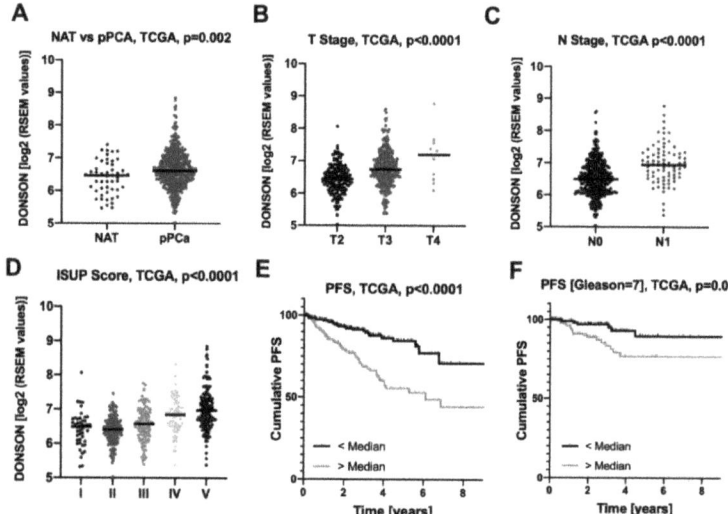

Figure 1. DONSON is associated with clinical-pathological parameters of malignancy and progression-free survival (PFS) using the PCa TCGA dataset (**A**) DONSON expression is enhanced in primary PCa compared to normal adjacent prostatic glands (NAT). DONSON is associated with locally advanced tumor expansion (T Stage), positive lymphonodal metastatic status (N Stage) and the dedifferentiation ISUP score (**B**–**D**). (**E**,**F**) DONSON overexpressing PCa exhibit a shortened PFS when analyzing the whole (**E**) or only the clinically relevant (**F**) subgroup of Gleason 7 carcinomas of the PCa TCGA cohort.

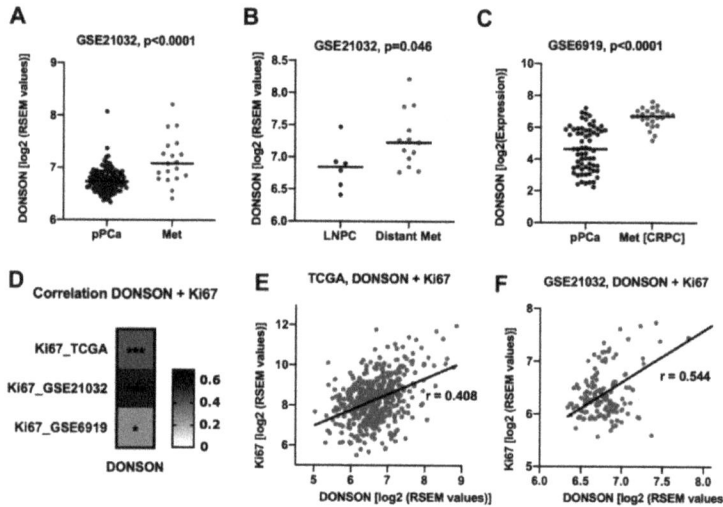

Figure 2. (**A**–**C**), DONSON expression is significantly increased in metastatic samples compared to primary PCA, which was particularly evident in distant (**B**) and androgen-deprivation resistant metastases (Met [CRPC], (**C**). (**D**), Correlation heatmap depicting DONSON's significant correlation to the proliferative activity of PCa in three cohorts. (**E**,**F**), Scatter plots with regression line included visualize the distribution of the TCGA and GSE21032 cohort with regard to the DONSON and Ki67 expression (parametric Pearson´s r is specified). * $p < 0.05$, *** $p < 0.001$.

2.2. DONSON Protein Expression on a PCa Tissue Microarray (TMA)

To test the prognostic potential of DONSON at the protein level, we stained and evaluated a large PCa TMA cohort immunohistochemically against DONSON. DONSON was expressed in the cytoplasm, which is in accordance with the staining pattern observed in the PCa and normal prostate gland specimens of The Human Protein Atlas cohort (HPA, www.proteinatlas.org) [20,21] (Figure 3A). Immunocytochemical DONSON staining in PC-3 cells with and without DONSON knockdown, induced via transfection of specific antisense oligonucleotides, was performed to confirm the cytoplasmic staining pattern and antibody specificity (Supplementary Figure S2). Interestingly, DONSON revealed a heterogeneous expression throughout the investigated cohort (DONSON expression negative/weak $n = 48$; DONSON expression moderate/strong $n = 68$). Of note, enhanced DONSON expression was associated with an advanced pT-stage (Figure 3B). In addition, the aggressive Gleason ≥ 8 PCa (ISUP IV+V) exhibited a significantly increased DONSON expression compared to Gleason ≤ 7 (ISUP I-III) (Figure 3C). No further significant associations between DONSON and clinical pathological parameters were evident, which may be due to the low sample size.

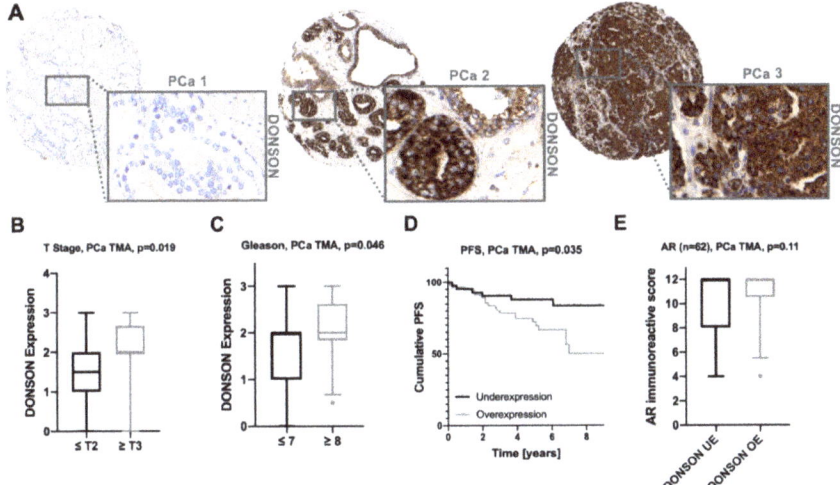

Figure 3. Immunohistochemical staining (IHC) against DONSON on a comprehensive PCa TMA with subsequent expression analysis (**A**), Representative images of the heterogeneous DONSON expression throughout the primary PCa cohort are depicted in three cases; 10× and 40× objective magnification. PCa 1 represents a well-differentiated DONSON-negative carcinoma. PCa 2 + 3 represent cases with particularly strong DONSON protein expression, wherein PCa 3 additionally exhibits an aggressive phenotype with fusing glands and components of a solid carcinoma. (**B,C**), DONSON expression is associated with advanced T Stage and Gleason score. (**D**), DONSON overexpression, defined as DONSON moderate/high (Score ≥ 2), predicts shortened PFS compared to the negative/low expression subgroup. (**E**), A strong statistical tendency for an increased nuclear AR expression was evident in the DONSON overexpressing subgroup; overexpression = OE, underexpression = UE.

In line with its potential as a risk stratifier in the PCa TCGA cohort, DONSON overexpression also showed a significant association with progression-free survival (PFS) at the protein level in the investigated cohort (Figure 3D). Further, a strong statistical trend was seen for DONSON to be an independent predictor of unfavorable PFS ($p = 0.13$; HR 1.48, 95% CI (0.89; 2.47); Table 1) measured by multivariate Cox regression co-adjusting the TNM stage and age.

The androgen receptor (AR) signaling pathway plays a crucial role in the progression of PCa, and nuclear expression of AR predicts an unfavorable clinical outcome and shorter time to the development of castration resistance [22]. Interestingly, in the examined PCa cohort, a strong trend for increased AR expression (studied earlier in [23]) in the DONSON overexpressing subgroup was evident (Figure 3E). In accordance with this, in both PCa progression cohorts a significant correlation of AR and DONSON mRNA expression was observed (GSE21032: Pearson's r = 0.204, p-value = 0.012; GSE6919: Pearson's r = 0.549, p-value < 0.0001).

2.3. Functional Characterization of DONSON In Vitro

In order to investigate the functional role of DONSON in vitro, we used the antisense locked nucleic acid (LNA) GapmeR system to induce efficient and specific DONSON-knockdowns in established PCa cell culture models. The prostate cancer cell lines PC-3, LNCaP, C4-2B, and DU-145 were screened for their DONSON baseline expression under standard conditions (Figure 4A). As LNCap and PC-3 expressed the highest DONSON protein levels, they have been chosen for further investigations. Thus, via transfection of the specific antisense oligonucleotides, we were able to induce efficient DONSON-depletion assessed by qRT-PCR, Western blotting, and immunocytochemistry (Figure 4B,C, Figure S2).

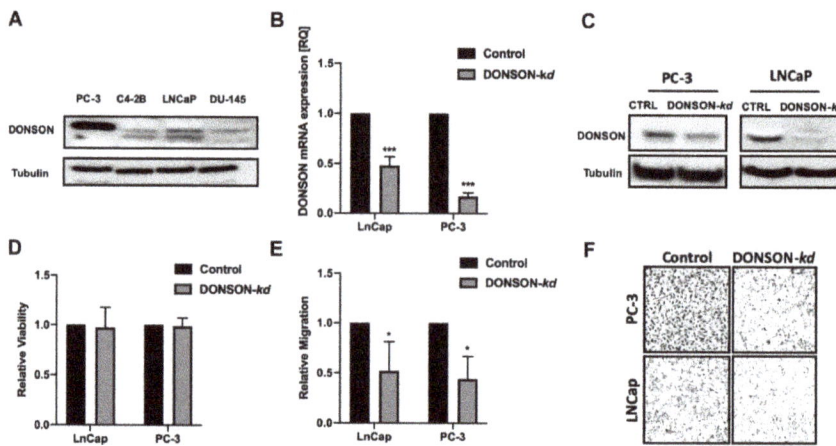

Figure 4. Effect of specific DONSON-depletion in the PCa cell lines LNCaP and PC-3. (**A**), Screening Western Blot for DONSON in four broadly used PCa cell lines. (**B,C**), Induction of efficient Antisense LNA GapmeR-mediated DONSON knockdowns in LNCaP and PC-3 with subsequent validation via qPCR (**B**) and Western Blotting (**C**). (**D,E**) DONSON-depletion did not affect cell viability but specifically reduced the cellular motility in a Boyden Chamber Migration Assay. (**F**), Membranes depicted in 10× objective magnification. Each experiment was performed in biological triplicates. * $p < 0.05$, *** $p < 0.001$.

After establishing efficient DONSON-depletion in both cell culture models, we aimed to investigate the dependence of important parameters of malignancy towards DONSON. In the conducted cell proliferation and cytotoxicity assay, no growth effects were evident in die DONSON-depleted PCa cells compared to the negative control (Figure 4D). Next, we explored the impact of DONSON-knockdown on the migration capacity of the investigated metastasizing PCa cells via Boyden chamber migration assays. Of note, a strong impairment of their migration capacity was seen after DONSON-knockdown (Figure 4E,F), which is thought to be an essential trait for metastatic spread and an important attribute conferring to an aggressive phenotype.

3. Discussion

To date, the role of DONSON in PCa has not been explored. In this study, we were able to identify the relatively unknown gene DONSON as a promising risk stratifier with oncogenic properties in the PCa cell culture model. DONSON was an independent predictor of a shortened PFS in the comprehensive PCa TCGA cohort and correlated with the clinical-pathological parameters (pT-stage, lymphonodal status, ISUP/Gleason score). In the group of Gleason 7 carcinomas, which plays a crucial role clinically due to the intermediate aggressiveness with regard to the prognosis and need for therapy, DONSON also shows an additive prognostic potential in the multivariate Cox analysis.

The prognostic potential of DONSON has been validated at the protein level in a large PCa TMA cohort, highlighting its potential as a robust biomarker. Of note, the DONSON protein was localized in the cytoplasm of the PCa samples, which was in accordance with the staining pattern observed in The Human Protein Atlas and as described previously for clear cell renal cell carcinoma tissue [7,8]. Staining specificity was confirmed via immunocytochemistry in PC-3 cells with and without DONSON knockdown. Nevertheless, due to its function in DNA replication and repair, an additional nuclear expression would have been expected. During the S phase, nuclear DONSON foci were observed [9]. However, the DNA replication and S phase only describes a small part of the cell cycle, and thus the localization of DONSON could differ during the G1 phase [24]. Furthermore, as the overall knowledge regarding DONSON is sparse, it may have additional functions, also inside the cytoplasm. As this was not the scope of our study, further investigations regarding its subcellular localization, trafficking, and exact biological function are needed to clarify this.

Interestingly, the PCa TMA cohort showed a heterogeneous picture, with some tumors being DONSON-negative while others, especially Gleason 8 and higher carcinomas, strongly overexpressed DONSON. It has to be mentioned that only a strong statistical trend was seen for DONSON to be an independent predictor of unfavorable PFS in this cohort (HR 1.46, 95% CI; 0.86–2.48; $p = 0.17$), which may be due to a relatively low sample size compared to the PCa TCGA cohort (PFS Follow-up PCa TMA cohort $n = 103$ (29 events); PCa TCGA cohort $n = 497$ (93 events)).

In addition, two independent PCa progression cohorts showed a significant increase in DONSON expression in the metastatic samples compared to pPCA, which was particularly evident in distant metastases and androgen-deprivation resistant metastases. The crucial step in PCa progression is displayed by the development of metastases and a castration-resistant status during androgen-deprivation therapy (ADT). Among the different mechanisms of CRPC development, aberrant androgen receptor (AR) signaling is thought to be a major player [22,25]. An association between DONSON and AR expression was observed in the PCa progression and the PCa tissue microarray (TMA) cohorts on both transcriptional and translational levels. However, the exact interaction of DONSON and the AR signaling pathway and a possible link between DONSON and the development of castration-resistance requires further functional investigations. In addition, the proliferative activity measured by Ki67 expression, which is also an established prognostic biomarker in PCa and other cancers [18,19], was significantly correlated with DONSON expression, which seems comprehensible due to the predicted function of DONSON as part of the replisome [10,26]. Thus, renal cell carcinoma cell lines showed decreased proliferative capacity after oligonucleotide-mediated DONSON knockdown [7,8]. However, in our PCa cell culture model, no influence on proliferation could be detected after DONSON-depletion, which suggests an additional unknown function of DONSON, but this requires further investigation. In our cell culture model, DONSON-depletion led to potent inhibition of cell motility, which is recognized as a surrogate for the metastatic capacity in vitro. This provides evidence that DONSON plays a role during the metastatic process, which could ultimately explain its significant upregulation in the metastatic samples in both PCa progression cohorts and the N+ pPCa samples (PCa TCGA).

Taxane-based therapy is a backbone of PCa therapy and preferentially attacks tumor cells with an increased cell division rate as well as limited DNA damage repair capacity. As DONSON plays a pivotal role in both cellular processes, replication, and maintaining genome stability, it could be an interesting therapeutic target for combination therapies [10,11]. Therefore, we think that our study on DONSON in PCa, as well as the fact that DONSON overexpression seems to mediate tumor-independent oncogenic properties, could be a starting point for further basic and oncological research on DONSON.

Thus, the results of our comprehensive expression analyses, as well as the functional data obtained after DONSON-depletion, lead us to the conclusion that DONSON is a promising prognostic biomarker with oncogenic properties in PCa.

4. Materials and Methods

4.1. Transcriptome Data Assembly

Log2 transformed RNA sequencing data generated by IlluminaHiSeq (Illumina, San Diego, CA, USA) and publicly available by the TCGA Research Network were downloaded via the UCSC Xena browser (http://xena.ucsc.edu, PCa $n = 497$, plus normal adjacent kidney tissue (NAT) $n = 52$; Table S1) [4,5].

Microarray data (Affymetrix Human Genome U95C Array; Affymetrix, Santa Clara, CA, USA) from the first prostate cancer progression cohort for DONSON, KI67, and AR were downloaded via Gene Expression Omnibus (GEO, http://www.ncbi.nlm.nih.gov/geo/, GSE6919) [15]. The expression profiles of 25 androgen-deprivation resistant metastatic samples derived from four patients were obtained from different metastatic sites and were thereby used as individual samples (pPCa $n = 66$, Met(CRPC) $n = 25$). Normalized log2 mRNA (DONSON, Ki67, AR) expression data and the clinical features of the second investigated progression cohort were obtained from http://cbio.mskcc.org/cancergenomics/prostate/, which included primary PCa and metastatic samples (GSE21032, pPCa $n = 131$, Met $n = 19$) [14].

4.2. Immunohistochemistry

A tissue microarray (TMA) from paraffin-embedded prostate tissue was assessed as described previously [23,27,28] (Supplementary Table S2). Paraffin sections of 5 µm thickness were cut and stained with the polyclonal DONSON-antibody (HPA039558, Atlas Antibodies, dilution 1:50; Sigma Aldrich, St. Louis, MO, USA) with the Ventana Benchmark automated staining system (Ventana Medical System, Tuscon, AZ, USA) [7,29–31]. The staining quality and specificity were confirmed by experienced uropathologists, and subsequently, the TMA cohort was stained. Two experienced observers independently scored the DONSON staining intensity with a score ranging negative, weak, moderate, or strong DONSON protein expression (score values 0 to 3) as previously described for PCa specimens [27]. Androgen receptor (AR) expression data, already collected using the immunoreactive score, were also available for a subset of the examined cohort ($n = 62$) [23].

4.3. Antisense LNA GapmeR-Mediated Knockdown

Transfections in both cell lines were conducted using a final concentration of 150 nM in a ratio of 3:1 with the FuGENE HD-Transfection reagent (E2311, Promega Corporation, Madison, WI, USA) in accordance with the producers' instructions and as described previously [7,31]. DONSON GapmeR sequence: 5′-A*C*C*A*G*T*C*A*C*T*C*A*T*T*A*A-3′. Non-targeting negative control GapmeR sequence: 5′-*C*G*T*A**G*T*C*G*A*G*G*A*A*G*T*A-3′.

4.4. Immunocytochemistry

Briefly, 72 h post-transfection, PC-3 cells were harvested and transferred into Cellmatrix (Type I-A) (Fujifilm Wako Chemicals, Osaka, Japan). Subsequently, cells were fixed in 4% paraformaldehyde for 24 h and embedded into paraffin. Afterward, DONSON staining was performed as described in Section 4.2.

4.5. Real-Time PCR

Transcriptional knockdown efficiency was assessed 48 h post-transfection using quantitative real-time PCR. The following primer sequences were used: DONSON forward primer: 5′-gtccagcattgtagggcaac-3′ and reverse primer: 5′-ggctctgctggaaggtacaa-3′; β-Actin forward primer: 5′-CCAACCGCGAGAAGATGA-3′ and reverse primer: 5′-CCAGAGGCGTACAGGGATAG-3′.

4.6. Western Blot

DONSON knockdown efficiency was assessed 72h post-transfection. The following antibodies were used: Anti-DONSON (1:1000, LS-C167506, Rabbit, LSBio, Seattle, WA, USA); Anti-alpha-Tubulin (1:4000, A5316, Mouse, Sigma-Aldrich, St. Louis, MO, USA).

4.7. Cell Proliferation Assays

We used the EZ4U cell proliferation and cytotoxicity assay kit according to the manufacturer's protocol (EZ4U, Biomedica Group, Vienna, Austria).

4.8. Migration Assays

Boyden Chamber Migration Assays (8.0 µm pore size, 353097, Falcon, Corning, Amsterdam, The Netherlands) were performed to assess cell motility and migration. The cells were plated 48 h post-transfection in the upper chamber of the migration inserts with starved RPMI medium (0% FCS), whereas the lower chamber was filled with standard medium containing 10% FCS for chemotactic attraction. The experiment was stopped after 48 h of incubation, the cells being fixed with 4% formaldehyde and colored with hematoxylin. Membranes were scanned, and the cells were counted automatically by nucleus detection using the QuPath software (v0.2.0-m6) [7,32].

4.9. Statistical Analysis

Microsoft Excel (v16), SPPS (v25), and GraphPad Prism (v8) were used for statistical analyses and visualization of the data. The nonparametric Mann–Whitney U or Kruskal–Wallis test were used for group comparisons. Pearson´s correlation coefficients were calculated. Survival analyses were performed using Kaplan Meier estimate curves and log-rank tests. Thus, multivariate Cox regression analyses were performed after co-adjustment of the TNM stage (the only $n = 3$ M1 in PCa TCGA were excluded; in PCa TMA no cM1 cases) and age to evaluate an independent and additive prognostic value on patients' progression-free survival.

4.10. Ethical Approval and Consent to Participate

All patients gave written informed consent for the collection of biomaterials. The study was approved by the Ethics Committee at the Medical Faculty of the Rheinische Friedrich-Wilhelms-University Bonn (number: 273/18; 013/20).

5. Conclusions

In total, our study could show for the first time that DONSON expression is strongly enhanced in phenotypically aggressive PCa and advanced metastatic samples and represents an interesting and robust prognostic biomarker. Further, DONSON could play an important role in the PCa progression and metastatic process supported by functional in vitro analyses.

Supplementary Materials: The following are available online at http://www.mdpi.com/2072-6694/12/11/3439/s1, Figure S1: DONSON overexpression is associated with an unfavorable OS in the PCa TCGA cohort, Figure S2: A, Immunocytochemical staining of DONSON in PC-3 control cells (NegA) compared to DONSON-knockdown. Images depicted in 10x objective magnification. B. The DONSON knockdown efficacy of the respective stained cells was confirmed via qPCR, Figure S3: Uncropped Western Blot images, Table S1: Clinical-pathological characteristics of the Prostate Cancer TCGA Cohort, Table S2: Clinical-pathological characteristics of the Bonn Prostate Cancer Tissue Microarray.

Author Contributions: Conceptualization, N.K., A.A., and J.E.; methodology, N.K., M.v.D., J.S., D.S., A.S., A.A., and J.E.; validation, N.K., M.v.D., J.S., D.S., A.S., G.K., M.M., M.H., M.R., A.A., and J.E.; investigation, N.K., M.v.D., and J.S.; resources, G.K., M.H., M.R., A.A., and J.E.; writing, N.K., M.v.D., A.A., and J.E.; review and editing, J.S., D.S., A.S., G.K., M.M., M.H., and M.R.; supervision, A.A. and J.E. All authors have read and agreed to the published version of the manuscript.

Funding: This research was funded by a Ferdinand Eisenberger grant of the Deutsche Gesellschaft für Urologie (German society of Urology), grant ID KIN1/FE-19 (NK).

Acknowledgments: The tissue samples were collected within the framework of the Biobank of the Center for Integrated Oncology Cologne Bonn at the University Hospital Bonn.

Conflicts of Interest: The authors declare no conflict of interest.

References

1. Siegel, R.L.; Miller, K.D.; Jemal, A. Cancer statistics, 2019. *CA Cancer J. Clin.* **2019**, *69*, 7–34. [CrossRef]
2. Gillessen, S.; Attard, G.; Beer, T.M.; Beltran, H.; Bjartell, A.; Bossi, A.; Briganti, A.; Bristow, R.G.; Chi, K.N.; Clarke, N.; et al. Management of Patients with Advanced Prostate Cancer: Report of the Advanced Prostate Cancer Consensus Conference. 2019. *Eur. Urol.* **2020**, *77*, 508–547. [CrossRef] [PubMed]
3. Dellis, A.; Zagouri, F.; Liontos, M.; Mitropoulos, D.; Bamias, A.; Papatsoris, A.G. Management of advanced prostate cancer: A systematic review of existing guidelines and recommendations. *Cancer Treat. Rev.* **2019**, *73*, 54–61. [CrossRef] [PubMed]
4. The Cancer Genome Atlas Research Network; Weinstein, J.N.; Collisson, E.A.; Mills, G.B.; Shaw, K.R.M.; Ozenberger, B.A.; Ellrott, K.; Shmulevich, I.; Sander, C.; Stuart, J.M. The Cancer Genome Atlas Pan-Cancer analysis project. *Nat. Genet.* **2013**, *45*, 1113–1120. [CrossRef]
5. Cancer Genome Atlas Research Network The Molecular Taxonomy of Primary Prostate Cancer. *Cell* **2015**, *163*, 1011–1025. [CrossRef] [PubMed]
6. Uhlen, M.; Zhang, C.; Lee, S.; Sjöstedt, E.; Fagerberg, L.; Bidkhori, G.; Benfeitas, R.; Arif, M.; Liu, Z.; Edfors, F.; et al. A pathology atlas of the human cancer transcriptome. *Science* **2017**, *357*, eaan2507. [CrossRef]
7. Klümper, N.; Blajan, I.; Schmidt, D.; Kristiansen, G.; Toma, M.; Hölzel, M.; Ritter, M.; Ellinger, J. Downstream neighbor of SON (DONSON) is associated with unfavorable survival across diverse cancers with oncogenic properties in clear cell renal cell carcinoma. *Transl. Oncol.* **2020**, *13*, 100844. [CrossRef]
8. Yamada, Y.; Nohata, N.; Uchida, A.; Kato, M.; Arai, T.; Moriya, S.; Mizuno, K.; Kojima, S.; Yamazaki, K.; Naya, Y.; et al. Replisome genes regulation by antitumor miR-101-5p in clear cell renal cell carcinoma. *Cancer Sci.* **2020**. [CrossRef]
9. Zhang, J.; Bellani, M.A.; James, R.C.; Pokharel, D.; Zhang, Y.; Reynolds, J.J.; McNee, G.S.; Jackson, A.P.; Stewart, G.S.; Seidman, M.M. DONSON and FANCM associate with different replisomes distinguished by replication timing and chromatin domain. *Nat. Commun.* **2020**, *11*, 3951. [CrossRef]
10. Reynolds, J.J.; Bicknell, L.S.; Carroll, P.; Higgs, M.R.; Shaheen, R.; Murray, J.E.; Papadopoulos, D.K.; Leitch, A.; Murina, O.; Tarnauskaitė, Ž.; et al. Mutations in DONSON disrupt replication fork stability and cause microcephalic dwarfism. *Nat. Genet.* **2017**, *49*, 537–549. [CrossRef]
11. Fuchs, F.; Pau, G.; Kranz, D.; Sklyar, O.; Budjan, C.; Steinbrink, S.; Horn, T.; Pedal, A.; Huber, W.; Boutros, M. Clustering phenotype populations by genome-wide RNAi and multiparametric imaging. *Mol. Syst. Biol.* **2010**, *6*, 370. [CrossRef] [PubMed]
12. Hanahan, D.; Weinberg, R.A. Hallmarks of Cancer: The Next Generation. *Cell* **2011**, *144*, 646–674. [CrossRef] [PubMed]
13. Epstein, J.I.; Egevad, L.; Amin, M.B.; Delahunt, B.; Srigley, J.R.; Humphrey, P.A. Grading Committee The 2014 International Society of Urological Pathology (ISUP) Consensus Conference on Gleason Grading of Prostatic Carcinoma: Definition of Grading Patterns and Proposal for a New Grading System. *Am. J. Surg. Pathol.* **2016**, *40*, 244–252. [CrossRef] [PubMed]
14. Taylor, B.S.; Schultz, N.; Hieronymus, H.; Gopalan, A.; Xiao, Y.; Carver, B.S.; Arora, V.K.; Kaushik, P.; Cerami, E.; Reva, B.; et al. Integrative Genomic Profiling of Human Prostate Cancer. *Cancer Cell* **2010**, *18*, 11–22. [CrossRef] [PubMed]
15. Chandran, U.R.; Ma, C.; Dhir, R.; Bisceglia, M.; Lyons-Weiler, M.; Liang, W.; Michalopoulos, G.; Becich, M.; Monzon, F.A. Gene expression profiles of prostate cancer reveal involvement of multiple molecular pathways in the metastatic process. *BMC Cancer* **2007**, *7*, 64. [CrossRef] [PubMed]
16. Chandran, U.R.; Dhir, R.; Ma, C.; Michalopoulos, G.; Becich, M.; Gilbertson, J. Differences in gene expression in prostate cancer, normal appearing prostate tissue adjacent to cancer and prostate tissue from cancer free organ donors. *BMC Cancer* **2005**, *5*, 45. [CrossRef] [PubMed]
17. Yu, Y.P.; Landsittel, D.; Jing, L.; Nelson, J.; Ren, B.; Liu, L.; McDonald, C.; Thomas, R.; Dhir, R.; Finkelstein, S.; et al. Gene expression alterations in prostate cancer predicting tumor aggression and preceding development of malignancy. *J. Clin. Oncol. Off. J. Am. Soc. Clin. Oncol.* **2004**, *22*, 2790–2799. [CrossRef]

18. Inwald, E.C.; Klinkhammer-Schalke, M.; Hofstädter, F.; Zeman, F.; Koller, M.; Gerstenhauer, M.; Ortmann, O. Ki-67 is a prognostic parameter in breast cancer patients: Results of a large population-based cohort of a cancer registry. *Breast Cancer Res. Treat.* **2013**, *139*, 539–552. [CrossRef]
19. Hammarsten, P.; Josefsson, A.; Thysell, E.; Lundholm, M.; Hägglöf, C.; Iglesias-Gato, D.; Flores-Morales, A.; Stattin, P.; Egevad, L.; Granfors, T.; et al. Immunoreactivity for prostate specific antigen and Ki67 differentiates subgroups of prostate cancer related to outcome. *Mod. Pathol.* **2019**, *32*, 1310–1319. [CrossRef]
20. Uhlén, M.; Fagerberg, L.; Hallström, B.M.; Lindskog, C.; Oksvold, P.; Mardinoglu, A.; Sivertsson, Å.; Kampf, C.; Sjöstedt, E.; Asplund, A.; et al. Tissue-based map of the human proteome. *Science* **2015**, *347*, 1260419. [CrossRef]
21. Uhlén, M.; Björling, E.; Agaton, C.; Szigyarto, C.A.-K.; Amini, B.; Andersen, E.; Andersson, A.-C.; Angelidou, P.; Asplund, A.; Asplund, C.; et al. A human protein atlas for normal and cancer tissues based on antibody proteomics. *Mol. Cell. Proteom. MCP* **2005**, *4*, 1920–1932. [CrossRef] [PubMed]
22. Donovan, M.J.; Hamann, S.; Clayton, M.; Khan, F.M.; Sapir, M.; Bayer-Zubek, V.; Fernandez, G.; Mesa-Tejada, R.; Teverovskiy, M.; Reuter, V.E.; et al. Systems pathology approach for the prediction of prostate cancer progression after radical prostatectomy. *J. Clin. Oncol. Off. J. Am. Soc. Clin. Oncol.* **2008**, *26*, 3923–3929. [CrossRef] [PubMed]
23. Mang, J.; Korzeniewski, N.; Dietrich, D.; Sailer, V.; Tolstov, Y.; Searcy, S.; von Hardenberg, J.; Perner, S.; Kristiansen, G.; Marx, A.; et al. Prognostic Significance and Functional Role of CEP57 in Prostate Cancer. *Transl. Oncol.* **2015**, *8*, 487–496. [CrossRef]
24. Natsume, T.; Tanaka, T.U. Spatial regulation and organization of DNA replication within the nucleus. *Chromosome Res.* **2010**, *18*, 7–17. [CrossRef] [PubMed]
25. Hu, R.; Denmeade, S.R.; Luo, J. Molecular processes leading to aberrant androgen receptor signaling and castration resistance in prostate cancer. *Expert Rev. Endocrinol. Metab.* **2010**, *5*, 753–764. [CrossRef]
26. Rai, R.; Gu, P.; Broton, C.; Kumar-Sinha, C.; Chen, Y.; Chang, S. The Replisome Mediates A-NHEJ Repair of Telomeres Lacking POT1-TPP1 Independently of MRN Function. *Cell Rep.* **2019**, *29*, 3708–3725.e5. [CrossRef]
27. Stein, J.; Majores, M.; Rohde, M.; Lim, S.; Schneider, S.; Krappe, E.; Ellinger, J.; Dietel, M.; Stephan, C.; Jung, K.; et al. KDM5C Is Overexpressed in Prostate Cancer and Is a Prognostic Marker for Prostate-Specific Antigen-Relapse Following Radical Prostatectomy. *Am. J. Pathol.* **2014**, *184*, 2430–2437. [CrossRef]
28. Gevensleben, H.; Dietrich, D.; Golletz, C.; Steiner, S.; Jung, M.; Thiesler, T.; Majores, M.; Stein, J.; Uhl, B.; Muller, S.; et al. The Immune Checkpoint Regulator PD-L1 Is Highly Expressed in Aggressive Primary Prostate Cancer. *Clin. Cancer Res.* **2016**, *22*, 1969–1977. [CrossRef]
29. Klümper, N.; Syring, I.; Offermann, A.; Shaikhibrahim, Z.; Vogel, W.; Müller, S.C.; Ellinger, J.; Strauß, A.; Radzun, H.J.; Ströbel, P.; et al. Differential expression of Mediator complex subunit MED15 in testicular germ cell tumors. *Diagn. Pathol.* **2015**, *10*, 165. [CrossRef]
30. Klümper, N.; Syring, I.; Vogel, W.; Schmidt, D.; Müller, S.C.; Ellinger, J.; Shaikhibrahim, Z.; Brägelmann, J.; Perner, S. Mediator Complex Subunit MED1 Protein Expression Is Decreased during Bladder Cancer Progression. *Front. Med.* **2017**, *4*, 30. [CrossRef]
31. Blajan, I.; Miersch, H.; Schmidt, D.; Kristiansen, G.; Perner, S.; Ritter, M.; Ellinger, J.; Klümper, N. Comprehensive Analysis of the ATP-binding Cassette Subfamily B Across Renal Cancers Identifies ABCB8 Overexpression in Phenotypically Aggressive Clear Cell Renal Cell Carcinoma. *Eur. Urol. Focus* **2020**. [CrossRef] [PubMed]
32. Bankhead, P.; Loughrey, M.B.; Fernández, J.A.; Dombrowski, Y.; McArt, D.G.; Dunne, P.D.; McQuaid, S.; Gray, R.T.; Murray, L.J.; Coleman, H.G.; et al. QuPath: Open source software for digital pathology image analysis. *Sci. Rep.* **2017**, *7*. [CrossRef] [PubMed]

Publisher's Note: MDPI stays neutral with regard to jurisdictional claims in published maps and institutional affiliations.

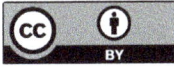

© 2020 by the authors. Licensee MDPI, Basel, Switzerland. This article is an open access article distributed under the terms and conditions of the Creative Commons Attribution (CC BY) license (http://creativecommons.org/licenses/by/4.0/).

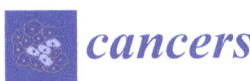

Review

Unusual Faces of Bladder Cancer

Claudia Manini [1] and José I. López [2,*]

1. Department of Pathology, San Giovanni Bosco Hospital, 10154 Turin, Italy; claudiamaninicm@gmail.com
2. Department of Pathology, Biocruces-Bizkaia Health Research Institute, Cruces University Hospital, Barakaldo, 48903 Bizkaia, Spain
* Correspondence: jilpath@gmail.com; Tel.: +34-94-600-6084

Received: 27 October 2020; Accepted: 7 December 2020; Published: 10 December 2020

Simple Summary: The spectrum of architectural and cytological findings in UC is wide, although transitional cell carcinoma, either papillary or flat, low- or high-grade, constitutes the majority of cases in routine practice. Some of these changes are just mere morphological variations, but others must be recognized since they have importance for the patient. The goal of this review is to compile this histological variability giving to the general pathologist a general idea of this morphological spectrum in a few pages. The review also updates the literature focusing specifically on the morphological and immunohistochemical clues useful for the diagnosis and some selected molecular studies with prognostic and/or diagnostic implications.

Abstract: The overwhelming majority of bladder cancers are transitional cell carcinomas. Albeit mostly monotonous, carcinomas in the bladder may occasionally display a broad spectrum of histological features that should be recognized by pathologists because some of them represent a diagnostic problem and/or lead prognostic implications. Sometimes these features are focal in the context of conventional transitional cell carcinomas, but some others are generalized across the tumor making its recognition a challenge. For practical purposes, the review distributes the morphologic spectrum of changes in architecture and cytology. Thus, nested and large nested, micropapillary, myxoid stroma, small tubules and adenoma nephrogenic-like, microcystic, verrucous, and diffuse lymphoepithelioma-like, on one hand, and plasmacytoid, signet ring, basaloid-squamous, yolk-sac, trophoblastic, rhabdoid, lipid/lipoblastic, giant, clear, eosinophilic (oncocytoid), and sarcomatoid, on the other, are revisited. Key histological and immunohistochemical features useful in the differential diagnosis are mentioned. In selected cases, molecular data associated with the diagnosis, prognosis, and/or treatment are also included.

Keywords: bladder cancer; diagnosis; differential diagnosis; prognosis; histopathology; immunohistochemistry

1. Introduction

Bladder cancer is a frequent neoplasm [1] in which tobacco use, pollution, and other varied agents have been directly implicated in its genesis and development [2]. Most of them are composed of transitional cells of low/intermediate grade, papillary architecture, and invasion limited to the lamina propria and submucosa. However, a smaller but significant number of cases do display dismal features like high-grade, non-papillary growth patterns, and muscularis propria invasion, with these patients pursuing an aggressive clinical course.

Aside from transitional cell carcinoma (TCC), other histological subtypes, like conventional squamous cell carcinoma, adenocarcinoma, and neuroendocrine carcinoma, are quite frequently seen in clinical practice, alone or in combination, particularly in the context of high-grade cases. These cases are not the subject of this review.

Although TCC is a histologically monotonous neoplasm composed in the vast majority of cases by easily recognizable transitional cells, a small subset of cases displays a broad spectrum of architectural and/or cytological characteristics that should be recognized since some of them carry diagnostic difficulties and/or prognostic implications [3] (Table 1). This recognition is increasingly important now that very promising advances linking morphological variants with genomic signatures are being identified [4].

Table 1. Unusual features in bladder cancer with prognostic profiles.

Architectural Changes	Prognostic Profiles
	Worse prognosis - Nested - Large nested - Micropapillary
	Not worse prognosis - Myxoid stromal change - Small tubules - Nephrogenic adenoma-like - Microcystic - Verrucous - Diffuse lymphoepithelioma-like
Cytological changes	
	Worse prognosis - Plasmacytoid - Signet-ring - Basaloid-squamous - Yolk-sac - Trophoblastic - Rhabdoid - Giant pleomorphic - Clear - Sarcomatoid
	Not worse prognosis - Lipid/lipoblast - Giant osteoclast-like - Eosinophilic (oncocytoid)

Clinical practice allows the pathologist to face unusual histological subtypes of urothelial carcinomas (UC), and conventional TCC displaying focal/extensive morphologic variations of uncertain significance. This narrative collects 25 years of personal experience of the authors in the routine diagnosis of bladder cancer.

2. Architectural Changes

2.1. Nested and Large Nested Architecture

Talbert and Young reported in 1989 three cases of a deceptively benign bladder carcinoma characterized by small packed cellular aggregates closely resembling von Brunn nests and nephrogenic adenoma [5]. Isolated cases of this histological subtype of bladder cancer had previously appeared in the literature, always being referred to as of von Brunn nest origin [6]. Now, nested UC is well recognized and fully characterized by histological, immunohistochemical, and molecular perspectives [7,8]. Under the microscope, nested UC appears as a non-papillary neoplastic growth of bland cells with scarce atypia arranged in small nests (Figure 1a) showing an evident infiltrating growth pattern at different levels of the bladder wall. Typically, the tumor does not induce a stromal reaction nor is accompanied by inflammatory infiltrates. Problems to recognize nested UC may arise in small superficial biopsies if crushing artifacts are present or if the infiltrative nature is not seen.

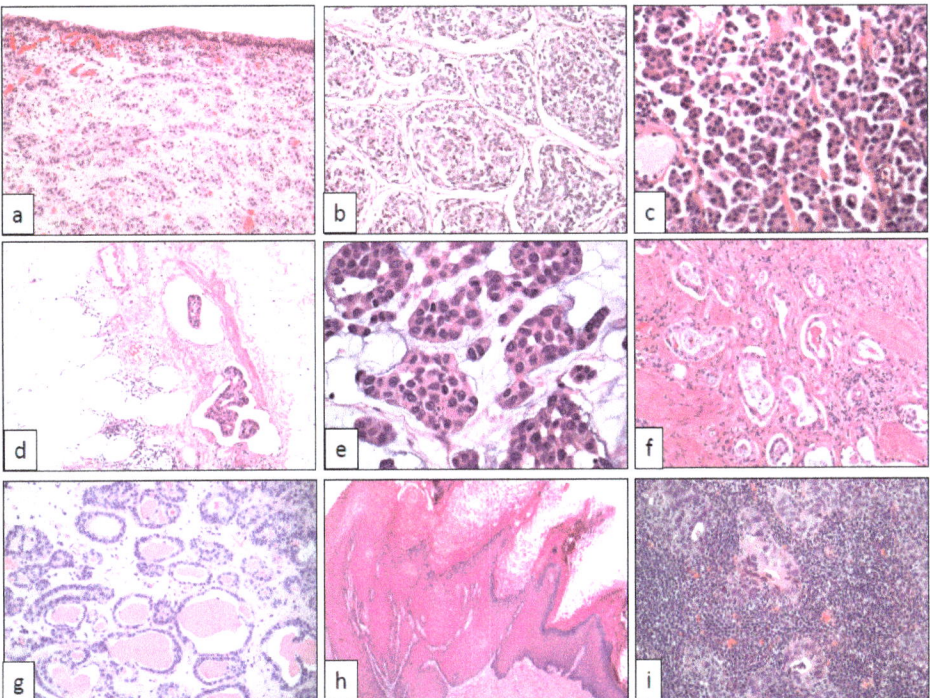

Figure 1. Architectural changes in bladder cancer (with original magnifications included). (**a**) Nested pattern (×100), (**b**) large nested pattern (×100), (**c**) micropapillary pattern (×250), (**d**) vascular invasion in the micropapillary pattern (×100), (**e**) myxoid basophilic stroma (×400), (**f**) small tubules (×100), (**g**) microcystic pattern (×100), (**h**) verrucous pattern (×40), and (**i**) lymphoepithelioma-like pattern (×250).

Cox and Epstein described in 2011 the large nested variant of UC reporting the characteristic histology of a tumor resembling large von Brunn nests with inverted growth in 23 patients [9]. Some isolated cases of this UC variant have been reported since then, and only two more series of cases have been published so far [10,11]. The large nested UC shares with the nested UC the same morphologic characteristics and clinical aggressiveness but the nests are larger (Figure 1b), with a growth pattern mimicking conventional inverted UC. These similarities have been advised to merge them into the same group in the last WHO classification of UC [12]. Interestingly, large nested UC displays a luminal phenotype, positive with FOXA1, GATA3, and CK 20 [12]. *FGFR3* and *TERT* genes are frequently mutated in this UC subtype [12].

2.2. Micropapillary Architecture

UC may sometimes display a micropapillary architecture. Delicate, thin, and fragile papillae without stromal axis are the hallmark of this morphological variant of UC (Figure 1c). To note, the invasive component of micropapillary UC shows nests with cells detached from the basal membrane, a typical artifact in this tumor that mimics lymphatic invasion and is associated with biological aggressiveness [13]. The vascular invasion is a very frequent histological finding (Figure 1d). Aside from rare pure examples, the majority of cases are mixed with a conventional transitional cell carcinoma, usually high grade. Like the rest of micropapillary carcinomas across the body [14], this histological subtype of UC has a dismal prognosis, even worse than conventional high-grade UC at the same stage [15], and typically presents with advanced stages at diagnosis. Although exceptional, micropapillary carcinomas from other sites may metastasize to the urinary bladder [16], making the correct diagnosis more difficult.

The first description of this variant of UC was made in 1994 by Amin et al. [17], where they stressed the histological similarities of this bladder tumor with the classic papillary serous carcinoma of the ovary. After that, many series have been published all along the urinary tract, including the renal pelvis and ureter [18,19].

Abundant immunohistochemical and molecular analyses have been performed in micropapillary UC [20–22] all confirming its aggressive potential. Although initially thought to be a variant of adenocarcinoma by some authors [23], Yang et al. have very recently reported that the micropapillary UC is not a variant of adenocarcinoma [22].

2.3. Myxoid Stromal Change

UC may display focal myxoid changes in the stroma (Figure 1e) mimicking the colloid adenocarcinomas seen in other sites. This change has been previously reported [24,25] and when observed in transurethral resection specimens, may lead to an erroneous interpretation of colonic adenocarcinoma invading the bladder wall. Solid cell nests immersed in a basophilic edematous stroma are the hallmark of this histological change, which is usually focal but can be generalized in some isolated cases. Again, immunohistochemistry is of much help in cases in which the transitional phenotype of the tumor is not evident on hematoxylin-eosin slides. GATA3 positivity, co-expression of CK7 and CK20, and CDX-2 negativity should resolve the diagnostic dilemma in doubtful cases [24]. Attention must be paid, however, to the occasional CK7 positivity of some colorectal adenocarcinomas, a finding that is a sign of dismal prognosis [26].

2.4. Small Tubules and Nephrogenic Adenoma-Like Architecture

Very occasionally, UC is composed of low-grade cells arranged in small tubules resembling *cystitis glandularis* or nephrogenic adenoma (Figure 1f) [27]. The bland cytologic features of this histologic subtype contrast with its frank infiltrative nature, even reaching the muscularis propria in some cases. Since nephrogenic adenoma may display also a concerning pseudo-infiltrative growth [28], an immunohistochemical study with PAX-8, CK7, p63, and napsin A [29] may be useful to make the differential diagnosis in problematic cases. The clinical significance of this histologic change is not established so far.

2.5. Microcystic Architecture

The microcystic histology has been rarely reported in the literature at UC. Aside from a handful of single case reports, the largest series published to date analyzes 20 cases [30]. The limited examples reported up to now show a bland histologic appearance, with round to oval cysts which often contain eosinophilic intraluminal secretion covered by low columnar or flattened urothelial cells (Figure 1g). Despite its deceptive bland histology, microcystic UC displays the same aggressiveness of conventional UC at the same stage. The main differential diagnosis is nephrogenic adenoma and adenocarcinoma of the bladder. In this sense, a basic immunohistochemical panel including p63 positivity and CK7/20 co-expression coupled with napsin A and PAX-8 negativities will resolve the eventual diagnostic troubles.

2.6. Verrucous Architecture

Genuine verrucous carcinoma is a rare tumor subtype in the urinary tract [31], however, conventional well-differentiated squamous cell carcinoma with "verrucous" architectural features is a much more common event. Since the difference between them has prognostic implications their correct identification by the pathologist matters. Verrucous carcinoma may recur but never metastasize. Some cases are related to HPV infection, others to schistosomiasis, but there are also cases unrelated to any known specific etiology [32].

The diagnosis of a verrucous carcinoma in the urinary tract, as elsewhere, is subjected to very strict histological criteria. Only low-grade keratinizing squamous cell carcinomas with superficial verrucous architecture should be considered (Figure 1h). Verrucous carcinomas may display a pushing border of growth into the lamina propria, but a true invasion is lacking. Noteworthy, any high-grade area across the tumor or frank stromal infiltration makes the diagnosis of verrucous carcinoma unsuitable.

2.7. Diffuse Architecture with Lymphoepithelioma-Like Changes

Lymphoepithelioma is the classical histological term referring to an undifferentiated carcinoma first described in the nasopharyngeal region of Asian patients [33]. Some of them are related to Epstein-Barr virus infection. Since then, analog histology has been described in many carcinomas widely distributed in the body. Aside from multiple case reports, several series of this tumor subtype in the bladder [33–36] and the upper urinary tract [37] have been published in the literature. Remarkably, the theoretical relationship of lymphoepithelioma-like UC with Epstein–Barr virus infection is no longer sustainable in cases arising in the urinary tract after the results obtained with FISH analyses in the largest series [35–37].

The tumor shows a diffuse growth of ill-defined islands of poorly-differentiated cells with badly defined cytoplasmic borders, large nuclei, and patent nucleoli. The stroma is heavily infiltrated by lymphocytes occasionally showing lymphoepithelial lesion (Figure 1i). By immunohistochemistry, GATA3, cytokeratins 34βE12, AE1-AE3, and CK7, p53 and p63 are positive in a variable number of cases, whereas TTF-1, CD30, and CK20 are negative [36,37]. The prognosis does not differ from conventional UC at the same stage.

3. Cytological Changes

3.1. Plasmacytoid Cells

Plasmacytoid UC is an aggressive tumor. This cytologic variant of UC can present as pure tumors or mixed with conventional UC and/or with other non-conventional UC. For example, mixed micropapillary and plasmacytoid UC cases have been occasionally reported [38]. Histological similarities with multiple myeloma were noticed since the first report by Sahin et al. in 1991 [39]. Since this original description, several large series have been published so far all of them confirming its dismal prognosis [40].

In its typical presentation, the tumor appears as flat, non-papillary, highly cellular masses growing diffusely in the urinary tract wall with infiltrative edges and frequent vascular invasion images. Neoplastic cells are non-cohesively arranged and show lateralized cytoplasm, nuclear atypia, and high mitotic count (Figure 2a). In doubtful cases, or patients with a previous history of plasma cell dyscrasia, immunohistochemistry is of help revealing its epithelial, non-plasmacytic, nature. Briefly, GATA-3 and CK7 are positive and CD 38 is negative. Positive immunostaining with CD 138 may be observed in this neoplasm, but this finding does not preclude the diagnosis of plasmacytoid UC [41].

HER2 overexpression has been observed by FISH in plasmacytoid UC [42]. Contrary to what happens in most UC, plasmacytoid variants do not seem to harbor TP53 gene mutations in a sequencing analysis [41]. On the other hand, TERT gene promoter mutations have been detected [43]. A study using whole-exome sequencing has detected somatic alterations in the CDH1 gene of 84% of plasmacytoid UC, a finding of clinical aggressiveness that seems to be specific to this tumor variant [44].

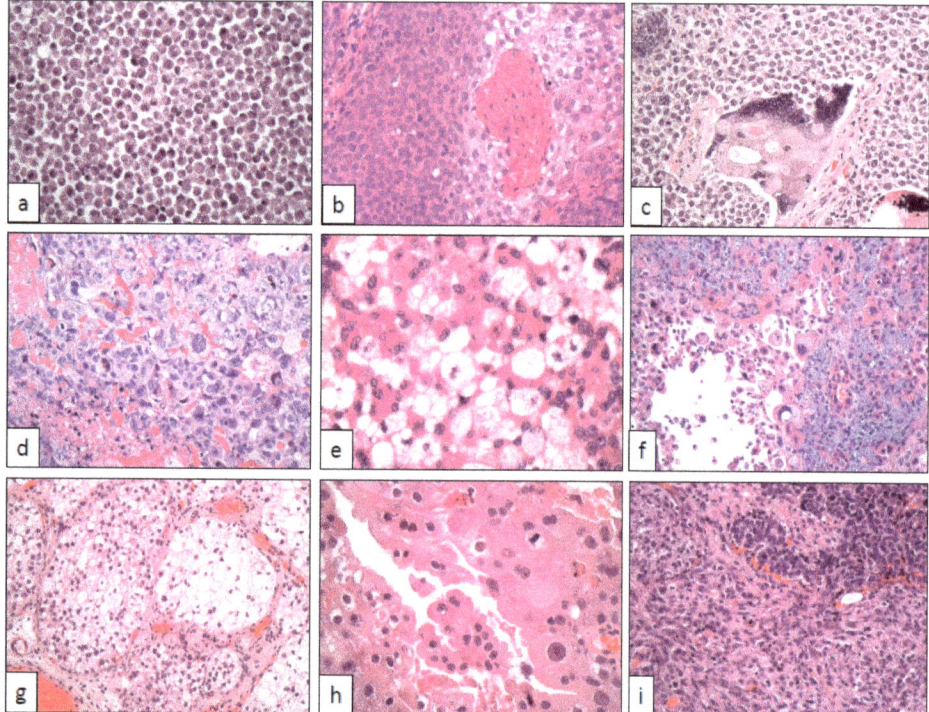

Figure 2. Cytological changes in bladder cancer. (**a**) Plasmacytoid cells (×250), (**b**) basaloid and squamous cells (×250), (**c**) syncytiotrophoblastic cells (×250), (**d**) trophoblastic cells (×250), (**e**) lipoblastic-like cells (×400), (**f**) pleomorphic giant cells (×250), (**g**) clear cells (×100), (**h**) eosinophilic (oncocytoid) cells (×400), and (**i**) sarcomatoid cells (×250).

3.2. Signet-Ring Cells

Since signet-ring cell features are very rare in UC, and their identification in transurethral resection specimens can raise the possibility of a metastatic seed from a neoplasm originating in the digestive tract. A careful search of the classical urothelial features (nests of transitional cells, papillae, in situ carcinoma in the surface epithelium, etc.) in the biopsy, if present, may be of help in the differential diagnosis. Otherwise, the clinical context of the patient and a basic immunohistochemical panel, for example, CK7/20, GATA-3, CDX-2, and p63, should resolve the dilemma. The analysis of the national Surveillance, Epidemiology, and End Results (SEER) database of 318 such cases confirms the worse prognosis of this histologic variant compared with conventional UC [45].

3.3. Basaloid-Squamous Cells

Basaloid-squamous cell carcinomas are aggressive neoplasms mainly located in the head and neck [46] and anal [47] regions. The tumor is extraordinarily uncommon in the urinary tract, with only a handful of single cases published to date [48–51]. Everywhere, most basaloid squamous cell carcinomas are associated with HPV infection [51].

Histologically, the tumor is deeply infiltrative and shows a typical biphasic pattern (Figure 2b). Basaloid atypical cells with high mitotic rate and scarce cytoplasm are arranged in lobes and nests showing peripheral palisading and stromal reaction. Basaloid nests are centered by squamous islands with evident keratinization. p16 is intensely positive in tumor cells.

3.4. Yolk Sac Cells

A very limited number of UC with yolk sac tumor differentiation has been reported in the literature [52–55]. The yolk sac differentiation represents an example of a somatic differentiation present in non-gonadal neoplasms [56]. A varied spectrum of patterns have been identified in these tumors: microcystic, vitelline, glandular enteric-like, hepatoid, solid, sarcomatoid, etc. An enteroblastic differentiation seems to be the most frequent histology in somatically derived yolk sac tumors [56].

Immunohistochemistry is useful to identify yolk sac differentiation in UC and other somatic tumors considering the wide spectrum of patterns that can be detected in this tumor. Alpha-fetoprotein and SALL4 are consistently positive. CK7, however, is negative. Markers of intestinal differentiation, like CDX2, are usually positive in enteroblastic areas and Her Par-1 in hepatoid ones. A polysomic abnormality in 12p has been detected in one recently published case [55].

3.5. Trophoblastic Cells

Trophoblastic differentiation is a rare event in UC that has been recently reviewed by Przybycin et al. in a series of 16 cases [57]. The spectrum includes isolated syncytiotrophoblast cells interspersed in a conventional UC, mixed choriocarcinoma and UC, and pure choriocarcinoma. Same as in the yolk sac differentiation, trophoblastic changes are examples of somatically derived differentiations in non-gonadal tumors.

Syncytiotrophoblasts are detected as isolated multinucleated giant cells immersed in high-grade UC (Figure 2c). Choriocarcinoma differentiation appears as hemorrhagic areas at low-power magnification. A closer view of these areas reveals the typical mixture of trophoblastic and syncytiotrophoblastic cells immersed in a necro-hemorrhagic background (Figure 2d).

By immunohistochemistry, β-hCG is expressed in trophoblastic and syncytiotrophoblastic cells, as well as in the malignant urothelial cells in a significant number of cases. Interestingly, increased levels of seric β-hCG in patients with UC is an independent prognostic factor [58]. GATA3 positivity has been detected in more than 70% of trophoblastic tumors in a large series [59] and appears as a useful marker to be included in the diagnostic panel. SALL4 is focally positive in less than 50% of the cases [57] and is negative in the larger syncytiotrophoblastic cells [60]. HSD3B1, a novel marker specific to trophoblastic differentiation [61], has been detected in 100% of the cases [57].

3.6. Rhabdoid Cells

Rhabdoid tumors have been documented in many different topographies across the body [62], always linked to biological aggressiveness and bad prognosis. Its histogenesis is still unclear. A handful of rhabdoid tumors of the bladder have been published, particularly in children and young adults [63–65]. There are, however, isolated cases reported in adulthood [66–68].

Aside from genuine rhabdoid tumors, a focal *rhabdoid* phenotype can be observed sometimes in UC [68], where large and ovoid cells with large atypical nuclei and lateralized eosinophilic cytoplasm may appear growing without any specific pattern usually in high-grade neoplasms. A possible rhabdomyoblastic dedifferentiation in the context of a sarcomatoid UC should be ruled out, at least theoretically, in these cases.

By immunohistochemistry, rhabdoid cells are positive for CK7, CK20, vimentin, E-cadherin, and β-catenin, p63, and INI-1 [68].

3.7. Lipid/Lipoblast-Like Cells

These two terms refer to a rare variant of UC composed of lipidic appearing tumor cells intermingled with transitional cells in variable proportions. It was first recognized by Mostofi et al. in 1999 [69]. Since then only single case reports and two short series [70,71] have been published. The longest series so far analyzes 27 cases collected from different international institutions [71]. Lipidic-appearing cells may resemble either adipocytes or adipoblasts (Figure 2e) and usually take part in a high-grade UC, not otherwise specified. Immunohistochemistry confirms the epithelial nature in all cases, including the co-expression of CK7 and CK20 [70,71].

3.8. Giant Cells

Giant cells are rarely observed in UC and only single case reports and a few short series have been published so far [72–74]. Two morphological variants have been described: osteoclast-like and giant pleomorphic cells, both of them associated with high-grade neoplasms. For practical purposes, these cells must be distinguished from trophoblastic and syncytiotrophoblastic cells appearing in some UC (see above). The presence of these giant cells in UC may be focal in the context of a high-grade UC or diffuse across the tumor, making difficult the correct diagnosis. A dedifferentiated sarcomatoid UC (see below) diagnosis can be considered in some of these cases.

Pleomorphic giant cell carcinoma have been described in many sites of the body and is a tumor subtype with dismal prognosis everywhere. Giant cell tumor areas in UC show a diffuse growth of cells with extreme pleomorphism and high mitotic count (Figure 2f). Cytoplasmic vacuolization and emperipolesis can be detected. Unusually, these tumors are at advanced stages at diagnosis, with deep infiltration in the bladder wall and frequent lymphatic dissemination [72]. Fifty percent of the patients reported in the series of Samaratunga et al. died of disease within the first year of follow-up [73]. By immunohistochemistry, the co-expression of CK7/20 and GATA3 positivity are retained in these tumors.

Osteoclast-like giant cells can be rarely observed in tumors originating in many sites of the body. In the bladder, they appear very occasionally in the context of high-grade UC. Contrary to the observed in pleomorphic giant cells, osteoclastic-like giant cells devoid of atypia and mitosis and show a reactive, non-neoplastic appearance. Whether these cells are truly neoplastic or reactive in the context of the tumor is a classical controversy that has been recently elucidated [74]. In this study, osteoclast-like giant cells are negative for GATA3, thrombomodulin, uroplakin II, and cytokeratin AE1/AE3, thus confirming their non-epithelial differentiation [74].

3.9. Clear Cells

Only single cases and a short series of 10 cases [75] of clear cell UC have been published so far. An advanced stage at diagnosis and an aggressive clinical course is the rule in these patients. Clear cell change, however, is regularly mentioned in several papers reviewing the varied morphology of UC in the bladder and upper urinary tract [76–80].

Clear cell change in UC reflects intracytoplasmic glycogen accumulation that in some cases is extreme this way resembling the typical clear cells observed in clear cell renal cell carcinoma. Usually, clear cell nests are intermingled in the tumor with conventional transitional cells (Figure 2g), which makes its correct identification easier. However, if the clear cell change is generalized or if transurethral resection specimens do not contain pieces of evidence of the urothelial origin of the tumor, the possibility of metastasis in the bladder of a clear cell renal cell carcinoma should be always taken into account [81].

3.10. Eosinophilic (Oncocytoid) Cells

An eosinophilic change can be observed in some UC resembling the cells of renal oncocytomas [82]. These cases show large granular and deeply eosinophilic elements with focal apocrinoid features (Figure 2h). Frequent nuclear pleomorphism is also seen, but true atypia is lacking. Mitoses are scarce, or absent, giving an overall impression of a low-grade tumor. Immunohistochemistry is that of the conventional UC, and neuroendocrine markers are negative. Anyway, further descriptions are needed to delineate better this histologic feature. At least for practical purposes, this histologic feature should be distinguished from oncocytic carcinoid tumors of the urinary bladder [83], an extraordinarily rare entity in the urinary bladder.

3.11. Sarcomatoid Cells

Sarcomatoid dedifferentiation is a relatively common finding in high-grade UC. Recent studies have approached the correlation between morphology and genomics in sarcomatoid bladder cancer through analyzing the epithelial to mesenchymal transition process concluding that UC developing sarcomatoid transformation are carcinomas of basal-type [84]. Practically all possible differentiations have been reported in the literature, from undifferentiated spindle cell (Figure 2i) to osteosarcoma. The epithelial component may be scarce or even not identified in some cases, so the diagnosis of primary sarcoma in the urinary bladder should be made with caution in transurethral resection specimens.

An excellent review of this topic based on a MEDLINE database study has been recently published [85].

4. Conclusions

This narrative collects the varied spectrum of morphological features that can be found in UC. These changes have been organized in architectural and cytological for didactic purposes, but mixtures of them are eventually found in real practice. The goal of this overview is to offer in a few pages the essentials for recognizing them giving diagnostic clues based on morphological and immunohistochemical keys.

Author Contributions: C.M. and J.I.L. have designed, reviewed, written, and approved the final version of the manuscript. Both authors have read and agreed to the published version of the manuscript.

Funding: José I. López is funded by MINECO, Spain grant ref. SAF2016-79847-R.

Conflicts of Interest: The authors declare no conflict of interest.

References

1. Siegel, R.L.; Miller, K.D.; Jemal, A. Cancer statistics, 2020. *CA Cancer J. Clin.* **2020**, *70*, 7–30. [CrossRef] [PubMed]
2. Teoh, J.Y.; Huang, J.; Ko, W.Y.; Lok, V.; Choi, P.; Ng, C.F.; Sengupta, S.; Mostafid, H.; Kamat, A.M.; Black, P.C.; et al. Global trends of bladder cancer incidence and mortality, and their associations with tobacco use and gross domestic products per capita. *Eur. Urol.* **2020**. [CrossRef]
3. Lobo, N.; Shariat, S.F.; Guo, C.C.; Fernandez, M.I.; Kassouf, W.; Choudhury, A.; Gao, J.; Williams, S.B.; Galsky, M.D.; Taylor III, J.A.; et al. What is the significance of variant histology in urothelial carcinoma? *Eur. Urol. Focus.* **2020**, *6*, 653–663. [CrossRef]
4. Al-Ahmadie, H.; Netto, G.J. Updates on the genomics of bladder cancer and novel molecular taxonomy. *Adv. Anat. Pathol.* **2020**, *27*, 36–43. [CrossRef]
5. Talbert, M.L.; Young, R.H. Carcinomas of the urinary bladder with deceptively benign-appearing foci. A report of three cases. *Am. J. Surg. Pathol.* **1989**, *13*, 374–381. [CrossRef] [PubMed]
6. Stern, J.B. Unusual benign bladder tumor of von Brunn nest origin. *Urology* **1979**, *14*, 288–289. [CrossRef]
7. Lin, O.; Cardillo, M.; Dalbagni, G.; Linkov, I.; Hutchinson, B.; Reuter, V.E. Nested variant of urothelial carcinoma: A clinicopathologic and immunohistochemical study of 12 cases. *Mod. Pathol.* **2003**, *16*, 1289–1298. [CrossRef] [PubMed]
8. Levy, D.R.; Cheng, L. The expanding molecular and mutational landscape of nested variant of urothelial carcinoma. *Histopathology* **2020**, *76*, 638–639. [CrossRef] [PubMed]
9. Cox, R.; Epstein, J.I. Large nested variant of urothelial carcinoma: 23 cases mimicking von Brunn nests and inverted growth pattern of noninvasive papillary urothelial carcinoma. *Am. J. Surg. Pathol.* **2011**, *35*, 1337–1342. [CrossRef] [PubMed]
10. Compérat, E.; McKenney, J.K.; Hartmann, A.; Hes, O.; Bertz, S.; Varinot, J.; Brimo, F. Large nested variant of urothelial carcinoma: A clinicopathological study of 36 cases. *Histopathology* **2017**, *71*, 703–710. [CrossRef]
11. Hacihasanoglu, E.; Behzatoglu, K. Large nested urothelial carcinoma: A clinicopathological study of 22 cases on transurethral resection materials. *Ann. Diagn. Pathol.* **2019**, *42*, 7–11. [CrossRef] [PubMed]

12. Weyerer, V.; Eckstein, M.; Compérat, E.; Juette, H.; Gaisa, N.T.; Allory, Y.; Stöhr, R.; Wullich, B.; Rouprêt, M.; Hartmann, A.; et al. Pure large nested variant of urothelial carcinoma (LNUC) is the prototype of an *FGFR3* mutated aggressive urothelial carcinoma with luminal-papillary phenotype. *Cancers* **2020**, *12*, 763. [CrossRef] [PubMed]
13. Shah, T.S.; Kaag, M.; Raman, J.D.; Chan, W.; Tran, T.; Kunchala, S.; Shuman, L.; DeGraff, D.J.; Chen, G.; Warrick, J.I. Clinical significance of prominent retraction clefts in invasive urothelial carcinoma. *Hum. Pathol.* **2017**, *61*, 90–96. [CrossRef] [PubMed]
14. Nassar, H. Carcinomas with micropapillary morphology. Clinical significance and current concepts. *Adv. Anat. Pathol.* **2004**, *11*, 297–303. [CrossRef] [PubMed]
15. Jin, D.; Jin, K.; Qiu, S.; Zhou, X.; Yuan, Q.; Yang, L.; Wei, Q. Prognostic values of the clinicopathological characteristics and survival outcomes in micropapillary urothelial carcinoma of the bladder: A SEER database analysis. *Cancer Med.* **2020**, *9*, 4897–4906. [CrossRef] [PubMed]
16. Ramalingam, P.; Middleton, L.P.; Tamboli, P.; Troncoso, P.; Silva, E.G.; Ayala, A.G. Invasive micropapillary carcinoma of the breast metastatic to the urinary bladder and endometrium: Diagnostic pitfalls and review of the literature of tumors with micropapillary features. *Ann. Diagn. Pathol.* **2003**, *7*, 112–119. [CrossRef]
17. Amin, M.B.; Ro, J.Y.; El-Sharkawy, T.; Lee, K.M.; Troncoso, P.; Silva, E.G.; Ordóñez, N.G.; Ayala, A.G. Micropapillary variant of transitional cell carcinoma of the urinary bladder. Histologic pattern resembling ovarian papillary serous carcinoma. *Am. J. Surg. Pathol.* **1994**, *18*, 1224–1232. [CrossRef]
18. Holmäng, S.; Thomsen, J.; Johansson, S.L. Micropapillary carcinoma of the renal pelvis and ureter. *J. Urol.* **2006**, *175*, 463–466. [CrossRef]
19. Perez-Montiel, D.; Hes, O.; Michal, M.; Suster, S. Micropapillary urothelial carcinoma of the upper urinary tract: Clinicopathologic study of five cases. *Am. J. Clin. Pathol.* **2006**, *126*, 86–92. [CrossRef]
20. Guo, C.C.; Dadhania, V.; Zhang, L.; Majewski, T.; Bondaruk, J.; Sykulski, M.; Wronowska, W.; Gambin, A.; Wang, Y.; Zhang, S.; et al. Gene Expression Profile of the Clinically Aggressive Micropapillary Variant of Bladder Cancer. *Eur. Urol.* **2016**, *70*, 211–220. [CrossRef]
21. Zinnall, U.; Weyerer, V.; Compérat, E.; Camparo, P.; Gaisa, N.T.; Knuechel-Clarke, R.; Perren, A.; Lugli, A.; Toma, M.; Baretton, G.; et al. Micropapillary urothelial carcinoma: Evaluation of HER2 status and immunohistochemical characterization of the molecular subtype. *Hum. Pathol.* **2018**, *80*, 55–64. [CrossRef] [PubMed]
22. Yang, Y.; Kaimakliotis, H.Z.; Williamson, S.R.; Koch, M.O.; Huang, K.; Barboza, M.P.; Zhang, S.; Wang, M.; Idrees, M.T.; Grignon, D.J.; et al. Micropapillary urothelial carcinoma of urinary bladder displays immunophenotypic features of luminal and p53-like subtypes and is not a variant of adenocarcinoma. *Urol. Oncol.* **2020**, *38*, 449–458. [CrossRef] [PubMed]
23. Johansson, S.L.; Borghede, G.; Holmäng, S. Micropapillary bladder carcinoma: A clinicopathological study of 20 cases. *J. Urol.* **1999**, *161*, 1798–1802. [CrossRef]
24. Tavora, F.; Epstein, J.I. Urothelial carcinoma with abundant myxoid stroma. *Hum. Pathol.* **2009**, *40*, 1391–1398. [CrossRef] [PubMed]
25. Gilg, M.M.; Wimmer, B.; Ott, A.; Langner, C. Urothelial carcinoma with abundant myxoid stroma. Evidence for mucinous production by cancer cells. *Virchows Arch.* **2012**, *461*, 99–101. [CrossRef] [PubMed]
26. Fei, F.; Li, C.; Cao, Y.; Liu, K.; Du, J.; Gu, Y.; Wang, X.; Li, Y.; Zhang, S. CK7 expression associates with the location, differentiation, lymph node metastasis, and the Dukes' stage of primary colorectal cancers. *J. Cancer* **2019**, *10*, 2510–2519. [CrossRef]
27. Young, R.H.; Oliva, E. Transitional cell carcinomas of the urinary bladder that may be underdiagnosed. A report of four invasive cases exemplifying the homology between neoplastic and non-neoplastic transitional cell lesions. *Am. J. Surg. Pathol.* **1996**, *20*, 1448–1454. [CrossRef] [PubMed]
28. Santi, R.; Angulo, J.C.; Nesi, G.; de Petris, G.; Kuroda, N.; Hes, O.; López, J.I. Common and uncommon features of nephrogenic adenoma revisited. *Pathol. Res. Pract.* **2019**, *215*, 152561. [CrossRef]
29. Sharifai, N.; Abro, B.; Chen, J.F.; Zhao, M.; He, H.; Cao, D. Napsin A is a highly sensitive marker for nephrogenic adenoma: An immunohistochemical study with a specificity test in genitourinary tumors. *Hum. Pathol.* **2020**, *102*, 23–32. [CrossRef] [PubMed]
30. Lopez-Beltrán, A.; Montironi, R.; Cheng, L. Microcystic urothelial carcinoma: Morphology, immunohistochemistry and clinical behaviour. *Histopathology* **2014**, *64*, 872–879. [CrossRef]

31. Park, S.; Reuter, V.E.; Hansel, D.E. Non-urothelial carcinomas of the bladder. *Histopathology* **2019**, *74*, 97–111. [CrossRef] [PubMed]
32. Flores, M.R.; Ruiz, M.R.; Florian, R.E.; De Leon, W.; Jose, L.S. Pan-urothelial verrucous carcinoma unrelated to schistosomiasis. *BMJ Case Rep.* **2009**, *2009*, bcr08.2008.0787. [CrossRef] [PubMed]
33. Holmäng, S.; Borghede, G.; Johansson, S.L. Bladder carcinoma with lymphoepithelioma-like differentiation: A report of 9 cases. *J. Urol.* **1998**, *159*, 779–782. [CrossRef]
34. López-Beltrán, A.; Luque, R.J.; Vicioso, L.; Anglada, F.; Requena, M.J.; Quintero, A.; Montironi, R. Lymphoepithelioma-like carcinoma of the urinary bladder: A clinicopathologic study of 13 cases. *Virchows Arch.* **2001**, *438*, 552–557. [CrossRef] [PubMed]
35. Tamas, E.F.; Nielsen, M.E.; Schoenberg, M.P.; Epstein, J.I. Lymphoepithelioma-like carcinoma of the urinary tract: A clinicopathological study of 30 pure and mixed cases. *Mod. Pathol.* **2007**, *20*, 828–834. [CrossRef] [PubMed]
36. Williamson, S.R.; Zhang, S.; Lopez-Beltran, A.; Shah, R.B.; Montironi, R.; Tan, P.H.; Wang, M.; Baldridge, L.A.; MacLennan, G.T.; Cheng, L. Lymphoepithelioma-like carcinoma of the urinary bladder: Clinicopathologic, immunohistochemical and molecular features. *Am. J. Surg. Pathol.* **2011**, *35*, 474–483. [CrossRef] [PubMed]
37. López-Beltrán, A.; Paner, G.; Blanca, A.; Montironi, R.; Tsuzuki, T.; Nagashima, Y.; Chuang, S.S.; Win, K.T.; Madruga, L.; Raspollini, M.R.; et al. Lymphoepithelioma-like carcinoma of the upper urinary tract. *Virchows Arch.* **2017**, *470*, 703–709. [CrossRef]
38. Park, S.; Cho, M.S.; Kim, K.H. A case report of urothelial carcinoma with combined micropapillary and plasmacytoid morphology in the urinary bladder. *Diagn. Cytopathol.* **2016**, *44*, 124–127. [CrossRef]
39. Sahin, A.A.; Myhre, M.; Ro, J.Y.; Sneige, N.; Dekmezian, R.H.; Ayala, A.G. Plasmacytoid transitional cell carcinoma. Report of a case with initial presentation mimicking multiple myeloma. *Acta Cytol.* **1991**, *35*, 277–280.
40. Kim, D.K.; Kim, J.W.; Ro, J.Y.; Lee, H.S.; Park, J.Y.; Ahn, H.K.; Lee, J.Y.; Cho, K.S. Plasmacytoid variant of urothelial carcinoma of the bladder: A systematic review and meta-analysis of clinicopathological features and survival outcomes. *J. Urol.* **2020**, *204*, 215–223. [CrossRef]
41. Raspollini, M.R.; Sardi, I.; Giunti, L.; Di Lollo, S.; Baroni, G.; Stomaci, N.; Menghetti, I.; Franchi, A. Plasmacytoid urothelial carcinoma of the urinary bladder: Clinicopathologic, immunohistochemical, ultrastructural, and molecular analysis of a case series. *Hum. Pathol.* **2011**, *42*, 1149–1158. [CrossRef] [PubMed]
42. Kim, B.; Kim, G.; Song, B.; Lee, C.; Park, J.H.; Moon, K.C. HER2 protein overexpression and gene amplification in plasmacytoid urothelial carcinoma of the urinary bladder. *Dis. Markers.* **2016**, *2016*, 8463731. [CrossRef] [PubMed]
43. Palsgrove, D.N.; Taheri, D.; Springer, S.U.; Cowan, M.; Guner, G.; Mendoza Rodriguez, M.A.; Rodriguez Pena, M.D.C.; Wang, Y.; Kinde, I.; Cunha, I.; et al. Targeted sequencing of plasmacytoid urothelial carcinoma reveals frequent TERT promoter mutations. *Hum. Pathol.* **2019**, *85*, 1–9. [CrossRef] [PubMed]
44. Al-Ahmadie, H.A.; Iyer, G.; Lee, B.H.; Scott, S.N.; Mehra, R.; Bagrodia, A.; Jordan, E.J.; Gao, S.P.; Ramirez, R.; Cha, E.K.; et al. Frequent somatic *CDH1* loss-of-function mutations in plasmacytoid-variant bladder cancer. *Nat. Genet.* **2016**, *48*, 356–358. [CrossRef] [PubMed]
45. Jin, D.; Qiu, S.; Jin, K.; Zhou, X.; Cao, Q.; Yang, L.; Wei, Q. Signet-Ring Cell Carcinoma as an Independent Prognostic Factor for Patients with Urinary Bladder Cancer: A Population-Based Study. *Front. Oncol.* **2020**, *10*, 653. [CrossRef] [PubMed]
46. Ereño, C.; Gaafar, A.; Garmendia, M.; Etxezarraga, C.; Bilbao, F.J.; Lopez, J.I. Basaloid squamous cell carcinoma of the head and neck. A clinicopathological and follow-up study of 40 cases and review of the literature. *Head Neck Pathol.* **2008**, *2*, 83–91. [CrossRef]
47. Graham, R.P.; Arnold, C.A.; Naini, B.V.; Lam-Himlin, D.M. Basaloid squamous cell carcinoma of the anus revisited. *Am. J. Surg. Pathol.* **2016**, *40*, 354–360. [CrossRef]
48. Vakar-Lopez, F.; Abrams, J. Basaloid squamous cell carcinoma occurring in the urinary bladder. *Arch. Pathol. Lab. Med.* **2000**, *124*, 455–459.
49. Hagemann, I.S.; Lu, J.; Lewis, J.S., Jr. Basaloid squamous cell carcinoma arising in [corrected] the renal pelvis. *Int. J. Surg. Pathol.* **2008**, *16*, 199–201. [CrossRef]
50. Neves, T.R.; Soares, M.J.; Monteiro, P.G.; Lima, M.S.; Monteiro, H.G. Basaloid squamous cell carcinoma in the urinary bladder with small cell carcinoma. *J. Clin. Oncol.* **2011**, *29*, e440–e442. [CrossRef]

51. Ginori, A.; Barone, A.; Santopietro, R.; Barbanti, G.; Cecconi, F.; Tripodi, S.A. Human papillomavirus-related basaloid squamous cell carcinoma of the bladder associated with genital tract human papillomavirus infection. *Int. J. Urol.* **2015**, *22*, 222–225. [CrossRef] [PubMed]
52. Samaratunga, H.; Samaratunga, D.; Dunglison, N.; Perry-Keene, J.; Nicklin, J.; Delahunt, B. Alpha-fetoprotein-producing carcinoma of the renal pelvis exhibiting hepatoid and urothelial differentiation. *Anticancer Res.* **2012**, *32*, 4987–4991. [PubMed]
53. Ravishankar, S.; Malpica, A.; Ramalingam, P.; Euscher, E.D. Yolk sac tumor in extragonadal pelvic sites: Still a diagnostic challenge. *Am. J. Surg. Pathol.* **2017**, *41*, 1–11. [CrossRef] [PubMed]
54. Melms, J.C.; Thummalapalli, R.; Shaw, K.; Ye, H.; Tsai, L.; Bhatt, R.S.; Izar, B. Alpha-fetoprotein (AFP) as a tumor marker in a patient with urothelial cancer with exceptional response to anti-PD-L1 therapy and an escape lesion mimic. *J. Immunother. Cancer* **2018**, *6*, 89. [CrossRef] [PubMed]
55. Espejo-Herrera, N.; Condom-Mundó, E. Yolk sac tumor differentiation in urothelial carcinoma of the urinary bladder: A case report and differential diagnosis. *Diagn. Pathol.* **2020**, *15*, 68. [CrossRef] [PubMed]
56. McNamee, T.; Damato, S.; McCluggage, W.G. Yolk sac tumours of the female genital tract in older adults derive commonly from somatic epithelial neoplasms: Somatically derived yolk sac tumours. *Histopathology* **2016**, *69*, 739–751. [CrossRef] [PubMed]
57. Przybycin, C.G.; McKenney, J.K.; Nguyen, J.K.; Shah, R.B.; Umar, S.A.; Harik, L.; Shih, I.M.; Cox, R.M. Urothelial carcinomas with trophoblastic differentiation, including choriocarcinoma. Clinicopathologic series of 16 cases. *Am. J. Surg. Pathol.* **2020**, *44*, 1322–1330.
58. Douglas, J.; Sharp, A.; Chau, C.; Head, J.; Drake, T.; Wheater, M.; Geldart, T.; Mead, G.; Crabb, S.J. Serum total hCGβ level is an independent prognostic factor in transitional cell carcinoma of the urothelial tract. *Br. J. Cancer* **2014**, *110*, 1759–1766. [CrossRef]
59. Banet, N.; Gown, A.M.; Shih, I.M.; Li, Q.K.; Roden, R.B.S.; Nucci, M.R.; Cheng, L.; Przybycin, C.G.; Nasseri-Nik, N.; Wu, L.S.F.; et al. GATA-3 expression in trophoblastic tissues. An immunohistochemical study of 445 cases, including diagnostic utility. *Am. J. Surg. Pathol.* **2015**, *39*, 101–108. [CrossRef]
60. Miettinen, M.; Wang, Z.; McCue, P.A.; Sarlomo-Rikala, M.; Rys, J.; Biernat, W.; Lasota, J.; See, Y.S. SALL4 expression in germ cell and non-germ cell tumors. A systematic immunohistochemical study of 3215 cases. *Am. J. Surg. Pathol.* **2014**, *38*, 410–420. [CrossRef]
61. Mao, T.L.; Kurman, R.J.; Jeng, Y.M.; Husng, W.; Shih, I.M. HSD3B1 as a novel trophoblast-associated marker that assists in the differential diagnosis of trophoblastic tumors and tumorlike lesions. *Am. J. Surg. Pathol.* **2008**, *32*, 236–242. [CrossRef] [PubMed]
62. Wick, M.R.; Ritter, J.H.; Dehner, L.P. Malignant rhabdoid tumors: A clinicopathologic review and conceptual discussion. *Sem. Diagn. Pathol.* **1995**, *12*, 233–248.
63. Warren, K.S.; Oxley, J.; Koupparis, A. Pure malignant rhabdoid tumor of the bladder. *Can. Urol. Assoc. J.* **2014**, *8*, e260–e262. [CrossRef] [PubMed]
64. Sterling, M.E.; Long, C.J.; Bosse, K.R.; Bagatell, R.; Shukla, A.R. A rapid progression of disease after surgical excision of a malignant rhabdoid tumor of the bladder. *Urology* **2015**, *85*, 664–666. [CrossRef] [PubMed]
65. Assadi, A.; Alzubaidi, A.; Lesmana, H.; Brennan, R.C.; Ortiz-Hernandez, V.; Gleason, J.M. Pure bladder malignant rhabdoid tumor successfully treated with partial cystectomy, radiation, and chemotherapy: A case report and review of the literature. *J. Pediatr. Hematol. Oncol.* **2020**. [CrossRef] [PubMed]
66. Parwani, A.V.; Herawi, M.; Volmar, K.; Tsai, S.H.; Epstein, J.I. Urothelial carcinoma with rhabdoid features: Report of 6 cases. *Hum. Pathol.* **2006**, *37*, 168–172. [CrossRef]
67. Fukumura, Y.; Fujii, H.; Mitani, K.; Sakamoto, Y.; Matsumoto, T.; Suda, K.; Yao, T. Urothelial carcinoma of the renal pelvis with rhabdoid features. *Pathol. Int.* **2009**, *59*, 322–325. [CrossRef]
68. Tajima, S. Rhabdoid variant of urotelial carcinoma of the urinary bladder: A case report with emphasis on immunohistochemical analysis regarding the formation of rhabdoid morphology. *Int. J. Clin. Exp. Pathol.* **2015**, *8*, 9638–9642.
69. Mostofi, F.K.; Davis, C.J.; Sesterhenn, I.A. *World Health Organization International Histological Classification of Tumours: Histological Typing of Urinary Bladder Tumours*, 2nd ed.; Springer: Berlin/Heidelberg, Germany, 1999.
70. Leroy, X.; Gonzalez, S.; Zini, L.; Aubert, S. Lipoid-cell variant of urothelial carcinoma: A clinicopathologic and immunohistochemical study of five cases. *Am. J. Surg. Pathol.* **2007**, *31*, 770–773. [CrossRef]

71. López-Beltrán, A.; Amin, M.B.; Oliveira, P.S.; Montironi, R.; Algaba, F.; McKenney, J.K.; de Torres, I.; Mazerolles, C.; Wang, M.; Cheng, L. Urothelial carcinoma of the bladder. Lipid cell variant: Clinicopathologic findings and LOH analysis. *Am. J. Surg. Pathol.* **2010**, *34*, 371–376. [CrossRef]
72. López-Beltrán, A.; Blanca, A.; Montironi, R.; Cheng, L.; Regueiro, J.C. Pleomorphic giant cell carcinoma of the urinary bladder. *Hum. Pathol.* **2009**, *40*, 1461–1466. [CrossRef] [PubMed]
73. Samatunga, H.; Delahunt, B.; Egevad, L.; Adamson, M.; Hussey, D.; Malone, G.; Hoyle, K.; Nathan, T.; Kerle, D.; Ferguson, P.; et al. Pleomorphic giant cells carcinoma of the urinary bladder: An extreme form of tumour de-differentiation. *Histopathology* **2016**, *68*, 533–540. [CrossRef] [PubMed]
74. Priore, S.F.; Schwartz, L.E.; Epstein, J.I. An expanded immunohistochemical profile of osteoclast-rich undifferentiated carcinoma of the urinary tract. *Mod. Pathol.* **2018**, *31*, 984–988. [CrossRef] [PubMed]
75. Mai, K.T.; Baterman, J.; Djordjevic, B.; Flood, T.A.; Belanger, E.C. Clear cell urothelial carcinoma: A study of 10 cases and meta-analysis of the entity. Evidence of mesonephric differentiation. *Int. J. Surg. Pathol.* **2017**, *25*, 18–25. [CrossRef]
76. Pérez-Montiel, D.; Wakely, P.E.; Hes, O.; Michal, M.; Suster, S. High-grade urothelial carcinoma of the renal pelvis: Clinicopathologic study of 108 cases with emphasis on unusual morphologic variants. *Mod. Pathol.* **2006**, *19*, 494–503. [CrossRef]
77. Amin, M.B. Histological variants of urothelial carcinoma: Diagnostic, therapeutic and prognostic implications. *Mod. Pathol.* **2009**, *24*, 6–15. [CrossRef]
78. Hayashi, H.; Mann, S.; Kao, C.S.; Grignon, D.; Idrees, M. Variant morphology in upper urinary tract urothelial carcinoma: A 14-year case series of biopsy and resection specimens. *Hum. Pathol.* **2017**, *65*, 209–216. [CrossRef]
79. López-Beltrán, A.; Henriques, V.; Montironi, R.; Cimadamore, A.; Raspollini, M.R.; Cheng, L. Variants and new entities of bladder cancer. *Histopathology* **2019**, *74*, 77–96. [CrossRef]
80. Rolim, I.; Henriques, V.; Rolim, N.; Blanca, A.; Marques, R.C.; Volavsek, M.; Carvalho, I.; Montironi, R.; Cimadamore, A.; Raspollini, M.R.; et al. Clinicopathologic analysis of upper urinary tract carcinoma with variant histology. *Virchows Arch.* **2020**, *477*, 111–120. [CrossRef]
81. Sim, S.J.; Ro, J.Y.; Ordonez, N.G.; Park, Y.W.; Kee, K.H.; Ayala, A.G. Metastatic renal cell carcinoma to the bladder: A clinicopathologic and immunohistochemical study. *Mod. Pathol.* **1999**, *12*, 351–355.
82. Tajima, S. Urothelial carcinoma with oncocytic features: An extremely rare case presenting a diagnostic challenge in urine cytology. *Int. J. Clin. Exp. Pathol.* **2015**, *8*, 8591–8597. [PubMed]
83. McCabe, J.E.; Das, S.; Dowling, P.; Hamid, B.N.; Pettersson, B.A. Oncocytic carcinoid tumour of the bladder. *J. Clin. Pathol.* **2005**, *58*, 446–447. [PubMed]
84. Genitsch, V.; Kollár, A.; Vandekerkhove, G.; Blarer, J.; Furrer, M.; Annala, M.; Herberts, C.; Pycha, A.; de Jong, J.J.; Liu, Y.; et al. Morphologic and genomic characterization of urothelial to sarcomatoid transition in muscle-invasive bladder cancer. *Urol. Oncol.* **2019**, *37*, 826–836. [CrossRef] [PubMed]
85. Malla, M.; Wang, J.F.; Trepeta, R.; Feng, A.; Wang, J. Sarcomatoid carcinoma of the urinary bladder. *Clin. Genitourin. Cancer* **2016**, *14*, 366–372. [CrossRef]

Publisher's Note: MDPI stays neutral with regard to jurisdictional claims in published maps and institutional affiliations.

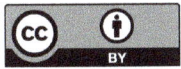

© 2020 by the authors. Licensee MDPI, Basel, Switzerland. This article is an open access article distributed under the terms and conditions of the Creative Commons Attribution (CC BY) license (http://creativecommons.org/licenses/by/4.0/).

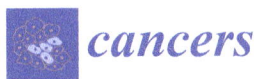

Article

Stroma Transcriptomic and Proteomic Profile of Prostate Cancer Metastasis Xenograft Models Reveals Prognostic Value of Stroma Signatures

Sofia Karkampouna [1], Maria R. De Filippo [1], Charlotte K. Y. Ng [2], Irena Klima [1], Eugenio Zoni [1], Martin Spahn [3], Frank Stein [4], Per Haberkant [4], George N. Thalmann [1,5,†] and Marianna Kruithof-de Julio [1,5,*,†]

1. Urology Research Laboratory, Department for BioMedical Research, University of Bern, Murtenstrasse 35, 3008 Bern, Switzerland; sofia.karkampouna@dbmr.unibe.ch (S.K.); mariarosaria.defilippo@unibas.ch (M.R.D.F.); irena.klima@dbmr.unibe.ch (I.K.); eugenio.zoni@dbmr.unibe.ch (E.Z.); george.thalmann@insel.ch (G.N.T.)
2. Oncogenomics Laboratory, Department for BioMedical Research, University of Bern, Murtenstrasse 40, 3008 Bern, Switzerland; charlotte.ng@dbmr.unibe.ch
3. Lindenhofspital Bern, Prostate Center Bern, 3012 Bern, Switzerland; martin.spahn@hin.ch
4. Proteomics Core Facility, EMBL Heidelberg, Meyerhofstraße 1, 69117 Heidelberg, Germany; frank.stein@embl.de (F.S.); per.haberkant@embl.de (P.H.)
5. Department of Urology, Inselspital, Anna Seiler Haus, Bern University Hospital, 3010 Bern, Switzerland
* Correspondence: marianna.kruithofdejulio@dbmr.unibe.ch
† These authors contributed equally to this work.

Received: 1 December 2020; Accepted: 10 December 2020; Published: 15 December 2020

Simple Summary: Currently, there is a need for prognostic tools that can stratify patients, who present with primary disease, based on whether they are at low or high risk for drug resistant and hormone-independent lethal metastatic prostate cancer. The aim of our study was to assess the potentially added value of tumor microenvironment (stroma) components for the characterisation of prostate cancer. By utilising patient derived-xenograft models we show that the molecular properties of the stroma cells are highly responsive to androgen hormone levels, and considerable ECM remodelling processes take place not only in androgen-dependent but also in androgen-independent tumor models. Transcriptomic mechanisms linked to osteotropism are conserved in bone metastatic xenografts, even when implanted in a different microenvironment. A stroma-specific gene list signature was identified, which highly correlates with Gleason score, metastasis progression and progression-free survival, and thus could potentially complement current patient stratification methods.

Abstract: Resistance acquisition to androgen deprivation treatment and metastasis progression are a major clinical issue associated with prostate cancer (PCa). The role of stroma during disease progression is insufficiently defined. Using transcriptomic and proteomic analyses on differentially aggressive patient-derived xenografts (PDXs), we investigated whether PCa tumors predispose their microenvironment (stroma) to a metastatic gene expression pattern. RNA sequencing was performed on the PCa PDXs BM18 (castration-sensitive) and LAPC9 (castration-resistant), representing different disease stages. Using organism-specific reference databases, the human-specific transcriptome (tumor) was identified and separated from the mouse-specific transcriptome (stroma). To identify proteomic changes in the tumor (human) versus the stroma (mouse), we performed human/mouse cell separation and subjected protein lysates to quantitative Tandem Mass Tag labeling and mass spectrometry. Tenascin C (TNC) was among the most abundant stromal genes, modulated by androgen levels in vivo and highly expressed in castration-resistant LAPC9 PDX. The tissue microarray of primary PCa samples (n = 210) showed that TNC is a negative prognostic marker of the clinical progression to recurrence or metastasis. Stroma markers of osteoblastic PCa bone metastases seven-up signature were induced in the stroma by the host organism in metastatic xenografts, indicating conserved mechanisms of tumor cells to induce a stromal premetastatic signature. A 50-gene list stroma signature was identified based on androgen-dependent responses, which shows a linear association with the Gleason score, metastasis progression and progression-free survival. Our data show that metastatic PCa PDXs, which differ in androgen sensitivity, trigger differential stroma responses, which show the metastasis risk stratification and prognostic biomarker potential.

Keywords: prostate cancer; stroma signature; patient-derived xenografts

1. Introduction

Bone metastases are detected in 10% of patients already at the initial diagnosis of prostate cancer (PCa) or will develop in 20–30% of the patients subjected to radical prostatectomy and androgen deprivation therapy and will progress to an advanced disease called castration-resistant prostate cancer [1]. Metastases are established when disseminated cancer cells colonize a secondary organ site. An important component of tumor growth is the supportive stroma: the extracellular matrix (ECM) and the nontumoral cells of the matrix microenvironment (e.g., endothelial cells, smooth muscle cells and cancer-associated fibroblasts). Upon interaction of the stroma compartment and tumor cells, the stroma responds by the secretion of growth factors, proteases and chemokines, thereby facilitating the remodeling of the ECM and, thus, tumor cell migration and invasion [2]. Therefore, tumor cell establishment requires an abnormal microenvironment. It is unclear whether the stroma is modulated by the tumor cells or by intrinsic gene expression alterations. Understanding the mechanisms of tumor progression to the metastatic stage is necessary for the design of therapeutic and prognostic schemes.

The bone microenvironment is favorable for the growth of PCa, as well as breast cancer, indicated by the high frequency of bone metastasis in these tumors. Studies have shown that cancer cell growth competes for the hematopoietic niche in the bone marrow with the normal residing stem cells [3], and depending on the cancer cell phenotype, this may lead to either osteoblastic or osteolytic lesions. The stroma signature of osteolytic PCa cells (PC-3) xenografted intraosseously in immunocompromised mice induce a vascular/axon guidance signature [4]. The stroma signature of osteoblastic lesions from human VCap and C4-2B PCa cell lines indicated an enrichment of the hematopoietic and prostate epithelial stem cell niche. A curated prostate-specific bone metastasis signature (Ob-BMST) implicated seven highly upregulated genes (*Aspn, Pdgrfb, Postn, Sparcl1, Mcam, Fscn1* and *Pmepa1*) [5], among which, *Postn* and *Fscn1* are bone-specific. Furthermore, *Aspn* and *Postn* expression is also increased in primary PCa cases [5], indicative of osteomimicry processes. The induction of osteoblastic genes in the stroma of primary tumors (PCa and breast), such as osteopontin and osteocalcin, has been suggested as a mechanism termed osteomimicry [6] to explain why the bone microenvironment is the preferential metastasis site. High stromal differences between benign, indolent and lethal PCa, combined with the enrichment of bone remodeling genes in high Gleason score cases [7], suggest that the stroma is an active player in PCa. During androgen deprivation, androgen-dependent epithelial cells will undergo apoptosis, while the supporting stroma is largely maintained or replaces the necrotic tissue areas [8]. Stromal cells do express androgen receptors (AR) and have active downstream signaling, while the absence of stromal AR expression is used as a prognostic factor of disease progression [9]. Furthermore, AR binds to different genomic sites in prostate fibroblasts compared to the epithelium [10] and to cancer-associated fibroblasts (CAFs) [11], indicating different roles of AR in epithelial or stroma cellular contexts. Prostate CAFs have tumor-promoting effects on marginally tumorigenic cells (LNCaP), irreversibly altering their phenotype and influencing their progression to androgen independence and metastasis [12,13].

In this study, we investigated whether metastatic PCa patient-derived xenograft models (PDXs) that differ in androgen sensitivity are triggering a differential stroma response. To elucidate the mechanisms of stroma contribution to tumor growth later on, we determined the unique gene expression profile of the stroma compared to the tumor compartment, the proteome changes of the tumor versus stroma. We identified androgen-dependent stroma gene expression signatures with potential disease progression prognostic values for primary PCa.

2. Results

2.1. Simultaneous Transcriptome Analysis of Human and Murine Signatures in PDXs Can Distinguish Androgen-Dependent Expression Changes in Tumor and Host-Derived Stroma

We analyzed the transcriptome of bulk PDX tumors grown subcutaneously in immunocompromised murine hosts by next-generation RNA-sequencing (RNA-Seq). Bone metastasis (BM)18 and LAPC9 PDXs were used in three different states: intact, post-castration (day 8 LAPCa9 and day 14 BM18) and androgen replacement (24 h) (Figure 1A). Tumor growth kinetics revealed the androgen-dependent phenotype of BM18, which regressed completely in two weeks post-castration (Figure 1B), and the androgen-independent phenotype of LAPC9 PDX tumors, which grew exponentially even after castration (Figure 1C), thus confirming the differential aggressiveness of the two models. The reduction of epithelial glands and proliferating Ki67+ cells in the BM18 castrated conditions (Figure 1D) was in contrast to the LAPC9 tumors (Figure 1E), which were morphologically indistinguishable among intact and castrated hosts. Bulk tumor tissues, which contain human tumor cells and mouse infiltrating stroma cells, were simultaneously analyzed from the same samples by RNA-Seq. To distinguish the transcriptome of the different organisms, the mouse and human reads were separated by alignment to a mouse and a human reference genome, respectively. Principal component analysis (PCA) of the human (tumor) 500 most variable genes showed that both castrated and replaced groups have altered expression profiles among each other and compared to the intact tumors. This was the case for the BM18 (Figure 2A) and the LAPC9 human transcriptomes (Figure 2B). The response to short-term androgen replacement showed a larger degree of variability in the BM18 (Figure 2A). However, the expression levels of direct AR target genes (*KLK3*, *NKX3.1* and *FKBP5*) identified by the RNA-Seq confirmed that androgen levels affected the activation of androgen receptor signaling in both BM18 (Figure 2C) and LAPC9 (Figure 2D, *KLK3* and *NKX3.1*). Differential expression analysis of the most variable human (tumor) genes, showed high variability among the castrated and intact groups, for both BM18 (Figure S1A) and LAPC9 (Figure S1B) transcript levels, while the LAPC9 replaced and castrated groups had similar profile among each other, discriminating them from the intact condition (Figure S1B).

PCA analysis of the BM18 mouse (stroma) transcriptome indicated that the majority of castrated samples (with and without 24-h androgen replacement) diverged from the intact tumor (Figure 2E). The LAPC9 mouse (stroma) transcriptome instead did not show specific clustering within or between the sample groups when plotting the top 500 most variably expressed genes (Figure 2F). The Ob-BMST signature of all seven genes (*Aspn*, *Pdgrfb*, *Postn*, *Aspn*, *Sparcl1*, *Mcam*, *Fscn1* and *Pmepa1*), which were upregulated in the bone stroma, as previously identified [5], were indeed expressed in the primary PCa TCGA cohort, as well as in both BM18 and LAPC9 PDXs (Figure S2A). *Pdgrfb*, *Postn*, *Aspn* and *Sparcl1*, specifically in the mouse RNA-Seq data, thus, are stroma-specific. Collectively, the Ob-BMST gene signature is expressed at equal levels in the BM18 and LAPC9 (intact) (Figure S2A). Some of these genes were differentially expressed upon castration in the BM18 (Figure 2G) but not in the LAPC9 (Figure 2H). A bone microenvironment-specific stroma signature induced by osteoblastic cell lines was conserved in bone metastasis PDXs maintained in other microenvironments and found in primary prostatic tissues.

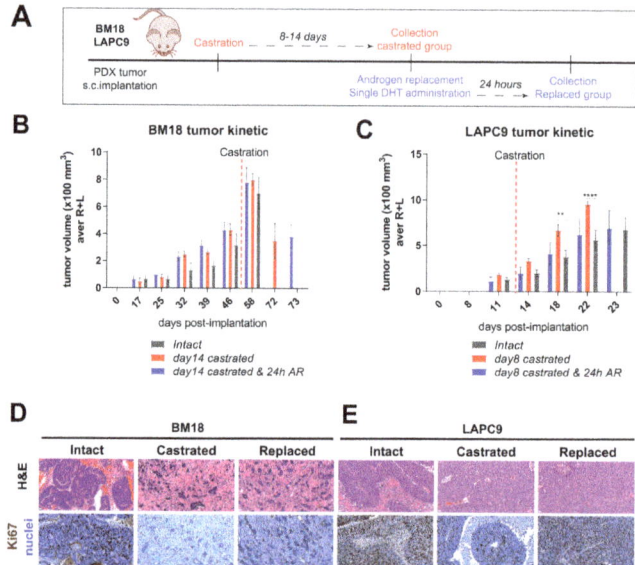

Figure 1. In vivo tumor growth properties of androgen-dependent BM18 versus androgen-independent patient-derived xenograft (PDX) models. (**A**) Scheme of in vivo BM18 and LAPC9 experiments, including the timeline of castration, androgen replacement (single dihydrotestosterone (DHT) administration) and collection of material for transcriptomic analysis. (**B**) BM18 PDX tumor growth progression in time. Groups: (1) intact tumors (collected at max size, $n = 3$), (2) castrated (day 14, $n = 4$) and (3) castrated, followed by testosterone readministration (castrated-testosterone) (day 15 since castration and 24 h since the androgen receptor (AR), $n = 3$). R; right tumor, L; left tumor per animal. (**C**) LAPC9 PDX tumor growth progression in time. Groups: (1) intact tumors (collected at max size, $n = 3$), (2) castrated (day 8, $n = 4$) and (3) castrated, followed by testosterone readministration (castrated-testosterone) (day 9 since castration and 24 h since AR, $n = 3$). Tumor scoring was performed weekly by routine palpation; values represent average calculations of the tumors of all animals per group (considering 2 tumors, left, L, and right, R, of each animal). Error bars represent SEM, calculated considering the no. of animals for each time point. Ordinary two-way ANOVA with Tukey's multiple comparison correction was performed, $p < 0.01$ (**) and $p < 0.0001$ (****). (**D**) Histological morphology of BM18 and (**E**) LAPC9 (from intact, castrated and androgen-replaced hosts), as assessed by Hematoxylin and Eosin staining (H&E, top). Scale bars: 20 µm, and proliferation marker Ki67 protein expression (bottom panel).

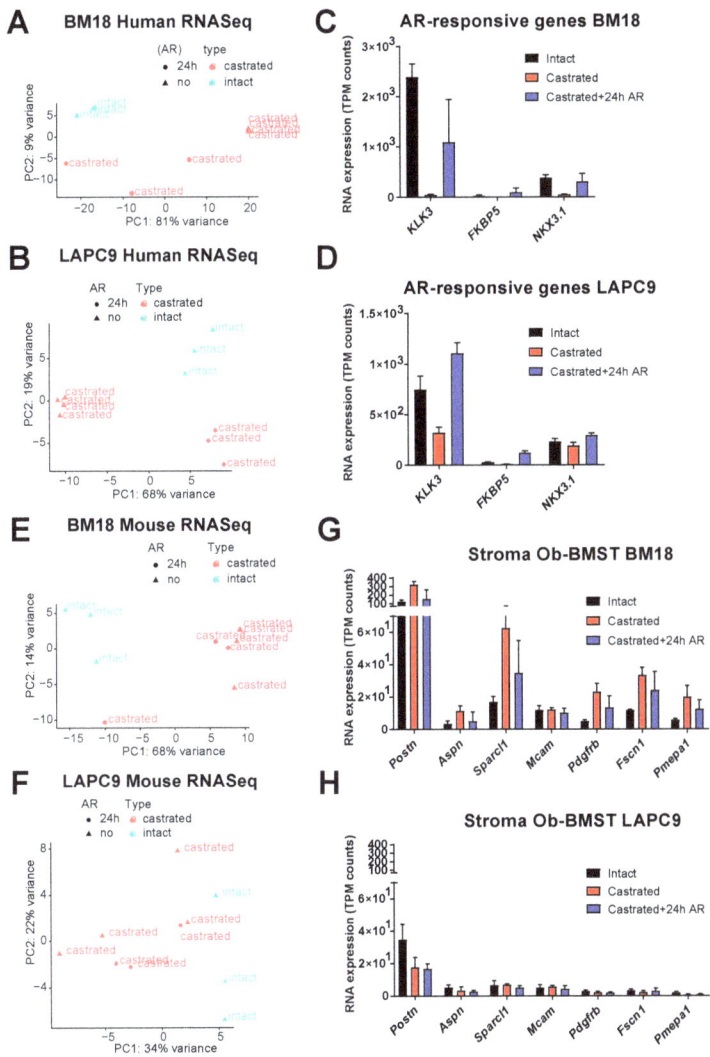

Figure 2. Separation of human (tumor) and mouse (stroma) transcriptomes of BM18 and LAPC9 tumors. (**A,B**) Principal component analysis plot of the gene expression of the 500 most variable genes on all samples; BM18 human transcripts (**A**) and LAPC9 human (**B**) at intact, castrated and replaced (castrated + 24 h AR) conditions. (**C,D**) Expression values of AR direct target genes as detected by RNA-Seq (transcript per million (TPM) counts) in the BM18 (**C**) or LAPC9 (**D**) tumors as confirmation of the effective repression of AR downstream signaling by castration. Intact ($n = 3$), castrated ($n = 4$) and replaced ($n = 3$). (**E,F**) Principal component analysis plot of the gene expression of the 500 most variable genes on all samples, BM18 mouse (**E**) and LAPC9 mouse (**F**) at intact, castrated and replaced (castrated + 24 h AR) conditions. (**G,H**) Expression values of the prostate-specific bone metastasis signature (Ob-BMST) seven upregulated stroma signature genes, as detected by RNA-Seq (TPM normalized counts) in the mouse transcriptome of BM18 (**E**) or LAPC9 (**F**) tumors.

2.2. Proteomic Analysis Provides Functional Information over the Identified Human/Mouse-Specific Transcriptome

To study the proteome of the tumor versus the stroma, human and mouse cell fractions were isolated by the magnetic cell sorting (MACS) mouse depletion method from tumor sample preparations: BM18 and LAPC9 each at the intact, castrated and replaced states. Protein lysates of either mouse or human origins (single replicate from a pool of $n = 3$ to 4 biological replicates per condition) were subjected to an in-solution tryptic digest following Tandem Mass Tag (TMT)-labeling of the resulting peptides and their mass spectrometric analysis (Figure 3A).

In addition to the initial experimental separation of the protein lysates, we further explored the species homologs of the identified proteins by computational analysis using a combined human and mouse protein sequence database. We identified 4198 proteins in the sample that were enriched for human cells. Thereof, 3154 were human-specific proteins, with 996 revealing a high homology shared among human and mouse, and only a fraction of 48 mouse-specific, peptides. (Figure 3B, left plot). For samples enriched in mouse cells, we identified, in total, 5192 proteins; thereof, 2486 mouse-specific proteins, 2379 shared homologs and 247 human-specific (Figure 3B, right plot). We searched for prostate specific markers such as KLK3, a prostate-specific antigen that is secreted by luminal cells. In the proteomic data, the human-specificity was confirmed, and the secreted protein was found also in the mouse fraction (Figure 3C). To further ensure that the proteomic data were indeed identifying real stromal-specific candidates, we searched specifically for the seven-gene Ob-BMST signature found also to be expressed in both BM18 and LAPC9. POSTN, PDGFRB and MCAM (Figure 3C) were indeed detected at the protein level, thus might have a functional role, and were found exclusively in the mouse fraction (Figure 3C, right plot) and hybridizing with mouse-specific sequences (Figure 3C, triangle indicates Mus Musculus species specificity).

2.3. Differential Expression Analysis Reveals Androgen-Dependent Stromal Gene Modulation in Androgen-Independent PDX Model

The relative ratio of human and mouse transcript reads reflected a higher stroma content in the BM18 compared to LAPC9 and significantly reduced human tumor content with enriched stroma content in the BM18 castrated group (Figure S2B). No major differences were observed in the LAPC9 castrated group (Figure S2C). We demonstrated that the human (tumor), as well as the mouse (stroma), transcriptomes follow androgen-dependent transcriptomic changes in the BM18 groups (intact versus castrated versus replaced) (Figure 2A,E). Venn Euler diagrams illustrate androgen level-dependent stromal gene expression modulation not only in the BM18 (Figure S2D and Table S1) but, also, in the androgen-independent (in terms of tumor growth) LAPC9 model (Figure S2E,F and Table S1). To identify the top-most significant AR-regulated stromal genes, we performed a differential expression analysis of BM18 tumors (Figure 4A) from castrated hosts and compared it to BM18 intact (the replaced tumors were not included here due to higher variability). Of the top-most variable genes, 50 were highly upregulated in BM18 tumors (z-score >1) and downregulated upon castration (Figure 4A). A differential expression analysis of LAPC9 tumors from castrated/replaced tumors versus intact tumors revealed the top-most differentially regulated genes: the 27 most upregulated genes in intact, which were downregulated in the castrated groups (Figure 4B). Among the 50 mouse genes that were highly upregulated in the intact BM18, and significantly modulated by castration, were 23 genes implicated in cell cycle/mitosis, 10 implicated in ECM and 3 related to spermatogenesis/hormone regulation, according to the Gene Ontology terms (Figure 4C). Two of these genes, *Tnc* and *Crabp1*, were also detected in the proteomic data (Figure 4C, highlighted in bold) and in both PDXs (Figure 4C,D, highlighted in red). Among the 27 mouse genes that were highly upregulated in the intact LAPC9, and significantly modulated by castration, seven genes were implicated in ECM/cell adhesion/smooth muscle function, and 14 were implicated in non-smooth muscle function and metabolism based on the Gene Ontology terms (Figure 4D). In the LAPC9 proteomic data, we detected 14 genes out of the 27 to be expressed in the mouse fractions (Figure 4D, bold), indicative of potential functional values. Of interest in potentially mediating tumor stroma extracellular interactions are a neural adhesion protein (*CD56*), implicated in cell–cell adhesion and migration by homotypic signaling, as well as Tenascin C (*Tnc*), an extracellular protein that is found abundantly in the reactive stroma of various cancer types, yet not expressed in normal stroma. Both genes were expressed at the protein level, exclusively in the mouse compartment of the BM18 and LAPC9, at all states (intact, castrated and replaced). Furthermore, Tnc was detected in both BM18 and LAPC9 at the transcriptional and proteomic levels and was reactivated after 24 h of androgen replacement (Figure 4B), indicative of AR-direct target gene modulation.

2.4. Cross Comparison of Stromal Transcriptome among Different PDXs Identifies ECM and Cell Adhesion Pathways in the LAPC9 Androgen-Independent Model

To assess the similarity between the stromal transcriptome of the androgen-independent LAPC9 and the BM18, a differential expression analysis was performed. In a panel of the 50 top-most variable genes comparing the tumors at their intact conditions, we identified several genes that follow the same pattern of modulation in intact tumors (Figure 5A) and in castrated tumors (Figure 5B). Of interest were the ECM-related genes downregulated in LAPC9 versus BM18; the Fibroblast Growth Factor receptor (*Fgfr4*), elastin microfibril interface (*Emilin3*) and upregulated collagen type 2 chain a1 (*Col2a1*).

The differential expression of LAPC9 castrated versus BM18 castrated highlighted genes that were identified in the analysis among LAPC9 castrated, replaced versus LAPC9 intact, such as Apelin (*Apln*), *Col2a1* and Tenascin C (*Tnc*).

To identify the biological processes ongoing in the LAPC9 compared to BM18, a pathway analysis was performed on the differentially expressed murine genes of the LAPC9 versus the BM18. Enrichment maps of the top 20 enriched GO biological pathways highly overlap pathways, such as ECM, focal tadhesion and cell adhesion/migration in the intact and castrated LAPC9 (Figure S3A,B). Similarly, among the KEGG pathway sets, there was an enrichment of stroma regulation (e.g., actin cytoskeleton, focal adhesion and cell adhesion) and bone and immune-related processes (e.g., osteoclast differentiation) (Figure S3C–F and Table S2). The enrichment of cancer-related pathways (e.g., PI3K/AKT, proteoglycans in cancer, pathways in cancer) was commonly found in the LAPC9 intact and castrated stroma transcriptomes (Figure S3E,F and Table S2).

Given that genes activated in a castrated state might be indicative of androgen resistance mechanism activation, we postulated that genes upregulated in the androgen-resistant LAPC9 over the androgen-dependent BM18 might be relevant for understanding the aggressive phenotype of LAPC9 and, therefore, of the advanced metastatic phenotype of similar tumors. One of those genes, Tenascin, is an ECM protein that is produced at the (myo)fibroblasts that is virtually absent in normal stroma in the prostate and other tissues and has been associated with the cancerous reactive stroma response in different cancers. We interrogated the expression of *Tnc* in the RNA-Seq data and found that it was highly upregulated in LAPC9 compared to BM18 both in intact ($\log_{FC}$ 4.23, $p < 0.001$) and among the castrated conditions ($\log_{FC}$ 6.9, $p < 0.001$) (Figure 5C). However, in both models, the *Tnc* levels significantly decreased upon castration (BM18, $p < 0.001$ and LAPC9, $p < 0.05$), indicating the potentially AR-mediated regulation of *Tnc* expression. In LAPC9 tumors, the TNC protein is expressed in the tumor-adjacent ECM and in the proximity of vessels (Figure 5D, intact and castrated) and co-expressed by smooth muscle actin (αSMA)- and collagen type I-positive myofibroblasts (Figure 5E). Instead, the intact BM18 tumors show TNC and collagen type I deposition in the ECM, but there is no overlap with αSMA-positive myofibroblasts (Figure 5D,E, BM18 intact). Castrated BM18 tumors have minimal TNC expression, found only in cells proximal to the remaining epithelial glands, yet with no typical fibroblast/stromal morphology (Figure 5D,E, BM18 intact), suggesting an altered phenotype of TNC upon androgen deprivation.

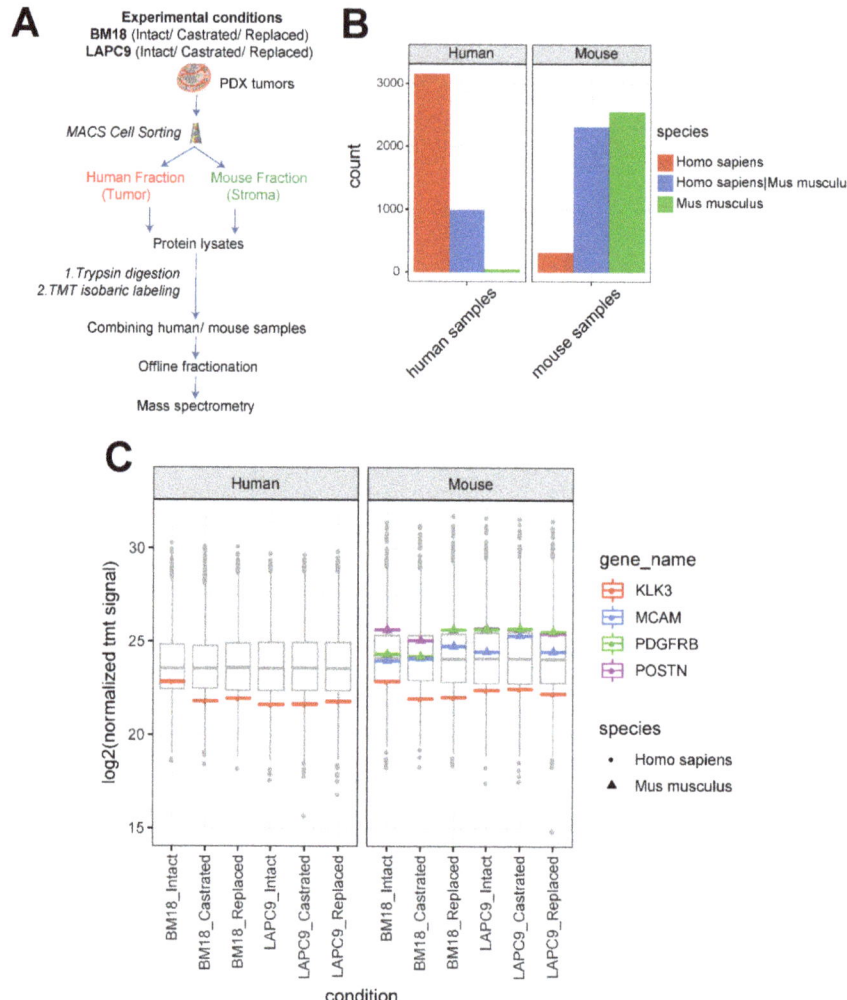

Figure 3. Proteomic analysis of human (tumor) versus mouse (stroma) of BM18 and LAPC9 tumors. (**A**) Experimental separation of human from mouse cell suspensions from fresh tumor isolations by MACS mouse depletion sorting. Cell fractions from intact/replaced ($n = 3$ each), castrated ($n = 4$) biological replicates were pooled into a single replicate ($n = 1$) to achieve an adequate cell number for the proteomic analysis (1×10^6 cells). Protein lysates from the different fractions of BM18/LAPC9 (intact, castrated and replaced) were subjected to Tandem Mass Tag (TMT) labeling (all-mouse or all-human samples were multiplexed in one TMT experiment each), followed by mass spectrometry. (**B**) Detected peptides from human and mouse fractions were searched against a combined human and mouse protein database. Number of species specific or shared proteins is indicated in different colors. (**C**) KLK3 (PSA; Prostate Serum Antigen) protein levels ($\log_2$ normalized TMT signal sum values) in human cell isolations (left) and in mouse cell isolations (right), and the protein sequence was predicted as human-specific (spheres indicate Homo Sapiens sequence). Seven-up Ob-BMST signature markers POSTN, PDGFRB and MCAM protein levels were absent in human cell isolations (left) and present in mouse cell isolations (right), while all the protein sequences were mouse-specific (triangles indicate Mus Musculus sequences).

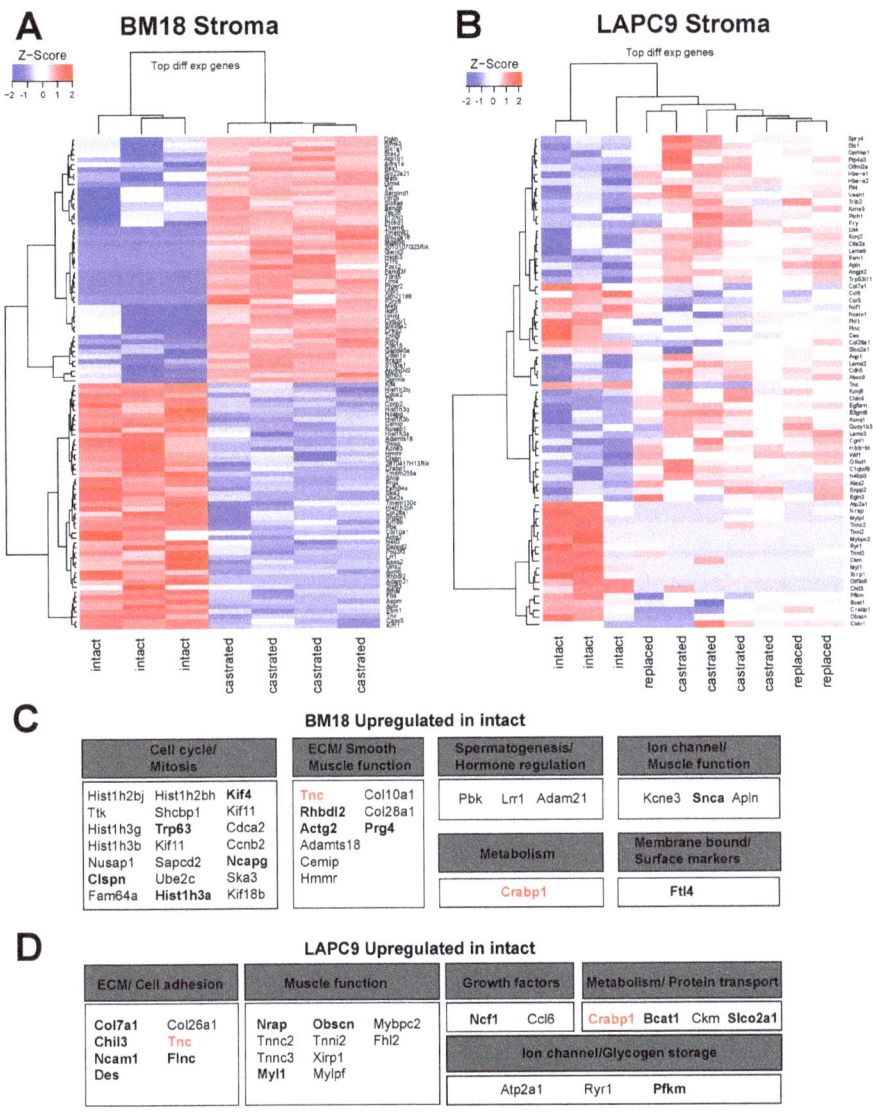

Figure 4. Differential expression analysis of the transcriptome indicates different expression profiles of stromal genes as response to androgen deprivation. (**A**) Heatmap represents a differential expression analysis of the most variable genes from the mouse transcriptome of BM18 castrated compared to BM18 intact tumors. Genes modulated by androgen deprivation due to castration in the up/downregulation compared to intact tumors are indicated in red or blue colors, respectively. (**B**) Heatmap represents Z-score of the differential expression analysis of most variable genes in the mouse transcriptome of LAPC9 castrated (with and without androgen replacement) compared to LAPC9 intact tumors. (**C**) Description of mouse genes found upregulated in BM18 intact tumors and the biological processes they are involved in, according to the Gene Ontology (GO) terms. (**D**) Description of the mouse genes found upregulated in LAPC9 intact tumors and the biological processes they are involved in, according to the GO terms.

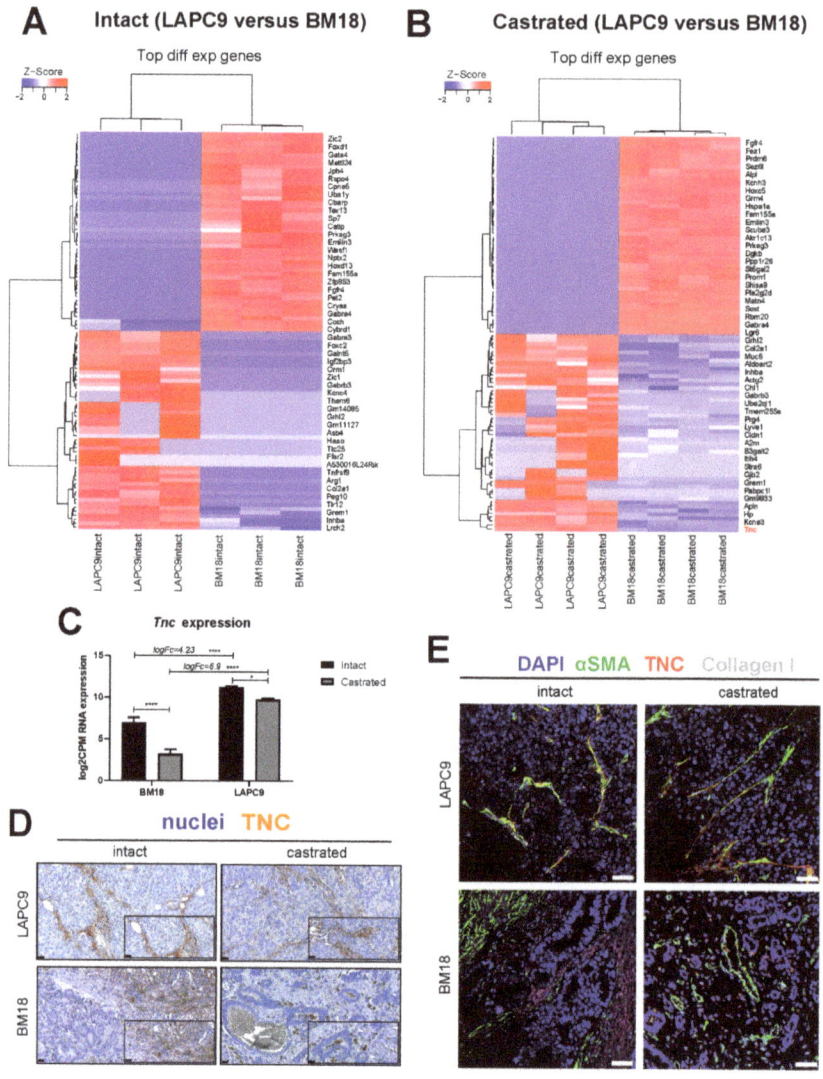

Figure 5. Cross-comparison of LAPC9 versus BM18 suggests stromal gene Tenascin C expression being associated with advanced PCa and regulated by androgen levels. (**A**) Heatmap represents the differential expression analysis of the top 100 most variable genes from the mouse transcriptome of LAPC9 intact tumors compared to BM18 intact tumors and (**B**) of LAPC9 castrated tumors compared to BM18 castrated tumors. (**A**) Subset of genes in LAPC9 samples have zero counts, leading to the same z-score, while the same genes are highly expressed in BM18 samples. (**C**) *Tnc* RNA expression (log$_2$CMP counts) in the stroma transcriptome. Log$_{FC}$ (fold change) enrichment of *Tnc* in LAPC9 over BM18 is indicated. Ordinary two-way ANOVA with Tukey's multiple comparison correction was performed, $p < 0.05$ (*) and $p < 0.0001$ (****). (**D**) Tenascin protein expression and stromal specificity assessed by immunohistochemistry in LAPC9 and BM18 tumors, both at the intact and castrated states. Scale bars: 20 μm. (**E**) Tenascin protein (indicated in red) colocalization with stromal markers, smooth muscle actin (αSMA, green) and collagen type I (gray) assessed by immunofluorescence in LAPC9 and BM18 tumors, both at the intact and castrated states. DAPI marks the nuclei. Scale bars: 50 μm.

2.5. Protein Expression of Tenascin and Its Interaction Partners

To assess whether the transcriptomic changes of *Tnc* in the PDX models corresponds to the functional protein and, thus, a relevant role in bone metastatic PCa, we performed a proteomic analysis. A mass spectrometry analysis of the human and mouse fractions indicated that the Tnc protein was expressed specifically in the mouse (stromal) fractions in BM18 and LAPC9 (Figure 6A). The isoform Tenascin X was also expressed at the protein level (Figure 6B). The interaction network of the mouse protein Tnc is based on experimental observations and prediction tools (STRING) and consists of laminins (Lamc1 and Lamb2); fibronectin (Fb1); integrins (Itga2, a7, a8 and a9) and proteoglycans (Bcan and Vcan) (Figure 6C). The human interactome is less-characterized, yet most of the interactome is conserved: laminins (LAMC1 and LAMB2); proteoglycans (NCAN and ACAN) and others such as interleukin 8 (IL-8), BMP4, ALB and SDC4 (Figure 6D). However, integrin interaction-binding partners in a human setting have not been confirmed. Given the importance of integrins for cell adhesion and migration known to be found in mesenchymal/stromal and epithelial tumor cells, we focused on the expression of human- and mouse-derived integrins. The *ITGA9*, *ITGA6* and *ITGA2* were all found to be expressed in both the RNA-Seq and proteomic data (Figure 6E, ITGA6, respectively); however, only the *ITGA2* protein was specifically found in the human counterpart and not overlapping with the mouse stroma (Figure 6F). Co-labeling both proteins indicated adjacent spatial localization with TNC deposition in close proximity to ITGA2-positive epithelial cells (Figure 6G); however, whether those cell populations acquired different properties compared to other epithelial cells has yet to be investigated. Overall, the tumor *ITGA2* and stromal *Tnc* is a potential molecular interaction, possibly part of the dual cellular communication among a tumor and its microenvironment cellular types and ECM.

2.6. Stromal Tenascin Expression as a Prognostic Factor of Disease Progression in High-Risk PCa

The detection of key mouse stromal genes in PCa PDXs gives the opportunity to evaluate the role and potential prognostic value of the human orthologs of these stromal genes. To validate the localization and stromal specificity of TNC protein expression, we performed immunohistochemistry on the primary PCa tissue sections. TNC is localized in the extracellular space (Figure 7A, primary cases). Next, we evaluated the TNC expression in a tissue microarray of 210 primary prostate tissues, part of the European Multicenter High Risk Prostate Cancer Clinical and Translational research group (EMPaCT) [14–16] (Figure 7B–G). Based on the preoperative clinical parameters of the TMA patient cases (Table 1, Table 2) and the D'Amico classification system [17], they represent intermediate (clinical T2b or Gleason n = 7 and PSA >10 and ≤ 20) and high-risk (clinical T2c-3a or Gleason score (GS) = 8 and PSA ≥ 20) PCa. The number of TNC-positive cells (Figure 7B) were quantified and averaged for all cores (four cores per patient case) in an automated way, including tissue selection, core annotation and equal staining parameters set. To investigate the association between the number of TNC-positive cells and patient survival or disease progression, we calculated the optimal cut-point for the number of TNC-positive cells by estimation of the maximally selected rank statistics [18]. Association between TNC-expressing cells and pT Stage indicated that the majority of cases cluster towards stages 3a and 3b (Figure 7C). A multiple comparison test among all groups showed no statistically significant association between the TNC expression and pathological stage (Table S3, $p > 0.05$). The overall survival probability between two patient groups with, respectively, high and low numbers of TNC-positive cells was indifferent ($p = 0.29$, Log-rank test) (Figure 7D). We focused on the probability of TNC expression in primary tumors to be a deterministic factor for clinical progression to local or metastasis recurrence. Clinical progression probability was higher in the TNC-low group compared the TNC-high group ($p = 0.04$ *, Log-rank test) (Figure 7E). Next, we examined the clinical progression in patients with pT Stage ≥3 (groups 3a, 3b and 4). The high T-Stage cases did separate into two groups based on the TNC expression, with the TNC low-expressing group exhibiting earlier a clinical progression (local or metastatic recurrence, $p = 0.013$ *, Log-rank test) (Figure 7F). The PSA progression probability in patients with pT Stage ≥3 indicated an association trend of a TNC-low group with earlier biochemical relapse events ($p = 0.07$, Log-rank test) (Figure 7G). Similarly, the TNC-low group correlated with a higher probability for PSA progression after radical prostatectomy among cases with carcinoma-containing (positive) surgical margins (Figure S4A, $p = 0.031$ *, Log-rank test) or positive lymph nodes (Figure S4B, $p = 0.092$, Log-rank test). A low number of TNC-expressing cells coincides with a poor prognosis in terms of metastasis progression, similarly to its downregulation upon castration in the bone metastasis PDXs (Figure 4B) based on the RNA-Seq analysis. To further evaluate the clinical relevance of this finding, in multiple clinical cohorts with available transcriptomic data and clinical information, a CANCERTOOL analysis was performed [19]. Similar to the protein TMA data (Figure 7), the *TNC* mRNA levels were significantly downregulated during the disease progression from primary to PCa metastasis, compared to the expression in the normal prostatic tissues in all five datasets tested (Figure 8A). The *TNC* expression shows a pattern of inverse correlations, with the Gleason score among GS6 to GS9; however, it significantly discriminated patient groups for the Gleason score in one out of three datasets tested (Figure 8B, TCGA dataset * $p = 0.049$, Glinsky $p = 0.06$, Taylor $p = 0.192$), with the highest expression found in a high GS10 group and indifferent among GS6-GS9. A disease-free survival analysis indicated that a low TNC expression is associated with a worse prognosis based on the Glinsky dataset (Q1 Glinsky et al. [20], * $p = 0.02$), while no statistically significant association was observed in the Taylor and TCGA dataset (Figure 8C). Overall, the TNC expression in tumor samples, both at the RNA and protein levels, becomes progressively less abundant in primary and metastasis PCa specimens, while a low TNC expression is significantly associated with the disease progression and poor disease-free survival (DFS) outcome.

2.7. Stroma Signatures from Androgen-Dependent and -Independent States Correlate with Disease Progression

In order to comprehensively map the stroma responses related to the disease severity, we analyzed the stroma gene signature lists associated to androgen dependency and aggressive androgen-independent states. The stroma signatures are categorized in clusters (C1–C4, Table S4) based on a differential expression analysis (Figures 4 and 5): C1 (50 highly upregulated genes in BM18 intact that get downregulated upon castration), C2 (27 highly upregulated genes in LAPC9 intact that get downregulated upon castration), C3 (32 highly upregulated genes in LAPC9 intact compared to BM18 intact) and C4 (24 highly upregulated genes in LAPC9 castrated compared to BM18 intact). Clusters C1 and C2 aim to identify the most responsive genes to androgen deprivation. C3 and C4 are designated to identify the genes/pathways enriched in the stroma of castration-resistant prostate cancer (CRPC) compared to the androgen-dependent tumor model. The TNC gene was among the signature list: C1, C3 and C4. The prognostic potential of the C1-C4 signatures in comparison to the bone signature Ob-BMST was tested on the TCGA cohort based on the Gleason score, gene expression and outcome data (Figure 9 and Table S5). The high signature scores of Ob-BMST, C1, C2 and C4 had statistically significant positive correlations with the high GS groups (Figure 9A, Ob-BMST and C1 ($p < 0.001$), C2 and C4 ($p < 0.01$)). In terms of gene expression, the C1 signature was significantly higher in primary tumors versus normal tissues (Figure 9B, $p < 0.001$), while the C2, C3 and C4 have lower signature scores in the tumor samples compared to normal (Figure 9B, C2 and C3 ($p < 0.001$) and C4 ($p < 0.01$)). Kaplan-Meier plots of progression-free survival (PFS) stratified as the bottom 25% (Q1), middle 50% (Q2 and 3) and top 25% (Q4) showed significant correlations among the high signature scores (Q4) of the C1 gene set and PFS (Figure 9C, $p < 0.001$), while none of the other gene lists showed significant correlations.

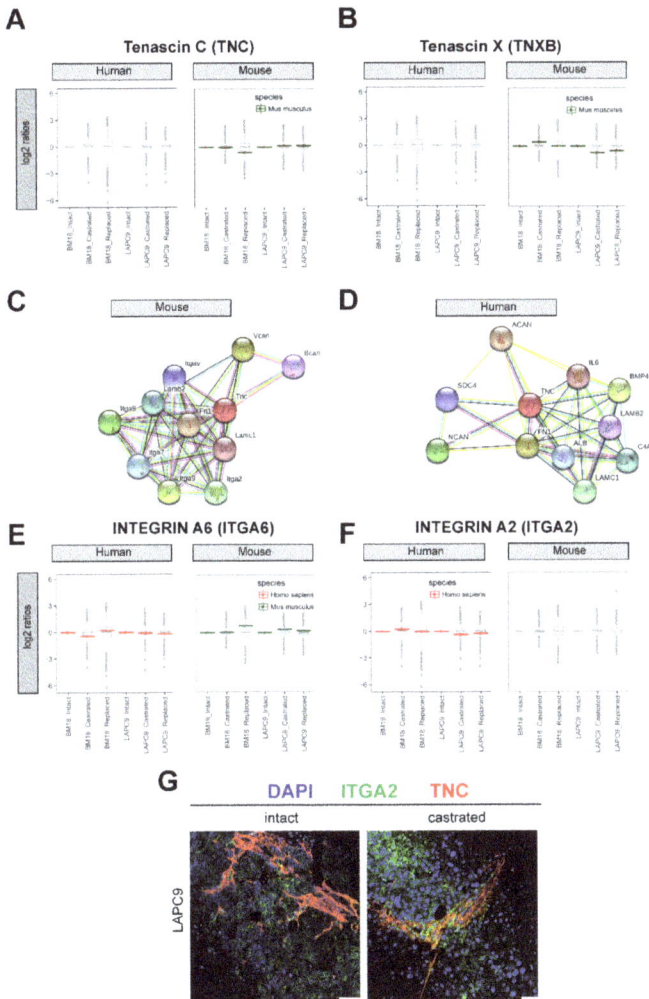

Figure 6. Tenascin C and its predicted interaction partners analyzed by mass spectrometry. (**A**) Tenascin C (TNC) and (**B**) alternative isoform Tenascin X (TNXB) protein relative abundance (log$_2$ ratios; single replicates per sample from a pool of n = 3 to 4) in human cell isolations (left) and present in mouse cell isolations (right). The variance stabilization normalization (vsn)-corrected TMT reporter ion signals were normalized by the intact conditions of either BM18 or LAPC9. The protein sequences were predicted as mouse-specific (green). (**C**) Protein interaction network of the mouse TNC protein based on the STRING association network (https://string-db.org/). (**D**) Protein interaction network of the human TNC protein based on the STRING association network https://string-db.org/. (**E**) Predicted TNC-binding partner integrin A6 (ITGA6) was detected by mass spectrometry in both the human and mouse protein lysates and matching the organism-specific protein sequence based on the bioinformatics analysis (red for human and green for mouse). (**F**) Predicted TNC-binding partner integrin A2 (ITGA2) was detected by mass spectrometry, specifically in the human protein lysates, and matched the human-specific protein sequence. (**G**) Spatial localization of the Tenascin protein (TNC, indicated in red) and integrin A2 (ITGA2, green) assessed by immunofluorescent co-labeling in LAPC9 intact and castrated tumors. DAPI marks the nuclei. Scale bars: 50 µm.

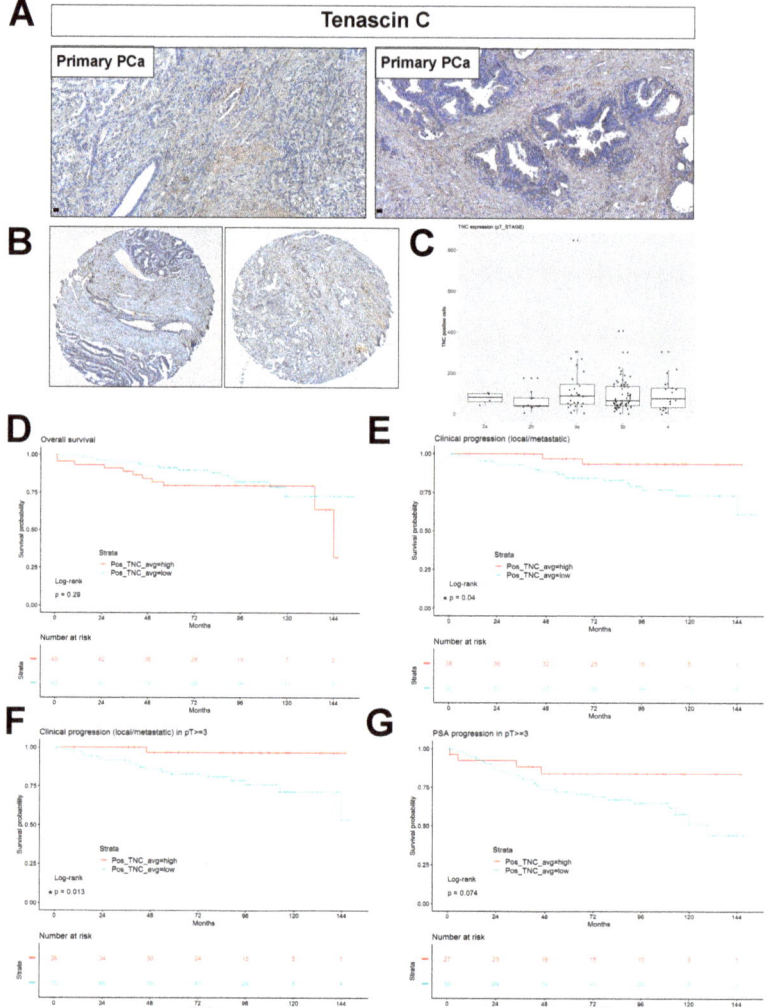

Figure 7. TNC protein expression is a negative metastasis prognostic factor in primary, high-risk PCa. (**A**) Validation of the protein expression and stromal specificity of TNC by immunohistochemistry in primary PCa cases. (**B**) Representative cases of TNC staining on primary PCa Tissue Microarray (TMA) from European Multicenter Prostate Cancer Clinical and Translational Research Group (EMPaCT). (**C**) TNC expression levels in terms of the no. of positive cells in the pT Stage classification. Statistical multiple comparison test, the Wilcoxon rank sum test, was performed; $p > 0.05$ (**D**) Overall survival probability in patient groups of TNC-high and TNC-low (no. of positive, TNC-expressing cells) ($p = 0.29$, ns—non significant). Average value represents the mean of four cores per patient case. (**E**) Clinical progression to the local recurrence or metastasis probability in patient groups of TNC-high and TNC-low expressions ($p = 0.04$ and * < 0.05). (**F**) Clinical progression to the local recurrence or metastasis probability among patients of pT Stages 3a, 3b and 4 based on TNC-high and TNC-low expressions ($p = 0.013$ and * < 0.05). (**G**) PSA progression probability among patients of pT Stages 3a, 3b and 4 based on the TNC-high and TNC-low expressions ($p = 0.074$, ns).

Table 1. Clinical parameters of the EMPaCT TMA patient cases.

Descriptive Statistics	Age at Surgery	PSA at Surgery	PSA Progression Time (Months)	Clinical Progression Time (Months)
Min	43	20	1	1
1st quartile	62	25.33	29.5	40.5
Median quartile	67	36.99	63.5	75.5
Mean quartile	66.18	50.56	63.47	70.89
3rd quartile	71	61.9	90	95.75
Max quartile	81	597	151	153

Table 2. Pathological staging, PSA and Clinical Progression of the EMPaCT TMA patient cases.

PSA Progression	Clinical Progression	Pathological Staging (No. of Patient Cases)				
		2a	2b	3a	3b	4
no	no	6	15	37	63	26
	yes	0	0	0	1	0
yes	no	0	5	7	11	7
	yes	1	7	9	9	6

To further assess the prognostic performance of the signatures, we correlated the C1-C4 gene signatures with PCa-specific stroma signatures identified by Tyekucheva et al. [7] and Mo et al. [21] (Table S4) across two cohorts containing both primary and metastatic PCa that were used [22,23]. The C3 and C4 showed the strongest linear correlations with the Tyekucheva and the Mo_up (upregulated in metastases) signatures when tested across the Grasso dataset (Figure S5A, r > 0.64), while the C4 signature also had positive correlations when tested across the Taylor et al. dataset (Figure S5B, r > 0.6). The C1 signature did not significantly correlate with the gene lists tested (Figure S5A, C1 $p > 0.05$). The low signature score of the C2 and C3 were significantly associated with metastatic disease progression (Figure S5B, $p < 0.001$) in both cohorts tested, and C4 showed a similar pattern (Figure S5B, C4 $p = 0.062$). A common pattern of the stroma signatures is a similar or enriched signature score at the primary stage compared to benign/normal tissue, and lower/depleted signature scores at the metastasis stage (Figure S5C,D; C2, C3 and C4, Tyekucheva and Mo and Figure 9B; C2-C4). Only a significant correlation with the Gleason score was observed by the C1 signature list, with a high signature score found at the high GS patient groups (Figure S5E, $p \leq 0.001$), which is in concordance to the linear correlation with metastatic disease in all clinical cohorts tested (Figure S5C,D, $p \leq 0.001$ and Figure 9, TCGA).

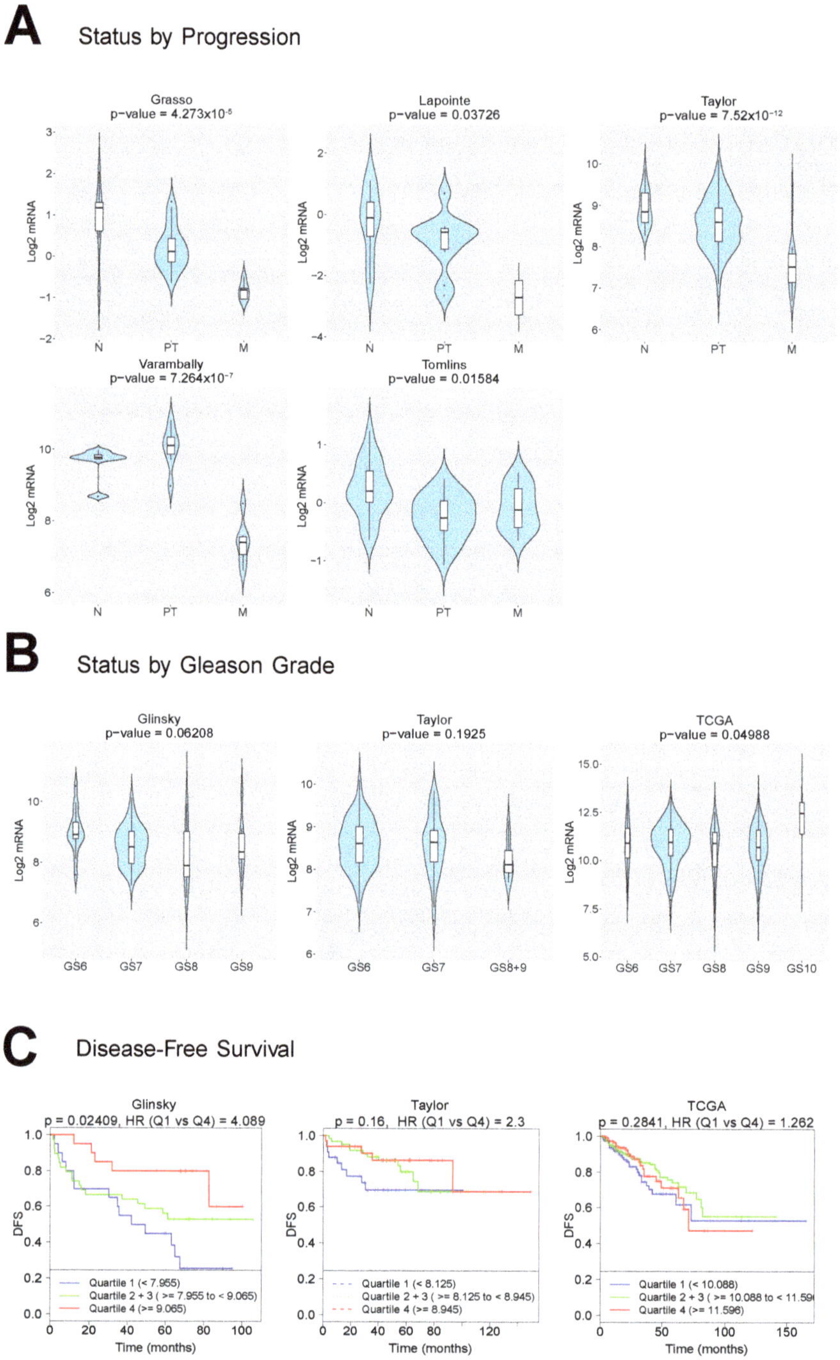

Figure 8. *TNC* RNA expression is inversely correlated with the disease progression, Gleason score and survival. (**A**) Violin plots depicting the expression of *TNC* among nontumoral (N), primary tumor (PT)

and metastatic (M) PCa specimens in the indicated datasets. The Y-axis represents the Log_2-normalized gene expression (fluorescence intensity values for microarray data or sequencing read values obtained after gene quantification with RNA-Seq Expectation Maximization (RSEM) and normalization using the upper quartile in case of RNA-seq). An ANOVA test is performed in order to compare the mean gene expression among two groups (nonadjusted *p*-value), obtained by a CANCERTOOL analysis. (**B**) Violin plots depicting the expression of *TNC* among PCa specimens of the indicated Gleason grade in the indicated datasets. The Gleason grades are indicated as GS6, GS7, GS8, GS8+9, GS9 and GS10. An ANOVA test is performed in order to compare the mean among groups (nonadjusted *p*-value), obtained by a CANCERTOOL analysis. (**C**) Kaplan-Meier curves representing the disease-free survival (DFS) of patient groups selected according to the quartile expression of *TNC*. Quartiles represent ranges of expression that divide the set of values into quarters. Quartile color code: Q1 (Blue), Q2 plus Q3 (Green) and Q4 (Red). Each curve represents the percentage (Y-axis) of the population that exhibits a recurrence of the disease along the time (X-axis, in months) for a given gene expression distribution quartile. Vertical ticks indicate censored patients. Quartile color code: Q1 (Blue), Q2 plus Q3 (Green) and Q4 (Red). A Mantel-Cox test is performed in order to compare the differences between curves, while a Cox proportional hazards regression model is performed to calculate the hazard ratio (HR) between the indicated groups. Nonadjusted *p*-values are shown. Analysis obtained by CANCERTOOL.

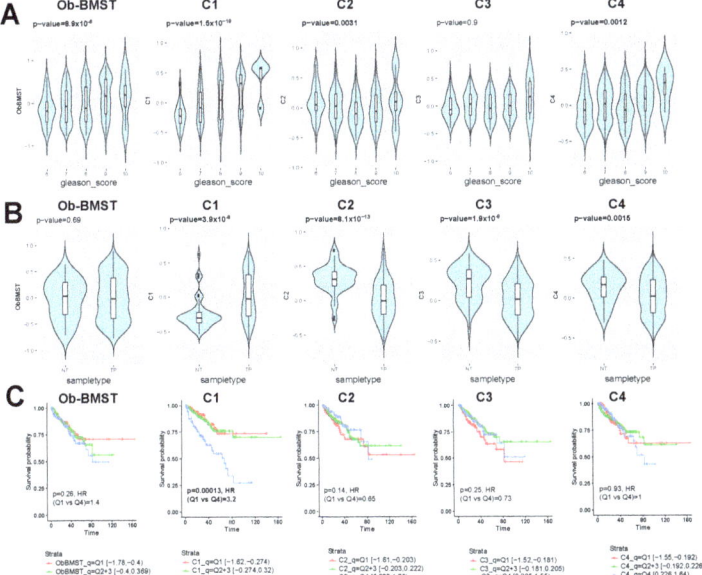

Figure 9. Stroma signatures identified from bone metastatic PDXs as prognostic biomarkers in primary PCa. (**A**) Violin plots showing Gene Set Variation Analysis (GSVA) signature scores of the Ob-BMST, C1-C4 gene sets, stratified by Gleason score from the TCGA cohort. Box-and-whisker plots illustrating median (midline), inter-quartile range (box), with the whiskers extending to at most 1.5 IQR from the box. Outliers beyond the range of the whiskers are illustrated as dots. P-values computed by Spearman correlation tests. (**B**) Violin plots showing GSVA signature scores of the Ob-BMST and C1-C4 gene sets stratified by sample types (NT: nontumor and TP: primary tumor) from the TCGA cohort. Box-and-whisker plots illustrating the median (midline) and interquartile range (box), with the whiskers extending to at most 1.5 IQR from the box. Outliers beyond the range of the whiskers are illustrated as dots. *P*-values computed by Mann-Whiney U tests. (**C**) Kaplan-Meier plots of progression-free survival (PFS) stratified as the bottom 25% (Q1), middle 50% (Q2 and 3) and top 25% (Q4) of the signature scores of the Ob-BMST and C1-C4 gene sets. *P*-values and hazard ratios computed by Cox proportional hazard regression.

3. Discussion

The role of the microenvironment upon cancer formation and progression to metastasis is supported by numerous studies [24,25]; however, the current knowledge is not sufficient to reconstruct the chain events from primary to secondary tumor progression. The normal stroma microenvironment is considered to halt tumor formation; however, after interactions with tumor cells, it also undergoes a certain "transformation" at the transcriptomic, and even at the genetic, levels [26–29]. The processes by which PCa tumor cells affect stroma and, in turn, stroma impacts primary PCa tumor growth or metastasis are complex and remain largely unclear.

We utilized well-established bone metastasis PDX models, which can be propagated subcutaneously and have different aggressiveness in terms of androgen dependency: the CRPC model LAPC9 representing complete androgen-independent advanced disease [30] and the BM18 that mimics human luminal PCa [31,32] and uniquely retains androgen sensitivity, typically seen in the primary and treatment-naïve stages. The androgen-independent stem cell populations that survive castration are well characterized in both models [31,33,34]; yet, the contribution of the stroma in those district tumor phenotypes has not been investigated. In vivo PDX models grafted in immunocompromised mice, although they lack the complexity of a complete immune system, represent the stroma compartment (endothelial cells, smooth muscle cells, myofibroblasts and cancer-associated fibroblasts). Due to the subcutaneous growth of BM PCa PDXs, the human stroma is replaced by mouse-infiltrating stromal cells and vasculature [35,36]. Mouse cell infiltration allows the discrimination of organism-specific transcripts, human-derived transcripts representing the tumor cells and mouse-derived transcripts representing the mouse stroma compartment. Using next-generation RNA-Seq, MACS-based human and mouse cell sorting, mass spectrometry and organism-specific reference databases, we have identified the tumor-specific (human) from the stroma-specific (mouse) transcriptomes and proteomes of bone metastasis PCa PDXs. The dynamics of AR signaling in the stroma are best represented in an in vivo setting [11]; therefore, to specifically examine the stroma changes dictated by PCa cells, we subjected the PDXs in androgen and androgen-deprived conditions. By imposing this selection pressure, we could identify androgen-dependent gene expression patterns.

We demonstrated that the human (tumor), as well as the mouse (stroma), transcriptomes follow androgen-dependent transcriptomic changes in the BM18 groups (intact versus castrated versus replaced). Despite the androgen-independent tumor growth of LAPC9, at the gene expression level, the LAPC9 tumor cells do follow AR-responsive patterns (human transcriptomes). However, the principal component analysis showed that, although castrated and replaced LAPC9 groups separate adequately based on the human transcriptome, they appear to have overall uniform stromal transcriptomes.

We report that transcriptomic mechanisms linked to osteotropism were conserved in bone metastatic PDXs, even in nonbone environments, and differential stroma gene expressions are induced by different tumors, indicating the tumor specificity of stroma reactivity. The Ob-BMST signature of all seven genes (*Aspn*, *Pdgrfb*, *Postn*, *Sparcl1*, *Mcam*, *Fscn1* and *Pmepa1*), which were upregulated in bone stroma previously identified [5], were indeed expressed in both BM18 and LAPC9 PDXs, specifically in the mouse RNA-Seq and, also, expressed at the protein level, as identified by mass spectrometry. The gene expression modulation of mouse stroma is, ultimately, an important evidence of the effects of tumor cells in their microenvironment, where they induce favorable conditions for their growth.

The differential expression analysis of the LAPC9 stroma signature from intact, castrated and replaced hosts highlighted the most significantly variable genes, which were modulated by androgen levels, despite the androgen-independent tumor growth phenotype. Focusing on the genes that were highly activated in intact but strongly modulated by castration, we categorized these genes based on Gene Ontology terms. We found that LAPC9 stromal genes were ECM remodeling components and genes involved in smooth muscle function or even in striated muscle function. Of interest are *CD56*, *Tnc* and *Flnc*. Among the BM18 most abundant stromal transcripts are genes involved in cell cycle regulation and cell division. Interrogating the differences among the two models, we focused on the transcriptome of LAPC9 normalized versus the less aggressive, androgen-dependent BM18. In particular, *Tnc* is expressed in both PDXs, higher in LAPC9, yet downregulated upon castration, suggesting a direct AR gene regulation. The differential expression analysis among both the PDXs after castration indicated that *Tnc* is upregulated more in LAPC9 than BM18, suggesting an association with disease aggressiveness. Genes that become upregulated in castrated conditions are likely to be linked to androgen resistance; thus, we studied *Tnc* for its potential role in metastasis progression.

TNC is an extracellular glycoprotein absent in normal prostates and postnatally silenced in most tissues. TNC is re-expressed in reactive stroma in human cancers, and there is evidence of its expression in low-grade tumors (Gleason 3) of human PCa [37] and, possibly, already activated at the prostatic intraepithelial neoplasia (PIN) stage [38,39]. In particular, high molecular weight TNC isoforms are expressed in cancer due to alternative mRNA splicing [38]. We examined whether an abundance of TNC-positive cells in primary PCa TMA can predict the metastatic progression and overall survival (12 years follow-up after radical prostatectomy). A high number of TNC-positive cells did not correlate with the overall survival or histological grade, in agreement with previous data [38]. The PSA progression after radical prostatectomy occurred earlier in the TNC-low group compared to the TNC-high group when high stage cases (pT ≥ 3), surgical margin-positive or lymph node-positive cases were investigated. In terms of clinical progression, the TNC-low group in the total number of cases and among the high stage (pT ≥ 3) cases showed a worse prognosis in terms of local recurrence/metastasis. This finding is in contrast to the study of Ni et al., showing that high levels of TNC are significantly linked to lymph node metastasis and the clinical stage [40] but in agreement with another study that reported a weak TNC expression in high-grade PCa [39]. No low-risk cases or metastasis tissues were used in our study, and we focused on TNC-producing cells, not the overall TNC expression in the matrix. Therefore we can only conclude that the TNC is indeed expressed in intermediate- and high-risk primary PCa as assessed at the preoperative diagnosis based on the D′Amico criteria [17] and that a high number of TNC-positive cells is inversely correlated with clinical progression.

More evidence points to the direction that the TNC might be degraded upon local recurrence in lung cancer [41,42], while high TNC is found in lymph and bone metastases sites [38] or even in certain types of bone metastasis [43]. In the TMA of PCa bone metastasis, San Martin et al. demonstrated a high TNC expression in trabeculae endosteum, the site of osteoblastic metastasis, and yet, a low TNC expression in the adjacent bone marrow sites [43]. Osteoblastic PCa cell lines proliferate rapidly in vitro and adhere to TNC protein, while osteolytic PC3 or lymph node-derived PCa lines do not show this phenotype, suggesting an association of TNC with osteoblastic but not osteolytic metastases. One of the ligands of TNC highly upregulated in VCap cells was α9 integrin, which binds directly TNC and a modulate expression of collagen [43], providing evidence for TNC-integrins in human PCa. Our RNA-Seq data indicate, also, the expression of α9 integrin, along with α6 and α2, and based on the proteomic human–mouse separation, we found integrin α2 to be the only one human-specific and, thus, tumor-specific for the PDXs used in this study. Although the molecular mechanism among TNC-ITGA2 should be further characterized, evidence on the correlation among α2 and α6 expressions in primary PCa and bone metastasis occurrence has been previously reported [44].

The reactivation of TNC expression is relevant for reactive stroma regulation, while TNC downregulation might be relevant for recurrence or metastasis initiation, which remains to be further investigated. Indeed, TNC is known to have pleiotropic functions in different cellular contexts, with both autocrine TNC expression in tumor cells and paracrine TNC from stroma in different stages of metastasis [45]; however, the cellular source of TNC in primary PCa was not addressed in our study. Our data demonstrate that androgens regulate stromal TNC expression, evident by the reduced TNC expression upon castration (even in the castration-resistant LAPC9) and immediate increased expression upon androgen replacement; thus, the TNC expression should be further evaluated in CRPC samples. Genomic amplification in the TNC gene associated with highly aggressive neuroendocrine PCa occurrence [46]. In a multi-omics approach study, the TNC protein was one of the panels of four markers detected in preoperative serum samples and, collectively, predict the biochemical relapse events with high accuracy [47].

In summary, we identified the stroma signature of bone metastatic PDXs, and by analyzing androgen-dependent versus androgen-independent tumors, we could demonstrate that the tumor-specific stroma gene expression changes. We could show that there are AR-regulated stromal genes modulated upon castration, even in the androgen-independent, for tumor growth, like the LAPC9 model. The osteoblastic bone metastasis stromal seven-gene signature was induced in the mouse-derived stroma compartment of BM18 and LAPC9, indicating conserved tumor mechanisms that can induce the transcriptomic "transformation" of mouse-infiltrating stroma (even in subcutaneous sites) to bone microenvironment-like stroma. The prognostic value of stroma signatures has been also demonstrated by another study utilizing PDXs associated with the metastasis prognosis from different lesions from a single PCa case and demonstrated the strong predictability of 93-gene stroma signatures to metastasis phenotypes in different clinical cohorts [21]. We identified androgen-dependent Tenascin C expression in the stroma of PDX models, which is downregulated in the conditions mimicking an aggressive disease (upon castration), similarly to the high clinical progression probability of a low TNC group in the primary PCa TMA. The higher stromal *Tnc* mRNA levels in the aggressive LAPC9 compared to BM18 may suggest that it would be relevant to examine the TNC mRNA and protein expressions in human bone metastasis or ideally matched primary metastasis cases in order to understand the kinetics of TNC in terms of disease progression. Given that TNC expression was found elevated from 0% in benign prostatic hyperplasia (BPH) stroma to 47% in tumor-associated stroma [29], its detection in circulation [47] and its immunomodulatory role [48] indicate TNC as a promising drug target and disease-determining factor. The TNC clinical progression predictive value performs best in an earlier stage, low-risk PCa, while our data show that, in high-risk PCa, a low number of TNC-producing cells were associated with poor prognosis, possibly due to changes in tissue remodeling and, thus, variable TNC levels.

These findings were corroborated by the external clinical cohorts of patients [22,23,49,50] (Grasso et al., Lapointe et al., Taylor et al. and Varambally et al.) showing that TNC levels are downregulated during the disease progression from primary to metastasis. Based on differential expression analysis, we identified clusters of stroma signatures based on androgen-(in)dependent responses (C1-C4). TNC is a component of the C1, C3 and C4 signatures. In silico validation of the identified prostate cancer-specific stroma expression signatures on additional clinical cohorts showed the potential for patient stratification. A common feature of the majority of the four clusters of gene lists tested indicated a low stroma signature score in the advanced disease stage and a correlation with disease progression (metastasis). This was the case also for previously published stroma signatures [7,21] (Tyekucheva et al. 2017 and Mo et al. 2017) when compared to our gene sets, perhaps due to the reduced stroma content in low-differentiated, advanced PCa stage. The signature most related to the androgen-independent stage (C4) positively correlated with the Gleason score in primary tissues from TCGA but not in the metastatic cohort of the Taylor dataset. Instead, we identified a 50-gene stroma signature (C1, derived from the most androgen-responsive stroma genes), which positively correlates with the disease progression, Gleason score and poor prognosis survival, consistently on all patient cohorts evaluated, both the primary and metastasis stages.

The regime that a metastatic, stroma-specific molecular signature may be detectable in the PCa site either prior to or during metastasis will most likely require not a single marker approach but a combination of biochemical and histological markers, taking into consideration dual tumor–stroma interactions in order to provide prognostic tools for improved patient stratification after the initial PCa diagnosis and preventive surveillance for metastasis risk.

4. Materials and Methods

4.1. Tumor Sample Preparation and Xenograft Surgery Procedure

LAPC9 and BM18 xenografts were maintained subcutaneously in 6-week-old CB17 SCID male mice under anesthesia (Domitor® 0.5 mg/kg, Dormicum 5 mg/kg and Fentanyl 0.05 mg/kg). All animal experiments were approved by the Ethical Committee of Canton Bern (animal licenses BE55/16 and BE12/17). Castration was achieved by bilateral orchiectomy. For androgen replacement, testosterone propionate dissolved in castor oil (86541-5G, Sigma-Aldrich, Buchs, Switzerland) was administered by single subcutaneous injection (2 mg per dosage, 25-G needle).

4.2. RNA Isolation from Tissue Samples

Tissue RNA was extracted using the standard protocol of Qiazol (79306, Qiagen AG, Hombrechtikon, Switzerland) tissue lysis by TissueLyser (2 min, 20 Hz). Quality of RNA was assessed by Bioanalyzer 2100 (Agilent Technologies, Basel, Switzerland). RNA from formalin-fixed-paraffin embedded (FFPE) material was extracted using the Maxwell® 16 LEV RNA FFPE Purification Kit (AS1260, Promega AG, Dübendorf, Switzerland).

4.3. RNA Sequencing

RNA extracted from BM18, and LAPC9 whole PDX tumor extracts (300 ng) were subjected to RNA sequencing. Specimens were prepared for RNA sequencing using Tru-Seq RNA Library Preparation Kit v2 or riboZero, as previously described [51]. RNA integrity was verified using the Bioanalyzer 2100 (Agilent Technologies, Basel, Switzerland). Complementary cDNA was synthesized from total RNA using Superscript III reverse transcriptase (18080093, Thermo Fisher Scientific, Basel, Switzerland). Sequencing was then performed on GAII, Hi-Seq 2000 or Hi-Seq 2500. The sample preparation was performed according to the protocol "NEBNext Ultra II Directional RNA Library Prep Kit (NEB #E7760S/L, Illumina GmbH, Zürich, Switzerland). Briefly, mRNA was isolated from total RNA using the oligo-dT magnetic beads. After fragmentation of the mRNA, a cDNA synthesis was performed. This was used for ligation with the sequencing adapters and PCR amplification of the resulting product. The quality and yield after sample preparation was measured with the Fragment Analyzer. The size of the resulting products was consistent with the expected size distribution (a broad peak between 300–500 bp). Clustering and DNA sequencing using the NovaSeq6000 was performed according to manufacturer's protocols. A concentration of 1.1 nM of DNA was used. Image analysis, base calling and quality check was performed with the Illumina (Illumina GmbH, Zürich, Switzerland) data analysis pipeline RTA3.4.4 and Bcl2fastq v2.20.

Sequence reads were aligned using STAR two-pass to the human reference genome GRCh37 [52] and mouse reference genome GRCm38. Gene counts were quantified using the "GeneCounts" option. Per-gene counts-per-million (CPM) were computed and $\log_2$-transformed, adding a pseudo-count of 1 to avoid transforming 0. Genes with $\log_2$ CPM <1 in more than three samples were removed. Differential expression analysis was performed using the edgeR package [53]. Normalization was performed using the "TMM" (weighted trimmed mean) method, and differential expression was assessed using the quasi-likelihood F test. Genes with false discovery rate FDR <0.05 and >2-fold were considered significantly differentially expressed. RNA-Seq Expectation Maximization (RSEM) was used to obtain TPM (transcripts per million) counts.

Pathway analysis (over-representation analysis) was performed using clusterProfiler R package [54] for Gene Ontology biological processes and KEGG. For Venn Euler diagram analysis, expressed genes were identified using the zFPKM transformation [55]. For the comparison between the states of the BM18 and LAPC9 models, genes were considered expressed if a gene had zFPKM values > −3 [55] in all samples.

4.4. Signature Validation on TCGA and Other Publically Available Datasets

TCGA gene expression, Gleason scores and outcome data were obtained from the PanCanAtlas publications supplemental data site (https://gdc.cancer.gov/about-data/publications/pancanatlas) [56,57]. For the Gene Set Variation Analysis (GSVA) analysis, RSEM expected counts in the upper quartile normalized to 1000 (i.e., the same normalization as TCGA) were used for BM18/LAPC9 gene expression. Mouse genes in gene signature lists were mapped to human homologs using the biomaRt R package (Table S5), using the "mmusculus_gene_ensembl" dataset and selecting only homologs with hsapiens_homolog_orthology_confidence = 1. Signature scores were calculated using the GSVA R package using the GSVA method [58].

Validation of the C1-C4 stroma signatures on publicly availably cohorts was performed using the Taylor (GSE21034) and the Grasso (GSE35988) datasets. Gene expression and sample information, including Gleason scores, were obtained via the GEOquery Bioconductor package. Mouse genes in the C1-C4 gene signature lists were mapped to human homologs using the biomaRt R package, using the "mmusculus_gene_ensembl" dataset and selecting only homologs with hsapiens_homolog_orthology_confidence = 1. Other gene sets are either human genes or include info on human homologs. Signature scores were calculated using the GSVA R package using the GSVA method [58].

4.5. Tissue Dissociation and MACS

Tumor tissue was collected in a basis medium (advanced Dulbecco Modified Eagle Medium F12 serum-free medium (12634010, Thermo Fisher Scientific, Basel, Switzerland) containing 10-mM Hepes (15630080, Thermo Fisher Scientific, Basel, Switzerland), 2-mM GlutaMAX supplement (35050061, Thermo Fisher Scientific, Basel, Switzerland) and 100 µg/mL Primocin (ant-pm-1, InVivoGen, LabForce AG, Muttenz, Switzerland). After mechanical disruption, the tissue was washed in the basis medium (220 relative centrifugal force (rcf), 5 min) and incubated in the enzyme mix for tissue dissociation (collagenase type II enzyme mix (17101-015, Gibco, Thermo Fisher Scientific, Basel, Switzerland) 5 mg/mL dissolved in the basis medium and DNase: 15 µg/mL (10104159001, Sigma-Aldrich, Buchs, Switzerland) and 10-µM Y-27632-HCl rock inhibitor (S1049, Selleckchem, Zürich, Switzerland). Enzyme mix volume was adjusted so that the tissue volume did not exceed 1/10 of the total volume, and tissue was incubated at 37 °C for 1 to 2 h, with mixing every 20 min. After the digestion of large pieces was complete, the suspension was passed through a 100-µm cell strainer (21008-950, Falcon®, VWR International GmbH, Dietikon, Switzerland) attached to a 50-mL Falcon tube, then using a rubber syringe to crash tissue against the strainer and wash in 5-mL basic medium (220 rcf, 5 min). Cell pellet was incubated in 5-mL precooled red blood cell lysis buffer (150-mM NH_4Cl, 10-mM $KHCO_3$ and 0.1-mM EDTA), incubated for 10 min and washed in equal volume of basis medium, followed by centrifugation (220 rcf, 5 min). Pellet was resuspended in 2–5 mL accutase™ (StemCell Technologies, 07920), depending on the sample amount; biopsies versus tissue and incubated for 10 min at room temperature. The cell suspension was passed through a 40-µm pore size strainer (21008-949, Falcon®, International GmbH, Dietikon, Switzerland), and the strainer was washed by adding 2 mL of accutase on the strainer. Single-cell suspension was counted to determine the seeding density and washed in 5 mL of basis medium and spun down 220 rcf, 5 min. Magnetic cell sorting was performed to separate purified human versus mouse cell fractions using the Mouse Cell Depletion Kit (130-104-694, Miltenyi Biotek, Solothurn, Switzerland). For the proteomic experiments, cell fractions from tumor tissues (n = 3 to 4 per condition) were pooled together in order to suffice for 10^6 cells, representing one technical replicate per sample.

4.6. Proteomics

4.6.1. Sample Preparation

Approx. 10^6 cell pellets ($n = 1$ technical replicate per condition deriving from $n = 3$ to 4 biological replicate samples) were resuspended in 50 µL PBS following the addition of 50 µL 1% SDS in 100-mM Hepes/NaOH, pH 8.5 supplemented with protease inhibitor cocktail EDTA-free (11836170001, Sigma-Aldrich, Buchs, Switzerland). Samples were heated to 95 °C for 5 min, transferred on ice, and benzonase (71206-3, Merck AG, Zug, Switzerland) was added to degrade DNA at 37 °C for 30 min. Samples were reduced by the addition of 2 µL of a 200-mM DTT solution in 200-mM Hepes/NaOH, pH 8.5 and, subsequently, alkylated by the addition of 4 µL of a 400-mM chloroacetamide (CAA, #C0267, Sigma-Aldrich, Buchs, Switzerland) solution in 200 mM Hepes/NaOH, pH 8.5. Samples were incubated at 56 °C for 30 min. Access CAA was quenched by the addition of 4 µl of a 200-mM DTT solution in 200 mM Hepes/NaOH, pH 8.5. Lysate were subjected to an in-solution tryptic digest using the single-pot solid phase-enhanced sample preparation (SP3) protocol [59,60]. To this end, 20 µL of Sera-Mag Beads (#4515-2105-050250 and 6515-2105-050250, Thermo Fisher Scientific, Basel, Switzerland) were mixed, washed with H_2O and resuspended in 100 µL H_2O. Two microliters of freshly prepared bead mix and 5 µl of an aqueous 10% formic acid were added to 40 µL of lysates to achieve an acidic pH. Forty-seven microliters of acetonitrile were added, and samples were incubated for 8 min at room temperature. Beads were captured on a magnetic rack and washed three times with 70% ethanol and once with acetonitrile. Sequencing grade-modified trypsin (0.8 µg; V5111, Promega AG, Dübendorf, Switzerland) in 10 µL 50 mM Hepes/NaOH, pH 8.5 were added. Samples were digested overnight at 37 °C. Beads were captured and the supernatant transferred and dried down. Peptides were reconstituted in 10 µL of H_2O and reacted with 80 µg of TMT10plex (#90111, Thermo Fisher Scientific, Basel, Switzerland) [61] label reagent dissolved in 4 µL of acetonitrile for 1 h at room temperature. Excess TMT reagent was quenched by the addition of 4 µL of an aqueous solution of 5% hydroxylamine (438227, Sigma-Aldrich, Buchs, Switzerland). Mixed peptides were subjected to a reverse-phase clean-up step (OASIS HLB 96-well µElution Plate, 186001828BA, Waters Corporation, Milford, MA, USA) and analyzed by LC-MS/MS on a Q Exactive Plus (Thermo Fisher Scientific, Basel, Switzerland), as previously described [62].

4.6.2. Mass Spectrometric Analysis

Briefly, peptides were separated using an UltiMate 3000 RSLC (Thermo Scientific, Basel, Switzerland) equipped with a trapping cartridge (Precolumn; C18 PepMap 100, 5 Lm, 300 Lm i.d. × 5 mm, 100 A°) and an analytical column (Waters nanoEase HSS C18 T3, 75 Lm × 25 cm, 1.8 Lm, 100 A°). Solvent A: aqueous 0.1% formic acid and Solvent B: 0.1% formic acid in acetonitrile (all solvents were of LC-MS grade). Peptides were loaded on the trapping cartridge using solvent A for 3 min with a flow of 30 µL/min. Peptides were separated on the analytical column with a constant flow of 0.3 µL/min applying a 2 h gradient of 2–28% of solvent B in A, followed by an increase to 40% B. Peptides were directly analyzed in positive ion mode, applied with a spray voltage of 2.3 kV and a capillary temperature of 320°C using a Nanospray-Flex ion source and a Pico-Tip Emitter 360 Lm OD × 20 Lm ID;, 10 Lm tip (New Objective, Littleton, MA, USA). MS spectra with a mass range of 375–1.200 m/z were acquired in profile mode using a resolution of 70,000 (maximum fill time of 250 ms or a maximum of 3×10^6 ions (automatic gain control, AGC)). Fragmentation was triggered for the top 10 peaks with 2–4 charges on the MS scan (data-dependent acquisition), with a 30 s dynamic exclusion window (normalized collision energy was 32). Precursors were isolated with a 0.7 m/z window and MS/MS spectra were acquired in profile mode with a resolution of 35,000 (maximum fill time of 120 ms or an AGC target of 2×10^5 ions).

4.6.3. Raw MS Data Analysis

Acquired data were analyzed using IsobarQuant [63] and Mascot V2.4 (Matrix Science, Chicago, IL, USA) using either a reverse-UniProt FASTA Mus musculus (UP000000589) or Homo sapiens (UP000005640) database. Moreover, a combined database thereof was generated and used for the analysis. These databases also included common contaminants. The following modifications were taken into account: Carbamidomethyl (C, fixed), TMT10plex (K, fixed), Acetyl (N-term, variable), Oxidation (M, variable) and TMT10plex (N-term, variable). The mass error tolerance for full-scan MS spectra was set to 10 ppm and for MS/MS spectra to 0.02 Da. A maximum of 2 missed cleavages were allowed. A minimum of 2 unique peptides with a peptide length of at least seven amino acids and a false discovery rate below 0.01 were required on the peptide and protein levels [64].

4.6.4. MS Data Analysis

The raw output files of IsobarQuant (protein.txt files) were processed using the R programming language (ISBN 3-900051-07-0). As a quality filter, only proteins were allowed that you were quantified with at least two unique peptides. Human and mouse samples were searched against a combined human and mouse database and annotated as unique for human or mouse or mixed. Raw signal-sums (signal_sum columns) were normalized using vsn (variance stabilization normalization) [65]. In order to try to annotate each observed ratio with a *p*-value, each ratio distribution was analyzed with the locfdr function of the locfdr package [66] to extract the average and the standard deviation (using the maximum likelihood estimation). Then, the ratio distribution was transformed into a z-distribution by normalizing it by its standard deviation and mean. This z-distribution was analyzed with the fdrtool function of the fdrtool package [67] in order to extract *p*-values and false discovery rates (fdr, *q*-values).

4.7. Tissue Microarray

Tissue microarray core annotations and quantification of positive staining were performed by QuPath software version v0.2.0-m8 [68] using the TMA map function. Kaplan–Meier curves to calculate the association between TNC-positive cells and disease progression were calculated using the "survfit" function and the global Log-Rank test using the Survival R package [69,70]. To estimate the survival, we used the function "surv_cutpoint", which employs maximally selected rank statistics (maxstat) to determine the optimal cut-point for continuous variables [18]. For pairwise comparison, the *p*-value was estimated by the Log-Rank test and adjusted with the Benjamini–Hochberg (BH) method. If no information on patient outcome was available, information at the last follow-up was used for all parameters. Clinical progression was defined as metastasis or local recurrence. Disease progression was defined by combining any form of recurrence (PSA and clinical progression). Data representation and graphical plots were generated using the ggplot2 R package [71]. Data analyses were done using RStudio version 1.1.463 [72] and R version 3.5.3 [73].

4.8. Immunohistochemistry

FFPE sections (4 µm) were deparaffinized and used for heat-mediated antigen retrieval (citrate buffer, pH 6, Vector Labs). Sections were blocked for 10 min in 3% H_2O_2, followed by 30 min, RT incubation in 1% BSA in PBS–0.1%Tween 20. The following primary antibodies were used (Table 3):

Table 3. Primary antibodies used for Immunohistochemistry

Dilution	Antibody	Company	Catalog No.
1 to 500	Ki67	Gene Tex	GTX16667
1 to 100	Tnc	R&D	MAB2138

Secondary anti-rabbit antibody Envision HRP (DAKO, Agilent Technologies, Basel, Switzerland) for 30 min or anti-rat HRP (Thermo Scientific, Basel, Switzerland). Signal detection with AEC substrate

(DAKO, Agilent Technologies, Basel, Switzerland). Sections were counterstained with Hematoxylin and mounted with Aquatex.

4.9. Immunofluorescence

After deparaffinization, heat-mediated antigen retrieval (citrate buffer, pH 6, Vector Labs) was performed. Sections were blocked in 1% BSA in PBS–0.1% Tween 20 for 30 min, RT incubation. The primary antibodies used (Table 4), were incubated overnight in blocking solution at 4 °C:

Table 4. Primary antibodies used for Immunofluorescence

Dilution	Antibody	Company	Catalog No.
1 to 500	αSMA	Sigma	A2547
1 to 500	ITGA2	Abcam	ab181548
1 to 500	Collagen type I	Southern Biotech	1310-01
1 to 50	Tnc	R&D	MAB2138

Secondary anti-rabbit/mouse/goat/rat antibodies coupled to Alexa Fluor®-488, 555 or 647 fluorochrome conjugates (Invitrogen, Thermo Scientific, Basel, Switzerland) were incubated for 90 min at 1:250 dilution in PBS. Sections were counterstained with DAPI solution (Thermo Scientific, Basel, Switzerland, final concentration 1 μg/mL in PBS, 10 min), washed and mounted with prolonged diamond antifade reagent (Invitrogen, Thermo Scientific, Basel, Switzerland).

5. Conclusions

In this proof-of-concept study, the molecular profile of the stroma in prostate cancer was shown to be responsive to androgen deprivation even in advanced, androgen-independent bone metastasis prostate cancer. We identified a stroma-specific gene expression signature that correlates with the Gleason score and metastatic disease progression of prostate cancer. Given the inevitable drug resistance to androgen deprivation therapies, stroma biomarker identification associated with resistance acquisition may complement standard histopathology and genomic evaluations for improved stratification of patients at high risk.

Supplementary Materials: The following are available online at http://www.mdpi.com/2072-6694/12/12/3786/s1: Figure S1. Related to Figure 2. Human transcriptomic profile of BM18 and LAPC9 tumors. Figure S2. Related to Figure 2. Human and mouse ratios of RNA-Seq transcript levels in intact and castrated settings. Figure S3. Related to Figure 5. Pathways enriched in the stroma of the CRPC LAPC9 compared to the BM18. Figure S4. Related to Figure 7. PSA progression in cases with positive surgical margins or lymph nodes status. Figure S5. Related to Figure 9. Correlations and prognostic performances of the C1, C2, C3 and C4 signatures compared to the previously identified stroma signatures. Table S1. Venn Euler diagrams. Table S2: Lists of enriched GO and KEGG pathways (attached as an Excel file). Table S3. Statistical test TNC expression in patient groups of different pT Stage classification in the high risk PCa TMA. Table S4. Stroma signature gene lists. Table S5. Human gene lists of Ob-BMST and C1-C4 signatures.

Author Contributions: Conceptualization, S.K. and M.K.d.J.; formal analysis, S.K., M.R.D.F., C.K.Y.N., E.Z., F.S. and P.H.; funding acquisition, S.K., G.N.T. and M.K.d.J.; investigation, S.K. and I.K.; methodology, E.Z. and P.H.; project administration, M.K.d.J.; resources, M.S., G.N.T. and M.K.d.J.; software, P.H.; supervision, M.K.d.J.; writing—original draft, S.K., F.S. and M.K.d.J. and writing—review and editing, M.R.D.F., C.K.Y.N., E.Z. and G.N.T. All authors have read and agreed to the published version of the manuscript.

Funding: This project received funding from the European Union's Horizon 2020 Research and Innovation Programme under the Marie Skłodowska-Curie Individual Fellowship (S.K.), grant agreement no. 748836 (STOPCa) and additional funding from the Swiss National Science Foundation (320030L_189369 to G.N.Thalmann).

Acknowledgments: The authors would like to thank the Microscopy Facility of the University of Bern, Francesco Bonollo, Peter C Gray, Salvatore Piscuoglio and all the members of the DBMR Urology laboratory for critical discussions and technical support.

Conflicts of Interest: The authors declare no conflict of interest.

Data Availability: The sequencing data have been submitted to the European Genome-Phenome Archive under the accession number EGAS00001004770.

References

1. Heidenreich, A.; Bastian, P.J.; Bellmunt, J.; Bolla, M.; Joniau, S.; van der Kwast, T.; Mason, M.; Matveev, V.; Wiegel, T.; Zattoni, F.; et al. EAU guidelines on prostate cancer. Part II: Treatment of advanced, relapsing, and castration-resistant prostate cancer. *Eur. Urol.* **2014**, *65*, 467–479. [CrossRef] [PubMed]
2. Malanchi, I.; Santamaria-Martinez, A.; Susanto, E.; Peng, H.; Lehr, H.A.; Delaloye, J.F.; Huelsken, J. Interactions between cancer stem cells and their niche govern metastatic colonization. *Nature* **2011**, *481*, 85–89. [CrossRef] [PubMed]
3. Shiozawa, Y.; Pedersen, E.A.; Havens, A.M.; Jung, Y.; Mishra, A.; Joseph, J.; Kim, J.K.; Patel, L.R.; Ying, C.; Ziegler, A.M.; et al. Human prostate cancer metastases target the hematopoietic stem cell niche to establish footholds in mouse bone marrow. *J. Clin. Invest.* **2011**, *121*, 1298–1312. [CrossRef] [PubMed]
4. Hensel, J.; Wetterwald, A.; Temanni, R.; Keller, I.; Riether, C.; van der Pluijm, G.; Cecchini, M.G.; Thalmann, G.N. Osteolytic cancer cells induce vascular/axon guidance processes in the bone/bone marrow stroma. *Oncotarget* **2018**, *9*, 28877–28896. [CrossRef] [PubMed]
5. Ozdemir, B.C.; Hensel, J.; Secondini, C.; Wetterwald, A.; Schwaninger, R.; Fleischmann, A.; Raffelsberger, W.; Poch, O.; Delorenzi, M.; Temanni, R.; et al. The molecular signature of the stroma response in prostate cancer-induced osteoblastic bone metastasis highlights expansion of hematopoietic and prostate epithelial stem cell niches. *PLoS ONE* **2014**, *9*, e114530. [CrossRef] [PubMed]
6. Rucci, N.; Teti, A. Osteomimicry: How the seed grows in the soil. *Calcif. Tissue Int.* **2018**, *102*, 131–140. [CrossRef]
7. Tyekucheva, S.; Bowden, M.; Bango, C.; Giunchi, F.; Huang, Y.; Zhou, C.; Bondi, A.; Lis, R.; Van Hemelrijck, M.; Andrén, O.; et al. Stromal and epithelial transcriptional map of initiation progression and metastatic potential of human prostate cancer. *Nat. Commun.* **2017**, *8*, 420. [CrossRef]
8. Setlur, S.R.; Rubin, M.A. Current thoughts on the role of the androgen receptor and prostate cancer progression. *Adv. Anat. Pathol.* **2005**, *12*, 265–270. [CrossRef]
9. Leach, D.A.; Need, E.F.; Toivanen, R.; Trotta, A.P.; Palenthorpe, H.M.; Tamblyn, D.J.; Kopsaftis, T.; England, G.M.; Smith, E.; Drew, P.A.; et al. Stromal androgen receptor regulates the composition of the microenvironment to influence prostate cancer outcome. *Oncotarget* **2015**, *6*, 16135–16150. [CrossRef]
10. Leach, D.A.; Panagopoulos, V.; Nash, C.; Bevan, C.; Thomson, A.A.; Selth, L.A.; Buchanan, G. Cell-lineage specificity and role of AP-1 in the prostate fibroblast androgen receptor cistrome. *Mol. Cell. Endocrinol.* **2017**, *439*, 261–272. [CrossRef]
11. Nash, C.; Boufaied, N.; Mills, I.G.; Franco, O.E.; Hayward, S.W.; Thomson, A.A. Genome-wide analysis of AR binding and comparison with transcript expression in primary human fetal prostate fibroblasts and cancer associated fibroblasts. *Mol. Cell. Endocrinol.* **2018**, *471*, 1–14. [CrossRef] [PubMed]
12. Thalmann, G.N.; Rhee, H.; Sikes, R.A.; Pathak, S.; Multani, A.; Zhau, H.E.; Marshall, F.F.; Chung, L.W.K. Human prostate fibroblasts induce growth and confer castration resistance and metastatic potential in LNCaP Cells. *Eur. Urol.* **2010**, *58*, 162–171. [CrossRef]
13. Thalmann, G.N.; Anezinis, P.E.; Chang, S.M.; Zhau, H.E.; Kim, E.E.; Hopwood, V.L.; Pathak, S.; von Eschenbach, A.C.; Chung, L.W. Androgen-independent cancer progression and bone metastasis in the LNCaP model of human prostate cancer. *Cancer Res.* **1994**, *54*, 2577–2581. [PubMed]
14. Briganti, A.; Spahn, M.; Joniau, S.; Gontero, P.; Bianchi, M.; Kneitz, B.; Chun, F.K.; Sun, M.; Graefen, M.; Abdollah, F.; et al. Impact of age and comorbidities on long-term survival of patients with high-risk prostate cancer treated with radical prostatectomy: A multi-institutional competing-risks analysis. *Eur. Urol.* **2013**, *63*, 693–701. [CrossRef] [PubMed]
15. Tosco, L.; Laenen, A.; Briganti, A.; Gontero, P.; Karnes, R.J.; Bastian, P.J.; Chlosta, P.; Claessens, F.; Chun, F.K.; Everaerts, W.; et al. The EMPaCT classifier: A validated tool to predict postoperative prostate cancer-related death using competing-risk analysis. *Eur. Urol. Focus.* **2018**, *4*, 369–375. [CrossRef] [PubMed]
16. Chys, B.; Devos, G.; Everaerts, W.; Albersen, M.; Moris, L.; Claessens, F.; De Meerleer, G.; Haustermans, K.; Briganti, A.; Chlosta, P.; et al. Preoperative risk-stratification of high-risk prostate cancer: A multicenter analysis. *Front. Oncol.* **2020**, *10*, 246. [CrossRef] [PubMed]

17. D'Amico, A.V.; Whittington, R.; Malkowicz, S.B.; Schultz, D.; Blank, K.; Broderick, G.A.; Tomaszewski, J.E.; Renshaw, A.A.; Kaplan, I.; Beard, C.J.; et al. Biochemical outcome after radical prostatectomy, external beam radiation therapy, or interstitial radiation therapy for clinically localized prostate cancer. *JAMA* **1998**, *280*, 969–974.
18. Kassambara, A. Survminer: Drawing Survival Curves Using 'ggplot2'. 2018. Available online: http://www.sthda.com/english/rpkgs/survminer/ (accessed on 1 January 2016).
19. Cortazar, A.R.; Torrano, V.; Martín-Martín, N.; Caro-Maldonado, A.; Camacho, L.; Hermanova, I.; Guruceaga, E.; Lorenzo-Martín, L.F.; Caloto, R.; Gomis, R.R.; et al. CANCERTOOL: A visualization and representation interface to exploit cancer datasets. *Cancer Res.* **2018**, *78*, 6320–6328. [CrossRef]
20. Glinsky, G.V.; Glinskii, A.B.; Stephenson, A.J.; Hoffman, R.M.; Gerald, W.L. Gene expression profiling predicts clinical outcome of prostate cancer. *J. Clin. Invest.* **2004**. [CrossRef]
21. Mo, F.; Lin, D.; Takhar, M.; Ramnarine, V.R.; Dong, X.; Bell, R.H.; Volik, S.V.; Wang, K.; Xue, H.; Wang, Y.; et al. Stromal gene expression is predictive for metastatic primary prostate cancer. *Eur. Urol.* **2018**, *73*, 524–532. [CrossRef]
22. Grasso, C.S.; Wu, Y.M.; Robinson, D.R.; Cao, X.; Dhanasekaran, S.M.; Khan, A.P.; Quist, M.J.; Jing, X.; Lonigro, R.J.; Brenner, J.C.; et al. The mutational landscape of lethal castration-resistant prostate cancer. *Nature* **2012**, *487*, 239–243. [CrossRef] [PubMed]
23. Taylor, B.S.; Schultz, N.; Hieronymus, H.; Gopalan, A.; Xiao, Y.; Carver, B.S.; Arora, V.K.; Kaushik, P.; Cerami, E.; Reva, B.; et al. Integrative genomic profiling of human prostate cancer. *Cancer Cell.* **2010**, *18*, 11–22. [CrossRef] [PubMed]
24. Sahai, E.; Astsaturov, I.; Cukierman, E.; DeNardo, D.G.; Egeblad, M.; Evans, R.M.; Fearon, D.; Greten, F.R.; Hingorani, S.R.; Hunter, T.; et al. A framework for advancing our understanding of cancer-associated fibroblasts. *Nat. Rev. Cancer* **2020**, *20*, 174–186. [CrossRef] [PubMed]
25. Corn, P.G. The tumor microenvironment in prostate cancer: Elucidating molecular pathways for therapy development. *Cancer Manag. Res.* **2012**, *4*, 183–193. [CrossRef]
26. Bissell, M.J.; Hines, W.C. Why don't we get more cancer? A proposed role of the microenvironment in restraining cancer progression. *Nat. Med.* **2011**, *17*, 320–329. [CrossRef]
27. Petersen, O.W.; Rønnov-Jessen, L.; Howlett, A.R.; Bissell, M.J. Interaction with basement membrane serves to rapidly distinguish growth and differentiation pattern of normal and malignant human breast epithelial cells. *Proc. Natl. Acad. Sci. USA.* **1992**, *89*, 9064–9068. [CrossRef]
28. Weaver, V.M.; Petersen, O.W.; Wang, F.; Larabell, C.A.; Briand, P.; Damsky, C.; Bissell, M.J. Reversion of the malignant phenotype of human breast cells in three-dimensional culture and in vivo by integrin blocking antibodies. *J. Cell. Biol.* **1997**, *137*, 231–245. [CrossRef]
29. Sung, S.-Y.; Hsieh, C.-L.; Law, A.; Zhau, H.E.; Pathak, S.; Multani, A.S.; Lim, S.; Coleman, I.M.; Wu, L.-C.; Figg, W.D.; et al. Coevolution of prostate cancer and bone stroma in three-dimensional coculture: Implications for cancer growth and metastasis. *Cancer Res.* **2008**, *68*, 9996–10003. [CrossRef]
30. Craft, N.; Chhor, C.; Tran, C.; Belldegrun, A.; DeKernion, J.; Witte, O.N.; Said, J.; Reiter, R.E.; Sawyers, C.L. Evidence for clonal outgrowth of androgen-independent prostate cancer cells from androgen-dependent tumors through a two-step process. *Cancer Res.* **1999**, *59*, 5030–5036.
31. Germann, M.; Wetterwald, A.; Guzman-Ramirez, N.; van der Pluijm, G.; Culig, Z.; Cecchini, M.G.; Williams, E.D.; Thalmann, G.N. Stem-like cells with luminal progenitor phenotype survive castration in human prostate cancer. *Stem Cells* **2012**, *30*, 1076–1086. [CrossRef]
32. McCulloch, D.R.; Opeskin, K.; Thompson, E.W.; Williams, E.D. BM18: A novel androgen-dependent human prostate cancer xenograft model derived from a bone metastasis. *Prostate* **2005**, *65*, 35–43. [CrossRef] [PubMed]
33. Li, Q.; Deng, Q.; Chao, H.-P.; Liu, X.; Lu, Y.; Lin, K.; Liu, B.; Tang, G.W.; Zhang, D.; Tracz, A.; et al. Linking prostate cancer cell AR heterogeneity to distinct castration and enzalutamide responses. *Nat. Commun.* **2018**, *9*, 3600. [CrossRef] [PubMed]
34. Chen, X.; Li, Q.; Liu, X.; Liu, C.; Liu, R.; Rycaj, K.; Zhang, D.; Liu, B.; Jeter, C.; Calhoun-Davis, T.; et al. Defining a population of stem-like human prostate cancer cells that can generate and propagate castration-resistant prostate cancer. *Clin. Cancer Res.* **2016**, *22*, 4505–4516. [CrossRef] [PubMed]

35. Cutz, J.-C.; Guan, J.; Bayani, J.; Yoshimoto, M.; Xue, H.; Sutcliffe, M.; English, J.; Flint, J.; LeRiche, J.; Yee, J.; et al. Establishment in severe combined immunodeficiency mice of subrenal capsule xenografts and transplantable tumor lines from a variety of primary human lung cancers: Potential models for studying tumor progression–related changes. *Clin. Cancer Res.* **2006**, *12*, 4043–4054. [CrossRef] [PubMed]

36. Hidalgo, M.; Amant, F.; Biankin, A.V.; Budinská, E.; Byrne, A.T.; Caldas, C.; Clarke, R.B.; de Jong, S.; Jonkers, J.; Mælandsmo, G.M.; et al. Patient-derived xenograft models: An emerging platform for translational cancer research. *Cancer Discov.* **2014**, *4*, 998–1013. [CrossRef] [PubMed]

37. Tuxhorn, J.A.; Ayala, G.E.; Smith, M.J.; Smith, V.C.; Dang, T.D.; Rowley, D.R. Reactive stroma in human prostate cancer. Induction of myofibroblast phenotype and extracellular matrix remodeling. *Clin. Cancer Res.* **2002**, *8*, 2912–2923. [PubMed]

38. Ibrahim, S.N.; Lightner, V.A.; Ventimiglia, J.B.; Ibrahim, G.K.; Walther, P.J.; Bigner, D.D.; Humphrey, P.A. Tenascin expression in prostatic hyperplasia, intraepithelial neoplasia, and carcinoma. *Hum. Pathol.* **1993**, *24*, 982–989. [CrossRef]

39. Xue, Y.; Smedts, F.; Latijnhouwers, M.A.; Ruijter, E.T.; Aalders, T.W.; de la Rosette, J.J.; Debruyne, F.M.; Schalken, J.A. Tenascin-C expression in prostatic intraepithelial neoplasia (PIN): A marker of progression? *Anticancer Res.* **1998**, *18*, 2679–2684.

40. Ni, W.-D.; Yang, Z.-T.; Cui, C.-A.; Cui, Y.; Fang, L.-Y.; Xuan, Y.-H. Tenascin-C is a potential cancer-associated fibroblasts marker and predicts poor prognosis in prostate cancer. *Biochem. Biophys. Res. Commun.* **2017**, *486*, 607–612. [CrossRef]

41. Cai, M.; Onoda, K.; Takao, M.; Kyoko, I.-Y.; Shimpo, H.; Yoshida, T.; Yada, I. Degradation of tenascin-C and activity of matrix metalloproteinase-2 are associated with tumor recurrence in early stage non-small cell lung cancer. *Clin. Cancer Res.* **2002**, *8*, 1152–1156.

42. Kusagawa, H.; Onoda, K.; Namikawa, S.; Yada, I.; Okada, A.; Yoshida, T.; Sakakura, T. Expression and degeneration of tenascin-C in human lung cancers. *Br. J. Cancer* **1998**, *77*, 98–102. [CrossRef] [PubMed]

43. San Martin, R.; Pathak, R.; Jain, A.; Jung, S.Y.; Hilsenbeck, S.G.; Piña-Barba, M.C.; Sikora, A.G.; Pienta, K.J.; Rowley, D.R. Tenascin-C and integrin α9 mediate interactions of prostate cancer with the bone microenvironment. *Cancer Res.* **2017**, *77*, 5977–5988. [CrossRef] [PubMed]

44. Colombel, M.; Eaton, C.L.; Hamdy, F.; Ricci, E.; van der Pluijm, G.; Cecchini, M.; Mege-Lechevallier, F.; Clezardin, P.; Thalmann, G. Increased expression of putative cancer stem cell markers in primary prostate cancer is associated with progression of bone metastases. *Prostate* **2012**, *72*, 713–720. [CrossRef] [PubMed]

45. Lowy, C.M.; Oskarsson, T. Tenascin C in metastasis: A view from the invasive front. *Cell Adh. Migr.* **2015**, *9*, 112–124. [CrossRef]

46. Mishra, P.; Kiebish, M.A.; Cullen, J.; Srinivasan, A.; Patterson, A.; Sarangarajan, R.; Narain, N.R.; Dobi, A. Genomic alterations of Tenascin C in highly aggressive prostate cancer: A meta-analysis. *Genes Cancer* **2019**, *10*, 150–159. [CrossRef]

47. Kiebish, M.A.; Cullen, J.; Mishra, P.; Ali, A.; Milliman, E.; Rodrigues, L.O.; Chen, E.Y.; Tolstikov, V.; Zhang, L.; Panagopoulos, K.; et al. Multi-omic serum biomarkers for prognosis of disease progression in prostate cancer. *J. Transl. Med.* **2020**, *18*, 1–10. [CrossRef]

48. Jachetti, E.; Caputo, S.; Mazzoleni, S.; Brambillasca, C.S.; Parigi, S.M.; Grioni, M.; Piras, I.S.; Restuccia, U.; Calcinotto, A.; Freschi, M.; et al. Tenascin-C protects cancer stem–like cells from immune surveillance by arresting T-cell activation. *Cancer Res.* **2015**, *75*, 2095–2108. [CrossRef]

49. Lapointe, J.; Li, C.; Higgins, J.P.; van de Rijn, M.; Bair, E.; Montgomery, K.; Ferrari, M.; Egevad, L.; Rayford, W.; Bergerheim, U.; et al. Gene expression profiling identifies clinically relevant subtypes of prostate cancer. *Proc. Natl. Acad. Sci. USA* **2004**. [CrossRef]

50. Varambally, S.; Yu, J.; Laxman, B.; Rhodes, D.R.; Mehra, R.; Tomlins, S.A.; Shah, R.B.; Chandran, U.; Monzon, F.A.; Becich, M.J.; et al. Integrative genomic and proteomic analysis of prostate cancer reveals signatures of metastatic progression. *Cancer Cell.* **2005**. [CrossRef]

51. Beltran, H.; Eng, K.; Mosquera, J.M.; Sigaras, A.; Romanel, A.; Rennert, H.; Kossai, M.; Pauli, C.; Faltas, B.; Fontugne, J.; et al. Whole-exome sequencing of metastatic cancer and biomarkers of treatment response. *JAMA Oncol.* **2015**, *1*, 466–474. [CrossRef]

52. Dobin, A.; Davis, C.A.; Schlesinger, F.; Drenkow, J.; Zaleski, C.; Jha, S.; Batut, P.; Chaisson, M.; Gingeras, T.R. STAR: Ultrafast universal RNA-seq aligner. *Bioinformatics* **2013**, *29*, 15–21. [CrossRef] [PubMed]

53. Nikolayeva, O.; Robinson, M.D. Edger for differential RNA-seq and ChIP-seq analysis: An application to stem cell biology. *Methods Mol. Biol.* **2014**, *1150*, 45–79.
54. Yu, G.; Wang, L.G.; Han, Y.; He, Q.Y. clusterProfiler: An R package for comparing biological themes among gene clusters. *OMICS: J. Integr. Biol.* **2012**, *16*, 284–287. [CrossRef]
55. Hart, T.; Komori, H.K.; LaMere, S.; Podshivalova, K.; Salomon, D.R. Finding the active genes in deep RNA-seq gene expression studies. *BMC Genom.* **2013**, *14*, 778. [CrossRef]
56. Cancer Genome Atlas Research, N. The molecular taxonomy of primary prostate cancer. *Cell* **2015**, *163*, 1011–1025.
57. Hoadley, K.A.; Yau, C.; Hinoue, T.; Wolf, D.M.; Lazar, A.J.; Drill, E.; Shen, R.; Taylor, A.M.; Cherniack, A.D.; Thorsson, V.; et al. Cell-of-origin patterns dominate the molecular classification of 10,000 tumors from 33 types of cancer. *Cell* **2018**, *173*, 291–304.e6. [CrossRef] [PubMed]
58. Hänzelmann, S.; Castelo, R.; Guinney, J. GSVA: Gene set variation analysis for microarray and RNA-seq data. *BMC Bioinform.* **2013**, *14*, 7. [CrossRef]
59. Hughes, C.S.; Foehr, S.; Garfield, D.A.; Furlong, E.E.; Steinmetz, L.M.; Krijgsveld, J. Ultrasensitive proteome analysis using paramagnetic bead technology. *Mol. Syst. Biol.* **2014**, *10*, 757. [CrossRef]
60. Moggridge, S.; Sorensen, P.H.; Morin, G.B.; Hughes, C.S. Extending the compatibility of the SP3 paramagnetic bead processing approach for proteomics. *J. Proteome. Res.* **2018**, *17*, 1730–1740. [CrossRef]
61. Werner, T.; Sweetman, G.; Savitski, M.F.; Mathieson, T.; Bantscheff, M.; Savitski, M.M. Ion coalescence of neutron encoded TMT 10-plex reporter ions. *Anal. Chem.* **2014**, *86*, 3594–3601. [CrossRef]
62. Becher, I.; Andres-Pons, A.; Romanov, N.; Stein, F.; Schramm, M.; Baudin, F.; Helm, D.; Kurzawa, N.; Mateus, A.; Mackmull, M.T.; et al. Pervasive protein thermal stability variation during the cell cycle. *Cell* **2018**, *173*, 1495–1507.e18. [CrossRef] [PubMed]
63. Franken, H.; Mathieson, T.; Childs, D.; Sweetman, G.M.; Werner, T.; Togel, I.; Doce, C.; Gade, S.; Bantscheff, M.; Drewes, G.; et al. Thermal proteome profiling for unbiased identification of direct and indirect drug targets using multiplexed quantitative mass spectrometry. *Nat. Protoc.* **2015**, *10*, 1567–1593. [CrossRef] [PubMed]
64. Savitski, M.M.; Wilhelm, M.; Hahne, H.; Kuster, B.; Bantscheff, M. A scalable approach for protein false discovery rate estimation in large proteomic data sets. *Mol. Cell. Proteomics.* **2015**, *14*, 2394–2404. [CrossRef] [PubMed]
65. Huber, W.; von Heydebreck, A.; Sultmann, H.; Poustka, A.; Vingron, M. Variance stabilization applied to microarray data calibration and to the quantification of differential expression. *Bioinformatics* **2002**, *18* (Suppl. S1), S96–S104. [CrossRef]
66. Efron, B. Large-scale simultaneous hypothesis testing. *J. Am. Statist. Assoc.* **2004**, *99*, 96–104. [CrossRef]
67. Strimmer, K. fdrtool: A versatile R package for estimating local and tail area-based false discovery rates. *Bioinformatics* **2008**, *24*, 1461–1462. [CrossRef]
68. Bankhead, P.; Loughrey, M.B.; Fernández, J.A.; Dombrowski, Y.; McArt, D.G.; Dunne, P.D.; McQuaid, S.; Gray, R.T.; Murray, L.J.; Coleman, H.G.; et al. QuPath: Open source software for digital pathology image analysis. *Sci. Rep.* **2017**, *7*, 16878. [CrossRef]
69. Therneau, T. A Package for Survival Analysis in S. 2015. Available online: https://www.mayo.edu/research/documents/tr53pdf/doc-10027379 (accessed on 28 September 2020).
70. Therneau, T. *PMG: Modeling Survival Data: Extending the Cox Model*; Springer: New York, NY, USA, 2000.
71. Wickham, H. *ggplot2: Elegant Graphics for Data Analysis*; Springer: New York, NY, USA, 2016.
72. RStudio Team. *RStudio: Integrated Development for R.*; RStudio: Boston, MI, USA, 2016.
73. R Core Team. *R: A language and Environment for Statistical Computing*; ARFfSC: Vienna, Austria, 2019.

Publisher's Note: MDPI stays neutral with regard to jurisdictional claims in published maps and institutional affiliations.

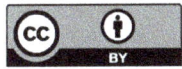

© 2020 by the authors. Licensee MDPI, Basel, Switzerland. This article is an open access article distributed under the terms and conditions of the Creative Commons Attribution (CC BY) license (http://creativecommons.org/licenses/by/4.0/).

MDPI
St. Alban-Anlage 66
4052 Basel
Switzerland
Tel. +41 61 683 77 34
Fax +41 61 302 89 18
www.mdpi.com

Cancers Editorial Office
E-mail: cancers@mdpi.com
www.mdpi.com/journal/cancers

www.ingramcontent.com/pod-product-compliance
Lightning Source LLC
LaVergne TN
LVHW070218100526
838202LV00015B/2058